Echocardiography in Practice

A Case-Oriented Approach

Echocardiography in Practice

A Case-Oriented Approach

Edited by

Susan E Wiegers MD
Director
Hospital of the University of Pennsylvania Cardiac Clinic
Associate Director
Non-invasive Imaging
Cardiovascular Imaging Program
University of Pennsylvania Medical Center
Philadelphia PA
USA

Ted Plappert CVT
Research Echocardiographer
University of Pennsylvania Medical Center
Philadelphia PA
USA

Martin St John Sutton MB BS FRCP
John Bryfogle Professor of Cardiovascular Diseases and Director
Cardiovascular Imaging Program
University of Pennsylvania Medical Center
Philadelphia PA
USA

MARTIN DUNITZ

© Martin Dunitz Ltd 2001

First published in the United Kingdom in 2001 by
Martin Dunitz Ltd
The Livery House
7–9 Pratt Street
London NW1 0AE

Tel: +44(0) 20 7482 2202
Fax: +44(0) 20 7267 0159
E-mail: info@mdunitz.globalnet.co.uk
Website: http://www.dunitz.co.uk

A CIP catalogue record for this book is available from the British
Library

ISBN 1-85317-723-7

Distributed in the United States by:
Blackwell Science Inc.
Commerce Place, 350 Main Street
Malden MA 02148, USA
Tel: 1-800-215-1000

Distributed in Canada by:
Login Brothers Book Company
324 Salteaux Crescent
Winnipeg, Manitoba R3J 3T2
Canada
Tel: 1-204-224-4068

Distributed in Brazil by:
Ernesto Reichmann Distribuidora de Livros, Ltda
Rua Coronel Marques 335, Tatuape 03440-000
São Paulo,
Brazil

Composition by Scribe Design, Gillingham, Kent, UK
Printed and bound in Hong Kong by Imago

Contents

Dedication

To my wonderful family: Barry, Ben, Peter and Aly.

To my friends and colleagues who assisted with many aspects of this endeavor and to the Tuesday writing group.

And finally to William L Morgan, MD who taught so many of us so much.

SEW

To Maureen with love

TJP

To Clare, Magali, Claire-Helene, Eleanor and Eugenie.

MSS

List of contributors

John Augoustides MD
Assistant Professor of Anesthesia, University of
Pennsylvania Medical Center, Philadelphia PA, USA

Gene Chang MD
Cardiovascular Division, Assistant Professor of
Medicine, University of Pennsylvania Medical Center,
Philadelphia PA, USA

Victor A Ferrari MD, FACC
Assistant Professor of Medicine, Cardiovascular Imaging
Section, University of Pennsylvania Medical Center,
Philadelphia PA, USA

Monali Gupta MD
Fellow in Radiology, Brigham & Women's Hospital,
Boston, MA, USA

Lilian P Joventino, MD
Cardiovascular Fellow, Beth Israel Deaconess Medical
Center, Boston, MA, USA

Martin G Keane MD, FACC
Assistant Professor of Medicine, Cardiovascular Imaging
Section, University of Pennsylvania Medical Center,
Philadelphia PA, USA

Jorge R Kizer MD, MSc
Fellow in Cardiovascular Medicine, University of
Pennsylvania Medical Center, Philadelphia PA, USA

Bruce D Klugherz MD
Assistant Professor of Medicine, Philadelphia VAMC,
University of Pennsylvania Medical Center, Philadelphia
PA, USA

Robert H Li MD
Fellow in Cardiovascular Medicine, University of
Pennsylvania Medical Center, Philadelphia PA, USA

Eileen MacDonald MD
Resident in Internal Medicine, University of
Pennsylvania Medical Center, Philadelphia PA, USA

Bonnie L Milas MD
Assistant Professor of Anesthesia, University of
Pennsylvania Medical Center, Philadelphia PA, USA

Riti Patel MD
Fellow in Cardiovascular Medicine, University of
Pennsylvania Medical Center, Philadelphia PA, USA

Vikas V Patel MD
Fellow in Cardiovascular Medicine, University of
Pennsylvania Medical Center, Philadelphia PA, USA

Muredach P Reilly MB
Instructor of Medicine, Cardiovascular Division,
University of Pennsylvania Medical Center, Philadelphia
PA, USA

Martin St John Sutton MB BS FRCP
John Bryfogle Professor of Cardiovascular Diseases and
Director, Cardiovascular Imaging, University of
Pennsylvania Medical Center, Philadelphia PA, USA

Frederick F Samaha MD, FACC
Chief, Cardiovascular Division, Philadelphia VAMC,
Assistant Professor of Medicine, University of
Pennsylvania Medical Center, Philadelphia PA, USA

Craig H Scott MD, FACC
Assistant Professor of Medicine, Cardiovascular Imaging
Section, University of Pennsylvania Medical Center,
Philadelphia PA, USA

Frank E Silvestry MD
Chief, Cardiovascular Division Philadelphia VAMC,
Assistant Professor of Medicine, University of
Pennsylvania Medical Center, Philadelphia PA, USA

Elizabeth A Tarka MD
Assistant Professor of Medicine, Cardiovascular Imaging
Section, University of Pennsylvania Medical Center,
Philadelphia PA, USA

Kuo-Yang Wang MD
Cardiovascular Division, Taichung Veterans General
Hospital, Taichung, Taiwan

Susan E Wiegers MD, FACC
Assistant Professor of Medicine, Cardiovascular Imaging
Section, University of Pennsylvania Medical Center,
Philadelphia PA, USA

Preface

Expertise in echocardiography requires not only a firm grasp of the technical and clinical aspects of the procedure, but an exposure to a broad variety of clinical situations. When Alan Burgess of the publishing company Martin Dunitz Ltd approached us to prepare this volume, we felt that a case-based approach would allow us to present our clinical studies in a format that would be helpful to a variety of professionals. In routine clinical practice, it may not be possible to accumulate exposure to the range of diagnoses demonstrated here. The book is directed not only at echocardiographers and cardiovascular trainees, but also at cardiologists, cardiothoracic anesthesiologists, internists and technologists who wish to improve their understanding of diagnostic non-invasive imaging. We have used a uniform format in presenting the cases; each case is composed of images from a single patient. However, the case presentations have been greatly simplified and in some cases are an amalgamation of several patients' experiences with these conditions. As such, they do not represent case reports.

We have attempted to present and discuss not only common clinical problems and their implications, but unusual cases and diagnostic dilemmas which have been seen in our laboratory over the past several years. Although the diagnosis in each case is given in its title, one way to use the book would be to read the case presentation and review the images generating an independent differential diagnosis prior to reading the figure legends and case discussion. The references at the end of each chapter provide further reading on the points discussed, rather than an exhausted bibliography of each subject.

Acknowledgements

The authors would like to acknowledge the technologists in the Echocardiographic Laboratory of the Hospital of the University of Pennsylvania. It is the expertise of these fine echocardiographers that has enabled us to present these images. We thank Karen Eberman, Lise Fishman, Eva Hungler, Kenneth Ruddell and Darlene Wright. We also thank the fellows and our colleagues on the attending staff at the hospital for their assistance. We appreciate the help and good humor of Alan Burgess of Martin Dunitz who made the book possible, and of Kate Roberts, our project editor, who helped to ensure this book's timely publication. Finally, we would like to gratefully acknowledge the superb editorial assistance of Dawn Riley who helped with many aspects of the manuscript preparation.

Susan E Wiegers
Ted Plappert
Martin St John Sutton
September 2000

SECTION I

Pericardial Disease

Mobile pericardial masses

Susan E Wiegers MD

A 33-year-old man was frequently non-compliant with dialysis. His end-stage renal disease was the result of glomerulonephritis. A small pericardial effusion had been noted on a previous echocardiogram one year earlier. The patient presented to the dialysis center complaining of worsening exercise tolerance and a cough. On examination, his blood pressure was 120/85 mmHg with 16 mmHg pulsus paradoxus. The heart rate was 100 bpm. The heart sounds were distant. A chest X-ray demonstrated a massively enlarged and rounded cardiac silhouette.

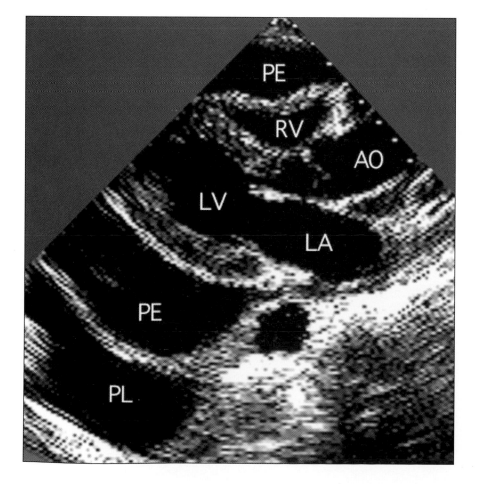

Figure 1.1
Parasternal long axis view of the heart in diastole. A large circumferential pericardial effusion (PE) is present. The anterior echo-free space is large and inversion of the anterior right ventricular free wall is evident in diastole. This is an echocardiographic sign of increased pericardial pressure. Posteriorly, the pericardial effusion is limited by the pericardial reflection posterior to the left atrium (LA) and anterior to the descending thoracic aorta. A large left pleural effusion (PL) is also present. LV, left ventricle.

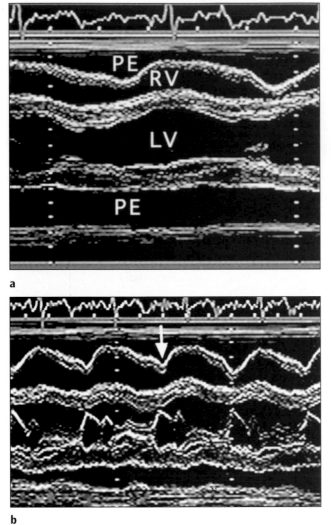

a

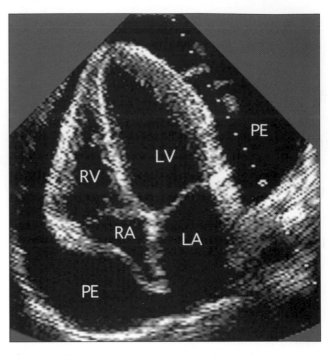

Figure 1.3
Off-axis apical four-chamber view. The transducer has been placed lateral to the left ventricular apex to demonstrate collapse of the right atrium (RA) which persisted for more than 40% of the cardiac cycle in real time. The very large pericardial effusion (PE) is seen to contain free floating masses, which swirled randomly within the pericardial space.

b

Figure 1.2
(a) M-mode from the parasternal position at the level of the papillary muscles. The pericardial effusion (PE) is present anteriorly and posteriorly to the heart. The left ventricle (LV) cavity size is small, consistent with decreased preload. The right ventricular (RV) dimension varies with respiration but collapses during diastole in some cycles.
(b) M-mode from the parasternal position at the level of the mitral valve. The arrow marks diastolic invagination of the right ventricular free wall in early diastole. The right ventricular dimension does increase in end diastole. These findings are consistent with increased intrapericardial pressure but are not diagnostic of tamponade.

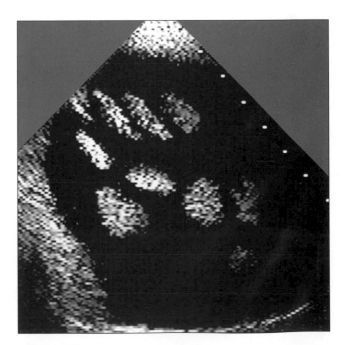

Figure 1.4
Posteriorly directed left axillary view of the massive pericardial effusion, demonstrating the pericardial 'fish' which were discrete masses floating within the fluid.

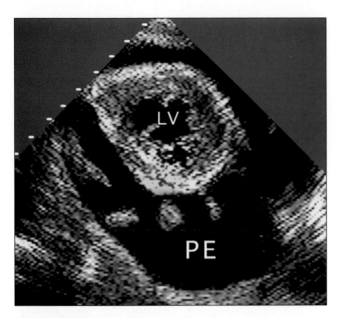

Figure 1.5
Parasternal short axis view of the left ventricle (LV) surrounded by the massive pericardial effusion (PE). The pericardial masses are again imaged. A large mass appears attached to the medial aspect of the parietal pericardium. The right ventricle is compressed in this frame and the right ventricular cavity cannot be seen.

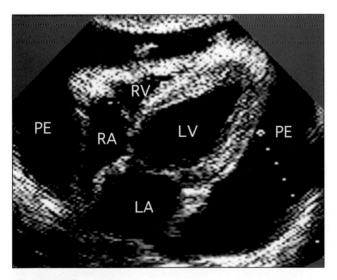

Figure 1.6
Subcostal four-chamber view directed towards the apex. Compression of the right atrium (RA) is again evidenced with reversal of the radius of curvature of the right atrial wall. The right ventricular cavity is very small and the free wall is compressed. Adequate clearance for percutaneous pericardiocentesis is demonstrated with >1 cm of free fluid at the level of the distal right ventricular free wall and apex.

Discussion

The patient had a massive chronic pericardial effusion which was due to uremia. The longstanding nature of the effusion was evidenced clinically by his stable hemodynamics.

The pericardium can accommodate a large amount of fluid if it accumulates slowly. However, even a small amount of rapidly accumulating pericardial fluid may cause hemodynamic collapse. The pericardial masses appeared to be collections of fibrinous debris within the effusion. Figure 1.1 demonstrates the relationship of the pericardial space to the pleural space and the descending thoracic aorta. The visceral pericardium which overlays the epicardium is reflected posteriorly at the level of the pulmonary veins to form the parietal pericardium. The pericardial space is normally a potential space between these two layers. A pericardial effusion occupies a space anterior to the descending thoracic aorta and terminates at the level of the atrioventricular groove. A pleural effusion may extend posteriorly to the aorta because it is not restricted by the pericardial reflections.

Echocardiography has replaced all other modalities for the evaluation of pericardial effusions.[1] Right atrial collapse is the most sensitive sign of increased intrapericardial pressure. Right ventricular diastolic collapse, left atrial collapse and finally left ventricular collapse may appear as the pericardial pressure rises. Respiratory variation of tricuspid valve inflow is also a sensitive sign of tamponade physiology.[2] This patient had increased intrapericardial pressure as evidenced by the right atrial collapse and the right ventricular compression. However, he did not have tamponade physiology either clinically or by echocardiographic signs. He was treated by percutaneous pericardiocentesis of 800 ml of fluid followed by daily dialysis.

References

1. Chandraratna PA. Echocardiography and Doppler ultrasound in the evaluation of pericardial disease. Circulation 1991;84:I303–10.

2. Appleton CP, Hatle LK, Popp RL. Cardiac tamponade and pericardial effusion: respiratory variation in transvalvular flow velocities studied by Doppler echocardiography. J Am Coll Cardiol 1988;11:1020–30.

2

Chronic tamponade

Frank E Silvestry MD

A 38-year-old woman presented to the emergency room with progressive cough, dyspnea and orthopnea. About 3 weeks prior to presentation, she began experiencing the symptoms of 'the worst cold of her life' with fevers and a dry cough. This gradually progressed to dyspnea on exertion, and later dyspnea at rest. She was unable to lie flat and noted 'a smothering sensation'. Her past medical and surgical history was unremarkable.

Physical examination revealed a well-developed woman in moderate distress. Her blood pressure was 110/90 mmHg and heart rate 115 bpm in sinus tachycardia. A pulsus paradoxus was measured at 24 mmHg. ECG demonstrated low voltage with non-specific ST and T wave changes. A chest X-ray revealed marked cardiomegaly with clear lungs. An urgent echocardiogram was obtained.

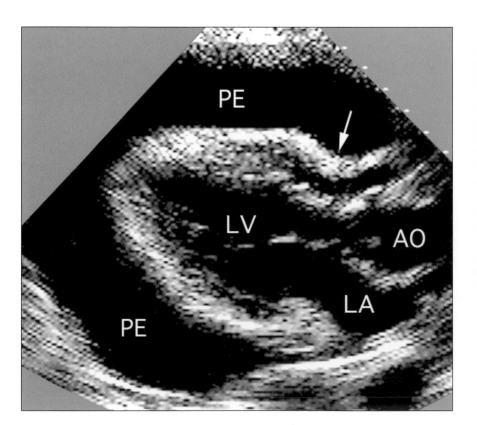

Figure 2.1
Parasternal long-axis view during early diastole demonstrating a large (>1000 ml) circumferential pericardial effusion surrounding the right and left ventricles, both anteriorly and posteriorly. The mitral valve is open indicating diastole, and the right ventricular free wall invagination (arrow) is evident. This represents right ventricular diastolic collapse and is indicative of increased intrapericardial pressure. The massive effusion is present posteriorly to the level of the pericardial reflection at the atrioventricular groove. Anteriorly, the effusion is seen to at least the level of the right ventricular outflow tract.

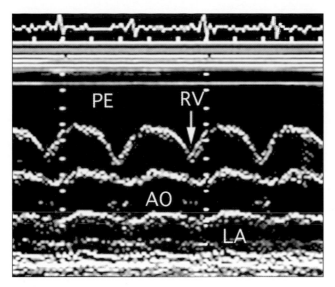

Figure 2.2
M-mode echocardiogram from the parasternal position at the level of the base of the heart. The wall of the right ventricular outflow tract (RV) is demonstrated at this level, anterior to the aortic root (AO) and left atrium (LA). The RV free wall collapses during diastole (arrow) and moves anteriorly only in late diastole, when the right ventricular pressure exceeds the intrapericardial pressure. M-mode echocardiography has an advantage in assessing RV wall motion, owing to its temporal resolution.

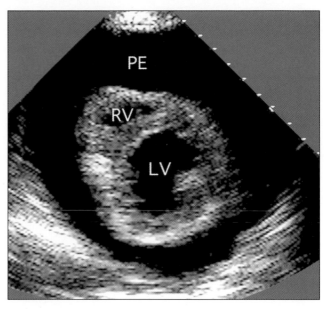

Figure 2.3
Parasternal short axis view of the left ventricle at the level of the papillary muscles, demonstrating a massive circumferential pericardial effusion, surrounding the left and right ventricles. The pericardium is indistinct and appears fuzzy. There are several areas that appear focally thickened, but no definite mass is appreciated.

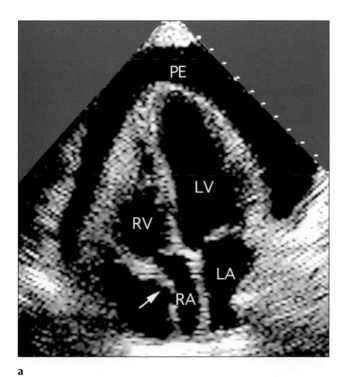

a

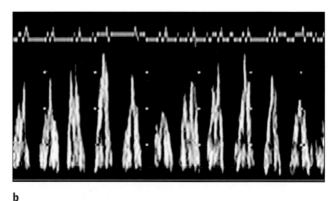

b

Figure 2.4
(a) Apical four-chamber view demonstrating a large circumferential pericardial effusion (PE) with right atrial collapse. An artifact from the right ventricular free wall extends along the ultrasound beam and might initially be mistaken for the right atrial wall. However, closer inspection demonstrates that the right atrial wall is severely compressed and has been invaginated towards the interatrial septum.
(b) Spectral display of transmitral pulsed-wave Doppler signal from the apical position. There is marked respiratory variation in flow velocities, corresponding to decreased transmitral filling with inspiration.

Discussion

This patient presented with clinical signs of chronic tamponade, and echocardiographic signs of increased intrapericardial pressure due to a large circumferential pericardial effusion. Tamponade occurs when a pericardial effusion causes a significant rise in intrapericardial pressure, and limits diastolic filling. The development of tamponade is related to the rate of the accumulation of intrapericardial fluid, and the extent to which the pericardium is able to stretch to accommodate the fluid. Acute tamponade can develop after the rapid introduction of only 150–200 ml of fluid into the pericardium, as is seen with acute cardiac trauma, aortic dissection with rupture into the pericardium, myocardial infarction with rupture, or following ventricular perforation during invasive procedures. This is a life-threatening disorder that typically presents with hypotension, tachycardia and elevated central venous pressures. A slowly developing effusion may produce chronic tamponade, and fluid accumulations may be quite large, often over 1000–1500 ml. Chronic tamponade typically presents in a less dramatic fashion, often without significant hypotension. In fact, patients with pre-existing hypertension typically present with a 'normal' or even elevated blood pressure. Tachycardia, a narrowing of the pulse pressure due to limitation of cardiac stroke volume, a pulsus paradoxus, and a widening of the cardiac silhouette on CXR may be the only signs of chronic tamponade.

Common etiologies of pericardial effusion with tamponade include malignancy, uremia, connective tissue disease and post-infectious pericarditis. After pericardiotomy, focal tamponade may develop because of compression of the right or the left atrium, or the right ventricle.

It should be emphasized that tamponade is a clinical syndrome, and is usually defined by clinical findings. Echocardiographic signs of increased intrapericardial pressure may precede the clinical syndrome and therefore are not specific for tamponade. With clinical tamponade a pericardial effusion is almost always seen on echocardiography. However, acute traumatic tamponade may result from a relatively small effusion, which may be difficult to demonstrate in all views. Collapse of the right atrium, right ventricle, and left atrium are commonly seen with increases in intrapericardial pressure. Right ventricular diastolic collapse is seen in over 80% of patients with tamponade.[1] Careful Doppler examination of both inflow and outflow velocities reveal respirophasic variation that is caused by abnormal ventricular interdependence.[2] An increase in right ventricular filling occurs upon inspiration, which results in shift of the interventricular septum towards the left, and reduces effective left ventricular filling. A decrease in the pressure gradient from the pulmonary veins to the left heart occurs as a result of increased intrapericardial pressure, and results in decreased mitral inflow velocities upon inspiration. This decrease in left ventricular preload thereby decreases stroke volume, and may result in respirophasic variation in aortic outflow velocities. Respiratory variation of flow is the hallmark of conditions associated with increased intrapericardial pressure, although it is not specific for tamponade, and may be seen in constrictive pericarditis and in conditions associated with increased negative intrathoracic pressures such as increased work of breathing, asthma, and pulmonary embolism.

Echocardiography may also be useful in choosing a therapeutic approach or monitoring during pericardiocentesis.[3] More than 1 cm of distance between the visceral and parietal pericardial surfaces is necessary for clearance for subxiphoid pericardiocentesis. This should be assessed only from the subcostal or epigastric window, since adherent pericardium may not be visualized from other views. Injection of contrast material or agitated saline after the needle is inserted into the pericardium can be used to confirm intrapericardial location. Failure to visualize echocardiographic contrast within the pericardium after injection of agitated saline into the pericardiocentesis needle or catheter should prompt immediate removal of the needle. Patients with predominantly loculated effusions may be referred for surgical drainage, through a small subxiphoid incision, by a video thoracoscopic approach, or via sternotomy.

The patient was taken to the catheterization laboratory where a percutaneous pericardiocentesis was performed. Over 1 liter of fluid was removed with prompt resolution of her symptoms. Cultures and cytology of the exudative fluid were negative. She remained well for several months but had a recurrence of her symptoms.

References

1. Reydel B, Spodick DH. Frequency and significance of chamber collapse during cardiac tamponade. Am Heart J 1990;119:1160–3.

2. Burstow DJ, Oh JK, Bailey KR, et al. Cardiac tamponade: characteristic Doppler observations. Mayo Clin Proc. 1989;64:312.

3. Chandratana PAN, Reid CL, Nimalasuriya A, et al. Application of two dimensional contrast studies during pericardiocentesis. Am J Cardiol 1983;52:1120–2.

3

Intrapericardial tumor with pericardial effusion

Frank E Silvestry MD

A 38-year-old woman presented to the emergency room with recurrent dyspnea and orthopnea. Three months earlier, she had begun experiencing similar symptoms and was found to have a large circumferential pericardial effusion with signs of increased intrapericardial pressure by echocardiography (see Chapter 2). Her physical examination and right heart catheterization at that time confirmed tamponade, and the effusion was drained by subxiphoid pericardiocentesis. Cultures and cytology of the pericardial fluid were negative. Her past medical and surgical history was otherwise unremarkable.

Physical examination upon presentation revealed a thin woman in moderate distress. Her blood pressure was 130/90 mmHg, and heart rate 108 bpm in sinus tachycardia. A pulsus paradoxus was measured at 18 mmHg. ECG demonstrated low voltage with non-specific ST and T wave changes. Her chest X-ray revealed cardiomegaly with clear lungs. An urgent echocardiogram was obtained.

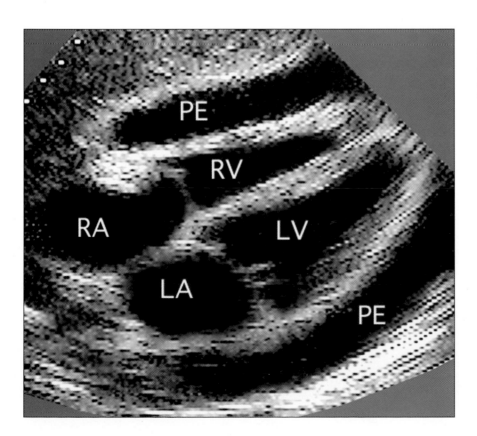

Figure 3.1
Subcostal four-chamber view demonstrating a moderate to large circumferential pericardial effusion (PE). There is no definite evidence of a mass in this view.

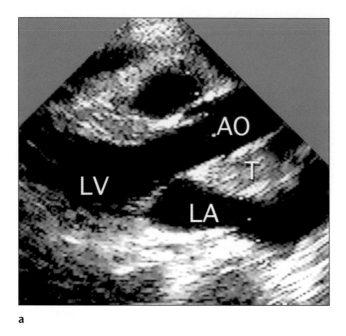

a

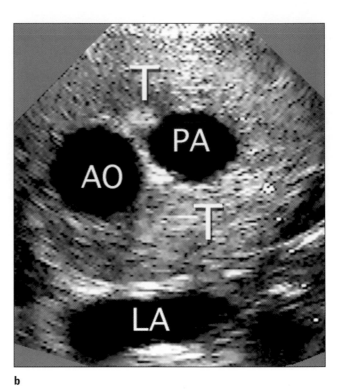

b

Figure 3.2

(a) Parasternal long axis view from high intercostal space. The usual anatomy has been distorted by a mass (T) which is best appreciated in this view posterior to the ascending aorta (AO). The mass compresses the left atrium (LA) to a small extent. There is a suggestion of the mass anterior to the aorta but this is not clearly seen.

(b) Parasternal short-axis view at the level of the pulmonary artery demonstrating a large tumor mass which encases the pulmonary artery (PA). The mass is over 7 cm in diameter and also surrounds the ascending aorta. The left atrium is clearly compressed by the mass in this view. This tumor's position is superior to the pulmonary artery as well, resulting in moderate pulmonary artery compression (see below).

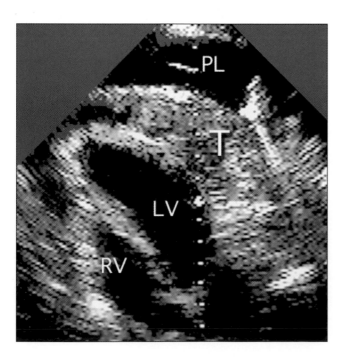

Figure 3.3

Off-axis apical four-chamber view demonstrating the extent of the tumor which is present within the pericardial space (PE) adjacent to the lateral wall of the left ventricle. There is a moderate amount of pericardial fluid seen at the left ventricular apex and surrounding the right ventricle. Note the left pleural effusion (PL), which is seen anterior to the left ventricle in this view. In comparison to the four-chamber subcostal view, the tumor is visualized by off-axis imaging but was not seen on the subcostal view.

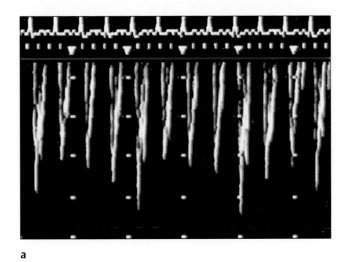

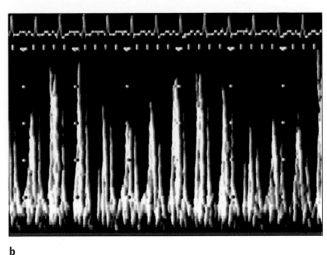

a   b

Figure 3.4

(a) Spectral display of pulsed-wave Doppler from the parasternal position across the pulmonary valve. The right ventricular filling normally increases with inspiration. Respirophasic variation in right ventricular outflow velocities is caused by the increased intrapericardial pressure from the tumor and fluid which is unable to accommodate the increased right ventricular volume.
(b) Spectral display of pulsed-wave Doppler from the apical position across the tricuspid valve. Again, respirophasic variation in diastolic inflow velocities confirms the presence of increased intrapericardial pressure.

Discussion

A large variety of extracardiac masses can been detected on two-dimensional echocardiography, including mediastinal tumors, pericardial tumors, intrathoracic neoplasms, and pericardial cysts. Clinical manifestations of malignant pericardial involvement include pericardial effusion with or without tamponade, neoplastic epicardial deposits, effusive–constrictive pericarditis, and constriction.

A pericardial effusion commonly results from neoplastic involvement of the visceral and parietal pericardium. Metastatic disease to the pericardium often results in thickening or nodular studding of the pericardium, although frank masses can be seen as well.[1] Pericardial thickening or nodular irregularity is not specific for neoplastic disease, and can also be seen with chronic effusions, or infectious pericardial processes. Other patterns of neoplastic disease include diffuse layering of echoes, tumor encasement, or pericardial metastases with intramyocardial extension.

When masses are seen within the pericardium, metastatic disease is often the etiology. Breast and lung carcinoma, lymphoma and leukemia, and malignant melanomas all commonly metastasize to the pericardium. Pericardial cysts, teratomas, angiosarcomas, and pheochromocytomas have all been detected by two-dimensional echocardiography within the pericardium. Transesophageal echocardiography may be superior to transthoracic echocardiography in identifying pericardial tumors, and determining their anatomic characteristics.[2] Whether this information contributes to clinical management is less clear, however.

This patient had undergone percutaneous drainage of the effusion three months previously without diagnosis, and chest computerized tomography was negative for masses at that time (Chapter 2). Owing to the recurrent nature of the problem, it was felt that a repeat pericardiocentesis would not be definitive. Therefore, the patient was taken to the operating room, where pericardial drainage and biopsy were performed through a video thoracoscopic approach. The biopsy revealed a granular cell tumor, a rare type of sarcoma. More commonly seen as a chest wall mass, this type of sarcoma is rarely seen in the pericardium. While not malignant per se, this tumor is locally invasive and was not resectable.

References

1. Chandaratna PAN, Aronow WS. Detection of pericardial metastases by cross-sectional echocardiography. Circulation 1981;63:197–9.

2. Smalling RG, Albornoz M, Tak T, et al. Role of transesophageal echocardiography in evaluating pericardial disease. Circulation 1992;86(Suppl 1):1726–29.

4

Thymoma

Susan E Wiegers MD

A 65-year-old woman complained of shortness of breath and difficulty performing normal daily activities. She became extremely fatigued and weak after walking one block. She noted that she could climb only half a flight of stairs without pulling herself on the hand rail. In the past month, she had also noted some double vision and difficulty swallowing. On physical examination, her lungs were clear. The cardiac examination was entirely normal. Her primary care doctor sent her for an echocardiogram to exclude cardiac dysfunction.

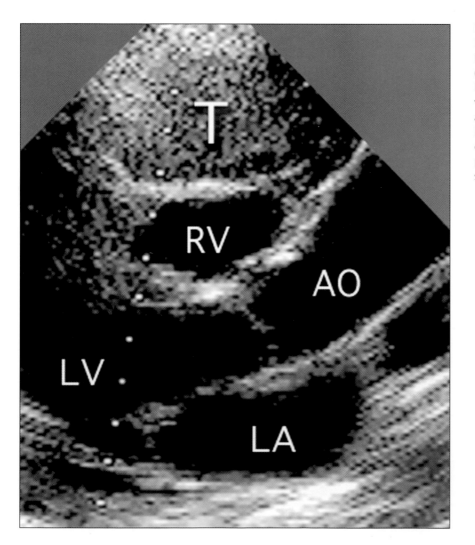

Figure 4.1
Parasternal long axis view taken from a high parasternal window. A large mass (T) fills the anterior mediastinal space between the chest wall and the right ventricular free wall (RV). The ascending aorta (AO) is normal, but the left atrium (LA) appears mildly compressed. The left ventricle (LV) is poorly seen from this high intercostal space.

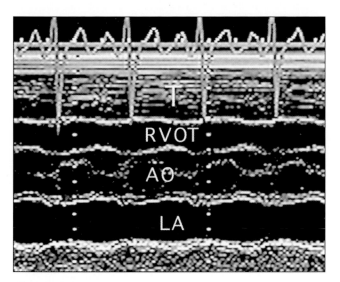

Figure 4.2
M-mode echocardiogram taken from the same high parasternal position. The tumor mass (T) in the anterior mediastinum is at least 3 cm in diameter. The right ventricular outflow tract (RVOT) is slightly compressed, although it is not narrowed enough to be hemodynamically significant.

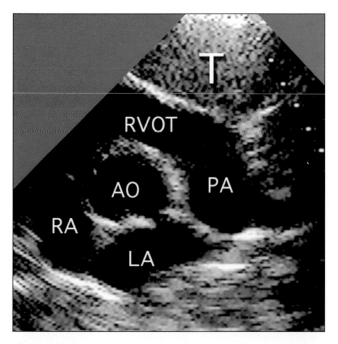

Figure 4.3
Parasternal short-axis view at the base of the heart. The large tumor mass (T) is again seen in the anterior mediastinum between the chest wall and the right ventricular outflow tract (RVOT). The pulmonary valve is not well visualized, but the pulmonary artery (PA) is normal. The left main pulmonary artery is seen to the right of the image at the bifurcation, but the right main pulmonary artery is not visualized in this view. The anterior mediastinum mass appears to surround the pulmonary artery down to the level of at least the mid-main artery. Its true extent is not well visualized in this image.

Discussion

The thymus is often visualized in neonatal echocardiograms in the anterior mediastinal space between the sternum and the right ventricle. In normal infants, the thymus may be as large as the heart itself and extend down to the level of the left ventricular apex. The thymic tissue has a homogeneous appearance. However, involution of the thymic tissue is expected in early childhood. By adulthood, the thymus is chiefly fat and is not usually imaged as a definite structure on echocardiogram. This patient had myasthenia gravis which accounted for her neuromuscular symptoms. This autoimmune disease is associated with abnormalities of the thymus in over 80% of patients. Hyperplasia of the thymus due to immune cell infiltration of the perivascular spaces in the organ is the most common abnormality. Non-malignant cortical thymomas and rarely invasive thymomas may be present in approximately 10% of patients.

On echocardiography, thymomas may be recognized as homogeneous echo-dense tissue in the anterior mediastinum. The anterior mediastinum is the small space between the sternum and the pericardium. Transthoracic echo may be more helpful than transesophageal echo in investigating these tumors, as they are in the far field in the transesophageal study. Thymomas may compress the heart and cause the superior vena caval syndrome as well as cardiac compression and localized tamponade. Posterior displacement of the heart, diminished dimensions of the left atrium and left ventricle, and pseudo-prolapse of the mitral valve have all been reported.[1] This patient had evidence of mild right ventricular outflow tract compression. However, there was no respiratory variation in the position of the interventricular septum or in the Doppler inflow velocities, thus ruling out localized tamponade.

Rarely thymomas may be invasive and penetrate the pericardium, pulmonary artery, or right atrium.[2,3] In this patient the thymoma was an incidental finding on the echocardiographic study. Cardiac disease was not the cause of her symptoms. However, the presence of the anterior mediastinal mass was confirmed by CAT scan. The patient's myasthenia responded to thymectomy.

References

1. Canedo M, Otken L, Stefadourous M. Echocardiographic features of cardiac compression by a thymoma stimulating cardiac tamponade in obstruction of the superior vena cava. Br Heart J 1997;39:1038–42.

2. Missault L, Duprez D, De Buyzere M, et al. Right atrial invasive thymoma with protrusion through the tricuspid valve. Eur Heart J 1992;13:1726–7.

3. Nishimura T, Kondo M, Miyazaki S, et al. Two-dimensional echocardiographic findings of cardiovascular involvement by invasive thymoma. Chest 1982;81:752–4.

5

Constrictive pericardial disease

Frank E Silvestry MD

A 42-year-old woman presented for liver transplant evaluation with a diagnosis of 'cryptogenic cirrhosis'. Following a bout of presumed 'viral hepatitis' one year previously, she had begun to experience increasing abdominal girth. Evaluation revealed elevated liver enzymes, an elevated prothrombin time, and ascites on abdominal ultrasonography. On careful questioning the patient recalled mild lower extremity edema and dyspnea. Clinical and laboratory evaluation revealed no evidence of viral hepatitis, malignancy, or collagen vascular disease.

The patient was thin. Her blood pressure was 110/80 mmHg, heart rate 93 bpm and regular. A pulsus was measured at 9 mmHg. Her jugular venous pressure was 15 cmH$_2$O, with a pronounced inspiratory rise (Kussmaul sign). Cardiac auscultation revealed a high-pitched late diastolic filling sound, prior to S1. The abdomen was distended with shifting dullness. There was mild lower-extremity edema. ECG demonstrated only non-specific ST and T wave changes. Chest X-ray revealed a normal-sized heart and clear lungs. An echocardiogram was obtained. The patient was diagnosed as having constrictive pericarditis and was taken to the operating room for pericardial stripping. A transesophageal echocardiogram was performed in the operating room.

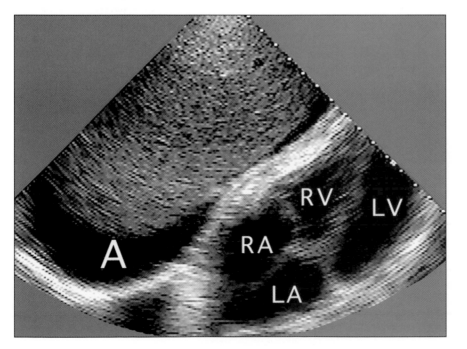

Figure 5.1
Transthoracic subcostal four-chamber view demonstrating marked thickening and fusion of the pericardial surfaces, best seen along the right ventricular free wall. The pericardium is very bright which is suggestive of scarring. A moderate amount of ascites (A) surrounds the liver. The shift of the interventricular septum to the left may be seen on this view, but must be confirmed from the apical position.

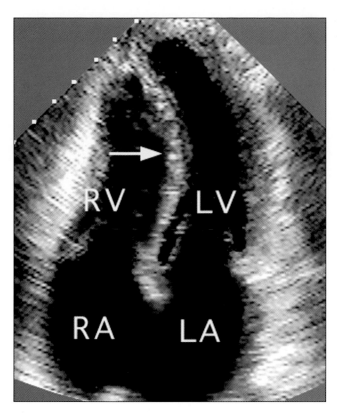

Figure 5.2
Transthoracic apical four-chamber view during diastole
demonstrating markedly abnormal diastolic septal motion
(arrow). The septum is bowed to the left during inspiration. This
finding is frequently seen with constriction and in real time is
appreciated as a sudden and vigorous shift to the left. Note the
echogenic, thickened, and tethered pericardium surrounding all
cardiac chambers. Both ventricles appear underfilled, as a result
of the pericardial constraint to diastolic filling.

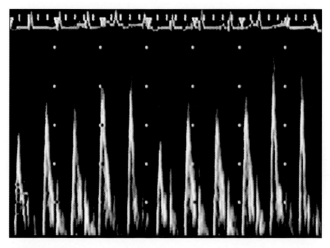

Figure 5.4
Spectral display of pulsed wave Doppler from the
transthoracic apical position. The sample volume has been
placed at the tips of the mitral valve leaflets. There is marked
inspiratory decline in mitral velocities consistent with
constriction (see Discussion).

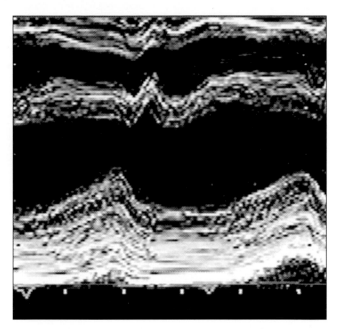

Figure 5.3
M-mode echocardiogram from the parasternal position. The
septal motion is markedly abnormal displaying the systolic
'bounce' in which there is sharp anterior motion of the
interventricular septum. The posterior wall motion is flat with
no posterior motion during diastole. These two findings are
highly suggestive of constrictive pericarditis.

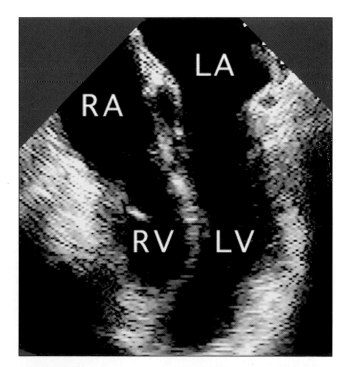

Figure 5.5
Transesophageal echocardiogram from the mid-esophageal
level in the transverse plane (imaging angle 0°). The four-
chamber view demonstrates the small ventricular chamber
sizes and the thickened and echo bright pericardium,
particularly overlaying the left ventricular lateral wall.

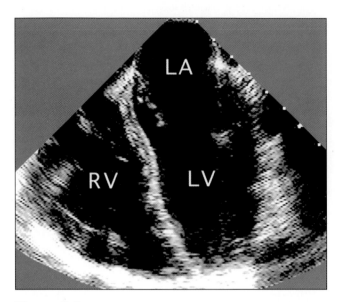

Figure 5.6
Transesophageal echocardiogram from the mid-esophageal level in the transverse plane (imaging angle 0°). This image was taken after the operation in which the pericardium was removed anteriorly and as far posteriorly as possible. The ventricular volumes have increased substantially.

Discussion

Constrictive pericardial disease can occur as a result of a wide variety of pericardial processes including post-viral pericarditis, tuberculous pericarditis, malignancy, post-uremic pericarditis, and post-pericardiotomy syndrome. It is characterized by pericardial thickening that impairs cardiac filling, resulting in right heart failure and low cardiac output. Chronic passive congestion of the liver can lead to 'cardiac cirrhosis'.

Thickening or calcification of the pericardial surfaces may be observed in constriction on transthoracic echocardiography, although this finding is neither reliably seen nor is it specific for constriction.[1] M-mode and two-dimensional echocardiography may demonstrate mid- to late diastolic flattening of the posterior wall, reflecting an abrupt cessation of ventricular filling after early diastole. On two-dimensional echocardiography, tethering of the pericardial surfaces results from adherence and fusion of the visceral and parietal pericardium. This lack of normal sliding motion of the pericardial surfaces is not specific for constriction, however. A dilated inferior vena cava (plethora) without respiratory variation is another common finding, but as it results from elevated right atrial pressure it is not specific for constriction per se.

Abnormal septal motion ('diastolic septal bouncing') results from abnormal interventricular dependence due to impaired expansion of the free walls of the ventricles caused by the constricting effect of the pericardium. This can be seen on M-mode or two-dimensional echocardiography as an exaggerated early diastolic notch with abrupt cessation of early passive filling, followed by a double component during atrial systole.[2] On M-mode, this double component comprises posterior displacement of the interventricular septum during atrial systole, followed by an abrupt anterior motion of the septum occurring at the end of atrial systole.

The hallmark of constriction is the demonstration of respiratory variation in mitral and tricuspid inflow.[3] These findings are similar to those seen with cardiac tamponade. In constriction, the thickened pericardium prevents changes in intrathoracic pressure with respiration from being transmitted to the cardiac chambers, thereby reducing the pressure gradient for flow from the pulmonary veins to the left atrium and ventricle. There is also an exaggerated shift of the interventricular septum towards the left ventricle with inspiration, further compromising left ventricular diastolic filling. Mitral inflow velocities are significantly reduced at the onset of inspiration, and the isovolumic relaxation time (IVRT) is prolonged. With expiration, mitral inflow velocities return to normal and IVRT shortens. A reciprocal relationship exists for tricuspid inflow. Both of these patterns have been demonstrated to become normal after pericardiectomy.

Often the echocardiographic diagnosis of constriction is made on the basis of eliciting a number of the findings described above, as no single finding itself is pathognomonic. The greater the number of associated findings identified, the higher the likelihood that constriction is present.[4] That said, other diagnostic measures, such as right heart catheterization and imaging of the pericardial surfaces with computerized tomography or magnetic resonance imaging, may be employed to corroborate the diagnosis and plan a therapeutic strategy.

This patient therefore had pericardial constriction rather than liver failure as a cause of her symptoms. She underwent pericardial stripping which was complicated by atrial fibrillation. Her symptoms resolved and she was able to return to normal activities.

References

1. Voelkel AG, Pietro DA, Folland ED, *et al*. Echocardiographic features of constrictive pericarditis. Circulation 1978;58:871–5.

2. Gibson TC, Grossman W, McLaurin LP, *et al*. An echocardiographic study of the interventricular system in constrictive pericarditis. Br Heart J 1976;38:738–43.

3. Hatle LK, Appleton CP, Popp RL. Differentiation of constrictive pericarditis and restrictive cardiomyopathy by Doppler echocardiography. Circulation 1989;79:357–70.

4. King SW, Pandian NG, Gardin JM. Doppler echocardiographic findings in pericardial tamponade and constriction. Echocardiography 1988;5:361–3.

6

Postoperative tamponade

Bonnie Milas MD

A 62-year-old man developed relative hypotension 12 hours postoperatively following myocardial revascularization (CABG). Hemodynamic monitoring revealed a progressive increase in the central venous pressure which was elevated at 25 mmHg, equal to the pulmonary artery diastolic pressure. The cardiac index was 2.1 l/m² and the systemic blood pressure 100/50 mmHg. The ECG demonstrated sinus tachycardia at 105 bpm. His chest drainage tube output had been a total of 1200 ml, but this had subsided. A transesophageal echocardiogram was performed to rule out cardiac tamponade.

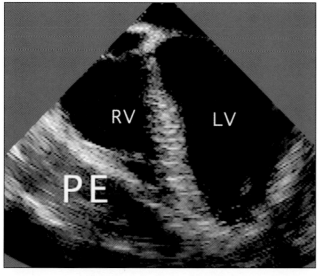

a

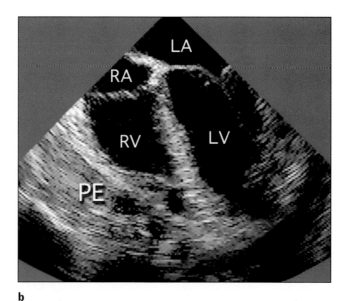

b

Figure 6.1
(a) Transesophageal four-chamber view in the transverse plane (imaging angle 0°) in diastole. A heterogeneous pericardial effusion (PE) is noted anterior to the right ventricle (RV) in the pericardial space. The hetergeneous nature (varying degrees of echodensity) of the effusion is due to the non-uniform clotting of blood that occurs in postoperative hemorrhage. The right ventricle appears to be extrinsically compressed by the adjacent pericardial clot. Although there is not complete right ventricular collapse or invagination during diastole, it is suspected that right ventricular diastolic filling is compromised. The left ventricle (LV) appears to be of normal size, suggesting adequate filling.
(b) Similar view in systole. Biventricular systolic function is normal.

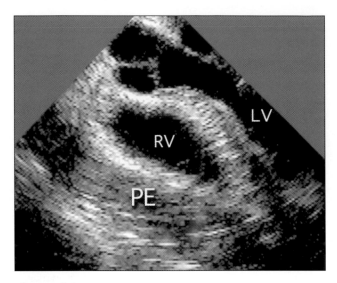

Figure 6.2
Transesophageal echocardiogram during diastole. The probe has been withdrawn and rotated to the patient's right compared to the previous image. The pericardial clot extends to the level of the atrioventricular groove.

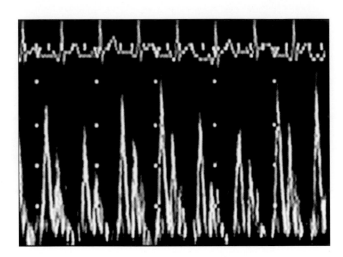

Figure 6.3
Spectral display of pulsed-wave Doppler of mitral valve inflow. The orientation has been inverted on the machine so that the flow away from the esophageal transducer is above the baseline. Variation in peak mitral valve inflow velocity is noted. The patient's cardiac rhythm is normal sinus and therefore the variance of inflow velocity is not due to variation in diastolic filling time from an irregular cardiac rhythm.

Discussion

Cardiac tamponade is not an uncommon complication following cardiac surgery. It can be attributed to coagulopathy, thrombocytopenia, hypothermia, qualitative platelet dysfunction, or inadequate surgical hemostasis. Tamponade occurs in non-operative settings owing to: cardiac chamber, coronary artery, or great vessel iatrogenic perforation; aortic dissection; myocardial infarction complicated by a free wall rupture; malignant effusion; uremia or hepatic failure, coagulopathy/thrombocytopenia; pneumopericardium secondary to esophageal rupture; or infection. Coexistent findings are dependent upon the inciting etiology.

Postoperatively, the diagnosis of pericardial tamponade may require a transesophageal examination. Following cardiac surgery, soft tissue changes and foreign bodies (epicardial pacing wires and chest evacuation tubes) may obscure echocardiographic windows.[1] Additionally, a pericardial clot may be highly localized and difficult to detect.[2] Two-dimensional echocardiographic findings that are consistent with pericardial tamponade include: early diastolic collapse of the right ventricle, late diastolic inversion of the right atrium, and inferior vena cava plethora with blunted respiratory variation. Right atrial collapse during late diastole is a sensitive sign of tamponade, but not a highly specific sign. Inversion of the right atrium for more than one-third of the R-R interval is considered sensitive (94%) and specific (100%) for a hemodynamically significant pericardial effusion. Since a pericardial clot may be very localized (as opposed to a circumferential pericardial

effusion), it may not present with typical findings of tamponade. Occasionally, the pericardial effusion will be partially clotted and it may be possible to detect flow within the collection. Spectral Doppler findings consistent with pericardial tamponade include: delayed mitral valve opening, demonstrated by an increased isovolumic relaxation time and decreased E velocity; marked respiratory variation and reciprocal changes in the mitral and tricuspid valve inflow Doppler tracings. Respiratory variation may be difficult to assess, or may be attenuated in the patient who is pharmacologically paralyzed and mechanically ventilated with positive pressure ventilation, in the postoperative setting. Accumulation of a hemodynamically significant pericardial effusion or clot is an indication for emergency mediastinal re-exploration.

This patient was urgently returned to the operating room and a large hematoma was evacuated. No specific bleeding site could be detected. The patient recovered without any further complications.

References

1. Reichert CL, Visser CA, Koolen JJ, *et al*. Transesophageal echocardiography in hypotensive patients after cardiac operations. Comparison with hemodynamic parameters. J Thorac Cardiovasc Surg 1992;104:321–6.

2. Chuttani K, Tischler MD, Pandian NG, *et al*. Diagnosis of cardiac tamponade after cardiac surgery: relative value of clinical, echocardiographic, and hemodynamic signs. Am Heart J 1994;127:913–18.

7

Pleural effusion causing cardiac tamponade

Susan E Wiegers MD

An elderly woman with a left lung mass had recently been diagnosed with metastatic bronchogenic carcinoma. There was a partial response to radiation therapy, but she developed increasing dyspnea on exertion. Chest X-ray revealed a very large left pleural effusion and the patient underwent thoracocentesis with some relief of symptoms. The left pleural effusion appeared slightly smaller on the immediate post-procedure radiograph. However, two weeks later she had an episode of exertional syncope and came to the emergency room. On physical examination, she was tachycardic with evidence of systemic hypoperfusion. The blood pressure was 85/65 mmHg with 20 mmHg of pulsus paradoxus. There were no breath sounds in the left posterior thorax. The heart sounds were distant and the jugular venous pressure was elevated. The cardiac impulse was not palpable. Given the patient's underlying malignant disease, cardiac tamponade due to a malignant pericardial effusion was suspected. An echocardiogram was performed in the emergency room.

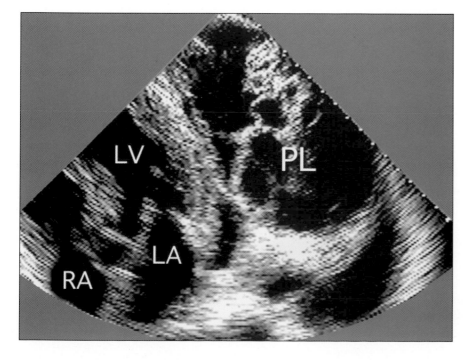

Figure 7.1
This diastolic image is taken from the standard apical transducer position for the four-chamber view. The heart is shifted to the right side of the chest by a massive left pleural effusion (PL). The pleural effusion consists of echolucent fluid interspersed with linear echodensities which are fibrinous debris within the effusion. The effusion is partially organized and probably loculated, although this cannot be determined on this echocardiographic image. There is thickening of the parietal pleura overlying the lateral wall of the left ventricle. This may be due to tumor infiltration of the pleura in this area or to pleural scarring. The cardiac chambers are small and left ventricular hypertrophy is present.

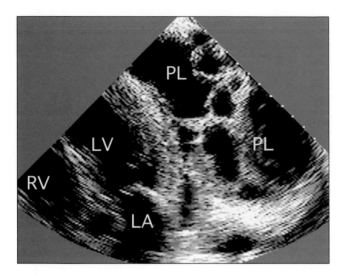

Figure 7.2
Leftward angulation of the transducer from the same position as in Figure 7.1 reveals further details of the left pleural effusion. Pockets of fluid appear to be walled off by the dense trabeculations, confirming that the effusion is loculated.

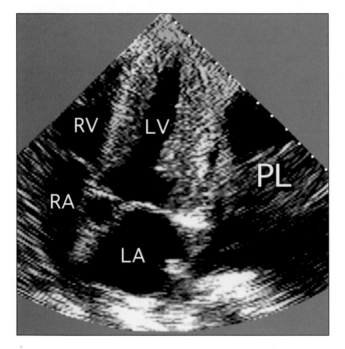

Figure 7.3
Four-chamber view of the heart in systole. This view was obtained by placing the transducer approximately 5 cm medial to the standard transducer position. The transducer is along the left lower sternal border rather than lateral to the mid-clavicular line. This change in position was necessary because of the shift in the cardiac position caused by the left pleural effusion (PL). Both ventricles have hyperdynamic function as evidenced by the small chamber areas in systole. The left atrium appears normal in size. The right atrial and ventricular chambers are small and are probably compressed by the shift in the left-sided chambers. The pleural effusion is again seen lateral to the left ventricle in the left chest. The loculations are less well seen in this view. There is no significant pericardial effusion evident on this image or in the subcostal image (not shown here).

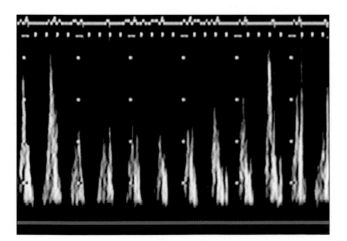

Figure 7.4
Pulsed-wave Doppler spectral display of mitral valve inflow. The sample volume has been placed at the mitral valve leaflet tips taken from the apical position. The rhythm was sinus tachycardia, but E and A waves have fused to a single diastolic filling wave, owing to the increased heart rate. There is marked respiratory variation in the inflow velocity. The minimum velocity of slightly less than 0.4 m/s is 50% of the maximum velocity, which is approximately 0.8 m/s. A variation of >30% of inflow velocity across the mitral valve is evidence of tamponade physiology. In this case, the limitation of cardiac filling is due to the pleural effusion that is compressing the heart rather than a pericardial effusion.

Discussion

Pericardial tamponade was originally suspected when the patient presented to the emergency room in shock because of the constellation of characteristic physical findings and the clinical setting. Appropriately, an emergency transthoracic echocardiogram was obtained to evaluate the cause of her hypotension. Echocardiography plays an increasing role in the emergency room, not only in trauma patients but also in acutely ill patients with hypotension or chest pain. Definitive diagnosis of the cause of the acute problem is usually possible. Transesophageal echocardiography may be necessary if the transthoracic images are inadequate.

This patient did in fact have cardiac tamponade. In this condition, limitation of diastolic filling leads to low ventricular volumes and decreased stroke volume. Compensatory tachycardia becomes insufficient to maintain cardiac output and shock ensues. Simultaneous limitation of right- and left-sided stroke volume results in fewer signs of pulmonary congestion than in other causes of cardiogenic shock. Small volumes of pericardial fluid that accumulate rapidly may cause tamponade. Malignant effusions generally accumulate very slowly, allowing gradual distension of the pericardium until the limit of the pericardial volume is reached and the intrapericardial pressure rises. In contrast, pleural effusions have rarely been reported to cause tamponade physiology.[1,2] However, an increase in intrapleural pressures can be transmitted to the intrapericardial space, resulting in a physiology indistinguishable from pericardial tamponade caused by a pericardial effusion. The pleural effusion must generally be left-sided and quite large to accomplish this degree of cardiac compression.

Some of the classic echocardiographic signs of tamponade are evident in this study. While diastolic chamber collapse is frequently seen and is a sensitive sign of tamponade, in some cases the ventricles are underfilled throughout the cardiac cycle without clear inversion of the radius of curvature of the chamber free walls. The resulting systolic function may be hyperdynamic or may be reduced, owing to the profound loss of preload. This patient had underfilled ventricular cavities and hyperdynamic systolic function. The respiratory variation in mitral inflow velocity was diagnostic of tamponade. The total cardiac volume is fixed throughout the cardiac cycle by the elevated left thoracic pressure and compression of the heart by the pleural effusion. With inspiration, venous return to the right side of the heart normally increases. The increased right ventricular volume forces the interventricular septum into the left ventricle with a resultant decrease in stroke volume. This is evidenced by a decrease in mitral inflow velocity during inspiration and a rise in expiration. Minor variation may normally be present but a change of more than 30% is considered significant on the left. The opposite pattern is seen on the right, with an increased velocity with inspiration and a fall with expiration. Variability is more common on the right side and tricuspid inflow variability must reach 50% to be considered significant.[3,4]

In order to appreciate the significant cardiac shift to the right in this patient, it is essential that the sonographer communicate the transducer position for each view to the interpreter. Most systems allow annotation directly on the image to this end. In this case, the echocardiographic images were helpful in revealing the dimensions of the pleural effusion as well as documenting the marked degree of organization. It was unlikely that this effusion could have been drained with simple thoracocentesis because it was highly organized and loculated. Therefore, the patient underwent closed drainage with a chest tube, and experienced prompt relief of her hemodynamic compromise.

References

1. Kaplan LM, Epstein SK, Stewards SL, *et al.* Clinical, echocardiographic, and hemodynamic evidence of cardiac tamponade caused by large pleural effusions. Am J Respir Crit Care Med 1995; 151:904–8.

2. Kisanuki A, Shono H, Kiyonaga K, *et al.* Two-dimensional echocardiographic demonstration of left ventricular diastolic collapse due to compression by pleural effusion. Am Heart J 1991;122:1173–5.

3. Leeman DE, Levine MJ, Come PC. Doppler echocardiography in cardiac tamponade: exaggerated respiratory variation in transvalvular blood flow velocity integrals. J Am Coll Cardiol 1988;11:572–8.

4. Appleton CP, Hatle LK, Popp RL. Cardiac tamponade and pericardial effusion: respiratory variation in transvalvular flow velocities studied by Doppler echocardiography. J Am Coll Cardiol 1988;11:1020–30.

8

Pericardial cyst

Susan E Wiegers MD

A 32-year-old woman went to see her primary care doctor complaining of palpitations. A 24-hour Holter recording demonstrated frequent bursts of supraventricular tachycardia at rates of 150 bpm and multiple premature atrial beats. She also complained of dyspnea on exertion but was able to carry out her normal activities. A chest X-ray demonstrated an enlarged cardiac silhouette with a round homogeneous mass along the right cardiac border. She was referred for an echocardiogram.

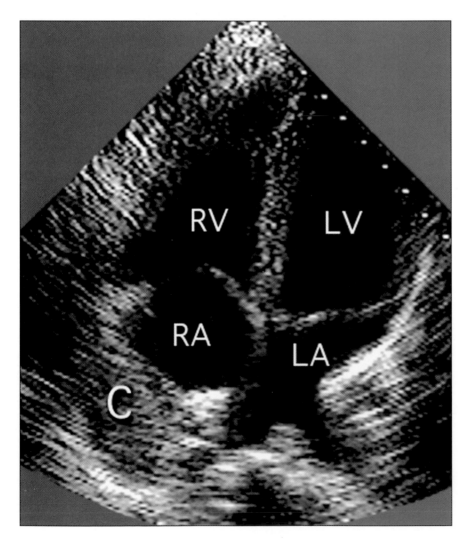

Figure 8.1
Apical four-chamber view. The transducer is medial to the standard apical position and has been placed at the right ventricular apex. The right ventricle and left ventricle appear normal in size, as do the atria. There is a large homogeneous mass (C) superior to the right atrium which is clearly extrinsic to the right atrium and does not appear to be compressing it. This was the only view in which this mass was detected, as the subcostal views in this patient were technically limited. The mass appears to be filled with homogeneous material which swirled slightly in real-time imaging.

Discussion

Pericardial cysts are benign, mediastinal masses that constitute 7–25% of all mediastinal tumors.[1] They are thought to be developmental cysts that arise because of failure of fusion of the embryonic layers of the pericardium. Pericardial cysts are usually asymptomatic and occur most frequently at the right costophrenic angle, as in this patient.[1,2] On chest X-ray, pericardial cysts usually appear as a round, sharply demarcated mass along the right cardiac silhouette. The radiographic appearance of the cysts can be considered to be pathognomonic and further workup is not recommended in the asymptomatic patient.

The availability of echocardiography has improved the diagnosis of pericardial cysts and allowed the differentiation from other malignant mediastinal masses. However, the location of the pericardial cyst may make diagnosis by transthoracic echocardiography difficult. Transesophageal imaging can be helpful in the assessment of masses posterior to the atria.[3] The echo usually reveals an echolucent mass adjacent to the right atrium, without evidence of infiltration or significant compression of cardiac structures. Pericardial cysts are generally echolucent and are not often filled with amorphous debris, as in this case. However, exudative-type fluid with a high protein content may produce the tissue characteristics present in this patient. A computerized tomography (CT) scan can confirm the water density of the mass if a low CT number is present, which would be consistent with the diagnosis of a pericardial cyst. Again, variable protein content and calcium content may cause some cysts to have a high CT number. Magnetic resonance imaging (MRI) can also be used to image the location of the cyst and to assess its composition.

Although the chest X-ray appearance, location and size of this patient's mass were all highly suggestive of a pericardial cyst, there was concern on the part of the treating physician that the mass was not echolucent. It did not appear to be a solid mass, because the contents moved during the cardiac cycle in a manner consistent with liquid. It appeared to be filled with proteinaceous debris, not specifically ruling out the mass as being a pericardial cyst. The patient underwent MRI, which was diagnostic of a pericardial cyst. The patient was reassured that the mass was not malignant. Over the next few months, her symptoms of arrhythmia progressed and failed to respond to beta-blockers. In addition, her dyspnea worsened although there was no evidence of tamponade. It was planned to undertake resection of the cyst via thoracoscopy. This technique has been described with good results in the occasional symptomatic patient and avoids the need for thoracotomy.[4] Percutaneous aspiration is also occasionally possible but was thought not to be an option in this patient, given the likely high density of the cyst fluid.[5]

References

1. Rice TW. Benign neoplasms and cysts of the mediastinum. Semin Thorac Cardiovasc Surg 1992;4:25–33.

2. Hynes JK, Tajik AJ, Osborn MJ, et al. Two-dimensional echocardiographic diagnosis of pericardial cyst. Mayo Clin Proc 1983;58:60–3.

3. Padder FA, Conrad AR, Manzar KJ, et al. Echocardiographic diagnosis of pericardial cyst. Am J Med Sci 1997;313:191–2.

4. Mouroux J, Padovani B, Maalouf J, et al. Pleuropericardial cysts: treatment by videothoracoscopy. Surg Laparosc, Endosc Percutan Tech 1996;6:403–4.

5. Ferguson MK. Thoracoscopic management of pericardial disease. Semin Thorac Cardiovasc Surg 1993;5:310–15.

9

Loculated pericardial effusion

Susan E Wiegers MD

A 74-year-old man was diagnosed with small cell carcinoma of the lung. He had minimal response to chemotherapy and was not a candidate for surgery. Mediastinal radiation resulted in severe esophagitis and fatigue. Four weeks after the initiation of therapy he presented with a disabling cough, which was much worse when supine. Severe dyspnea on exertion limited his activity and he became unable to move from bed to chair. He was brought to his doctor's office, where his blood pressure was 80/70 mmHg and the heart rate was 110 bpm. The heart sounds were muffled. There were decreased breath sounds at the left base and dullness to percussion halfway up the left posterior lung field. The patient was admitted to the hospital, where an echocardiogram was obtained to assess left ventricular function.

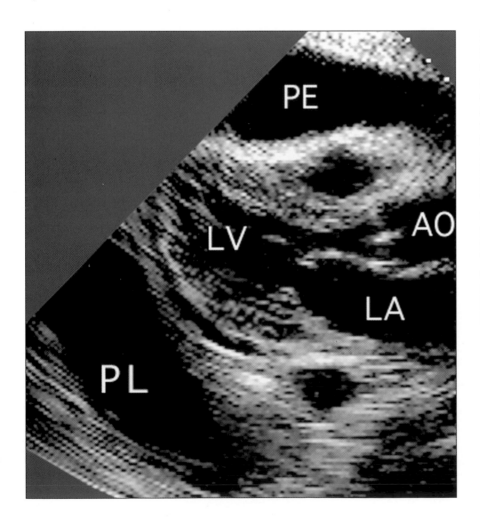

Figure 9.1
Parasternal long-axis view at maximum depth setting to record structures posterior to the heart. There is a large anterior pericardial effusion (PE) that appears to be compressing the right ventricular cavity. The right ventricular free wall which is unusually well seen owing to the presence of the effusion, is inverted in this diastolic image. The left ventricular chamber is small (LV). The left atrium (LA) and aorta (AO) are normal. There is a small posterior pericardial effusion seen between the epicardium and parietal pericardium. There is a large posterior pleural effusion (PL) that extends superiorly to the descending thoracic aorta, which is imaged in short axis posterior to the left atrium.

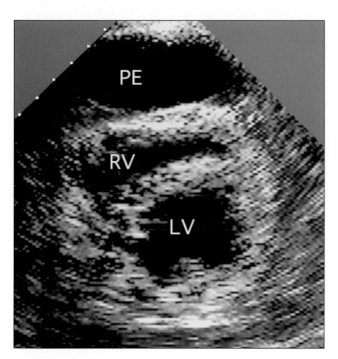

Figure 9.2
Parasternal short-axis view at the level of the papillary
muscles. A large anterior pericardial effusion (PE) is present
between the chest wall and the right ventricular free wall
(RV). The right ventricular cavity is small, owing to right
ventricular compression. The pericardial effusion is loculated.
There is no pericardial effusion surrounding the left ventricle
(LV). The posterior pericardium is thickened and appears to
be adherent to the left ventricular free wall.

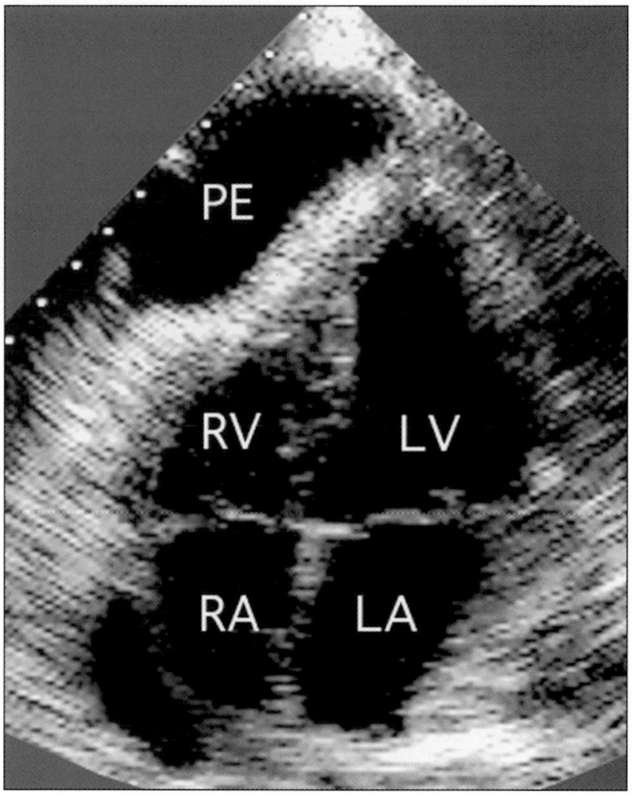

Figure 9.3
Apical four-chamber view in systole. The loculated pericardial
effusion (PE) is demonstrated overlying the right ventricular
free wall and apex. There is marked compression of the distal
right ventricular cavity. In addition, there is a significant
pericardial effusion seen adjacent to the right atrial free wall
(RA). There is no right atrial compression in this frame, but
inversion of the right atrial wall was noted throughout one-
half of the cardiac cycle.

Discussion

Metastatic pericardial disease may cause a large pericardial effusion that is most often circumferential. Slow
accumulation of the pericardial fluid allows the
pericardium to expand to accommodate the increased
volume. Thus, a large chronic effusion may be present
without clinical or echocardiographic signs of increased
intrapericardial pressure or tamponade. Adhesion of the
two layers of the pericardium, the parietal and visceral
pericardium, will limit the pericardial space available to
the fluid collection. Any process that involves inflammation of the pericardium may result in the formation of
scar tissue and fusion of the two layers. Transmural
myocardial infarction with associated pericarditis is a
common example. Previous cardiac surgery may also lead
to pericardial scarring and loss of the pericardial space.
Repeated viral infections or mycobacterial disease may
also result in pericardial scarring. This patient had infiltration of a tumor into the pericardium along the left

ventricular lateral wall. The tumor involved both layers of
the pericardium and had obliterated the pericardial space
at this level.

Loculated pericardial fluid may cause tamponade even
when the effusion is not large, if the pressure in the
pericardial space rises above the diastolic pressure of the
chamber and limits filling. The marked compression of
the right ventricle in this case caused a decrease in the
cardiac output with resultant hypotension and tachycardia. Inversion of the radius of curvature of the right
ventricle is a diagnostic sign of severe pericardial
compression. Respiratory variation of tricuspid inflow
velocities was present in this patient, although not shown
here. Loculated pericardial effusions may be misinterpreted as other mediastinal structures, particularly if they
are partially consolidated. Occasionally, use of another
imaging modality may be necessary to verify the
diagnosis.

This patient did not have adequate subcostal clearance for percutaneous drainage of the fluid. In this situation, open surgical drainage via sub-xiphoid pericardiectomy may relieve the tamponade. Recently, thorascopic procedures have successful drained loculated fluid and helped in the retrieval of biopsy specimens when the etiological diagnosis is in question.[1,2]

References

1. Geissbuhler K, Leiser A, Fuhrer J, *et al*. Video-assisted thoracoscopic pericardial fenestration for loculated or recurrent effusions. Eur J Cardio-Thorac Surg 1998;14:403–8.

2. Nugue O, Millaire A, Porte H, *et al*. Pericardioscopy in the etiologic diagnosis of pericardial effusion in 141 consecutive patients. Circulation 1996;94:1635–41.

10

Para-aortic lymphoma

Riti Patel MD

An 18-year-old male was referred by his primary-care physician to a cardiologist for evaluation of tachycardia. The workup included a transthoracic echocardiogram, which revealed a large pericardial effusion. Serial echocardiograms were performed during the week and the effusion was not resolving. A routine chest X-ray was remarkable for a large mediastinal mass. A computerized tomography (CT) scan of the chest confirmed the mass and pericardial effusion, and also revealed a left pleural effusion. Pathology of the mediastinal mass subsequently showed lymphoblastic lymphoma.

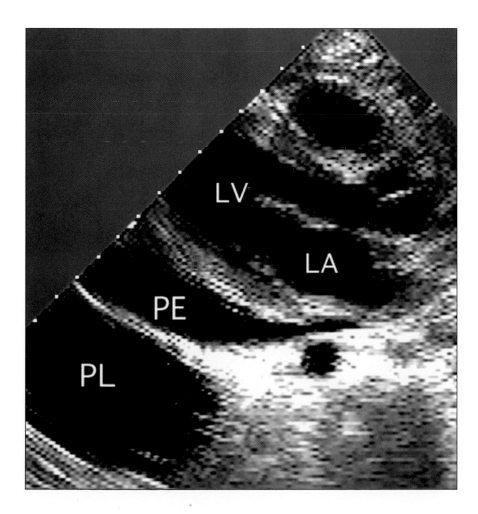

Figure 10.1
Parasternal long-axis view at a greater depth than the usual imaging field. There is pericardial effusion (PE), extending between the left atrium (LA) and the descending thoracic aorta. A large, left pleural effusion (PL) is visible posterior to the pericardial effusion. There is an ill-defined mass in the area of the descending thoracic aorta. The lumen of the aorta is unusually small, measuring less than 1 cm in diameter in this view.

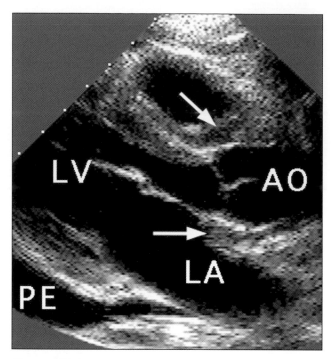

Figure 10.2
Parasternal long axis in diastole. The left ventricle (LV) and atrium (LA) are of normal size. There is marked thickening (arrows) of the walls of the aortic root and ascending aorta (AO). The thickening is a diffuse process that appears to be external to the walls of the aorta and does not narrow the lumen. The process projects into the left atrium. The posterior pericardial effusion is again visible.

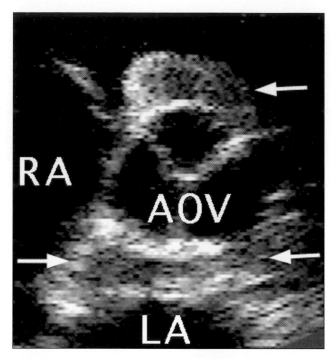

Figure 10.3
Close-up image of the aortic valve (AOV) from the parasternal short-axis view. A mass is present in the right ventricular outflow tract (single arrow) which appears to be extrinsic to the aortic root wall. There is also thickening of the posterior wall of the aortic root (double arrows) and it is less clear whether the process involves the wall of the aorta or is present between the aortic root and the left atrial wall.

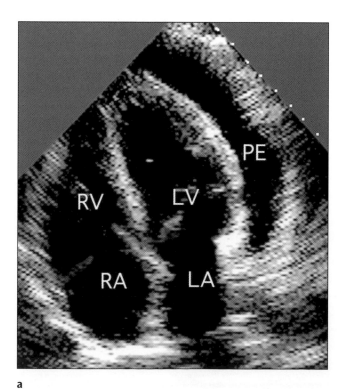

a

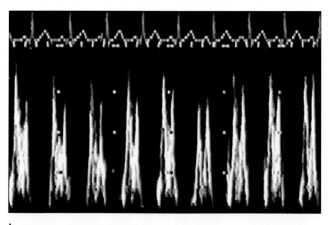

b

Figure 10.4
(a) Apical four-chamber view demonstrating the normal-sized chambers and the large lateral pericardial effusion (PE). In this view there is no definitive evidence of a mass or of any abnormality of the left atrial wall.
(b) Spectral display of pulsed-wave Doppler across the tricuspid valve. The diastolic inflow velocities are normal. There is minor respiratory variation in the peak velocity but far less than the 50% variation necessary for the diagnosis of increased intrapericardial pressure.

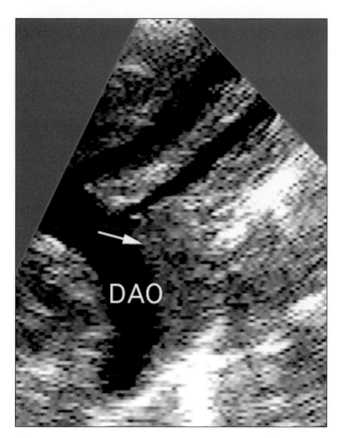

Figure 10.5
Suprasternal notch image of the descending thoracic aorta (DAO). The left common carotid and left subclavian arteries are also clearly seen. There is a mass along the lateral wall of the aorta (arrow) which appears to be compressing or invading the wall. The ostium of the subclavian artery is clearly narrowed by the process.

Discussion

Cardiac involvement by metastatic neoplasms is relatively uncommon and primary cardiac tumors are even more rare. Cardiac metastases are usually indicative of widely disseminated disease; the most common malignancies in order of decreasing frequency are lung, lymphoma, breast, leukemia, stomach, melanoma, liver, and colon.[1] The most common sites of involvement are the pericardium and epicardium. In a series of 744 necropsied patients with diffuse malignant disease, myocardial involvement was rarer and associated with cutaneous melanoma and lymphoma. Endocardial involvement was exceptionally uncommon.[2]

Cardiac manifestations of lymphoma often include effusions, as in this case, or conduction abnormalities. In a rare example of primary cardiac lymphoma, a 61-year-old woman was admitted with an effusion and complete atrioventricular block.[3] Echocardiography revealed several polypoid masses in the right atrium which resolved after three cycles of chemotherapy. In addition, infiltration of the conduction system by lymphoma may result in the need for temporary pacing.[4,5]

There is scanty literature describing imaging of primary cardiac tumors, particularly lymphomas. The available literature focuses on CT and magnetic resonance imaging (MRI) modalities.[6,7] Angiosarcoma is the most common primary cardiac malignancy and tends to involve the pericardium and right atrium. Valvular involvement is a hallmark of rhabdomyosarcoma, especially in children. Involvement of the left atrium, mitral valve and pulmonary veins is a feature of leiomyosarcoma. Primary and metastatic cardiac lymphoma occurs more commonly in immunocompromised hosts, and frequently involves the pericardium. The location of this mass along the aorta, extending to the descending thoracic aorta, is quite uncommon.

This patient was not otherwise immunocompromised and his disease manifested as an effusion as well as extensive ascending aortic and paravalvular thickening. No conduction disease was apparent. Treatment with Cytoxan, Adriamycin, vincristine, and prednisone was initiated and the patient received six cycles of chemotherapy. There was no evidence of tumor lysis. However, the hospital course was complicated by a pneumothorax that occurred after removal of a chest tube inserted to drain the large left pleural effusion. The patient was discharged 9 days after admission.

References

1. Abraham KP, Reddy V, Gattuso P. Neoplasms metastatic to the heart. Am J Cardiovasc Pathol 1990;3:195–8.

2. MacGee W. Metastatic and invasive tumors involving the heart in a geriatric population. Virchows Arch 1991;419:183–9.

3. Aleksic I, Herse B, Busch T, et al. Third degree atrioventricular block caused by malignant non-Hodgkin's lymphoma. Cardiovasc Surg 1999:7: 378–80.

4. Kamimura M, Tanabe N, Hojo M, et al. Malignant lymphoma demonstrating sick sinus syndrome. Intern Med 1998;37:463–6.

5. Nakayama Y, Uchimoto S, Tsumura K, Morii H. Primary cardiac lymphoma with infiltration of the atrioventricular node. Cardiology 1997;88:613–6.

6. Versluis PJ, Lamers RJ, Van Belle AF. Primary malignant lymphoma of the heart: CT and MRI features. Rofo Fortschr Geb Rontgenstr Neuen Bildgeb Verfahr 1995;162:533–4.

7. Araoz PA, Eklund HE, Welch TJ, Breen JF. CT and MRI imaging of primary cardiac malignancies. Radiographics 1999;19:1421–34.

SECTION II

The Right Heart

11

Superior vena cava mass

Susan E Wiegers MD

A 55-year-old man developed end-stage renal disease requiring dialysis. A subclavian catheter was placed for hemodialysis access prior to the maturation of the surgically created arteriovenous fistula in his left arm. Over the course of several weeks, the patient developed facial and right arm swelling. A transthoracic echocardiogram was unrevealing. A transesophageal echocardiogram was performed to evaluate the superior vena cava.

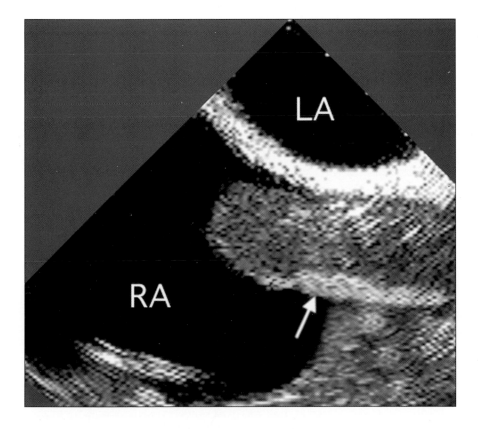

Figure 11.1
Transesophageal echocardiogram from the mid-esophagus in the longitudinal plane (imaging angle 90°). A large homogeneous mass (arrow) consistent with thrombus appears to fill the entire superior vena cava and projects into the right atrium (RA). An echodense linear structure in the anterior portion of the superior vena cava (towards the bottom of the screen) is the catheter in the superior vena cava. The catheter is followed to the junction of the superior vena cava and right atrium but does not appear to enter the right atrium. In this view, the thrombus appears to completely occlude the superior vena cava, which is moderately dilated. The interatrial septum and left atrium are normal.

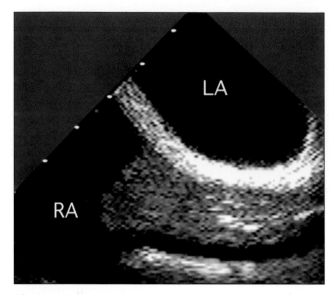

Figure 11.2
Transesophageal echocardiogram from the longitudinal axis (imaging angle 90°) with minimal rotation of the transducer towards the left side compared to Figure 11.1. The thrombus is once again visualized in the superior vena cava projecting into the right atrium. The superior vena cava is now seen to be partially patent and the catheter is out of plane. In this view, the distal edge of the thrombus appears more irregular than in the previous image.

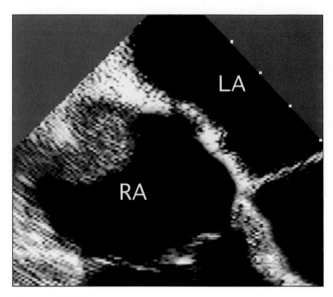

Figure 11.3
Transesophageal echocardiogram from the transverse plane (imaging plane 0°) of a modified four-chamber view. The right atrial thrombus is once again seen projecting from the area of the superior vena cava into the right atrium. In this view, withdrawal of the probe would demonstrate the short-axis view of the superior vena cava with the partially occlusive thrombus. The right atrium and tricuspid valve are normal.

Discussion

Catheter-associated thrombus is a well-described complication of temporary and longer-term indwelling catheters. Usually the thrombosis is asymptomatic, but the process may be complicated by infection, complete superior vena cava obstruction, embolization into the pulmonary vasculature, and rarely embolization across a patent fossa ovale to the systemic circulation. The superior vena cava is difficult to image in transthoracic studies but may be visualized in the subcostal view with anterior angulation of the transducer and in the right parasternal images. Occasionally, a thrombus may be large enough to project into the right atrium and appear as a right atrial mass on transthoracic study. However, another imaging modality is almost always required to determine the diagnosis. Doppler interrogation of the superior vena cava from the apical or subcostal position may reveal loss of the normal biphasic flow, turbulent flow and increased velocity.[1,2]

Transesophageal echocardiography is often diagnostic in the evaluation of catheter-associated thrombosis.[3,4] The thrombus is generally adherent and closely associated with the catheter, although at times the attachment site may not be easily visualized. Omniplane imaging from multiple levels is often necessary for full assessment of the superior vena cava. The short-axis of the superior vena cava from the transverse plane (not shown) is an underutilized view which can demonstrate turbulent flow with color Doppler imaging and is helpful for measurement of the degree of obstruction of the vessel. It is not possible to align the Doppler ultrasound beam along the direction of flow of the superior vena cava from the transesophageal position. Therefore, the Doppler demonstration of obstruction relies on detection of turbulent flow, which may be seen even in short-axis imaging. Serial studies can be used to assess the response to fibrinolytic therapy or systemic anticoagulation.[5]

Owing to concern that fibrinolytic therapy would induce embolization, it was not given to this patient. The patient was treated with intravenous heparin and showed improvement in his facial swelling after several days. The catheter was removed under transesophageal guidance and it was clear that the thrombus was adherent to the wall of the superior vena cava. The patient was dialyzed through the surgically created shunt and showed no evidence of pulmonary embolization.

References

1. Hammeril M, Meyer RA. Doppler evaluation of central venous lines in the superior vena cava. J Pediatr 1993;122:S104–8.

2. Nishino M, Tanouchi J, Ito T, *et al.* Echocardiographic detection of latent severe thrombotic stenosis of the superior vena cava and innominate vein in patients with a pacemaker: integrated diagnosis using sonography, pulse Doppler, and color flow. Pacing Clin Electrophysiol 1997;20:946–52.

3. Podolsky LA, Manginas A, Jacobs LE, *et al.* Superior vena caval thrombosis detected by transesophageal echocardiography. J Am Soc Echocardiogr 1991;4:189–93.

4. Weber T, Huemer G, Tschernich H, *et al.* Catheter-induced thrombus in the superior vena cava diagnosed by transesophageal echocardiography. Acta Anaesthesiol Scand 1998;42:1227–30.

5. Guindo J, Montagud M, Carreras F, *et al.* Fibrinolytic therapy for superior vena cava and right atrial thrombosis: diagnosis and follow-up with biplane transesophageal echocardiography. Am Heart J 1992;124:510–13.

12

Chiari network—normal variant

Susan E Wiegers MD

A 70-year-old man presented with the sudden onset of left hemiparesis. The magnetic resonance imaging angiogram was highly suggestive of a thrombus in the middle cerebral artery. Because the transthoracic echocardiogram did not reveal a potential cardiac source of embolus, he underwent transesophageal echocardiographic study. No cardiac source of embolism was demonstrated.

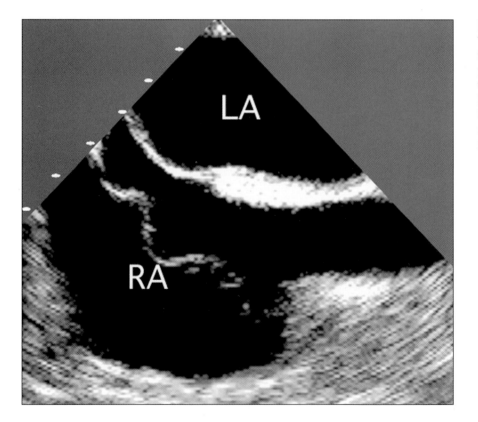

Figure 12.1
Transesophageal echocardiogram from the mid-esophagus in the longitudinal plane (imaging angle 90°). The superior vena cava is seen on the right of the image entering the right atrium. There is a thread-like structure within the right atrium (RA) which was highly mobile in real time.

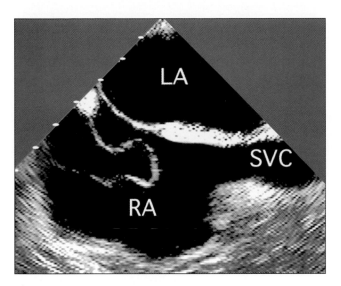

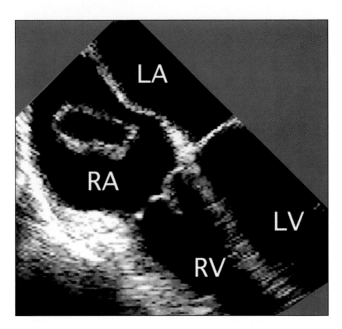

Figure 12.2
Similar transesophageal view to that in Figure 12.1, but the transesophageal probe has been advanced slightly. The attachment of the structure to the wall near the entrance of the inferior vena cava is evident. It is obvious from comparing Figures 12.1 and 12.2 that the structure is highly mobile. This represents a Chiari network, which is a normal structure, although in this patient it is particularly prominent.

Figure 12.3
Transesophageal echocardiogram from the level of the mid-esophagus in the transverse plane (imaging angle 0°). This view reveals that the network on some levels appears as a ring. The net-like structure has variable attachments in the right atrium. The whip-like motion and its thin thread-like characteristics distinguish it from a thrombus or other mass.

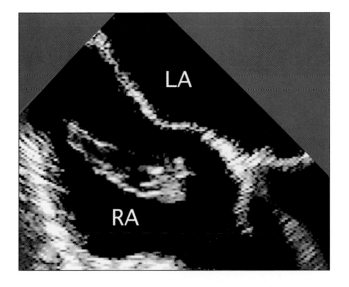

Figure 12.4
Close-up view of the right atrium from the transesophageal image in Figure 12.3. The Chiari network appears to be a latticework of threads. There appears to be thickening at the end of the network closest to the tricuspid valve. However, this represents an oblique cut of the multiple threads within the structure. In real time, it was easily appreciated that there was no thickening.

Discussion

The Chiari network was first described in 1897 in an autopsy series by Dr Chiari. It was noted to be present in 2–3% of the population. This embryonic remnant has no known purpose and is not pathological. Entrapment of right cardiac catheters has been reported. The Chiari network appears to be a web-like structure with a variable number of thread-like components. It is characterized by whip-like motion within the right atrium and attachment to the wall of the right atrium in close proximity to the entrance of the inferior vena cava.[1] It was detected in approximately 1.5% of transthoracic studies in a series in 1984.[2] However, technical improvements in image quality may have increased the incidence of its detection.

While the Chiari network has no clinical significance, it must be distinguished from other pathological masses in the right atrium including thrombus, vegetation, and myxoma. The characteristic features should allow this differentiation. Another embryonic remnant in the right atrium is a persistent sinus venosus valve or Eustachian valve. This ridge along the posterior wall of the right atrium runs from the right side of the inferior vena cava to the interatrial septum, where it joins the Thebesian valve at the fossa ovalis. In the fetal circulation, the Eustachian valve directs the oxygenated blood from the inferior vena cava across the interatrial septum to the left side of the heart. This membrane usually regresses, but can be prominent and can occasionally be mistaken for other masses.

References

1. Panidis I, Kotler M, Mintz G, *et al*. Clinical and echocardiographic features of right atrial masses. Am Heart J 1984;107:745–58.

2. Werner J, Cheitlin M, Gross B, *et al*. Echocardiographic appearance of the Chiari network. Differentiation from right heart pathology. Circulation 1981;63:1104–9.

13

Tricuspid valve injury after cardiac transplant

Susan E Wiegers MD

A 52-year-old man underwent a heart transplant for ischemic cardiomyopathy. He had frequent right-heart biopsies to rule out rejection, according to the transplant center protocol. New tricuspid regurgitation was demonstrated on his six-month post-transplant echocardiogram. At this time the patient was asymptomatic and doing well on an immunosuppressive regimen.

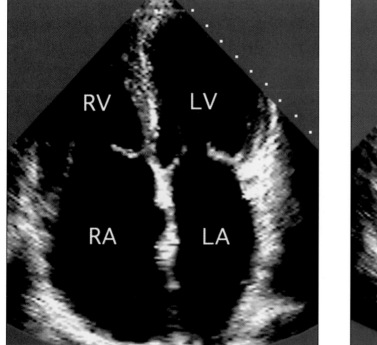

a

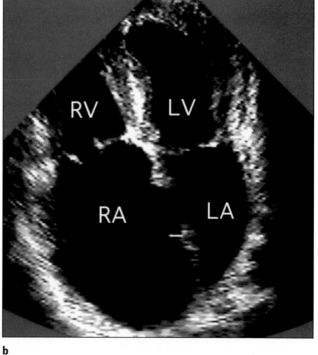

b

Figure 13.1
(a) Apical four-chamber view in diastole. There is biatrial enlargement consistent with orthotopic heart transplant. However, the right atrium (RA) is more severely dilated than the left atrium (LA). The level of the atrial anastomosis is visualized in the interatrial septum as an echodense area in the mid-interatrial septum. The left ventricle (LV) is of normal size but the right ventricle (RV) is dilated. Normally, the area of the right ventricle in the four chamber view should be two-thirds the area of the left ventricle. Although the lateral wall of the right ventricle is not clearly seen, the right ventricle is at least as large as the left ventricle in this view.
(b) Similar four-chamber view in systole. The left ventricular systolic function is normal. The right atrium expands with systole. This is consistent with significant tricuspid regurgitation. While the tricuspid valve is poorly seen in this view, the coaptation does not appear to be normal. The mitral valve appears to coapt normally.

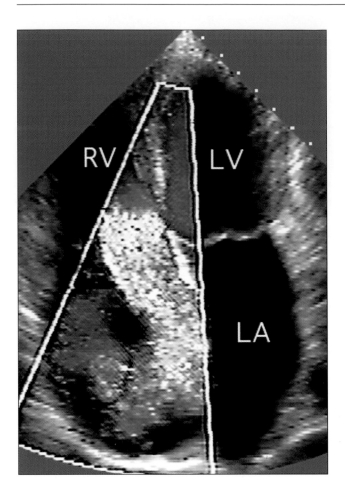

Figure 13.2
Apical four-chamber view in systole with color Doppler flow imaging. The presence of severe tricuspid regurgitation is confirmed. A turbulent jet fills the medial half of the right atrium and extends to the posterior wall.

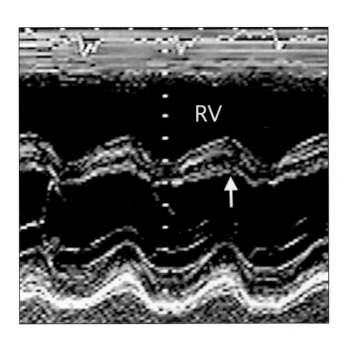

Figure 13.3
M-mode echocardiogram from the parasternal position. The right ventricle (RV) is dilated. The left ventricle is of normal size but there is marked paradoxical motion of the interventricular septum (arrow). During systole, the posterior wall moves anteriorly. However, the septum is paradoxical and moves anteriorly as well. Septal paradoxical motion may occur in patients with orthotopic heart transplant after their surgery. However, in this case, the severe RV volume overload contributed to the abnormal septal motion.

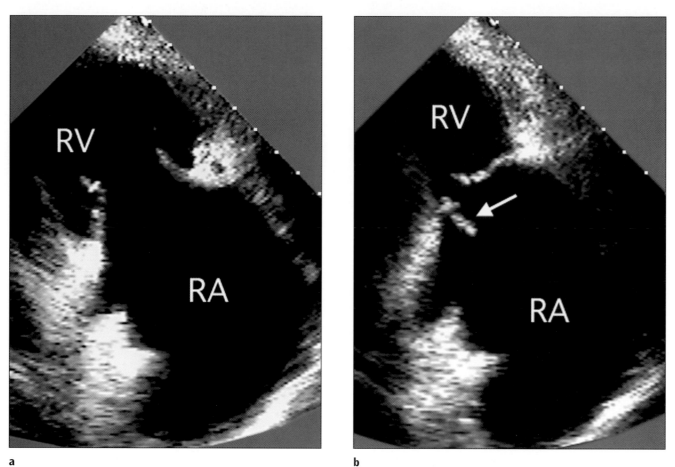

a   b

Figure 13.4

(a) Parasternal long-axis right ventricular (RV) inflow view in diastole. The tricuspid valve leaflets appear to be normal and open normally in diastole. The posterior leaflet of the tricuspid valve is imaged on the left of the screen and the anterior leaflet is imaged on the right of the screen. The right ventricular inflow view in the parasternal axis is the only standard view in which the posterior leaflet of the tricuspid valve is seen.

(b) Similar right ventricular inflow view in systole. Once again the right atrium (RA) is larger in systole than in diastole, consistent with severe tricuspid regurgitation. The posterior leaflet of the tricuspid valve is flail (arrow) and prolapses into the right atrium. Chords to this portion of the posterior leaflet were torn during biopsy, resulting in the flail leaflet.

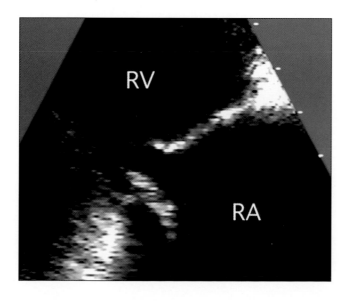

Figure 13.5

Close up image of the right ventricular inflow view from the parasternal long axis. Once again the flail portion of the posterior leaflet is visualized prolapsing into the right atrium in diastole. The anterior leaflet appears to be entirely normal.

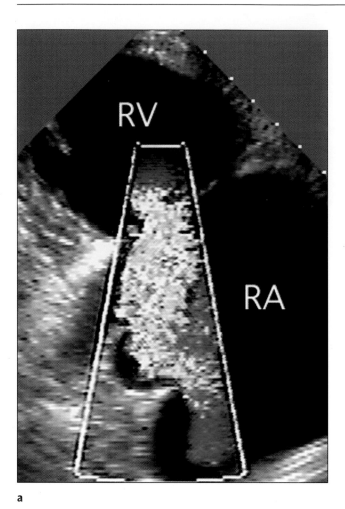

a

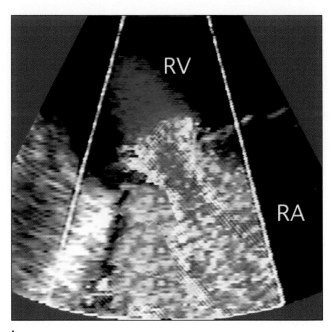

b

Figure 13.6

(a) Parasternal right ventricular inflow view with color Doppler flow imaging demonstrating significant tricuspid regurgitation. The regurgitation occurs at the level of the flail posterior leaflet and is the direct result of the failure of the valve leaflets to coapt.

(b) The proximal flow convergence in the right ventricle is noted on this close-up image of the tricuspid valve in systole with color Doppler flow imaging from the right ventricular inflow view. The diameter of the regurgitant jet is very wide, consistent with a large regurgitant orifice and severe tricuspid regurgitation.

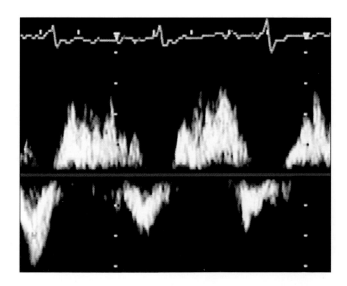

Figure 13.7

Spectral display of pulsed-wave Doppler velocities from the subcostal view in the middle hepatic veins. There is systolic flow into the hepatic veins, representative of severe tricuspid regurgitation. Normal forward flow from the hepatic veins into the inferior vena cava is demonstrated in diastole.

Discussion

A number of factors may result in tricuspid regurgitation after heart transplantation. The anastomosis of the right ventricle is more technically challenging than the anastomosis of the left atrium. The annulus of the tricuspid valve is non-planar and asymmetric. It is difficult to approximate the tricuspid annular geometry, therefore tricuspid regurgitation is more common than mitral regurgitation immediately after heart transplant.[1] Right ventricular dilatation from pulmonary hypertension will also result in tricuspid annular dilatation and subsequent regurgitation. The biotome forceps used to biopsy the right ventricle for diagnosis of cardiac rejection or for screening for this entity are sharp-toothed tools that have the potential to damage cardiac structures. Many reports of disruption of the tricuspid chordae have been published.[2] While mild tricuspid regurgitation may be due to surgical factors, severe tricuspid regurgitation is usually due to disruption of the tricuspid valve apparatus during right ventricular biopsy.[3] Many patients are asymptomatic after tricuspid valve injury and the precipitation of severe tricuspid regurgitation. In patients with low pulmonary artery pressures, the murmur associated with tricuspid regurgitation may be soft or inaudible. Severe tricuspid regurgitation may only be detected on routine echocardiographic examination. However, symptoms of right ventricular failure may eventually ensue, and medical therapy is usually ineffective.[4]

The posterior leaflet of the tricuspid valve is seen only in the parasternal long-axis right ventricular inflow view. This view is obtained by medial and inferior angulation of the transducer from the parasternal long-axis view of the left atrium and left ventricle. Inappropriate rotation of the transducer will lead to the septal leaflet, rather than the posterior leaflet, of the tricuspid valve being visualized. The other views in which the tricuspid valve is clearly seen are the parasternal short axis, the apical four-chamber view and the subcostal view. In all of these views, it is the septal and the anterior leaflets of the tricuspid valve that are imaged. Occasionally, it is possible to image the posterior leaflet of the tricuspid valve from the short axis, usually in the subcostal position. From this orientation, prolapse of the leaflet is difficult to discern. However, other abnormalities of the valve, such as attached vegetation, may be clearly visible.

References

1. Rees AP, Milani RV, Lavie CJ, *et al.* Valvular regurgitation and right-sided cardiac pressures in heart transplant recipients by complete Doppler and color flow evaluation. Chest 1993;104:82–7.

2. Braverman AC, Coplen SE, Mudge GH, *et al.* Ruptured chordae tendineae of the tricuspid valve as a complication of endomyocardial biopsy in heart transplant patients. Am J Cardiol 1990;66:111–13.

3. Stahl RD, Karwande SV, Olsen SL, *et al.* Tricuspid valve dysfunction in the transplanted heart. Ann Thorac Surg 1995;59:477–80.

4. Huddleston CB, Rosenbloom M, Goldstein JA, *et al.* Biopsy-induced tricuspid regurgitation after cardiac transplantation [see comments]. Ann Thorac Surg 1994;57:832–6; discussion 836–7.

14

Tricuspid valve vegetation associated with a pacemaker wire

Victor A Ferrari MD

A 70-year-old male underwent aortic valve replacement because of calcific aortic stenosis. Postoperatively he required a dual-chamber transvenous permanent pacemaker for high-grade atrioventricular block. One month after discharge, he complained of intermittent fevers to 102°F, fatigue, and an occasional non-productive cough. He denied other symptoms.

On physical examination, the sternum was stable but there was a small ballottable effusion within the left infraclavicular pacemaker pocket. There was minimal erythema at the incision site with no purulent discharge. The breath sounds were mildly decreased at the left base. On auscultation, the patient had normal and crisp prosthetic heart sounds, and a normally split S2. There was a grade I/VI systolic ejection murmur at the right upper sternal border with no diastolic murmur. The white blood cell count was 14 000. The chest X-ray showed left lower lobe atelectasis. A transthoracic echocardiogram (TTE) demonstrated normal left ventricular size with normal left ventricular function, and a normally functioning St Judes aortic valve prosthesis. There was a suggestion of abnormal thickening of the tricuspid valve, but artifact from the prosthetic valve prevented a complete evaluation of the leaflets. He underwent a transesophageal echocardiogram (TEE) for better assessment of the tricuspid valve and the pacemaker wire.

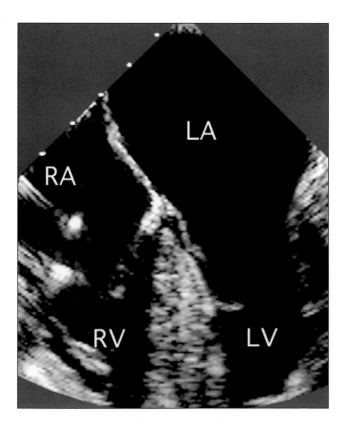

Figure 14.1
Transesophageal four-chamber view at the mid-esophageal level in the transverse plane (imaging angle 0°) demonstrates the four cardiac chambers (RA, right atrium; RV, right ventricle; LA, left atrium; LV, left ventricle). A portion of the pacemaker wire is seen in the right atrium and appears as a highly echogenic structure. There is shadowing from the wire that extends towards the lateral tricuspid annulus. Two leaflets of the tricuspid valve are seen in this diastolic frame: the anterior leaflet to the left, and the septal leaflet attached to the septum. In this plane, the lateral wall of the right ventricle is to the left of the image, and the interventricular septum is in the middle of the image. Though not appreciated in this view, the right atrium is moderately dilated.

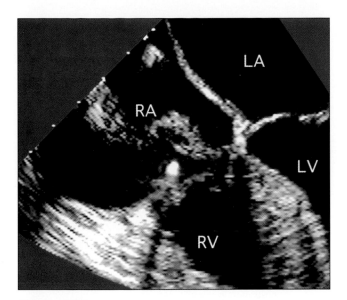

Figure 14.2
In the same plane, but with more retroflexion of the transducer, the right heart chamber sizes may be better visualized. Two pacemaker wires are present: one atrial and one ventricular. A small part of the atrial wire may be seen at the top of the right atrium, adjacent to the interatrial septum. The ventricular wire, which appears much thicker than normal, owing to a covering composed of thrombus or infected material, courses down the center of the right atrium, and is seen just proximal to the tricuspid valve plane again as a highly echogenic structure. Note the shadowing (dark angular line) distal to the wire indicative of a structure highly reflective of ultrasound energy. This artifact is more prominent in this image than in the previous figure. A pedunculated mass consistent with a large vegetation is attached to the atrial surface of the septal leaflet of the tricuspid valve, but appears to be closely associated with the pacemaker wire. The vegetation prolapses into the right atrium and measures approximately 2 cm × 1 cm. The pacemaker wire obscures the view of the anterior leaflet but it does appear to be thickened. There was no evidence in this view or others of an abscess of the valve ring.

Discussion

Endocarditis related to pacemaker wire infection is a rare but very serious complication of permanent transvenous pacer insertion. The incidence of infection varies from 0.13% to 7%.[1] The natural history of this type of infection is surprisingly poor, with a mortality rate close to 33%. Epidemiologically, early infections (within several months of insertion) are most often due to *Staphylococcus aureus*. Late or chronic infections are most frequently due to *Staphylococcus epidermidis*. The implantation site may be tender, erythematous, or have an effusion. However, even in the absence of local findings, the pacer pocket is frequently involved in the infectious process. In one

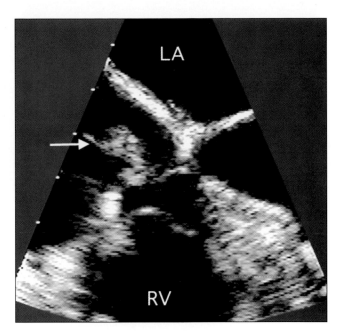

Figure 14.3
The highly mobile vegetation has several smaller satellite components (arrow) which are themselves freely mobile and can be seen only on TEE. This series of images underscores the usefulness of transesophageal imaging over transthoracic studies in the detection and depiction of tricuspid valve vegetations.

study,[1] 38% of patients had either clinical or radiographic evidence of pulmonary involvement—from cough or bronchitic symptoms to an infiltrate on chest X-ray, presumably due to septic embolization.

Echocardiography can detect abnormal masses associated with the pacemaker lead, but cannot differentiate thrombus from infected vegetation. A thrombus may also become secondarily infected, making the distinction even more difficult. Therefore, the diagnosis of pacemaker lead vegetation must be made in a clinical context consistent with an infectious process.[2] In the absence of signs or symptoms of systemic infection, a thrombus associated with a pacemaker wire may be treated with thrombolytic therapy to prevent an initial or recurrent pulmonary embolism.[3] Two recent studies have demonstrated the incidence of pulmonary embolism associated with tricuspid valve endocarditis using ventilation/perfusion scanning at a rate of 30–40%.[1,4]

Recent studies have proven the superiority of TEE over transthoracic echocardiography in this setting. Earlier studies showed equivalency of the techniques for right-sided infections, but were conducted in a limited population of intravenous drug abusers with large vegetations. TTE detected pacemaker lead vegetations in only 7–30% of patients, whereas transesophageal echocardiography demonstrated pacemaker lead vegetations in 85–95% of patients.[1,2] Three major factors account for the decreased sensitivity of transthoracic studies: there is an inadequate precordial acoustic window; pacemaker leads produce reverberations and artifacts in the transthoracic examination that can mask a vegetation close to these structures; and TEE is better for assessment of the superior vena cava and the upper right atrium. In some of the recent studies, only 10–15% of patients with infected leads also had tricuspid valve vegetations, despite the proximity of the infected wire to the leaflets. One major advantage of TEE is its ability to demonstrate tricuspid valve involvement.

As opposed to the standard medical therapy for isolated tricuspid valve endocarditis, conservative medical treatment alone is rarely successful, and several studies have suggested that the entire device (leads and generator) should be removed quickly for optimal management, provided the patient is a surgical candidate.[5] This technique, known as ablation, can be performed by use of percutaneous or open surgical techniques; the relative preference for these techniques is uncertain, but probably depends on the size of the vegetations and on the timing related to diagnosis. Percutaneous removal seems to be safer when vegetation size is ≤ 10 mm. A recent article underscores the difficulty of percutaneous pacemaker lead removal due to differing patterns of lead encapsulation and fibrosis associated with chronic lead implantation.[6]

References

1. Klug D, Lacroix D, Savoye C, *et al*. Systemic infection related to endocarditis on pacemaker leads: clinical presentation and management. Circulation 1997;95:2098–107.

2. Vilacosta I, Sarria C, San Roman JA, *et al*. Usefulness of transesophageal echocardiography for diagnosis of infected transvenous permanent pacemakers. Circulation 1994;89:2684–7.

3. Cooper CJ, Dweik R, Gabbay S. Treatment of pacemaker-associated right atrial thrombus with 2–hour rTPA infusion. Am Heart J 1993;126:228–9.

4. Cacoub P, Leprince P, Nataf P, *et al*. Pacemaker infective endocarditis. Am J Cardiol 1998;82:480–4.

5. Hajrula A, Jarvinen A, Virtanen KS, Mattila S. Pacemaker infections: treatment with total or partial pacemaker system removal. Thorac Cardiovasc Surg 1985;33:218–20.

6. Candinas R, Duru F, Schneider J, *et al*. Postmortem analysis of encapsulation around long-term ventricular endocardial pacing leads. Mayo Clin Proc 1999;74:120–5.

15

Ebstein's anomaly

Martin St John Sutton MBBS
Susan E Wiegers MD

A 41-year-old woman complained of sudden onset of rapid palpitations lasting 16 hours associated with fatigue on mild to moderate exertion. She went to her local emergency room where an ECG showed her to be in atrial flutter with a ventricular response of 148 bpm with 2 : 1 atrioventricular block and right bundle branch block. Before receiving any medication she spontaneously reverted to normal sinus rhythm. Further detailed history was non-contributory; she denied any previous illnesses and had never previously had any cardiac symptoms. She worked as a middle-school gym teacher.

On examination of her cardiovascular system, the only abnormality was a split first heart sound, a pansystolic murmur at the left fourth intercostal space which varied with respiration consistent with tricuspid regurgitation, but with no obvious 'v' wave in the jugular venous pulse, and a normally splitting second heart sound. Oxygen saturation in the room air was 97% at rest. The ECG showed sinus rhythm with right atrial enlargement and right bundle branch block. The chest X-ray showed mild cardiomegaly, right atrial enlargement, and normal pulmonary vasculature.

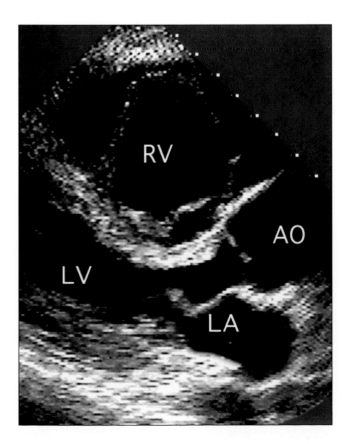

Figure 15.1
Parasternal long-axis view. The right ventricle is markedly dilated. The highly mobile structures in the right ventricular cavity are portions of the apically displaced tricuspid valve. The left ventricle is small and underfilled. The interventricular septum is bowed to the left in this early diastolic frame.

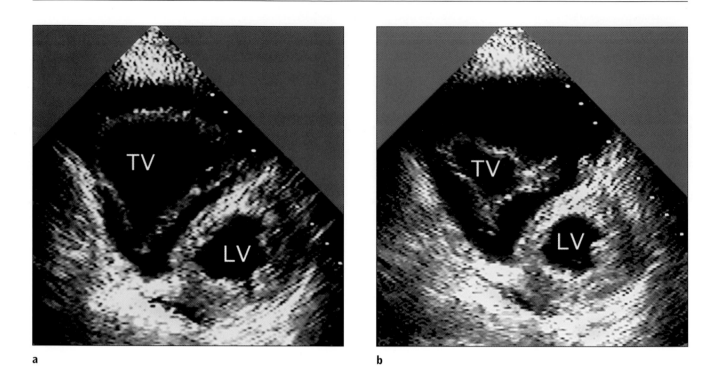

a   b

Figure 15.2

(a) Parasternal short-axis view at the level of the left ventricular papillary muscles. The tricuspid valve is apically displaced and very abnormal. The right ventricle is greatly enlarged.

(b) Similar view in systole. Left ventricular fractional shortening is normal, but the right ventricle is severely hypokinetic. The tricuspid valve leaflets do not fully coapt. The anterior leaflet moves towards the septum, but the septal and posterior leaflets are tethered and relatively immobile.

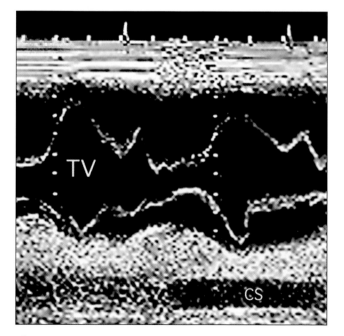

Figure 15.3

M-mode echocardiogram through the tricuspid valve with the transducer in the parasternal position. The tricuspid valve leaflets (TV) are markedly hyperexcursive. The dilated coronary sinus (CS) is also visible as the transducer is swept towards the base of the heart.

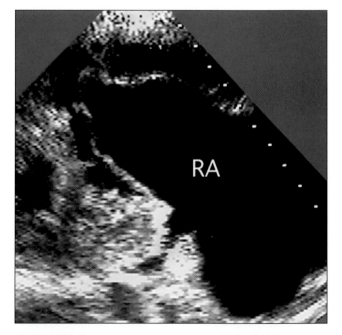

Figure 15.4

Right ventricular inflow view from a low parasternal window. The giant right atrium (RA) includes the atrialized portion of the right ventricle. The tricuspid leaflets are large and abnormal. Attachment of the elongated septal leaflet to the interventricular septum is seen.

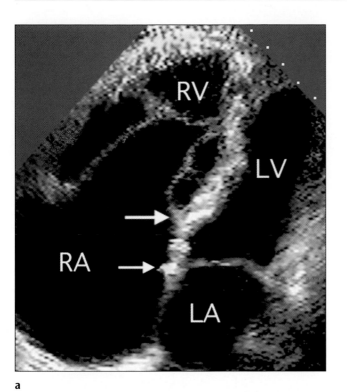

a

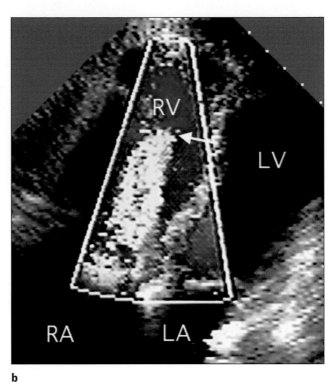

b

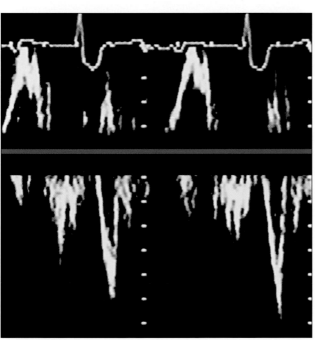

c

Figure 15.5

(a) Modified apical four-chamber view. The transducer is in the left mid-clavicular line, medial to the true apex of the heart. The tricuspid annulus (larger arrow) is apically displaced more than 2 cm from the mitral annulus (smaller arrow). The septal leaflet of the tricuspid valve appears to attach to the interventricular septum at multiple points. Only a small portion of the right ventricle, at the apex, is distal to the tricuspid inflow formed by the leaflets.

(b) Similar view with color flow Doppler imaging in systole. The origin of the tricuspid regurgitant signal (arrow) is displaced apically from the annulus. This point marks the apical extent of the atrialized right ventricle.

(c) Spectral display of pulsed-wave Doppler through the tricuspid valve. The sample volume has been placed in the atrialized portion of the right ventricle. The tricuspid regurgitation flow velocity is less than 1.5 m/s. This low velocity represents atrial hypertension but more importantly the inability of the right ventricle to generate pressure.

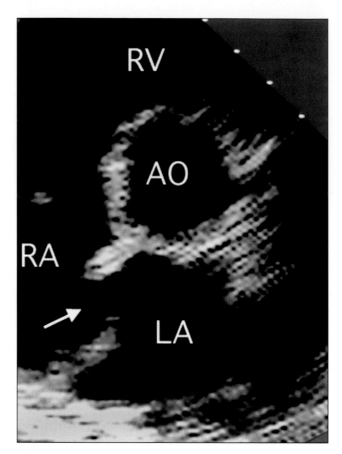

Figure 15.6
Parasternal short-axis view at the base of the heart with a
close-up of the interatrial septum. A moderate-sized
secundum type atrial septal defect is present.

importantly from downward displacement of the tricuspid
septal and mural anterior leaflets. This downward displacement is optimally demonstrated at the crux of the heart,
where the tricuspid septal leaflet takes origin from the
interventricular septum more than 8 mm apically
compared to the origin of the anterior mitral valve leaflet.
Although often not so obvious, the anterior leaflet of the
tricuspid valve takes origin from below the valve annulus.
The anterior and septal leaflets are adherent to the
endocardium being restrained by what appear to be super-
numerary chordae.[1] The residual right ventricle may be
rudimentary and dysfunctional. Furthermore, in Ebstein's
anomaly more than 50% of patients show a shunt from
right to left at the atrial level, most frequently via a defect
in the secundum atrial septum or through a stretched
patent foramen ovale. The size of the atrial septal defect
should be assessed by contrast injection or transesophageal
echocardiography and the magnitude of the shunt
estimated. Right atrial hypertension may result in significant right to left shunting through a large atrial septal
defect and cyanosis. Echocardiography is also important
for the evaluation of residual right ventricular function[2]
and the results of surgical correction.[3]

Antiarrhythmic therapy may be indicated for symptomatic atrial arrhythmias, which occur frequently in
patients who are otherwise asymptomatic. In patients with
Ebstein's anomaly who have undergone prosthetic tricuspid valve replacement, the tendency to develop thrombotic obstruction of the prosthesis is a known
complication which can be treated with thrombolytic
therapy. Ideally, the atrial septum would be intact, to
decrease the risk of paradoxical embolization.

Discussion

The diagnosis in this relatively asymptomatic patient was
Ebstein's anomaly. This congenital abnormality may vary
from minor abnormality of the tricuspid valve to gross
right heart abnormalities requiring surgical marsupializa-
tion of the atrialized ventricle and prosthetic valve replacement. Characteristic echocardiographic features are usually
easily demonstrated. The right atrium is markedly enlarged
in part due to the presence of tricuspid regurgitation but

References

1. Rusconi PG, Zuberbuhler JR, Anderson RH, *et al*. Morphologic-
    echocardiographic correlates of Ebstein's malformation. Eur Heart J
    1991;12:784–90.

2. Nihoyannopoulos P, McKenna WJ, Smith G, *et al*. Echocardio-
    graphic assessment of the right ventricle in Ebstein's anomaly:
    relation to clinical outcome. J Am Coll Cardiol 1986;8:627–35.

3. Marino JP, Mihaileanu S, el Asmar B, *et al*. Echocardiography and
    color-flow mapping evaluation of a new reconstructive surgical
    technique for Ebstein's anomaly. Circulation 1989;80:1197–202.

16

Right atrial thrombus

Susan E Wiegers MD

A 60-year-old man with a history of lung carcinoma treated with surgery and radiation developed sick sinus syndrome and had a permanent pacemaker placed. Several months later he was admitted with pleuritic chest pain and mild shortness of breath. A lung ventilation and perfusion scan was positive for multiple subsegmental defects. Due to the high probability of a pulmonary embolus, an echocardiogram was done to assess right ventricular function.

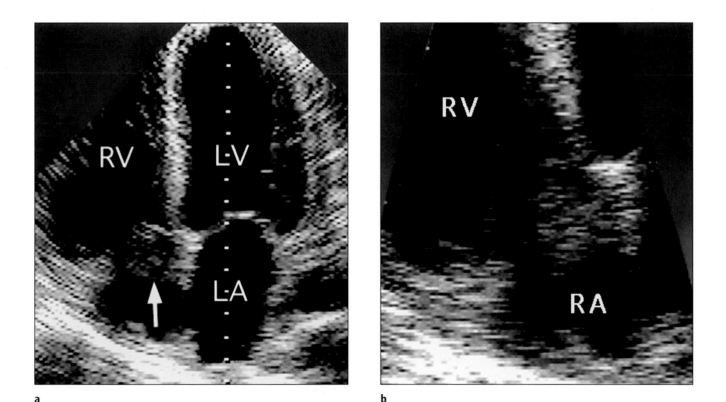

a   b

Figure 16.1
(a) Apical four-chamber view in systole demonstrates a moderately dilated left ventricle (LV) and left atrium (LA). The right ventricular cavity size (RV) is normal. A pacemaker wire is seen in the right ventricular cavity. There is a large mass (arrow) at the level of the tricuspid valve which appears to fill the tricuspid valve orifice.
(b) In diastole a magnified image of the same view shows apparent attachment of the right atrial mass to the interatrial septum. The posterior and lateral walls of the right atrium are not normal and contain tissue with an echodensity similar to that of the mass.

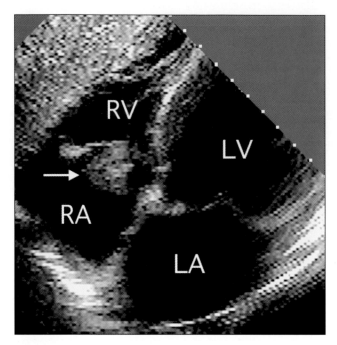

Figure 16.2
An off-axis subcostal view demonstrates an intact interatrial septum without definite attachment of the mass (arrow) to the septum. This image is obtained by angulation of the transducer from the standard sub-xiphoid position.

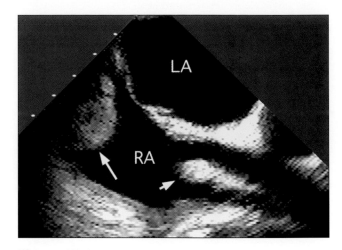

Figure 16.4
Transesophageal echocardiogram in the longitudinal axis (90°) in the mid-esophagus. The pacemaker (small arrow) is seen in the superior vena cava entering the right atrium (RA). The pacemaker acoustic shadow is thickened and in real time demonstrated chaotic motion at its edge. This finding is highly suggestive of thrombus or vegetation associated with the pacemaker wire. The right atrial mass (large arrow) does not appear to be attached to the pacemaker in this view. However, rotation of the transducer demonstrated the attachment of the large mass to the pacemaker wire at the level of the tricuspid annulus.

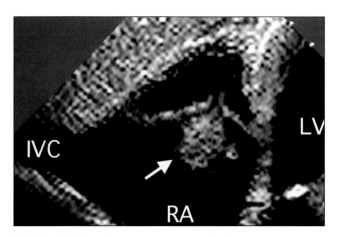

Figure 16.3
A close-up of the right atrium in the previous view demonstrates that the inferior vena cava (IVC) is widely patent and contains no masses. The nature of the mass (arrow) is not clearly defined.

Discussion

The differential diagnosis of the right atrial mass in this case includes myxoma, metastatic tumor, thrombus and vegetation. Initial images suggested the attachment of the mass to the interatrial septum, raising the question of atrial myxoma. However, additional views demonstrated that this was not the case. Off-axis images are especially important in evaluation of the interatrial septum since the septum is parallel to the ultrasound beam in the standard apical and parasternal short-axis views. Dropout of the image may occur in these views because optimal two-dimensional imaging requires structures to be perpendicular to the ultrasound beam. While chamber size cannot be accurately determined from off-axis views, certain anatomic information may be reliably obtained. A myxoma would almost certainly have an attachment to the interatrial septum, thus excluding this diagnosis. In addition, the mass was not present on the echocardiogram performed 3 months earlier, prior to the pacemaker placement. While a metastatic tumor might demonstrate such rapid growth, it is unlikely that this large, intracardiac mass represents a neoplasm.

It is clear from Figure 16.1a and b that the mass is not attached to the tricuspid valve leaflets, since it does not exhibit any motion between the systolic and diastolic frames. The mass is very large to be a vegetation, particularly in an afebrile patient with little history to suggest the diagnosis. Vegetations may be associated with pacemakers rather than valve leaflets. In this case, the presence of an additional mass along the posterior wall of the right atrium is highly suggestive of thrombus. The nature of the mass was confirmed by the transesophageal echocardiogram which demonstrated attachment of the thrombus to the pacemaker in the superior vena cava and right atrium. Both transthoracic and transesophageal echocardiography have occasionally demonstrated the presence of a right atrial clot in patients with acute pulmonary embolism.[1,2] Treatment must be individually tailored.

In this case, the patient was pacemaker-dependent but had a limited life expectancy, owing to the presence of recurrent lung carcinoma. Thrombolysis was contraindicated because it was feared that partial lysis of the clot would result in embolism of a large mass leading to acute compromise. He was treated with heparin followed by oral anticoagulation with partial resolution of the atrial mass and no further clinical sequelae.

References

1. Redberg RF, Hecht SR, Berger M. Echocardiographic detection of transient right heart thrombus: now you see it, now you don't [see comments]. Am Heart J 1991;122:862–4.

2. Adamick R, Zoneraich S. Echocardiographic visualization of a large mobile right atrial thrombus with sudden embolization during real-time scanning. Am Heart J 1990;120:699–701.

17

Carcinoid heart disease

Susan E Wiegers MD

Effort intolerance, pedal edema and increasing abdominal distension led a 62-year-old woman to see her physician. She had complained of diarrhea for several months and had noticed frequent uncomfortable flushing episodes. Her condition failed to improve with vigorous diuresis. The classic echocardiographic findings led to the search for carcinoid tumor and several small liver metastases were discovered. Because of intractable symptoms, she underwent tricuspid valve replacement for treatment of her severe right heart failure and tricuspid stenosis. However, postoperative right ventricular dysfunction and severe bleeding due to an uncontrollable coagulopathy led to her death 2 weeks after surgery.

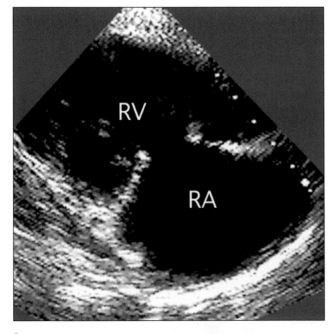

a

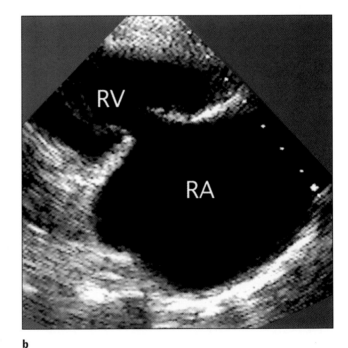

b

Figure 17.1
(a) Parasternal right ventricular (RV) inflow view. In diastole the tricuspid valve leaflets are thickened and shortened. The tips are rounded so that the leaflets resemble clubs. The valve is moderately stenotic. The abnormal leaflets fail to open completely but do not dome as in rheumatic tricuspid stenosis. Both the right ventricle (RV) and the right atrium (RA) are dilated.
(b) In the systolic view incomplete closure of the valve is demonstrated. The leaflets are fixed, demonstrating little movement during the cardiac cycle.

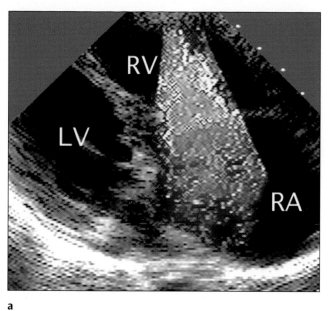 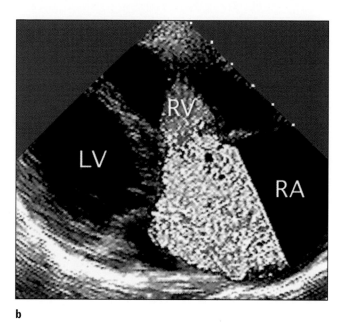

a   b

Figure 17.2

(a) Parasternal right ventricular inflow view with color Doppler flow imaging. Right ventricular inflow during diastole demonstrates the proximal flow convergence—proximal isovelocity surface area (PISA phenomenon)—characteristic of flow through stenotic lesions. The inflow jet on the right ventricular side is turbulent and aliases, also consistent with stenosis.

(b) In systole, torrential tricuspid regurgitation flows through the leaflets, which are fixed. The turbulent jet fills the right atrium. The PISA phenomenon can now be seen on the ventricular side of the valve.

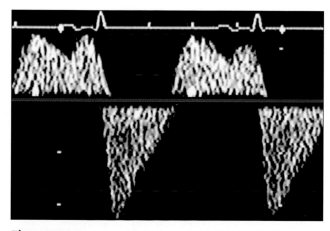

Figure 17.3

Spectral display of continuous-wave Doppler across the tricuspid valve from the apical position. The tricuspid regurgitant velocity tracing is dagger-shaped with an early peak pressure and rapid fall-off. This pattern is found with right ventricular systolic failure. There is torrential tricuspid regurgitation through the fixed tricuspid leaflets. The peak systolic velocity cannot be used to estimate the peak right ventricular systolic pressure because the right ventricle and right atrium are essentially common chambers during systole. The elevated diastolic velocity across the tricuspid valve (above the baseline) and the prolonged pressure half-time are evidence of the associated mild tricuspid stenosis.

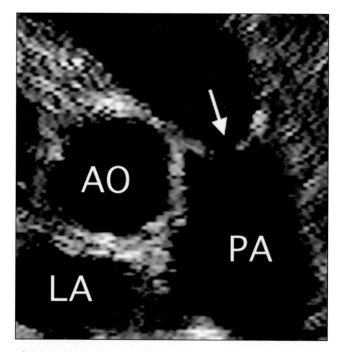

Figure 17.4

Parasternal short-axis view at the base of the heart during systole. The pulmonary valve (arrow) is thickened and stenotic. The leaflets do not dome but are fixed in position. The pulmonary artery is mildly dilated.

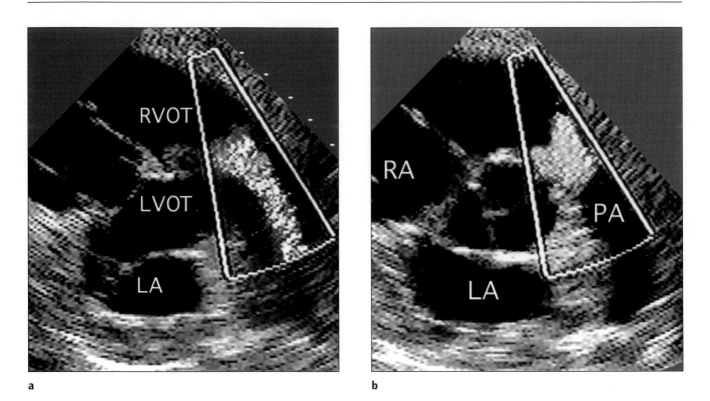

a   b

Figure 17.5
(a) Parasternal short axis view at the base of the heart during systole with color Doppler imaging. The turbulent jet across the pulmonary valve confirms the presence of important stenosis.
(b) Similar view in diastole. The color jet of pulmonary regurgitation is broad at the level of the valves and appears to fill the entire right ventricular outflow tract at its origin. The fixed leaflets are both stenotic and regurgitant. The severe pulmonary regurgitation demonstrated in this view does not appear to extend far into the right ventricle. This may be due to the right ventricular diastolic pressures, or to the distal portion of the jet being out of plane in this view.

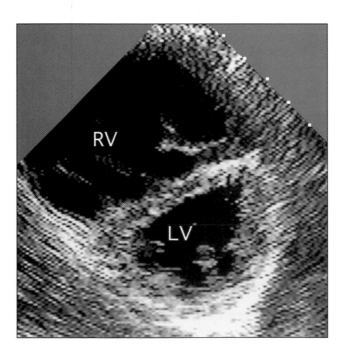

Figure 17.6
Parasternal short-axis view of the heart in diastole. The right ventricle (RV) is massively enlarged and is many times larger than the left ventricle (LV) in this view. The flattening of the interventricular septum is due to right ventricular volume overload.

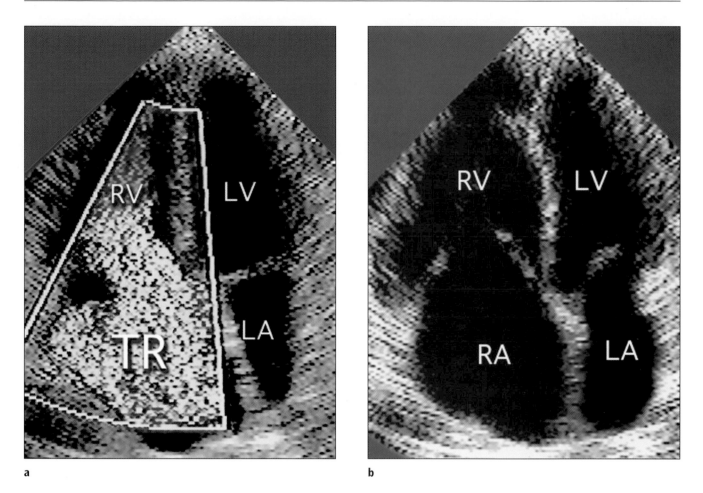

a   b

Figure 17.7
(a) Apical four-chamber view in systole with color flow Doppler imaging. The right ventricle (RV) is again demonstrated to be dilated compared to the left ventricle (LV). The jet of massive tricuspid regurgitation arises more distally in the right ventricle than is normal. This is due to the fact that the tricuspid leaflets are fixed open and the regurgitation commences at the leaflet tips. (b) Similar two-dimensional image in systole. The fixed position of the tricuspid leaflets is well seen. The right atrium is also massively enlarged.

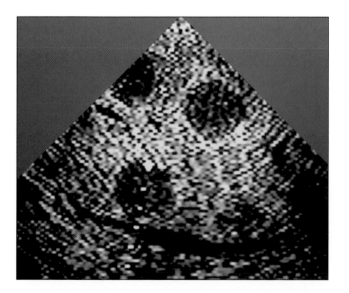

Figure 17.8
Subcostal view of the liver. The dilated hepatic vein is demonstrated in the inferior portion of the image. Several round nodules of metastatic carcinoid tumor are present within the hepatic tissue.

Discussion

Echocardiography is more sensitive than catheterization for demonstrating cardiac involvement in carcinoid disease.[1] This patient had the classic findings of right-sided involvement due to carcinoid syndrome. The tricuspid valve is involved in 90% of patients with carcinoid heart disease. The leaflets of the valve become fibrotic, thickened, and fixed. The etiology of these pathological changes are not clearly understood but are thought to be related to the effects of serotonin and other vasoactive substances secreted by the tumors. Interest in this entity has increased with the recent finding that several anorectic agents are possibly responsible for similar pathological changes in the left-sided valves.

Differentiation from rheumatic disease is straightforward. The entire tricuspid leaflet thickens and becomes immobile. In rheumatic disease, commissural fusion leaves the body of the leaflet relatively spared. The belly of the leaflet moves throughout the cardiac cycle but domes in diastole, resulting in stenosis. In contrast, the leaflets affected by carcinoid disease are thickened and completely immobile. Thus, severe regurgitation is always associated with the lesion.

The spectral velocity pattern of the tricuspid regurgitation has been previously described and is associated with 'wide open' regurgitation.[2] On pulsed-wave Doppler, the tricuspid regurgitation may appear laminar. The peak right ventricular systolic pressure cannot be estimated with torrential tricuspid regurgitation because the right atrial systolic pressure approaches that of the right ventricle. In this case, the presence of pulmonary stenosis further precludes extrapolation of the tricuspid jet velocity to peak pulmonary artery pressure. Pulmonary regurgitation and stenosis were also seen in this patient and have been reported to occur in 50% of the patients with carcinoid heart disease. Right ventricular failure may ensue from the volume and pressure load. Small pericardial effusions may also occur. Intracardiac metastases and left-sided valvular thickening[3] as well as marked thickening of the right atrial wall[4] may also be seen and are best diagnosed by transesophageal echocardiography. It is not uncommon to visualize hepatic abnormalities during the subcostal images. However, consultation with appropriate colleagues should be sought before a diagnosis is tendered.

References

1. Robiolio PA, Rigolin VH, Wilson JS, et al. Carcinoid heart disease. Correlation of high serotonin with valvular abnormalities detected by cardiac catheterization and echocardiography. Circulation 1995;92:790–5.

2. Pellikka PA, Tajik AJ, Khandheria BK, et al. Carcinoid heart disease. Clinical and echocardiographic spectrum in 74 patients. Circulation 1993;87:1188–96.

3. Le Metayer P, Constans J, Bernard N, et al. Carcinoid heart disease: two cases of left heart involvement diagnosed by transthoracic and transoesophageal echocardiography. Eur Heart J 1993;14:1721–3.

4. Lundin L, Landelius J, Andren B, et al. Transoesophageal echocardiography improves the diagnostic value of cardiac ultrasound in patients with carcinoid heart disease. Br Heart J 1990;64:190–4.

18

Right atrial mass—biopsy under echocardiographic guidance

Susan E Wiegers MD

Muredach P Reilly MB

A 74-year-old man with a history of severe emphysema required chronic oxygen therapy at home. The patient had recently noticed swelling in the ankles which progressed to pitting edema of the abdominal wall. He developed a distended abdomen but had no shortness of breath beyond his baseline. On the morning of admission he had an episode of syncope and thereafter was lethargic. He complained of chest pain and severe shortness of breath. The fire rescue team was called and the patient was transported to the emergency room. Physical examination revealed an obese elderly man who was hypotensive and tachycardic.

The chest was clear and the heart sounds were distant. Anasarca was present. The oxygen saturation was 80% with the patient breathing 100% O_2. An echocardiogram was performed to assess the presence of congestive heart failure.

The transthoracic study demonstrated a right atrial mass. No definite abnormality of the kidneys or pelvic organs was visualized on radiographic imaging. The patient's condition continued to deteriorate, requiring intubation. Therefore, a biopsy of the mass in the right atrium was performed under echocardiographic guidance to direct further therapy.

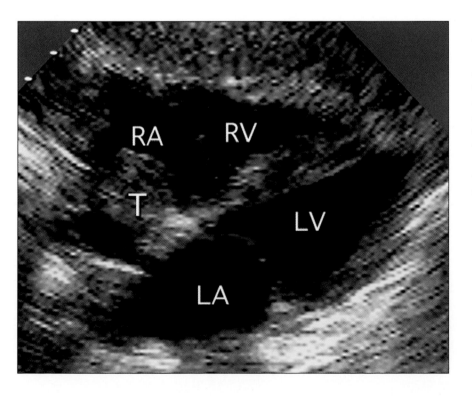

Figure 18.1
Transthoracic image from the subcostal position. The heart is imaged in a four-chamber view in systole. The right ventricular (RV) and left ventricular (LV) chambers are normal. There is a mass (T) in the right atrium (RA) which at first glance appears to be attached to the interatrial septum. However, the mass extends to the left of the screen towards the origin of the inferior vena cava.

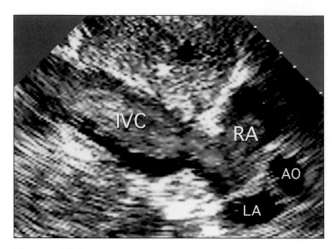

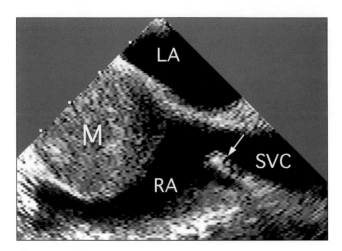

Figure 18.2
Angulation of the transducer towards the inferior vena cava (IVC) demonstrates the mass filling the IVC. The IVC is dilated and a small, echo-lucent lumen is seen in the inferior portion of the screen. The mass appears to have caused nearly complete obstruction of the intrahepatic portion of the IVC and the orifice to the right atrium. The mass extends from the IVC, across the right atrium to the interatrial septum. AO, aortic root.

Figure 18.3
Transesophageal echocardiogram from the mid-esophageal level in the longitudinal plane (imaging angle 90°) demonstrating the large tumor mass (M) filling the right atrium. The superior vena cava (SVC) is seen to the right of the image. The biotome forceps (arrow) is visualized within the superior vena cava approaching the mass which originates from the inferior vena cava. From the transesophageal image it is clear that the mass abuts the interatrial septum mildly distorting its position. However, it does not appear to have invaded or crossed the tissue of the septum. The edge of the homogeneous mass is smooth and slightly more echodense than the mass itself. This appearance is suggestive of the presence of a capsule.

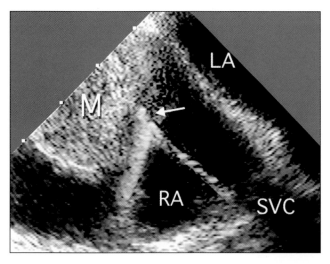

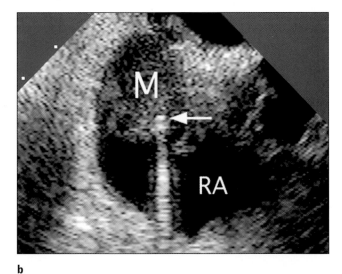

a   b

Figure 18.4
(a) Transesophageal image from the mid-esophageal level in the longitudinal plane (imaging angle 90°) with rotation of the entire probe towards the right side of the body. The biotome has been advanced and introduced into the mass (arrow). An echodense line originates from the tip of the biotome down towards the lower left of the image. This ring-down artifact is in the line of the ultrasound beam and is due to artifact created by the very dense biotome tips.
(b) Transesophageal image from the mid-esophagus in the transverse plane (imaging angle 0°). The presence of the biotome within the mass was verified in an orthogonal view prior to biopsy samples being taken. The actual course of the biotome catheter from the superior vena cava is out of plane in this image. Only the ring down artifact from the tip of the biotome catheter (arrow) is visualized extending down into the right atrium along the path of the ultrasound beam. The artifact is linear and echodense and must be distinguished from the image of the catheter itself.

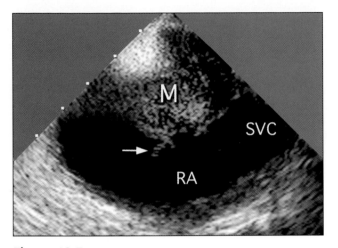

Figure 18.5
Transesophageal image from the mid-esophagus in the longitudinal plane (imaging angle 90°). The biotome has been removed from the superior vena cava. The site of the biopsy of the tumor is well visualized (arrow). The capsule of the mass has been disrupted and the discontinuity is seen in the surface of the mass where the biopsy specimen was taken. Echolucency is present immediately subjacent to the biopsy site, representing disruption of the mass by the biotome forceps and hemorrhage within the mass.

Discussion

Chronic obstruction of the inferior vena cava by a tumor mass may be mistaken clinically for right-sided valvular lesions or constrictive pericarditis. This patient had clinical evidence of right sided obstruction which on echocardiography was demonstrated to be at the level of the inferior vena cava and right atrium. The mass itself did not obstruct the superior vena cava or the tricuspid valve. The patient had slowly developing anasarca due to the inferior vena cava obstruction, but the acute decompensation appeared to have been due to a pulmonary embolism. Although tumor embolism has certainly been reported, the smooth encapsulated appearance of this mass makes that diagnosis somewhat unlikely. However, a thrombus might have formed in the inferior vena cava due to stasis and low flow with subsequent embolization. It appears improbable that a deep venous thrombosis from the lower extremities could have passed the high-grade obstruction and reached the pulmonary circulation. Transthoracic echocardiography from the subcostal position easily diagnosed the tumor mass and hemodynamic compromise.

The patient was acutely ill but had severe concomitant illness which made survival of a prolonged tumor resection unlikely. His physicians felt that a definitive tissue diagnosis would allow them to decide whether to be aggressive with the patient's treatment. There was also concern that the mass was simply a large thrombus which might be conservatively managed. The patient's systemic anticoagulation was discontinued and he underwent percutaneous biopsy under echocardiographic guidance to minimize the risk of perforation of the right atrium or inferior vena cava. In this situation transesophageal imaging allows real-time direction of the biotome forceps. The biopsy specimens are not taken until accurate placement is confirmed. As demonstrated in these images, the biotome is highly reflectile and experience is necessary to ensure that the tip of the biotome rather than the distal extent of the reverberation artifact is being visualized. Similar care must be taken in monitoring the progress of the percutaneous pericardiocentesis needle, because the artifact arising from the highly refractile needle may be seen out of the plane of the true tip of the needle. In this case successful biopsy was confirmed not only by the verification of the location of the needle but also by the change in the contour of the mass after specimens had been taken.

Transesophageal echocardiography has also been useful intraoperatively to monitor the removal of masses extending into the right atrium from the inferior vena cava. Multiplane imaging allows confirmation that all of the tumor has been removed and provides sensitive monitoring of right ventricular function which will acutely deteriorate with tumor embolization.[1,2] The biopsy was read as myosarcoma which was demonstrated to arise from the wall of the inferior vena cava. Although these tumors may not be as aggressive as the classical sarcoma tumor, the location of the tumor makes resection technically challenging. This patient's hemodynamics continued to deteriorate and he was not considered to be a surgical candidate.

References

1. Singh I, Jacobs LE, Kotler MN, et al. The utility of transesophageal echocardiography in the management of renal cell carcinoma with intracardiac extension. J Am Soc Echocardiogr 1995;8:245–50.

2. Koide Y, Mizoguchi T, Ishii K, et al. Intraoperative management for removal of tumor thrombus in the inferior vena cava or the right atrium with multiple transesophageal echocardiography. J Cardiovasc Surg 1998;39:641–7.

19

Persistent left superior vena cava

Susan E Wiegers MD

A 28-year-old woman presented to her primary care physician complaining of a 3-day history of fevers, rigors, and a cough productive of green sputum. She smoked two packs of cigarettes a day but was otherwise well. The physical examination was remarkable for consolidation at the right lower base. A chest X-ray demonstrated a right lower lobe infiltrate and an enlarged heart. The patient was treated as an outpatient with oral antibiotics. After the convalescence, an echocardiogram was undertaken to evaluate the enlarged heart.

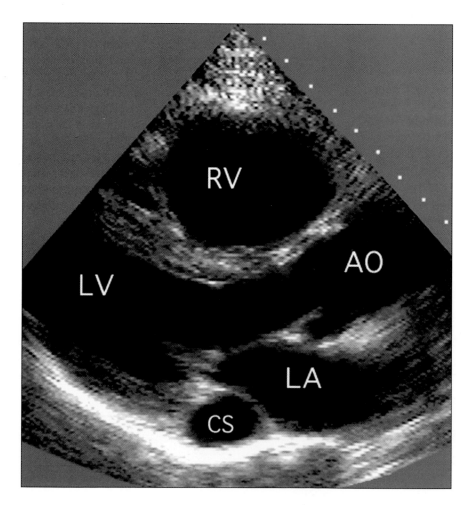

Figure 19.1
Parasternal long-axis view in systole. The coronary sinus (CS) is markedly enlarged. Although in its usual location, the coronary sinus is usually not visible posterior to the left atrium in the atrio-ventricular groove. The left atrium (LA) and left ventricle (LV) are of normal size and the valves appear normal. However, the right ventricle (RV) is enlarged.

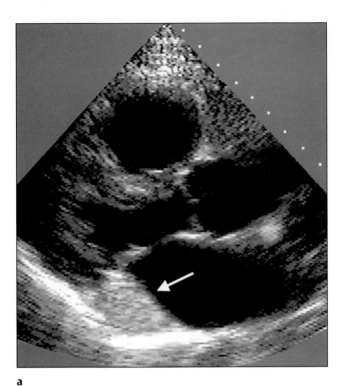

a

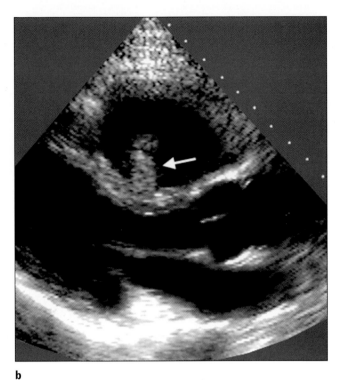

b

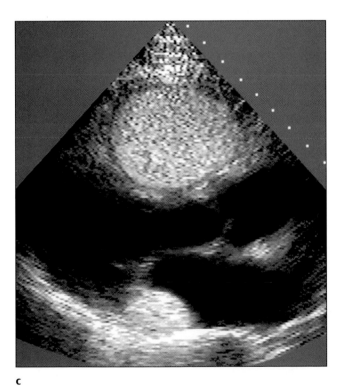

c

Figure 19.2

(a) Parasternal long axis view after injection of agitated saline into the left antecubital vein. Note the contrast (arrow) filling the coronary sinus. The coronary sinus fills prior to any opacification of the right side of the heart which is diagnostic of persistent left superior vena cava.

(b) Parasternal long-axis view in the next cardiac cycle after injection of the agitated saline. Contrast is now beginning to appear in the right ventricle (arrow). The coronary sinus (unmarked) continues to be opacified by the bubbles.

(c) Parasternal long-axis view several cardiac cycles after injection of agitated saline into the left ante-cubital vein. The coronary sinus and right ventricle are completely opacified. There is no contrast present in the left side of the heart. If the coronary sinus had an anomalous connection to the left atrium, there would be at least a few bubbles visualized in the left atrium.

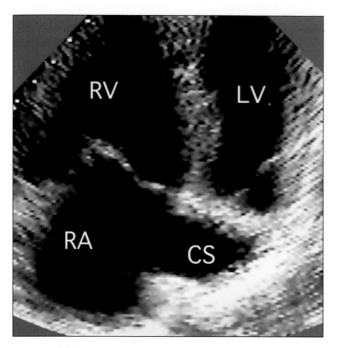

Figure 19.3
Close-up image from the apical four-chamber view which is slightly off axis, demonstrating the coronary sinus (CS) entering the right atrium (RA). The coronary sinus ostium is markedly enlarged as is the right side of the heart. Without the contrast injection it would not be possible to tell whether the dilated coronary sinus were due to elevated right-sided heart pressures or to a persistent left superior vena cava.

Discussion

This patient had the incidental finding of an enlarged heart demonstrated on a chest X-ray. Several abnormalities are present in this echocardiogram. The differential diagnosis of a dilated coronary sinus is persistent left superior vena cava and elevated right-sided pressures. It is rare for elevated right sided pressures to result in such marked dilatation of the coronary sinus. Several anatomical arrangements are possible with persistent left superior vena cava, which almost always empties into the coronary sinus and subsequently into the right atrium. Usually, the right superior vena cava empties directly into the right atrium in the standard arrangement. There is a variable involution of the brachiocephalic vein from the left. Injection of agitated saline from the right antecubital vein will result in opacification of the right atrium and right ventricle. On occasion, a few microbubbles may reflux into the coronary sinus. However, the degree of opacification will be mild. On contrast injection into the left antecubital vein, the agitated saline will pass into the left cephalic vein, into the left superior vena cava and then into the coronary sinus. Thus, the coronary sinus will be the first cardiac structure to opacify with left-sided injection. Injection into both the right and left antecubital veins is necessary to establish the diagnosis.[1] In this patient, right-sided injection did not result in opacification of the coronary sinus prior to contrast appearing in the right side of the heart. Transesophageal echocardiography can also be used to make the diagnosis. The connection of the left superior vena cava to the coronary sinus is usually outside the fields of view obtainable by both transthoracic and transesophageal imaging. However, the left superior vena cava may sometimes be visualized with the transthoracic transducer placed in the left supraclavicular fossa and angled caudad.

Persistent left superior vena cava is most often an incidental finding on echocardiogram. Although it is clinically benign, the anatomical arrangement makes placement of intravenous pacemakers and pulmonary artery catheters difficult from the left side. The right-sided approach should be used in all patients except in the most unusual of circumstances. Retrograde cardioplegia will also be complicated by the presence of left superior vena cava.[2]

Persistent left superior vena cava in itself does not cause right ventricular enlargement, as was present in this patient. There is no shunt in isolated persistent left superior vena cava and there is no hemodynamic effect. However, the lesion is associated with other congenital anomalies such as atrial septal defect and unroofed coronary sinus, in which there is a connection between the coronary sinus and the floor of the left atrium. The shunt in an unroofed coronary sinus is left to right: from the left atrium to the coronary sinus to the right atrium, similar in effect to an atrial septal defect. This patient had no evidence of an unroofed coronary sinus and there was no definite visualization of an atrial septal defect. However, the pulmonary artery flow velocities were elevated and the calculated Qp/Qs shunt ratio was greater than 2 : 1 which is consistent with a left to right intracardiac shunt. Magnetic resonance imaging demonstrated a sinus venosus atrial septal defect which could not be seen on transthoracic echocardiography.

References

1. Chaudhry F, Zabalgoitia M. Persistent left superior vena cava diagnosed by contrast transesophageal echocardiography. Am Heart J 1991;122:1175–7.

2. Roberts W, Risher W, Schwarz K. Transesophageal echocardiographic identification of persistent left superior vena cava: retrograde administration of cardioplegia during cardiac surgery. Anesthesiology 1994;81:760–2.

20

Cardiac neurofibroma

Susan E Wiegers MD

A 65-year-old man had a history of neurofibromatosis. Two of his six children, but none of his siblings, were also affected. He had otherwise been well and had no history of seizures, headaches, or abdominal pain and he had never been hospitalized. He developed atrial fibrillation at a rapid ventricular rate which precipitated his presentation to the emergency room. On physical examination his blood pressure was 140/90 mmHg and his pulse was 155 bpm. He had clear lungs and a normal cardiac examination except for the irregular tachycardia. Innumerable subcutaneous nodules consistent with neurofibromas were present. He spontaneously converted to normal sinus rhythm after intravenous beta-blockers had been used to slow the rate. An echocardiogram was obtained as an outpatient to assess his cardiac function.

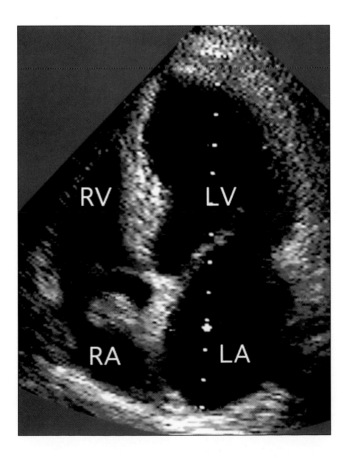

Figure 20.1
Apical four-chamber view in diastole. There is mild concentric left ventricular hypertrophy. The left ventricular chamber size is normal as was the systolic function, which is not demonstrated here. The right-sided chambers were also of normal size. The interatrial septum is thickened and there is a mobile mass which projects into the right atrium. The mass is attached to the interatrial septum. While it was mobile in real time, it did not occlude the tricuspid valve orifice and was not in proximity to the orifices of the vena cava.

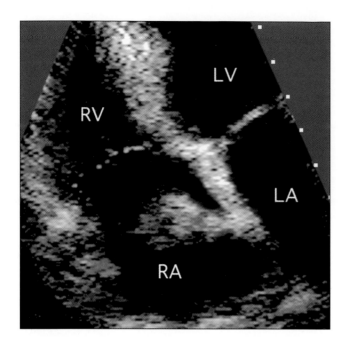

Figure 20.2
Close-up image of the mass taken from an off-axis apical four-chamber position. The mass arises from the interatrial septum, which is abnormally thickened in the portion closest to the atrioventricular valve planes. The mass appears to be contiguous with this area of thickening and appears to be part of the same process. The edges of the mass are indistinct and the mass itself was highly mobile. This appearance is atypical for a myxoma, which usually appears to have a well-defined border and to be more echodense. While myxomas most often arise from the interatrial septum, the septum itself is usually normal.

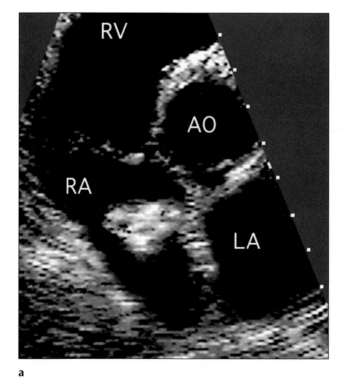

a

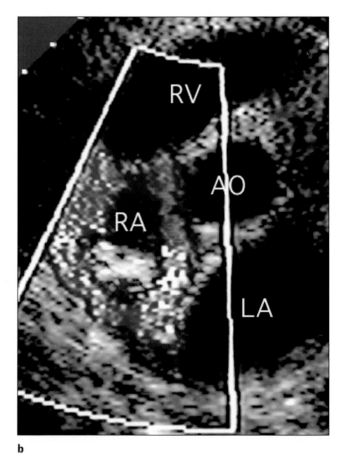

b

Figure 20.3
(a) Parasternal short-axis view at the base of the heart. The imaging sector has been narrowed to afford better resolution of the mass. The right atrium (RA) is of normal size but contains the mass, which appears to measure approximately 2.3 cm in diameter. Its attachment to the interatrial septum is again visualized. The right ventricle (RV) appears to be slightly enlarged but this off-axis image does not allow for true assessment of the chamber sizes. In fact, the right ventricle was not dilated as demonstrated in Figure 20.1. The aortic root (AO) and left atrium (LA) appear to be normal as well.
(b) Color flow Doppler imaging in a similar view. The inflow into the right atrium surrounds the right atrial mass. The flow has low velocity and is laminar which signifies that the mass is not causing any obstruction to flow.

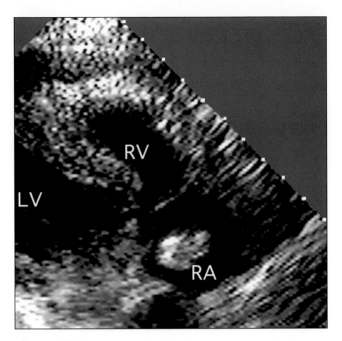

Figure 20.4
Parasternal long-axis right ventricular inflow view. This image is also taken off axis from the standard transducer position as demonstrated by the fact that the left ventricle (LV), rather than the posterior wall of the right ventricle, is seen on the left of the screen. This position allowed imaging of the mass in the right atrium (RA) but not its attachment to the septum which is out of plane. The interatrial septum is parallel to the plane of the image. In real time, the mass was mobile but did not cross the tricuspid valve annulus.

of the mass were indistinct which is also not characteristic of a myxoma. Finally, the abnormality of the interatrial septum is not usually seen in myxoma and is suggestive of another process.

Neurofibromas may arise in any cardiac chamber and have on occasion caused symptoms due to obstruction of the right ventricular outflow.[4,5] Unlike the situation in tuberous sclerosis, in which approximately 20% of affected adult patients have cardiac rhabdomyomas on echocardiographic study, cardiac neurofibromas are rarely present in patients with neurofibromatosis. There has been some speculation that involvement of cardiac nerves in patients with von Recklinghausen disease predisposes the patients to 'silent' myocardial ischemia and possibly to coronary artery spasm. Malignant transformation of cardiac neurofibromas to rhabdomyosarcomas has been reported.[6] The change in the interatrial septum is of concern, given this risk. The incidence of such a transformation is unknown. The patient did well on prophylactic oral beta blockers and has been followed for several years with no recurrence of atrial fibrillation and no change in the size of the mass.

This study demonstrates once again the importance of a flexible approach to the echocardiographic examination. Standard views are necessary to determine chamber size and valvular function. However, many abnormalities are best imaged in off-axis positions. Sufficient time should be allotted to each study to allow the scanner to fully delineate unusual findings that may require multiple non-standard views.

Discussion

The right atrial mass is presumably the cause of the patient's atrial fibrillation. The mass was highly mobile and may have irritated the atrial endocardium. The tumor is most likely to be a neurofibroma, which is a rare benign tumor of the heart accounting for less than 0.3% of cardiac tumors in large pathology series.[1–3] The differential diagnosis of the mass includes thrombus, myxoma, and malignant tumor. A thrombus is unlikely, given the attachment to the interatrial septum and the lack of predisposing conditions for thrombus formation. The mass is possibly a myxoma, but its appearance is not characteristic. A myxoma is a solid tumor that may be mobile and even prolapse through the tricuspid valve. However, myxomas rarely exhibit the high-frequency, chaotic motion of this mass which was apparent in real-time imaging. The edges

References

1. Tazelaar H, Locke T, McGregor C. Pathology of surgically excised primary cardiac tumors. Mayo Clin Proc 1992;67:957–65.

2. Molina J, Edwards J, Ward H. Primary cardiac tumors: experience at the University of Minnesota. Thorac Cardiovasc Surg 1990;38:183–91.

3. Blondeau P. Primary cardiac tumors: French studies of 533 cases. Thorac Cardiovasc Surg 1990;38:192–5.

4. Henderson W, Huckell V, English J, et al. Right outflow tract obstruction by a pedunculated neurofibroma: case report and literature review. Can J Cardiol 1997;13:387–90.

5. Rosenquist G, Krovetz L, Haller JJ, et al. Acquired right ventricular outflow obstruction in a child with neurofibromatosis. Am Heart J 1970;79:103–8.

6. Mata M, Wharton M, Geisinger K, et al. Myocardial rhabdomyosarcoma in multiple neurofibromatosis. Neurology 1981;31:1549–51.

21

Rheumatic valvular disease

Susan E Wiegers MD

A 55-year-old woman presented to the emergency room with severe shortness of breath and edema. She was visiting her family from a tropical country, where she had always had a limited exercise capacity due to an unspecified heart condition. In the 2 months since her arrival, she initially improved but then began to develop increasing pedal edema and orthopnea. In the past few days, she had slept in a chair because of profound shortness of breath.

On physical examination, she was thin and dyspneic. The patient was in atrial fibrillation at a rate of 130 bpm and the blood pressure was 110/70 mmHg. There was dullness to percussion half-way up both lung fields and rales at the apices. The first heart sound was quiet. There was a loud systolic murmur at the apex and a harsh systolic murmur at the left upper sternal border. The P_2 component of S_2 was loud. A diastolic rumble was audible at the apex and at the right lower sternal border. This diastolic murmur and the systolic murmur audible in this area increased with inspiration. The patient was treated with oxygen and diuretics, with improvement in her symptoms. An echocardiogram was performed to assess the valvular heart disease.

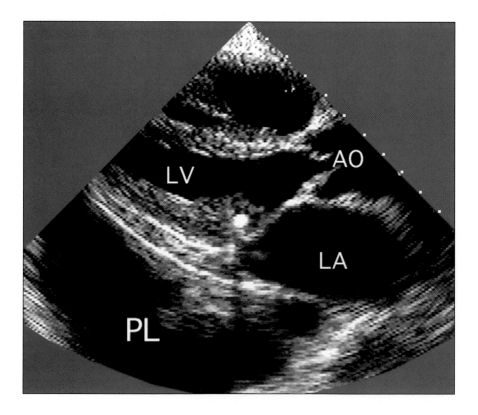

Figure 21.1
Parasternal long axis view in systole. The depth of field is intentionally set to image the structures posterior to the heart. There is a large left pleural effusion (PL) with a mass along the pleura which probably represents atelectatic lung. Mild left ventricular hypertrophy is present but the left ventricular cavity size is small in systole, suggesting normal left ventricular systolic function. The right ventricle appears to be enlarged and the radius of curvature of the interventricular septum has been reversed. This is evidence of both right ventricular pressure and volume overload. The left atrium (LA) is enlarged. The mitral valve appears thickened and calcified although the posterior leaflet is poorly seen. The normal chordal attachments to the valve are obscured by dense thickening and calcification of the subvalvular structures. The aortic valve (AO) is thickened and does not open completely in systole. However, the doming of the leaflets is not particularly evident in this image.

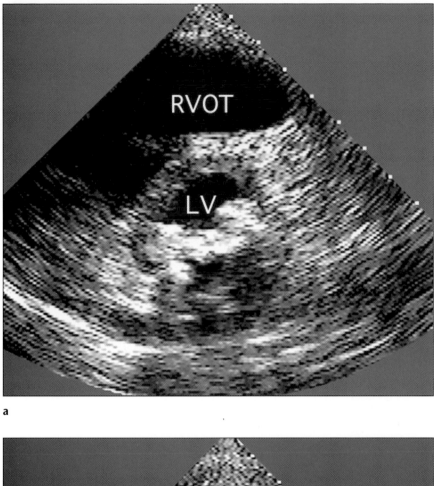

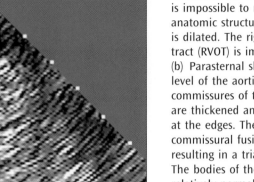

a

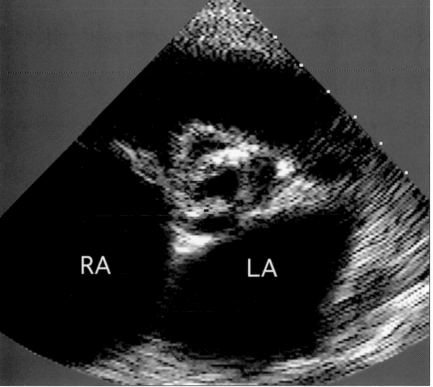

b

Figure 21.2
(a) Parasternal short axis view at the level of the mitral valve orifice. The mitral valve is densely calcified and it is impossible to make out the normal anatomic structures. The right ventricle is dilated. The right ventricular outflow tract (RVOT) is imaged at this level.
(b) Parasternal short-axis view at the level of the aortic valve. The commissures of the aortic valve cusps are thickened and retracted or curled at the edges. There has been commissural fusion at the annulus resulting in a triangular valvular orifice. The bodies of the coronary cusps are relatively normal. The commissural involvement distinguishes the rheumatic process present in this patient from the more common senile calcific aortic stenosis which tends to involve the body of the leaflets.

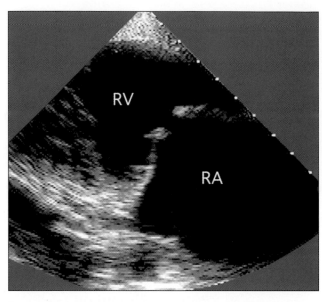

a

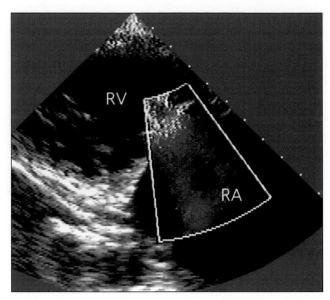

b

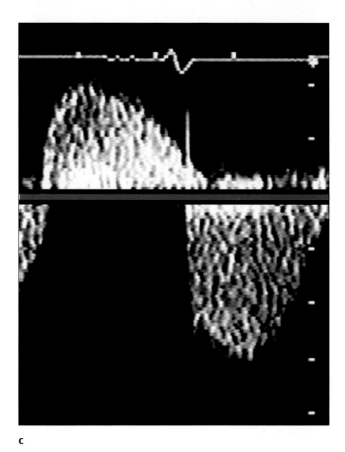

c

Figure 21.3

(a) Parasternal right ventricular inflow view of the tricuspid valve. Both leaflets are thickened especially at the tips and dome in diastole. This frame represents their maximum opening during diastole. The right atrium is clearly dilated although this view is not routinely used to assess chamber size.

(b) Similar diastolic view with color flow Doppler imaging. The color Doppler inflow jet aliases at the level of the valve leaflets resulting in turbulent flow into the right ventricle. Proximal acceleration of flow is noted on the right atrial side of the flow. Both phenomena are consistent with significant tricuspid stenosis.

(c) Spectral display of continuous-wave Doppler across the tricuspid valve. The peak diastolic velocity of the inflow signal, represented as flow above the baseline, is approximately 1.8 m/s, which is much higher than the normal tricuspid inflow velocity. The spectral envelope was traced using the standard ultrasound machine software. Analysis of the spectral tracing via the modified Bernoulli equation yielded a peak gradient of 16 mmHg and a mean of 5 mmHg.

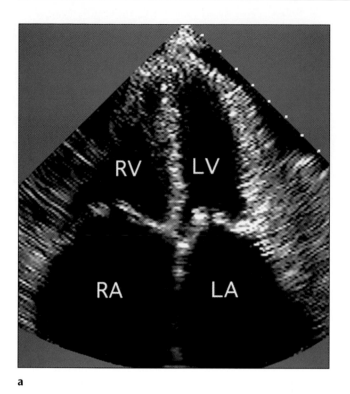

a

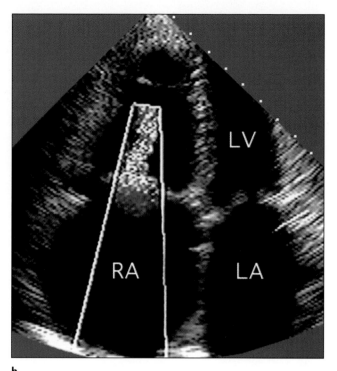

b

c

Figure 21.4

(a) Apical four-chamber view in diastole. The left ventricular cavity is small and underfilled. The left atrium (LA) is moderately enlarged and the right atrium (RA) severely so. The mitral valve and the tricuspid valves are thickened and calcified more prominently at the tips than the body of the leaflets. This image alone is diagnostic of rheumatic heart disease with mitral and tricuspid stenosis. The pattern of thickening of the leaflets and the diastolic doming are pathognomonic of a rheumatic process. The right ventricle is enlarged and hypertrophied. A portion of the left pleural effusion is visible at the top of the screen on the right side of the image, adjacent to the left ventricle. Note that the tricuspid valve is slightly apically displaced compared to the mitral valve which is the normal anatomical relationship.

(b) Apical four-chamber view in diastole with color flow Doppler imaging. The transducer has been moved medially over the right ventricular apex. The change in position may be deduced by identifying the structure that is located immediately below the apex of the triangle in the two-dimensional display. In this image, the right ventricular apex, rather than the left ventricular apex, is now in this position. The distal lateral wall of the left ventricle and the left pleural effusion are no longer imaged. The off-axis imaging allows alignment of the ultrasound beam with the tricuspid inflow and regurgitation jets. Note that the right ventricle appears larger than in the previous figure. It is important to judge the right ventricular size from the true apical position demonstrated in the previous figure. Even normal-sized right ventricles may appear enlarged with placement of the transducer over the right ventricular apex, rather than in the standard view. The color flow Doppler jet of the tricuspid inflow is again diagnostic of tricuspid stenosis. Normally the tricuspid inflow is laminar and of low velocity. In this case, the jet becomes turbulent and aliases at the level of the valve. The jet in the right ventricle is of high velocity and turbulent. Proximal acceleration of the jet on the right atrial surface is noted.

(c) Spectral display of continuous-wave Doppler across the mitral valve taken from the apical position. The peak velocity is over 2 m/s, which is markedly abnormal for this valve. Analysis of the spectral envelope reveals the peak gradient to be 22 mmHg and the mean gradient to be 11 mmHg.

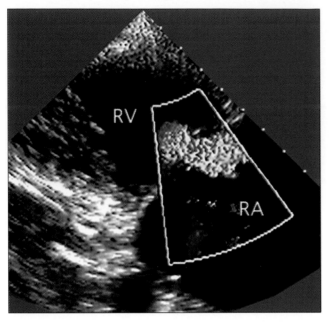
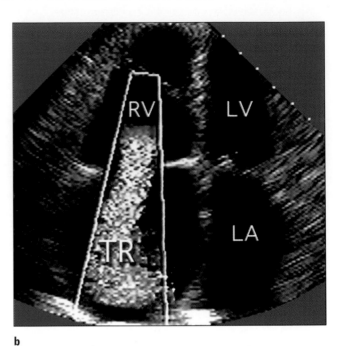

a   b

Figure 21.5

(a) Parasternal right ventricular inflow view of the tricuspid valve in systole. The tricuspid regurgitation jet arises at the level of the valve and extends for a short distance into the dilated right atrium. Although the jet is wide at the level of the tricuspid valve, it does not appear to be severe in this view.

(b) Off-axis apical four-chamber view in systole with color flow Doppler imaging of the tricuspid regurgitation jet. The position of the transducer is the same as in Figure 21.4b. The width of the jet at the level of the valve is similar to that in the previous figure. However, the jet appears to fill much of the right atrium. The disparity in the area of the jet is due, not to beat-to-beat differences in the severity of regurgitation, but to alignment of the ultrasound beam with the jet. The peak velocity of the tricuspid regurgitation jet was 2.9 m/s which yields an estimated peak pulmonary artery systolic pressure of 49 mmHg, assuming a right atrial pressure of 15 mmHg.

Discussion

Rheumatic heart disease is characterized by progressive commissural fusion and fibrosis of the valves. In tropical climates, the disease appears to progress more rapidly, with severe stenosis developing sooner than in temperate climates. Involvement of the tricuspid valve is rare but multivalvular involvement is characteristic of rheumatic disease. Both regurgitation and stenosis are the result of this pathological process.

Commissural fusion leads to the characteristic echocardiographic features of rheumatic disease. The leaflets themselves do not become fixed until late in the disease. Rather, the rheumatic process tends to involve the edges and the tips of the valve leaflets. The commissures thicken and eventually fuse, but the bodies of the leaflet remain mobile. This accounts for doming of the valves, which are tethered along the commissures but still retain mobility. Rheumatic heart disease is the only process that will result in diastolic doming of both the tricuspid and the mitral valves. The aortic involvement demonstrated in this

patient is also characteristic of rheumatic disease. The commissures of the aortic valve cusps are thickened and have begun to fuse at the annular level. With time, this fusion would be expected to extend along the commissures toward the tips of the leaflets resulting in more and more severe stenosis. The aortic valve cusps also tend to become fixed, resulting in an orifice that is both regurgitant and stenotic.

Tricuspid stenosis is generally due to rheumatic disease. Other, rarer, causes include congenital abnormalities and carcinoid heart disease. In carcinoid disease, the leaflets become thickened but do not dome in diastole. The entire leaflet, rather than the commissures and the tips of the leaflets, is affected by the carcinoid process. The thickened, abnormal leaflets become immobile but do not dome. The pattern of tricuspid valve motion is thus very useful in diagnosing the cause of tricuspid stenosis.[1,2] Congenital abnormalities of the valve are ruled out in this case by the normal arrangement and location of the leaflets. Rheumatic involvement of the mitral and aortic valves should prompt careful examination of the tricuspid valve as well. Signs and symptoms due to tricuspid stenosis may be erroneously attributed to other valvular lesions. Tricuspid valve replacement should be considered at the time of mitral or aortic valve surgery if severe tricuspid stenosis is present. Therefore, it is most important to establish the diagnosis.

There are no methods for estimating tricuspid valve area in clinical practice at present. The orifice area of the tricuspid valve is considerably larger than the mitral valve, usually 6–7 cm^2. A small decrease in the valve area may lead to some degree of hemodynamic obstruction. Doppler echocardiography can be used to measure the peak and mean gradients across the valve. While the pressure half time of the spectral envelope would be expected to be longer with more severe stenosis, the Hatle equation has not been validated for the tricuspid valve. Large series are lacking because of the relative rarity of the diagnosis. Even a mean gradient of 2 mmHg is enough to diagnose tricuspid stenosis. Provocation of the gradient with fluid loading may be useful in equivocal cases.[3] While rheumatic tricuspid stenosis is generally well tolerated, hepatomegaly, pedal edema and ascites may eventually develop.[4]

The variation in the size of the color flow Doppler jet, depending on the angle of incidence of the ultrasound beam, is a well-known phenomenon. The right ventricular inflow view is important for determining the morphology of the tricuspid valve and is the only view in which the posterior leaflet of the valve is imaged. However, the ultrasound beam is not as well aligned with the inflow jet across the tricuspid valve or with most central jets of tricuspid regurgitation from this view. Not only will the velocity measured by continuous-wave Doppler generally be lower in the right ventricular inflow view than in the apical four-chamber view, but the size of the color

Doppler jet itself will appear smaller. Once again, interpretation of the echocardiogram requires the synthesis of data from multiple views.

This patient was found to have severe mitral stenosis, mild aortic stenosis with moderate regurgitation and severe tricuspid stenosis and regurgitation. Moderate pulmonary hypertension was present, owing to the mitral stenosis. It was thought that the acute decompensation had been precipitated by the development of rapid atrial fibrillation. The patient underwent replacement of all three involved valves with bileaflet mechanical valves. Her course was complicated by complete heart block, requiring the placement of a permanent pacer with epicardial leads, and postpericardiotomy syndrome, which responded to anti-inflammatory agents. She remains in atrial fibrillation but has done extremely well with a marked improvement in her exercise tolerance.

References

1. Pearlman A. Role of echocardiography in the diagnosis and evaluation of severity of mitral and tricuspid stenosis. Circulation 1991;84:1193–7.

2. Shimada R, Takeshita A, Nakamura M, et al. Diagnosis of tricuspid stenosis by M-mode and two-dimensional echocardiography. Am J Cardiol 1984;53:164–8.

3. Ribeiro P, al Zaibag M, Sawyer W. A prospective study comparing the haemodynamic with the cross-sectional echocardiographic diagnosis of rheumatic tricuspid stenosis. Eur Heart J 1989;10:120–6.

4. Roguin A, Rinkevich D, Milo S, et al. Long-term follow-up of patients with severe rheumatic tricuspid stenosis. Am Heart J 1998;136:103–8.

22

Tricuspid valve endocarditis

Susan E Wiegers MD

A 25-year-old woman presented to the emergency room with a high fever, chills, and myalgias. She had been ill for 3 days before seeking medical treatment. On the morning of presentation, she had a shaking chill and felt weak. The patient was an active intravenous drug user, injecting heroin at least once a day. Several attempts at detoxification programs and methadone maintenance had resulted in temporary abstinence. The patient had begun injecting drugs again approximately 6 months prior to this presentation. A recent HIV test was negative.

On physical examination the patient was febrile with a temperature of 103.5°F. The blood pressure was 120/70 mmHg and the pulse was 125 bpm. The patient looked acutely ill with a respiratory rate of 20 but the physical examination was essentially unremarkable except for skin lesions consistent with intravenous drug use. There was a soft flow murmur at the right upper sternal border but no other murmurs were present. The chest X-ray showed four rounded opacities bilaterally which were consistent with embolic phenomenon. An echocardiogram was ordered to rule out endocarditis.

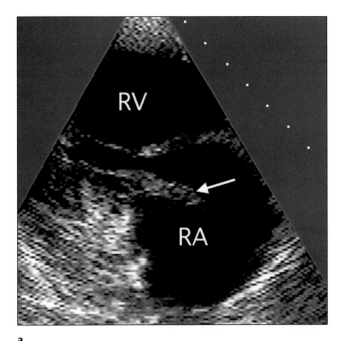

a

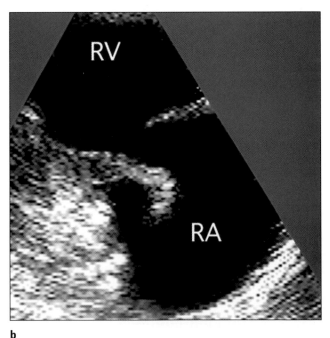

b

Figure 22.1
(a) Parasternal right ventricular inflow view of the tricuspid valve. There is a large mass (arrow) measuring approximately 3 cm attached to the posterior leaflet of the tricuspid valve. Normal chordal attachments from the papillary muscles are visible to the tips of both the posterior and anterior leaflets. The mass flails into the right atrium (RA) in this systolic view. The tricuspid leaflets do not coapt completely, owing to the flail posterior leaflet. This resulted in severe tricuspid regurgitation (not shown here).
(b) Further posterior angulation of the transducer in this subsequent systolic frame, demonstrates that the entire posterior leaflet is thickened from the annulus to the tip of the leaflet. It is impossible to determine where the leaflet ends and the vegetation begins. Note that the portion of the anterior leaflet imaged in this view appears to be uninvolved and is relatively normal.

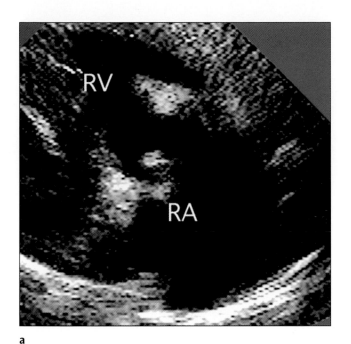

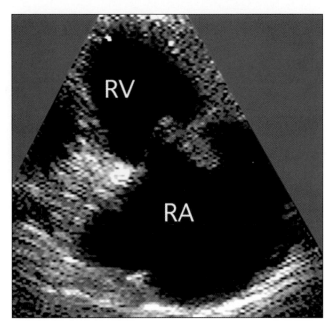

a   b

Figure 22.2

(a) Clockwise rotation of the transducer brings the septal leaflet into view on the left of the screen. The right ventricular posterior wall is no longer imaged on the left of the screen; the interventricular septum is seen with a small portion of the left ventricular cavity visible to the left of the septum. The leaflet seen on the left is therefore the septal leaflet rather than the posterior leaflet. The septal leaflet of the tricuspid valve appears markedly abnormal from the annulus to the tip of the leaflet. In addition, there is a small mass attached to the tip of the leaflet. Again, it is not possible to distinguish where the valve structure ends and the vegetation begins. The annulus is thickened and is more echodense than the surrounding myocardium. This is suggestive of involvement of the annulus with the infection, if not frank abscess formation. Note that, in comparison to the previous image, the portion of the anterior leaflet of the tricuspid valve imaged in this frame has a large vegetation attached to its tip.

(b) Systolic image in the same plane. The septal leaflet appears somewhat more normal in this frame, but there is a vegetation attached to the anterior leaflet which appears in the right atrium in systole. This portion of the leaflets appear to coapt and neither leaflet is flail.

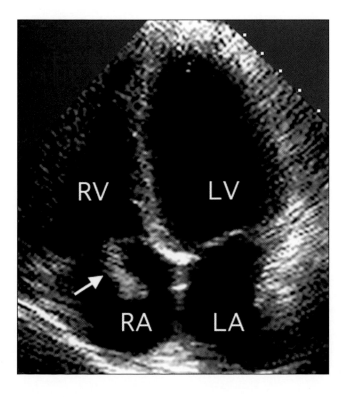

Figure 22.3

Apical four-chamber view demonstrating a large vegetation attached to the tricuspid valve leaflet seen in this systolic frame. The mass represents the confluence of several vegetations which are attached to the tips of the septal and anterior leaflets. This mass was highly mobile in real time.

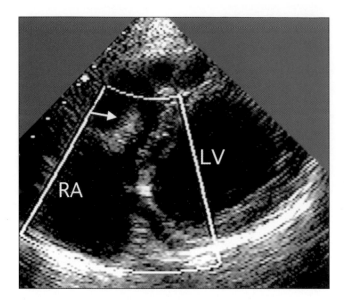

Figure 22.4
Off-axis parasternal short-axis view of the anterior leaflet of the tricuspid valve. The large mass (arrow) is seen in the right ventricular cavity in this diastolic image. The mass flailed into the right atrium in systole and was present in the right ventricle in diastole. This highly mobile characteristic increases the likelihood of embolism to the pulmonary artery. Note the mildly enlarged coronary sinus seen emptying into the right atrium at the level of the atrioventricular groove at the bottom of the screen.

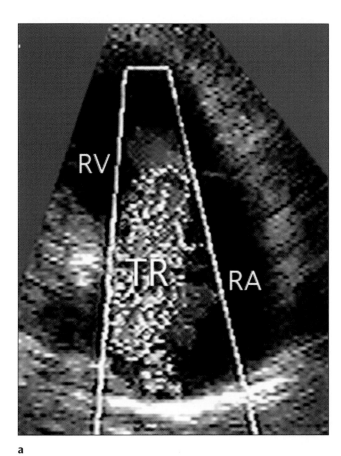

a

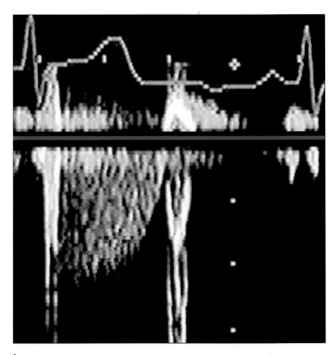

b

Figure 22.5
(a) Parasternal right ventricular inflow view with color flow Doppler imaging of the tricuspid valve in systole. There is a large jet of tricuspid regurgitation that obscures the presence of the vegetation. The severe regurgitation is due to the flail portion of the leaflet and the resultant incompetency.
(b) Spectral display of continuous-wave Doppler across the tricuspid valve from the apical position. The peak velocity is 2 m/s (each calibration mark represents 1 m/s). This predicts a normal peak pulmonary artery systolic pressure of 26 mmHg, assuming a right atrial pressure of 10 mmHg.

Discussion

Endocarditis is a common complication of intravenous drug use. Tricuspid valve endocarditis is generally more common than left-sided endocarditis in this situation. It is thought that the patients are particularly susceptible to right-sided infection, owing to the repeated introduction of contaminated substances into the venous system. Echocardiography is frequently performed in febrile intravenous drug users with a systemic illness and no localizing findings, even prior to the results of the blood cultures being available. This patient had radiographic evidence of septic pulmonary emboli, increasing the likelihood that vegetations would be detected.

The most important view in this patient's echocardiographic examination was the parasternal view of the right ventricular inflow which imaged the tricuspid valve. This view is sometimes left out of routine studies but is an important part of the complete echocardiographic examination. From the parasternal long axis view of the left ventricle, posterior and medial angulation of the transducer brings the right ventricle inflow into view. This is the only plane in which the posterior leaflet of the tricuspid valve is imaged. The retrosternal location of the tricuspid valve makes it more difficult to visualize than the other cardiac valves from the parasternal window. The posterior leaflet is particularly difficult to image, as it is the smallest of the three leaflets and curves around the diaphragmatic surface of the heart from the inferolateral wall of the right ventricle to its septal insertion. Often, the right ventricular inflow view is incorrectly obtained and the septum rather than the right ventricular posterior free wall is imaged on the left of the screen. It may be particularly difficult to obtain the correct orientation in patients who cannot assume the left lateral decubitus position or in those with dilated right ventricles. If it is the interventricular septum rather than the posterior wall of the right ventricle that is imaged, the septal leaflet of the tricuspid valve rather than the posterior leaflet is visible. The tricuspid valve has a surface area and annulus that are considerably larger than the mitral valve. Therefore, multiple off-axis views are necessary to fully image the tricuspid valve leaflets. In this case, the anterior leaflet appears to be normal in some views but clearly has a large vegetation attached to the tip in other views. The echocardiographic image intersects the valve in a single plane and the geometry of the tricuspid valve may lead to erroneous conclusions unless the entire valve is inspected.

Extremely large vegetations involving the tricuspid valve are not uncommon in right-sided endocarditis in intravenous drug users.[1,2] *Staphylococcus aureus* is the most common infecting organism, although multiple organisms may be isolated from the blood cultures.

Although the short-term prognosis is generally good for intravenous drug users with bacteremia and tricuspid valve vegetations, vegetations greater than 2 cm are associated with an increased risk of death. One study reported a mortality of 33% in patients with extremely large vegetations. Surgery for tricuspid endocarditis is recommended in this setting only for intractable infection. Excision of the tricuspid valve without valve replacement has been the surgery of choice.[3] Immunosuppression may influence the development of tricuspid valve endocarditis, but intravenous drug use is a risk factor for both HIV infection and endocarditis. Left-sided but not right-sided endocarditis has a higher mortality rate in HIV-positive patients compared to HIV-negative controls.[4]

Recent interest was focused on short-course antibiotic therapy for right-sided endocarditis in patients with *Staphylococcus aureus* infection in intravenous drug users.[5,6] A 2-week course of penicillinase-resistant penicillin and gentamicin intravenously has been shown to cure many patients with uncomplicated tricuspid valve endocarditis caused by methicillin-sensitive *Staphylococcus aureus*. However, patients should be monitored by echocardiography to rule out the progression of disease and the development of metastatic infection to other valves or the free wall of the right ventricle. Patients with vegetations larger than 2 cm are best treated with longer antibiotic courses.

This patient had blood cultures positive for *Staphylococcus aureus*. She was treated for 1 week in the hospital with intravenous antibiotics but then signed out against medical advice and was lost to follow-up.

References

1. Hecht SR, Berger M. Right-sided endocarditis in intravenous drug users. Prognostic features in 102 episodes. Ann Intern Med 1992;117:560–6.

2. Mathew J, Addai T, Anand A, *et al*. Clinical features, site of involvement, bacteriologic findings, and outcome of infective endocarditis in intravenous drug users. Arch Intern Med 1995;155:1641–8.

3. Arbulu A, Holmes RJ, Asfaw I. Surgical treatment of intractable right-sided infective endocarditis in drug addicts: 25 years experience. J Heart Valve Dis 1993;2:129–37; discussion 138–9.

4. Ribera E, Miro JM, Cortes E, *et al*. Influence of human immunodeficiency virus 1 infection and degree of immunosuppression in the clinical characteristics and outcome of infective endocarditis in intravenous drug users. Arch Intern Med 1998;158:2043–50.

5. Torres-Tortosa M, de Cueto M. Vergara A, *et al*. Prospective evaluation of a two-week course of intravenous antibiotics in intravenous drug addicts with infective endocarditis. Grupo de Estudio de Enfermedades Infecciosas de la Provincia de Cadiz. Eur J Clin Microbiol Infect Dis 1994;13:559–64.

6. DiNubile MJ. Short-course antibiotic therapy for right-sided endocarditis caused by *Staphylococcus aureus* in injection drug users. Ann Intern Med 1994;121:873–6.

23

Prosthetic tricuspid valve obstruction

Martin St John Sutton MBBS

A 32-year-old woman was admitted complaining of short-ness of breath for 5 days progressing to the point that she was extremely dyspneic at rest. She had noted abdominal bloating and mild ankle edema for several days prior to the onset of the symptoms. At the age of 5 years she had been limited in her exercise capacity and was noticed to be mildly cyanosed on exercise. Cardiac catheterization was complicated by rapid atrial tachycardia with hypoten-sion but established the diagnosis of Ebstein's anomaly, moderate tricuspid regurgitation and a secundum atrial septal defect. She was managed conservatively until the age of 16 when she underwent tricuspid bioprosthetic replacement and reconstruction of the atrioventricular annulus. She was symptom free for 6 years but then developed increasing fatigue and was shown by two-dimensional echocardiography to have calcified the bioprosthesis, which was both stenotic and regurgitant.

She underwent tricuspid valve replacement with a St Jude's prosthesis and was orally anticoagulated. Two weeks before her recent symptomatic deterioration she developed profuse vaginal bleeding; a blood count revealed a hemoglobin level of 6.8 g/dl and her warfarin was temporarily discontinued.

On examination she was markedly breathless at rest with air hunger; her systolic blood pressure was 90 mmHg and her heart rate 118 bpm. The jugular venous pressure was elevated to above the angle of the jaw with a promi-nent 'a' wave. There was mild bilateral ankle edema and hepatic enlargement. The apical impulse was unremark-able, and on auscultation the tricuspid prosthetic closing sounds were not audible, suggesting thrombotic occlusion of the tricuspid prosthesis. ECG demonstrated sinus tachycardia and right bundle branch block. Chest X-ray showed cardiomegaly and clear lung fields.

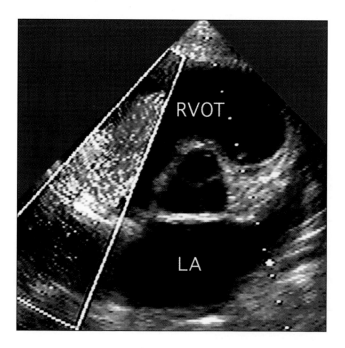

Figure 23.1
Left parasternal short-axis view at aortic valve level. The right ventricular outflow tract (RVOT) is enlarged. There is a mechanical prosthesis in the tricuspid valve position with an aliased color flow Doppler velocity signal in diastole consistent with right ventricular inflow tract obstruction. The aortic valve, pulmonary valve, left atrium and left atrial appendage are all normal.

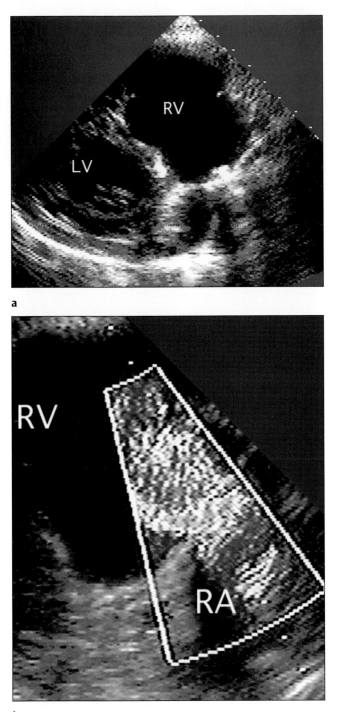

a

b

Figure 23.2
(a) Left parasternal view of the right ventricular inflow tract demonstrated no prosthetic valve disc motion from systole to diastole. The prosthetic valve produces significant shadowing of the right atrium which prevents evaluation of right atrial size and the presence of thrombus.
(b) Similar view with color flow Doppler imaging. The diastolic flow is markedly turbulent across the valve which is consistent with valvular obstruction. There is proximal acceleration on the atrial side of the valve which also signifies obstruction to flow.

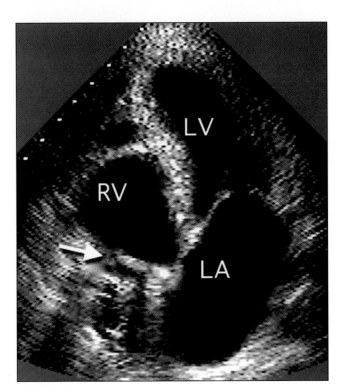

Figure 23.3
Apical four-chamber view showing a normal left ventricle, a dilated left atrium and right ventricle and a prosthesis in the tricuspid position (arrow) which in real time failed to show leaflet motion. The right atrium appears to be filled with a mass. However, this is an artifact due to reverberations from the prosthetic valve rather than a right atrial mass.

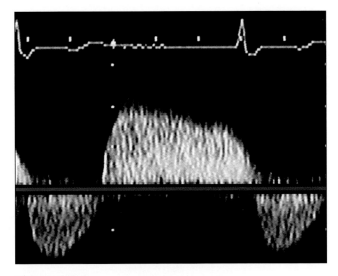

Figure 23.4
Continuous-wave Doppler across the tricuspid valve demonstrating the characteristic high peak velocity and slow decay in diastole with minor regurgitant flow, confirming the presence of prosthetic malfunction. The peak velocity is 2.1 m/s predicting an initial diastolic gradient across the valve of 18 mmHg, which is very abnormal for the tricuspid valve. (Each calibration mark represents 1 m/s.)

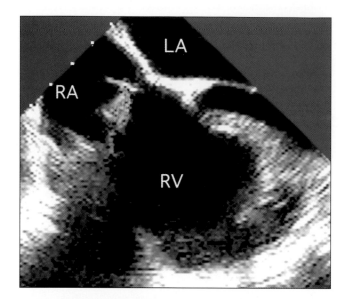

Figure 23.5
Transesophageal echocardiogram from the mid-esophageal level in the transverse plane. There is thrombus encapsulating and partially occluding the tricuspid St Jude prosthesis. The right ventricle is enlarged and abnormal owing to the Ebstein's anomaly.

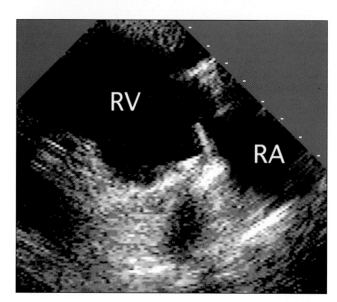

a

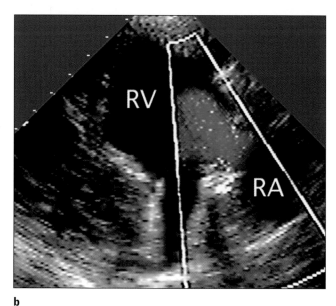

b

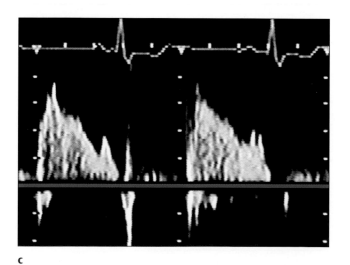

c

Figure 23.6
(a) The day following thrombolytic therapy with front-loaded tPA these right ventricular inflow images were obtained from the left parasternal region. One of the mechanical leaflets of the St Jude prosthesis is visible projecting into the right ventricle in diastole. The other leaflet is out of plane in this view.
(b) Similar view with color flow Doppler imaging. The diastolic jet has low velocity and is not turbulent. There is no obstruction to flow through the prosthetic valve.
(c) Spectral display of pulsed-wave Doppler across the tricuspid prosthesis. The sample volume has been placed in the right ventricle at the tips of the tricuspid prosthesis leaflets. Comparison with Figure 23.4 now reveals that the flow is normal, and of low velocity. The deceleration slope is rapid. The peak velocity is now less than 0.8 m/s (80 cm/s) consistent with a trivial gradient across the prosthetic valve. (Each calibration mark represents 20 cm/s.) There has been a change in the slope of the spectral envelope which signifies relief of the obstruction.

Discussion

The diagnosis was quickly established to be thrombotic encapsulation of the mechanical prosthetic valve due to the discontinuation of oral anticoagulant therapy. The rapid onset of symptoms of dyspnea and air hunger was due to extreme reduction in pulmonary blood flow and cardiac output. The high venous pressure, dependent edema, and hepatic engorgement were indicative of resistance to filling of the right heart; the prominent 'a' wave suggested that the obstruction was at tricuspid valve level, because the right atrium was contracting against a partially closed tricuspid valve. The continuous wave Doppler demonstrated extremely high gradients across the valve and very slow decay in the gradient throughout diastole.

The treatment of Ebstein's anomaly is by tricuspid valve replacement and closure of defects in the atrial septum which are present in approximately 50% of patients. A tricuspid bioprosthesis, rather than a mechanical prosthesis, was initially chosen because the patient wanted to have children without committing to oral anticoagulation. The bioprosthesis predictably calcified and became stenotic and regurgitant. The replacement with a St Jude prosthetic valve was expected to be more durable. However, thrombotic occlusion is a well recognized complication of tricuspid valve replacement when anticoagulation is inadequate. International normalized ratio (INR) levels between 3.0 and 4.0 are necessary at all times. Cessation of warfarin for vaginal bleeding down to a hemoglobin level of 6 g was understandable but inappropriate. Thrombolytic therapy for tricuspid valve occlusion has been successful.[1] We were not anticipating thromboembolism to the systemic circulation because the atrial septum was intact following surgical closure, but we were concerned regarding further bleeding due to the thrombolytic therapy. The patient responded to the thrombolytic therapy with a relief of her symptoms and a decrease in the velocity across the tricuspid valve. Thus, a third operation was avoided.

Reference

1. Hurrell D, Schaff H, Tajik A. Thrombolytic therapy for obstruction of mechanical prosthetic valves. Mayo Clin Proc 1996;71:605–13.

24

Multivalvular endocarditis

Jorge R Kizer MD
Susan E Wiegers MD

A 44-year-old man was transferred to the hospital from the chronic care facility where he resided because of a fever to 104.1°F. He had undergone repair of a Dandy-Walker cranial malformation which required placement of a ventriculoperitoneal shunt. Four months prior to his admission the shunt had been revised but had subsequently become infected with methicillin-sensitive *Staphylococcus aureus*. A new shunt was placed. The patient was started on intravenous oxacillin via a chronic indwelling intravenous catheter. One week prior to his admission the antibiotics had been discontinued but the fever promptly recurred and the oxacillin was restarted.

Physical examination was remarkable for fever, blood pressure of 100/60 mmHg, pulse of 110 bpm and a room air oxygen saturation of 91%. The jugular venous waveform had a prominent V-wave. Diffuse crackles were auscultated in both lung fields. There was a soft holosystolic murmur at the lower left sternal border and an early diastolic murmur at the upper left sternal border. Splinter hemorrhages were present in the left index and middle digits. Laboratory examination revealed leukocytosis with a left shift. Multiple bilateral air-space densities consistent with septic emboli were evident on chest X-ray. Four out of four blood cultures were positive for methicillin resistant *Staphylococcus aureus*. The patient received intravenous vancomycin and gentamicin after removal of the indwelling venous catheter. However, he remained febrile. Transthoracic echocardiography revealed vegetations on the tricuspid, pulmonary, and aortic valves. Because of failure to respond to medical therapy, he was taken to the operating room, where this transesophageal study was performed.

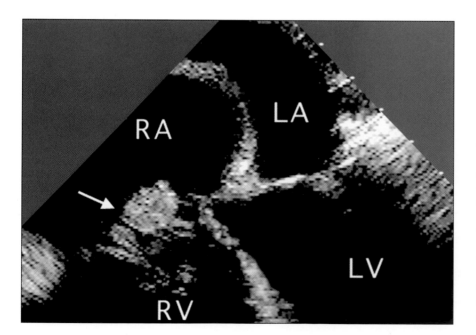

Figure 24.1
Transesophageal echocardiogram from the mid-esophageal level in the transverse plane (imaging angle 0°). The left atrium (LA) is small. The right atrium (RA) is enlarged and the intra-atrial septum bulges into the left atrium consistent with elevated right atrial pressures. The tricuspid valve (arrow) imaged between the right atrium and the right ventricle (RV) contains a multi-lobulated mass consistent with a large vegetation. This mass involves the septal leaflet of the tricuspid valve as well as the anterior leaflet which is imaged on the left of the screen. Parts of the mass extend into the right ventricle. The mitral valve between the left atrium and left ventricle (LV) is not well seen in this view.

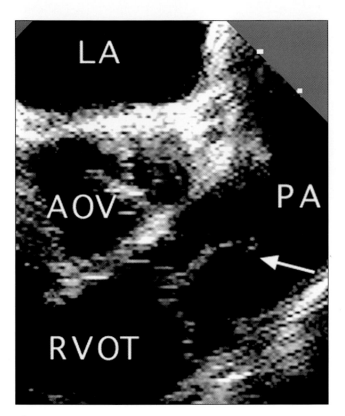

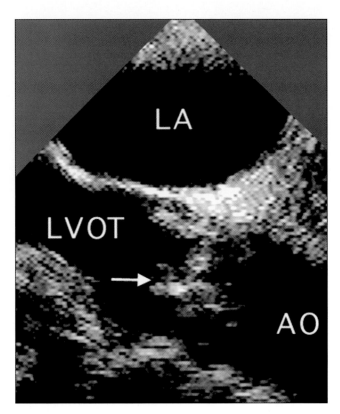

Figure 24.2
Transesophageal echocardiogram from a high esophageal level in a modified transverse plane (imaging angle 30°). The pulmonary valve, located between the right ventricular outflow tract (RVOT) and the pulmonary artery (PA) contains a pedunculated mass (arrow) that extends into the pulmonary artery. This vegetation was highly mobile in real time. In addition, the aortic valve (AOV) appears to be abnormal although it is poorly seen in this off-axis image.

Figure 24.3
Transesophageal echocardiogram from the mid-esophageal level in the longitudinal plane (imaging angle 135°). The aortic valve (arrow) contains a multi-lobulated vegetation which involves all of the valve leaflets imaged in this view. In addition, there is marked thickening of the posterior aortic root which is highly suggestive of aortic root abscess. There was severe aortic regurgitation associated with this vegetation which is not shown in this image.

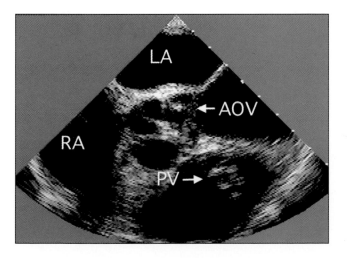

Figure 24.4
Transesophageal echocardiogram from the mid-esophageal level in the transverse plane (imaging angle 0°). The transducer has been withdrawn slightly from the modified four-chamber view. The aortic valve (AOV) is very abnormal with multiple vegetations (arrow) involving all of the leaflets. A multi-lobulated vegetation (PV) is attached to the ventricular surface of the pulmonary valve and prolapses into the right ventricular outflow tract. This mass was out of plane in Figure 24.2 and so was not imaged. This indicates the necessity for visualization of the valves in multiple planes.

Discussion

Right-sided endocarditis in patients without congenital heart disease is predominantly observed in the setting of intravenous drug use, chronic indwelling venous catheters, alcoholism, generalized sepsis, immunocompromised hosts, and dermal infections.[1-3] The pulmonary valve is much less frequently involved than the tricuspid valve. Infective endocarditis of the pulmonary valve is typically an acute process, which is reflected by the fact that *Staphylococcus aureus* is the most common offending pathogen. Multi-valvular endocarditis may occur with virulent organisms such as *Staphylococcus aureus*, which have a well-described propensity to attack normal heart valves. The patient's multi-valvular infective endocarditis developed because of colonization of the indwelling intravenous cannula by resistant bacterial strains typically found in chronic care facilities and hospitals. One such strain, methicillin-resistant *Staphylococcus aureus*, seeded his chronic indwelling catheter and the resultant high-grade bacteremia with the aggressive pathogen presumably led to involvement of his tricuspid valve with metastatic spread to his pulmonary and aortic valves. The transesophageal echocardiogram raises the concern of aortic root abscess because of the thickening of the posterior root. There was no evidence of direct spread across the intervalvular fibrosa from the pulmonary valve to the aortic valve. At surgery, the aortic root was debrided but there was no definitive abscess. The patient required replacement of his tricuspid valve which was almost completely destroyed, resulting in torrential tricuspid regurgitation which is not shown here. In addition, the aortic valve required replacement. The pulmonary valve was debrided of multiple vegetations. The patient then received 6 weeks of antibiotic therapy with vancomycin. His ventriculo-peritoneal shunt was not replaced and he has been subsequently stable off antibiotic therapy.

The finding of a mass consistent with a vegetation on an echocardiography study required careful examination of all the other valves in multiple planes. Metastatic lesions are not uncommon in endocarditis. The presence of multi-valvular infection markedly changes both the prognosis of response to medical therapy and the planned surgical approach.

References

1   Saccente M, Cobbs C. Clinical approach to infective endocarditis. Cardiol Clin 1996;14:351–62.

2. Terpenning M, Buggy B, Kauffman C. Infective endocarditis: clinical features in young and elderly patients. Am J Med 1987;83:626–34.

3. Panidis I, Kotler M, Mintz G. Right-heart endocarditis: clinical and echocardiographic features. Am Heart J 1984;107:759–64.

25

Right ventricular enlargement—normal finding

Susan E Wiegers MD

A 20-year-old student underwent a routine athletic screening physical examination. She participated in collegiate long-distance running and volleyball. She had no symptoms and no significant past medical history. A systolic murmur was heard and an echocardiogram ordered.

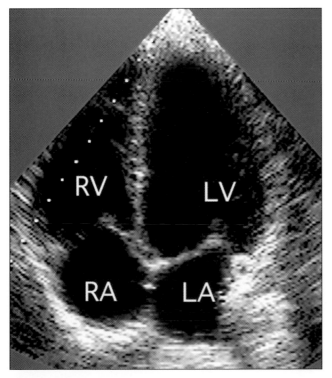

Figure 25.1
Apical four-chamber view in diastole. The left ventricle and atrium are of normal size. The right atrium and ventricle are mildly dilated. There is dropout in the interatrial septum. The pulmonary veins are not well visualized.

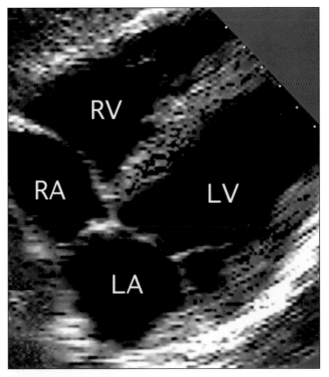

Figure 25.2
Subcostal view demonstrating mild enlargement of the right side. No tricuspid regurgitation was present. The interatrial septum is intact but the pulmonary veins could not be identified.

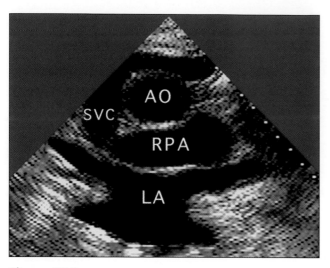

Figure 25.3

Two-dimensional image from the suprasternal notch. The transducer is rotated so that the aorta (AO) is seen in short axis. The right pulmonary artery (RPA) is seen in long axis as it passes beneath the aortic arch. The brachiocephalic vein (not labelled) at the top of the screen connects to the superior vena cava (SVC) to the right of the aorta (left of the screen). The transducer has been angulated posteriorly to image the posterior portion of the left atrium (LA) including all four pulmonary venous connections. The right superior vein is imaged on the left of the screen immediately below the SVC and the right inferior vein is seen below. The left pulmonary veins similarly enter the left atrium on the right of the screen.

Discussion

This patient had mild right-sided enlargement. A pulmonary flow murmur was present and the echocardiographer was initially concerned that a left to right shunt was present. The interatrial septum and the interventricular septum were intact. However, anomalous pulmonary venous return can be difficult to detect and will cause significant right-sided dilatation due to the shunt flow. The suprasternal notch should be a standard imaging position in every echocardiographic study. The images may be technically limited in adults, although this is a variable finding. Typically, the aorta is imaged in the long axis with the descending thoracic aorta on the right of the screen and the right pulmonary artery in the short axis. Rotation of the transducer with posterior angulation produces the 'crab view' of the left atrium, so named for the configuration of the pulmonary veins. Demonstration of the pulmonary venous connections helps exclude partial anomalous pulmonary venous return and should be attempted on every patient.

26

Severe pulmonary hypertension

Susan E Wiegers MD

A patient with a 10-year history of active sarcoidosis underwent serial echocardiograms to evaluate progressive pulmonary hypertension. The patient had initially been fairly well controlled on systemic steroids but her condition had deteriorated over the preceding year. She was now dependent on supplemental oxygen and was dyspneic on mild exertion.

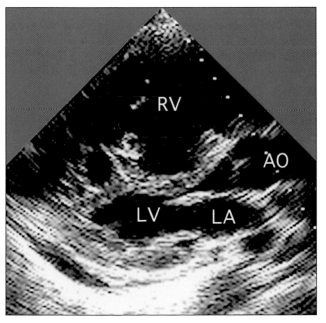

a

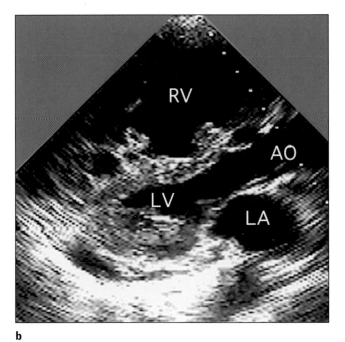

b

Figure 26.1
(a) Parasternal long-axis view in diastole. The right ventricle is massively enlarged, compressing the left ventricular cavity. The moderator band of the right ventricle is inserted into the mid-septum on the right ventricular side, but passes out of the plane of the image; its attachment to the right ventricular free wall is not seen. A small posterior pericardial effusion is present.
(b) Similar view in systole. The interventricular septum has moved anteriorly into the right ventricle. The posterior wall of the left ventricle has thickened and moved anteriorly, which accounts for most of the change in the left ventricular cavity dimension. Although the left ventricular fractional shortening is reduced by the paradoxical motion of the interventricular septum, right ventricular ejection is augmented by this motion. The interventricular septum does thicken, which distinguishes this finding from a region of dyskinesis due to infarction.

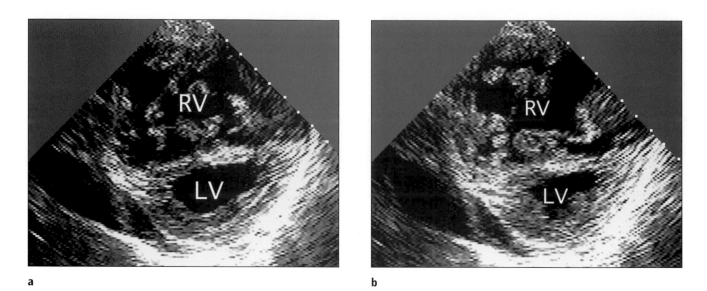

a
b

Figure 26.2
(a) Diastolic image from the parasternal short axis of the right ventricle and the left ventricle. The massive dilatation and hypertrophy of the right ventricle is noted. The left ventricular cavity is oval, rather than round, due to the interventricular septal flattening.
(b) Systolic image of the same view. The interventricular septum is flattened in systole and diastole, a pattern consistent with right ventricular volume and pressure overload.

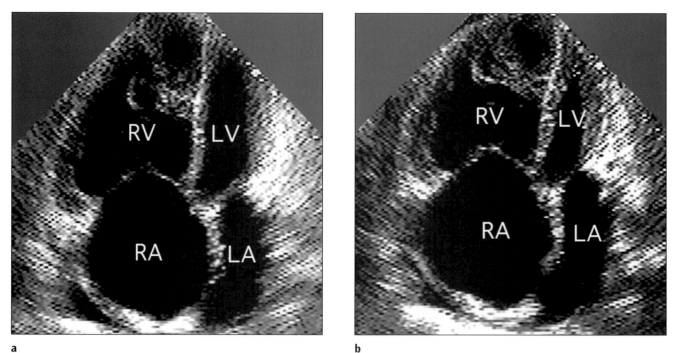

a
b

Figure 26.3
(a) Apical four-chamber view in diastole demonstrates a severely enlarged right ventricle (RV) and atrium (RA). Severe right ventricular hypertrophy is present. The moderator band in the mid-right ventricular cavity is massively hypertrophied. The echodensities at the right ventricular apex probably represent trabeculations, but apical thrombi cannot be excluded. The left ventricle (LV) and atrium (LA) are compressed by the right-sided chambers. A small pericardial effusion is observed overlying the right atrium and ventricle.
(b) Systolic frame of the same view. The area of the right ventricle has changed only slightly which is indicative of profound right ventricular dysfunction. Incomplete closure of the tricuspid valve is demonstrated with tenting of the tricuspid valve leaflets into the right ventricle. The tricuspid annulus is extremely dilated which prevents the anatomically normal leaflets from closing properly.

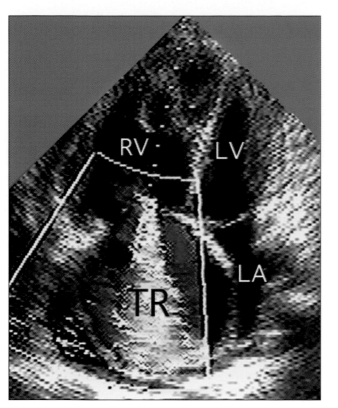

a

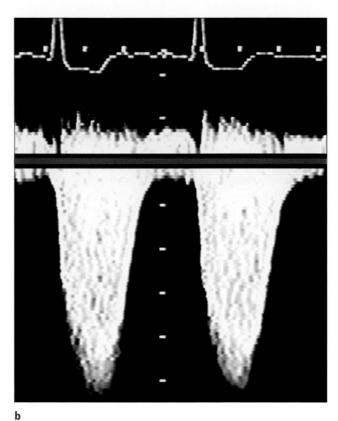

b

Figure 26.4

(a) Color Doppler flow imaging in systole from the apical four-chamber view. Severe tricuspid regurgitation (TR) is visualized in the right atrium extending to the posterior wall. The tricuspid regurgitation is due to annular dilatation and severe pulmonary hypertension.
(b) Spectral display of continuous-wave Doppler flow velocities of tricuspid regurgitation taken from the apical position. The peak velocity of the TR jet is approximately 5 m/s. Each calibration mark represents 100 cm/s or 1 m/s. The predicted peak systolic gradient is 100 mmHg. An estimated right atrial pressure of 20 mmHg is added to the systolic gradient to arrive at a peak pulmonary artery pressure of 120 mmHg, suprasystemic levels. Note the asymmetry of the TR spectral envelope with a rapid deceleration after the peak velocity is achieved, as opposed to the more rounded envelope typical of regurgitant jets. This pattern is evidence of right ventricular failure, with inability to maintain the peak pressure and a rapid fall in generated systolic pressure.

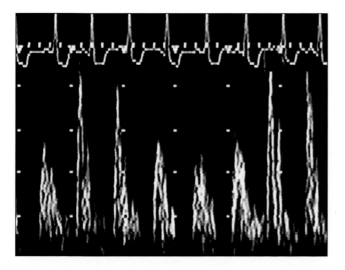

Figure 26.5

Spectral flow velocity display of pulsed-wave Doppler across the tricuspid valve. There is significant respiratory variation of the inflow velocity. Pericardial constraint due to the massive right ventricular enlargement causes the pattern which, in a different setting, would be evidence of tamponade physiology or at least of elevated intrapericardial pressure.

Discussion

The markedly elevated right-sided pressure, along with the severe right ventricular hypertrophy, speaks to the chronicity of the process. A normal right ventricle which has been operating against normal pulmonary artery pressures would not be able to mount such an elevated right ventricular pressure acutely. Sarcoidosis results in pulmonary hypertension by scarring and destruction of pulmonary parenchyma as well as direct involvement of the branch pulmonary arteries. Improvement with corticosteroid treatment has been reported.[1] Pulmonary hypertension due to veno-occlusive disease by non-caseating granulomas has also been reported.[2] Some authors have suggested that the elaboration of the pulmonary vasoconstricting eicosanoid thromboxane may contribute to pulmonary hypertension. It is, however, a rare complication of sarcoidosis, occurring in less than 4% of patients.

Calculation of the peak pulmonary artery pressure uses the modified Bernoulli equation to relate the velocity of the tricuspid regurgitation jet to the gradient between the right ventricle and atrium in systole. The relationship is given by the equation:

$$PG = 4v^2$$

where *PG* is the difference between the right ventricular and right atrial systolic pressures and *v* is the velocity of the tricuspid regurgitation jet measured by continuous-wave Doppler. An estimated right atrial pressure is then added to the gradient to obtain the pulmonary artery pressure.[3] A common convention is to add 10 mmHg if the right atrium is normal in size, 15 mmHg if the right atrium is dilated, and 20 mmHg if the inferior vena cava is dilated and does not demonstrate a 50% decrease in diameter with inspiration. This method assumes that the right ventricular peak pressure is equal to the peak pulmonary artery pressure. This will obviously not be the case in the presence of pulmonary stenosis whether valvular, infundibular or supravalvular. In these cases, the tricuspid jet velocity can be used to calculate only the peak right ventricular systolic pressure. Most ultrasound systems allow measurement of the tricuspid valve regurgitant jet velocity on-line. However, a casual measurement may result in a large propagated error since the value is squared to obtain the pressure gradient. Care should be taken to measure the jet velocity at the peak of the clearly defined spectral envelope and not at an extrapolated peak. If the spectral envelope is technically limited, the minimum estimated pulmonary artery systolic pressure may be reported with the note that the true value may be

significantly higher. In the setting of torrential tricuspid regurgitation, such as is seen with a flail leaflet, the right ventricle and atrium become essentially a single chamber in systole. The pressure gradient between the two chambers is necessarily reduced without any change in the peak right ventricular systolic pressure. In this case again, the minimum pulmonary artery pressure is reported with the note that it may be a significant underestimate of the true systolic pressure.

In this patient, the pattern of interventricular septal motion is highly suggestive of severe pulmonary hypertension. Diastolic flattening, as best seen from the parasternal short axis, is most consistent with right ventricular volume overload, usually due to severe tricuspid regurgitation. The degree of systolic flattening has been shown to correlate with the level of right ventricular pressure overload, usually due to pulmonary hypertension. Severe tricuspid regurgitation will result from tricuspid annular dilatation. A tricuspid annular dimension greater than 3.4 cm in diastole correlates with the presence of severe tricuspid regurgitation.[4]

The respiratory variation in Doppler inflow velocities in this case is evidence of ventricular interdependence. The extreme right ventricular dilatation results in compromise of left ventricular filling which is exaggerated during the normal increase in right-sided volume with inspiration.

This patient continues to be managed with corticosteroids, but is doing poorly. Sarcoidosis, like other systemic diseases, has been reported to recur in lung transplants. This option is under consideration in this patient, given her serious clinical situation.

References

1. Rodman D, Lindenfeld J. Successful treatment of sarcoidosis-associated pulmonary hypertension with corticosteroids. Chest 1990;97:500–2.

2. Hoffstein V, Ranganathan N, Mullen J. Sarcoidosis simulating pulmonary veno-occlusive disease. Am Rev Respir Dis 1986;134:809–11.

3. Yock PG, Popp RL. Noninvasive estimation of right ventricular systolic pressure by Doppler ultrasound in patients with tricuspid regurgitation. Circulation 1984;70:657–62.

4. Fisher EA, Goldman ME. Simple, rapid method for quantification of tricuspid regurgitation by two-dimensional echocardiography. Am J Cardiol 1989;63:1375–8.

27

Right ventricular mass

John Augoustides MD
Susan E Wiegers MD

A 45-year-old man with a 6-month history of treatment for a high-grade abdominal wall sarcoma developed presyncope and severe exercise intolerance. The clinical examination was remarkable for peripheral edema and high jugular venous pressure. Metastatic nodules were evident on the chest wall. Echocardiography at another institution was interpreted as demonstrating severe pulmonary hypertension. He was referred to the pulmonary service for evaluation of pulmonary emboli.

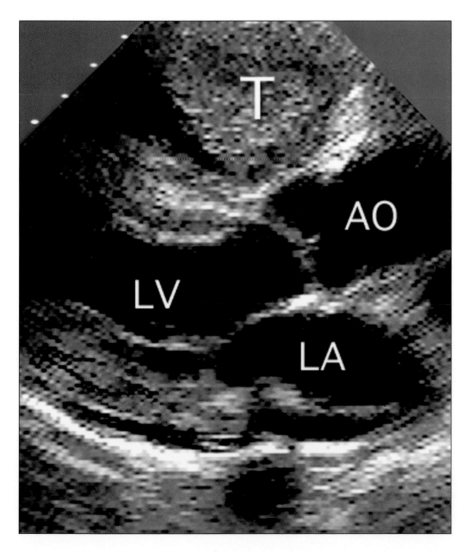

Figure 27.1
The normal anatomy of the parasternal long-axis view is distorted by the large mass occupying most of the right ventricular cavity. The tumor (T) completely fills the high right ventricular outflow tract. There is a small pericardial effusion posterior to the left ventricle (LV) and left atrium (LA). AO, aorta.

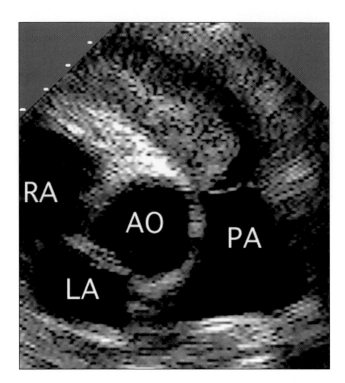

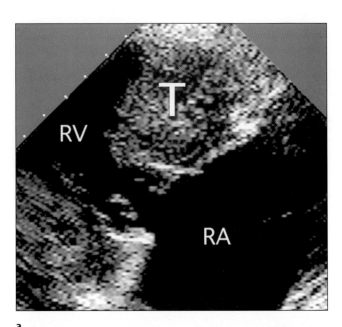

a

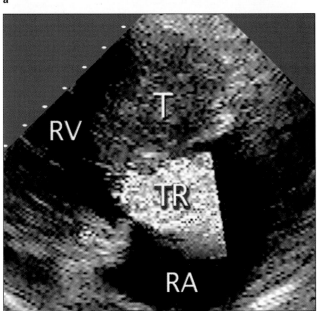

b

Figure 27.2

In the parasternal short-axis view, the tumor mass again is seen to fill the high right ventricular outflow tract to the level of the pulmonary valve, which is visualized in diastole at the distal extent of the mass. The mass is causing severe outflow obstruction. The pulmonary artery (PA) appears to be clear of tumor but is severely dilated. This raises the concern of previous pulmonary embolization and elevated pulmonary artery pressures.

Figure 27.3

(a) The tumor mass restricts the opening of the anterior leaflet of the tricuspid valve in diastole. The posterior leaflet is seen to open normally. The right atrium (RA) is dilated.
(b) Disruption of the architecture of the tricuspid valve results in severe tricuspid regurgitation which is here visualized as a turbulent systolic jet in the right atrium.
(c) Spectral display of continuous-wave Doppler across the tricuspid valve from the apical position. The high tricuspid regurgitation velocity (approximately 4.7 m/s) predicts a peak right ventricular systolic pressure of 88 mmHg greater than the right atrial pressure. This elevated pressure is due to the right ventricular outflow tract obstruction (subvalvular stenosis caused by the tumor) and not to pulmonary hypertension.

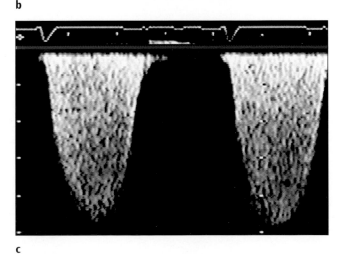

c

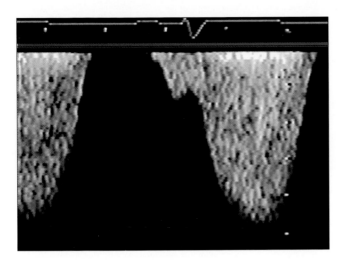

Figure 27.4
Spectral display of continuous-wave Doppler across the right ventricular outflow tract from the parasternal position. Note the difference in contour of the velocity flow envelope compared to that of the tricuspid regurgitation. The peak velocity is similar, with a peak gradient between the right ventricle and pulmonary artery of 88 mmHg. Note that forward flow in the right ventricular outflow tract begins with atrial systole. This indicates that the very high right ventricular diastolic pressures open the pulmonary valve prior to ventricular contraction.

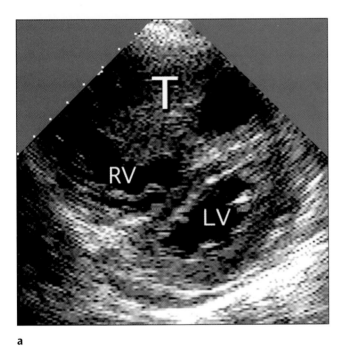

a

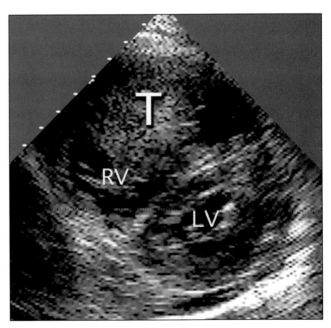

b

Figure 27.5
(a) Short-axis parasternal view in diastole. The right ventricular pressure is higher than the left ventricular pressure in both systole and diastole. In this diastolic view the flattening of the interventricular septum is evident. The tumor mass fills much of the right ventricular cavity, which is dilated.
(b) In systole, the left ventricular cavity is smaller but the interventricular septum remains flattened. The small pericardial effusion is again seen posterior to the left ventricle.

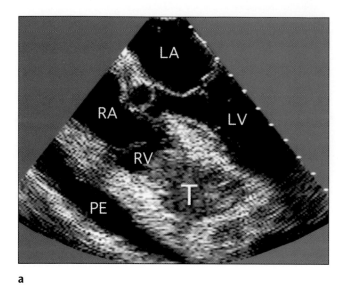

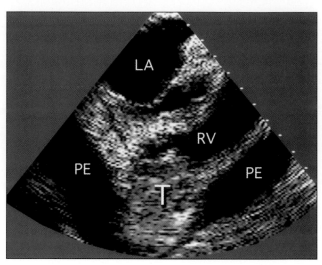

a   b

Figure 27.6

(a) Transesophageal four-chamber view from the transverse plane (imaging angle 0°). The transducer has been rotated towards the right of the patient to obtain this image. The tumor mass (T) fills the right ventricular cavity from the apex to near the level of the tricuspid valve. Careful examination of the image demonstrates that the main portion of the mass has an echocardiographic appearance which is different from that of the uninvolved myocardium.

(b) Transesophageal image from the longitudinal plane (imaging angle 135°) with the transducer rotated to the right. The tumor mass (T) fills the right ventricular cavity and is encroaching on the right ventricular outflow, tract which is seen on the right of the screen (RV). At the right ventricular apex, the tumor mass has infiltrated the myocardial wall and appears to have completely penetrated the myocardium to reach the epicardium. There is a large circumferential pericardial effusion. It should be noted that this study was performed several weeks later in the patient's course when a pericardial effusion had appeared. The anterior mitral valve leaflet (AMVL) is visible between the left atrium (LA) and a small portion of the left ventricular outflow tract which is visualized in this image.

Discussion

The initial echocardiographic approach to a cardiac mass is to analyze its morphology, position and hemodynamic effects. A large ventricular mass is either a thrombus or a tumor. A right ventricular thrombus, usually apical in location, is associated with significant right ventricular failure from infarction, contusion, cardiomyopathy, or cor pulmonale. This mass extends well beyond the apex and the clinical history and echocardiographic assessment are negative for the aforementioned causes of right ventricular failure.

A right ventricular tumor is either primary or secondary. Primary tumors are either benign or malignant. The differential diagnosis of this right ventricular mass is focused by the clinical history of high-grade abdominal wall sarcoma and metastatic chest wall nodules. Malignant involvement of the heart is most commonly from metastatic spread.[1] This secondary involvement may be by direct extension (e.g. esophageal carcinoma), lymphatic spread (e.g. bronchogenic carcinoma), venous extension (e.g. renal cell carcinoma), or hematogenous dissemination (e.g. melanoma, sarcoma, and leukemia).[2]

Malignant tumors may metastasize to involve the pericardium, myocardium, and/or endocardium. The echocardiographic examination in this case does not determine whether the origin of the mass is myocardial or pericardial with extension into the ventricle. Either scenario may be accompanied by a pericardial effusion. A malignant effusion may accumulate rapidly to cause cardiac tamponade; percutaneous drainage offers symptomatic relief. In this case, the hemodynamic compromise was due to severe right ventricular outflow obstruction by the metastatic sarcoma and resultant symptoms of low cardiac output and right heart failure. The effusion may also have contributed to decreased filling of the ventricles. The prognosis in such a case is extremely poor, given the high-grade tumor and the severe degree of myocardial compromise already present. Surgical resection is contraindicated since the sarcoma has metastasized systemically. The possible therapeutic options would include appropriate chemotherapy and/or radiation therapy. Unfortunately, cardiac transplantation, an option for primary cardiac tumors, is not possible in uncontrolled metastatic disease.

Transthoracic echocardiography sufficiently characterizes this massive right ventricular involvement. Transesophageal echocardiography may offer better delineation of location and extent of metastatic extension in less severe cases. Transesophageal echocardiography is clearly contraindicated in the presence of malignant involvement of the esophagus.

References

1. Salcedo EE, White RD, Cohen GI, Davison, MB. Cardiac tumours: diagnosis and management. Curr Probl Cardiol 1992;17:75–137.

2. Kutalek SP, Panidis IP, Kotler MN, *et al.* Metastatic tumors of the heart detected by two-dimensional echocardiography. Am Heart J 1985;109:343–9.

28

Right ventricular dysplasia

Martin St John Sutton MBBS
Vikas V Patel MD

A 24-year-old male was referred for assessment of cardiomegaly detected on chest X-ray obtained as part of a routine physical investigation. At the time of presentation he had experienced no symptoms of chest pain, dyspnea, palpitations, or syncope. He had no family history of congenital heart disease. Six months later he was admitted to hospital complaining of fatigue, effort intolerance, and bilateral lower extremity edema.

Physical examination revealed sinus tachycardia, a systolic blood pressure of 100 mmHg, edema of both legs to mid-calf and marked elevation of the jugular venous pressure. The apical impulse was diffuse and laterally displaced. Right- and left-sided third heart sounds and bilateral lower zone crackles suggested biventricular failure. An ECG showed sinus rhythm, low voltage and right atrial enlargement.

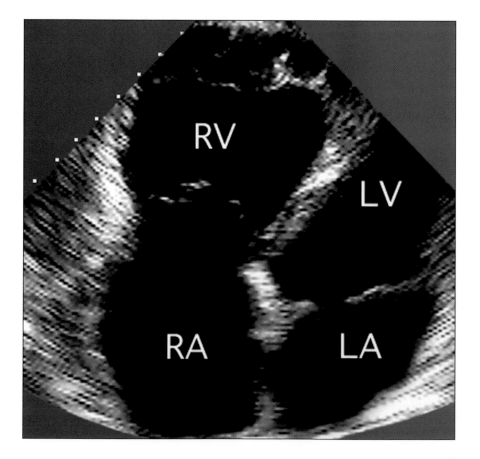

Figure 28.1
Apical four-chamber view demonstrating massive enlargement of the right atrium and right ventricle. The left ventricle was of normal to small size and posteriorly located, with moderately impaired contractile function. The relationship of the tricuspid valve annulus to the mitral annulus is normal, which excludes Ebstein's anomaly.

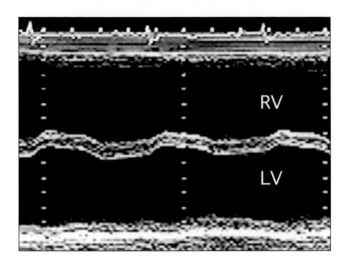

Figure 28.2
M-mode echocardiogram from the parasternal position. The right ventricle is severely enlarged but biventricular systolic dysfunction is present. Paradoxical systolic motion of the interventricular septum due to right ventricular volume overload is also well demonstrated.

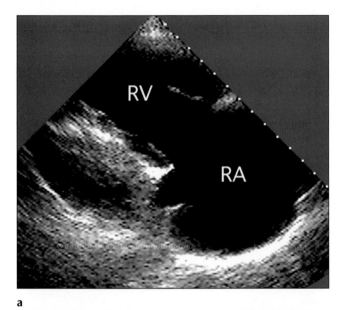

a

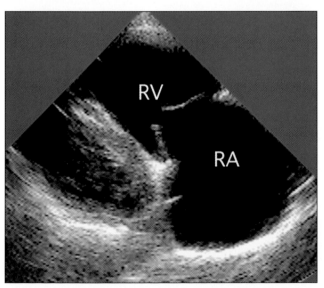

b

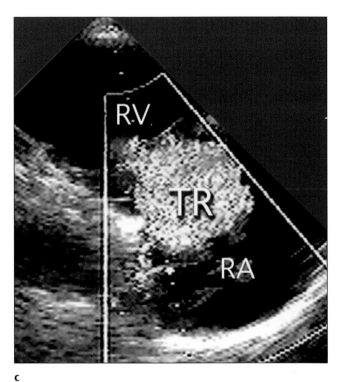

c

Figure 28.3
(a) Parasternal right ventricular inflow view in diastole. Both the right ventricle and the right atrium are severely enlarged. The tricuspid valve leaflets are normal.
(b) Similar view in systole. The annular dilatation results in incomplete closure of the tricuspid valve. The leaflets are unable to coapt. It is clear that the tricuspid valve takes its origin from the annulus and has unrestricted motion which again excludes Ebstein's anomaly from the echocardiographic differential diagnosis.
(c) Free tricuspid valve regurgitation is present through the partially open tricuspid valve leaflets in systole.

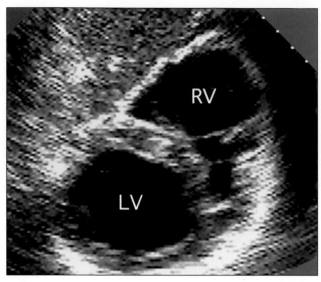
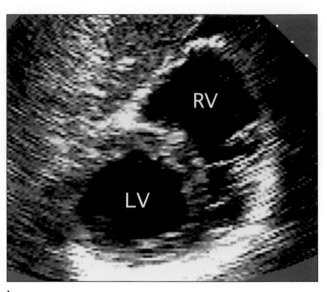

a   b

Figure 28.4
(a) Subcostal short-axis view of the ventricles in diastole. The right ventricular wall thickness especially of the free wall towards the apex appears unusually thin and scarred, with no systolic thickening.
(b) Similar view in systole. There is decreased left ventricular function but the walls all thicken and the cavity area is decreased. The right ventricular wall fails to demonstrate any motion and the right ventricular area remains unchanged in this view.

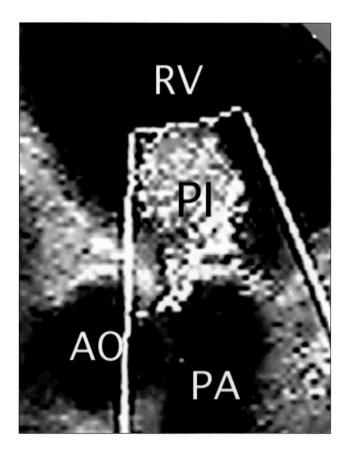

Figure 28.5
Parasternal view of the pulmonary valve and pulmonary artery with color flow Doppler imaging. Severe pulmonary insufficiency (PI) arises from the level of the pulmonary valve and extends into the severely enlarged right ventricular cavity. The pulmonary artery is of normal size.

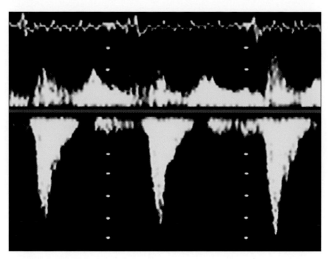

a

Figure 28.6

(a) Spectral display of continuous-wave Doppler flow velocities of the tricuspid regurgitation, taken from the apical position. (Each calibration mark represents 20 cm/s.) The velocity of the tricuspid regurgitation is exceptionally low. This, along with the normal pulmonary trunk, excludes pulmonary hypertension as a cause of the patient's condition.

(b) Spectral display of pulsed wave Doppler in the pulmonary artery. Right atrial contraction opens the pulmonary valve prematurely. The flow velocity is greater during atrial systole than during ventricular systole, which follows (arrow). Right atrial pressure exceeds pulmonary diastolic pressure, causing the late diastolic flow in the pulmonary artery. Right ventricular power failure is indicated by the comparison between the ability of the right atrium and that of the right ventricle to generate pressure.

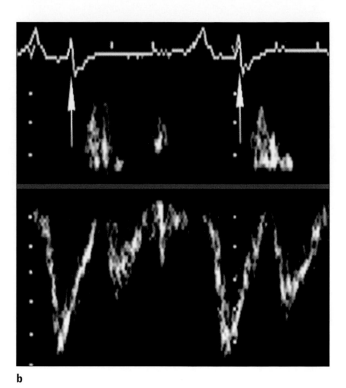

b

Discussion

The diagnosis in this patient was right ventricular dysplasia. Histopathological confirmation was obtained when the patient underwent orthotopic heart transplantation one year later for rapidly progressive symptomatic biventricular heart failure, which was minimally responsive to angiotensin converting enzyme (ACE) inhibitor therapy, diuretics, and digitalis. The right ventricular walls were so thin that they were transparent and transilluminated. The unusual features in this case included no family history (right ventricular dysplasia has a strong familial prevalence), no palpitations, syncope, or documented arrhythmia. Left ventricular involvement is also rare.[1]

The key echocardiographic features are recognition of the 'relative absence of right ventricular free wall muscle' and the fine fibrous echo-bright trabeculations taking origin from the moderator band and free wall at the right ventricular apex.[2] Other causes of right ventricular enlargement and severe right ventricular contractile dysfunction must be excluded. This was done by documenting low right ventricular systolic pressure, normal tricuspid valve origin, unrestricted leaflet mobility, and near normal left ventricular size. Importantly, there is a wide spectrum of abnormalities that, when severe, are as described above, but may be subtle and consist of regional right ventricular thinning and dysfunction that is easily overlooked.

References

1. Nava A, Thiene G, Canciani B, *et al.* Familial occurrence of right ventricular dysplasia; study of nine families. J Am Coll Cardiol 1988;12:1222–8.

2. Kullo IJ, Edwards WD, Seward JB. Right ventricular dysplasia: the Mayo Clinic experience. Mayo Clin Proc 1995;70:541–8.

29

Pectus excavatum

Martin St John Sutton MBBS
Susan E Wiegers MD

A 38-year-old man with systemic sclerosis complained of shortness of breath on mild to moderate exertion of 3 months' duration with an exercise capacity of eight blocks on the flat. He denied chest pain, palpitations, or syncope. His systemic sclerosis had been in remission since beginning treatment with corticosteroids. He had no risk factors for coronary heart disease.

On examination he was not dyspneic at rest, he was thin and tall with a marked pectus excavatum but he had no other stigmata of Marfan's syndrome. His blood pressure, heart rate, jugular venous pressure, and peripheral pulses were all normal. The apical impulse was unremarkable but on auscultation there was an ejection systolic murmur at the upper left sternal border which varied in intensity with respiration, a normally splitting second heart sound and no ejection click, suggesting right ventricular outflow tract obstruction either at subvalvular or supravalvular level. The ECG showed sinus rhythm and normal intervals and morphology. The chest X-ray showed a pectus, normal heart size and configuration, and normal lung parenchyma.

Owing to the patient's pectus excavatum the standard parasternal long-axis views and apical views were technically limited.

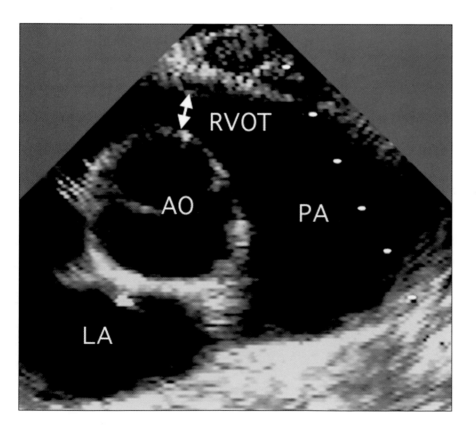

Figure 29.1
Parasternal short-axis view of the aorta demonstrated normal aortic and pulmonary valves but narrowing of the right ventricular outflow tract (RVOT; double-headed arrow) by the depressed sternum due to the pectus. The impact of compression and narrowing of the right ventricular outflow tract was reflected in the increased velocity of blood flow proximal to the pulmonary valve (not shown). The pulmonary artery is imaged off axis but is enlarged.

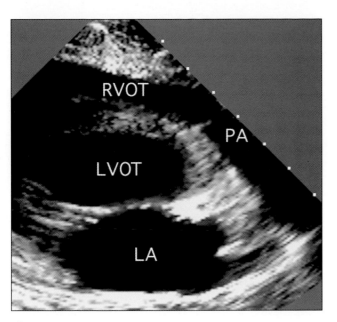

Figure 29.2
Parasternal short-axis view at the level of the left ventricular outflow tract (LVOT). The mild narrowing of the right ventricular outflow tract (RVOT) is again apparent.

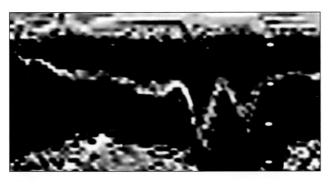

Figure 29.3
M-mode echocardiogram of the pulmonary valve from the parasternal position in systole. Early closure of the valve is demonstrated; this is suggestive of pulmonary hypertension. However, a similar M-mode finding may be seen in idiopathic dilatation of the pulmonary artery.

Discussion

The etiology of the cardiac murmur was the partial compression of the right ventricular outflow tract by the depressed sternum (pectus). Left and right ventricular size and function were normal. The outflow tract compression was mild and did not contribute to the patient's dyspnea or recent decrease in exercise capacity. Posterior displacement of the right ventricular outflow tract by the sternum is optimally seen in the left parasternal long-axis view of the left ventricle. In the apical four-chamber view, the body of the right ventricle has an hourglass deformity. Anteroposterior compression of the right ventricle causes apparent dilatation at the apex and the base of the ventricle. Pectus excavatum is a skeletal abnormality associated with Marfan's syndrome and, when present, should initiate echocardiographic examination of the aorta to exclude dilatation of the ascending aorta and of the mitral valve, to exclude systolic prolapse. These constitute the cardiovascular stigmata of Marfan's syndrome.[1]

This patient's dyspnea was related to pulmonary fibrosis from systemic sclerosis. The pulmonary process had resulted in mild pulmonary hypertension. This was not the result of the thoracic deformity in this case. Although surgical repair of thoracic abnormalities can be accomplished, the surgery is generally not indicated for mild pectus excavatum.[2] Cardiac compression by the deformed thoracic cage does not alter hemodynamics, although pulmonary compression can in some cases produce symptoms.

References

1. Seliem M, Duffy C, Gidding S, *et al.* Echocardiographic evaluation of the aortic root and mitral valve in children and adolescents with isolated pectus excavatum: comparison with Marfan's patients. Pediatr Cardiol 1992;13:20–3.

2. Garcia V, Seyfer A, Graeber G. Reconstruction of congenital chest-wall deformities. Surg Clin North Am 1989;69:1103–18.

30

Persistent pulmonary hypertension after thromboendartectomy

Victor A Ferrari MD

A 49-year-old woman had a history of systemic hypertension and antiphospholipid antibody syndrome. She had a 7-year history of severe pulmonary hypertension due to chronic unresolved pulmonary emboli. Right heart catheterization had revealed pulmonary artery systolic pressures of 80–90 mmHg. She had undergone pulmonary thromboendarterectomy with successful evacuation of a moderate amount of bilateral thrombus and chronic organized fibrinous material. Her pulmonary artery pressures were effectively unchanged after surgery. Signs and symptoms of right ventricular failure occurred within 1 month of surgery and required the institution of continuous intravenous prostacyclin therapy, with only modest improvement in symptoms. Recently, she developed worsening of her chronic dyspnea and, despite supplemental oxygen therapy, was unable to walk more than 10 feet without severe breathlessness. A transthoracic echocardiogram was ordered to evaluate her ventricular function.

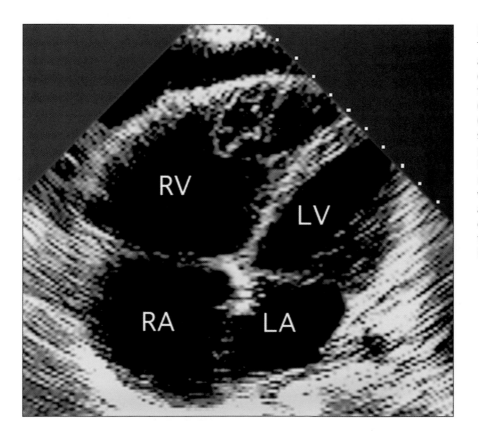

Figure 30.1
Transthoracic echocardiogram from the apical four-chamber view at end diastole. There is severe dilatation of the right atrium (RA) and right ventricle (RV) which compresses the left ventricle (LV). The tricuspid valve annulus is severely dilated which results in loss of proper coaptation of the tricuspid valve leaflets and severe tricuspid regurgitation (see below). The right ventricle is moderately hypertrophied and a moderate-sized pericardial effusion (PE) is present. There were no two-dimensional or Doppler signs of increased intrapericardial pressure.

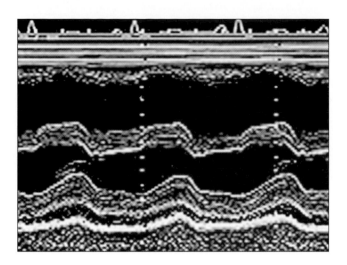

Figure 30.2
M-mode echocardiogram from the parasternal position at the mid-ventricular level. The right ventricular cavity is dilated and the free wall is thickened. There is marked paradoxical motion of the interventricular septum with the septum moving anteriorly in systole. This pattern is due to elevated right ventricular pressures and can be differentiated from dyskinesis due to infarction of the septum by the normal dimension and the preserved systolic thickening.

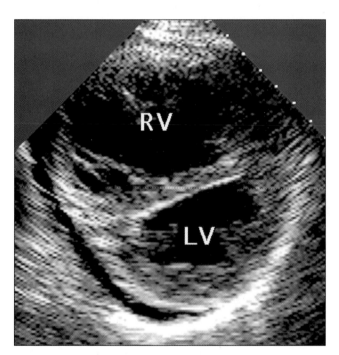

a

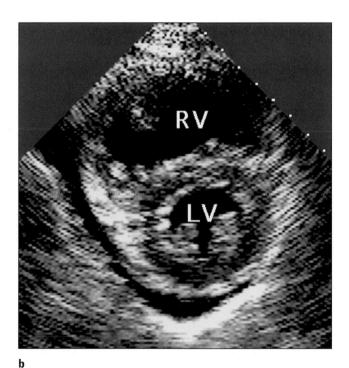

b

Figure 30.3
(a) Parasternal short axis view at the mid-ventricle showing the relationship of the right ventricle and left ventricle in diastole. There is severe dilatation and moderate hypertrophy of the right ventricle with a pronounced shift or flattening of the interventricular septum toward the left ventricle, indicating that right ventricle end-diastolic pressure significantly exceeds left ventricle end-diastolic pressure. This finding can be seen in either right ventricle volume or right ventricle pressure overload states. It is usually present when right ventricle pressure overload is accompanied by significant tricuspid regurgitation (TR). Again, note the presence of the small to moderate pericardial effusion.
(b) At end systole in the same view, the right ventricular cavity area has decreased, but not nearly to normal size, indicating a moderate degree of right ventricular dysfunction. Note that the septum has lost its flattened appearance and has become more rounded. Owing to the patient's systolic hypertension, the difference between the left and right ventricular systolic pressures is not as great as the difference between the diastolic pressures. In many patients with severe pulmonary hypertension but without systemic hypertension, the septum will retain its flattened (or 'D-shaped') appearance during systole.

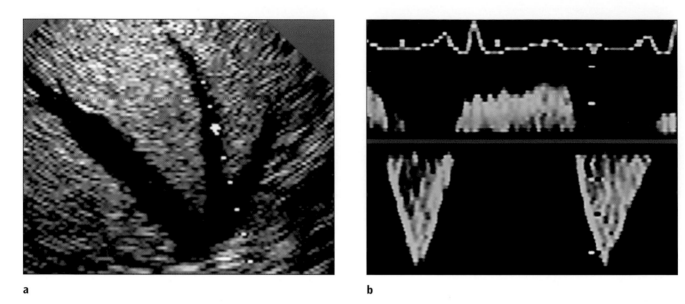

a   b

Figure 30.4

(a) This is a subcostal view of the liver with numerous severely dilated hepatic veins due to the severely elevated right atrial pressure and reflux of blood into the inferior vena cava and the hepatic veins secondary to severe TR. The cursor indicates the sampling site for Doppler interrogation in the next figure.

(b) Pulsed-wave Doppler examination of the hepatic veins indicates systolic reversal of flow due to the severe TR. The systolic signal is towards the transducer, indicating flow away from the right atrium. Normally, biphasic flow towards the heart is present in the hepatic veins.

Discussion

Pulmonary hypertension may develop as a result of both acute and chronic unresolved pulmonary embolism. The hemodynamic effects of pulmonary emboli depend on the degree of embolic pulmonary vascular obstruction, the patient's history of cardiopulmonary disease, and the chronicity of the embolic disease.[1] Acute pulmonary embolism can cause acute pulmonary hypertension through a combination of pulmonary vascular obstruction, alveolar hypoxia due to splinting from pleuritic chest pain, or direct vasoconstriction from vasoactive substances.[2] Even massive embolism cannot acutely raise the peak pulmonary artery systolic pressure to more than 50–60 mmHg in a normal right ventricle that has not gradually adapted to the increased load.[3]

Chronic pulmonary embolism may occur in two forms—in situ thrombosis and chronic unresolved thromboembolic occlusion of the proximal pulmonary arteries. In situ thrombosis develops from local endothelial dysfunction of the pulmonary microvasculature due to high pulmonary artery pressures and flows, which result in a local hypercoagulable state. These microthrombi are not detectable on pulmonary angiography. On echocardiography, only the results of the chronic pulmonary hypertension are evident. The pulmonary arteries may be

dilated but laminated thrombus or other filling defects are not seen. The syndrome of chronic unresolved pulmonary embolism occurs because of partial obstruction of the proximal pulmonary vessels by organized, but incompletely lysed, thromboemboli. Vascular obstruction can be due to luminal blockage by a large fibrinous mass, or to fibrous webs or rings that partially occlude the vessels. These obstructions are visible using both invasive and non-invasive testing methods, and remain present even after prolonged anticoagulation therapy. It is important to diagnose this disorder, as it is surgically remediable, frequently with marked reductions in pulmonary artery pressures and significant improvement in clinical status.[4,5] This patient was diagnosed late in the course of her disease, and by the time of her surgery had developed a fixed and irreversibly elevated pulmonary vascular resistance.

Transthoracic echocardiography with pulsed-wave, continuous-wave, and color Doppler imaging is the best initial study for the evaluation of patients with pulmonary hypertension. Patients with right ventricular hypertrophy have evidence of a chronic process that has developed over months to years, depending on the degree of hypertrophy. Regional wall motion abnormalities or wall thinning suggestive of ischemic heart disease can also be detected. Doppler imaging can provide accurate estimates of the pulmonary artery systolic pressures (provided tricuspid regurgitation is present) and rule out the presence of pulmonary stenosis, which can be erroneously diagnosed as pulmonary hypertension by the unwary. Echocardiography can also guide further testing to distinguish those with chronic pulmonary emboli from those with primary pulmonary hypertension. Right ventricular pulse pressure can be estimated from the TR and pulmonic regurgitation (PR) jet velocities. Patients with chronic thromboembolic disease appear to have wider pulse pressures than patients with primary pulmonary hypertension.[6] Transesophageal echocardiography may provide better assessment of the intracardiac structures and rule out intracardiac shunts or significant mitral valve disease that may cause secondary pulmonary hypertension. Echocardiography can also provide important prognostic information. For example, the presence of a pericardial effusion associated with severe pulmonary hypertension, as in this patient, is a prognostic indicator of a poor outcome.[7]

Treatment options are limited in patients with this type of advanced lung disease. Patients with severe fixed pulmonary hypertension are frequently placed on systemic anticoagulation and oxygen. Most patients are followed with clinical examinations and echocardiography to assess their pulmonary artery pressure and right ventricular function over time. Some patients may be candidates for continuous prostacyclin therapy, but the response to treatment is variable, and the associated costs are high. While lung transplantation is an option in some patients, it is not uncommon for programs to have waiting periods of 2 years or more. This patient's condition continued to deteriorate clinically despite prostacyclin therapy. She was listed for lung transplantation, but died suddenly during the waiting period.

References

1. Elliott C. Pulmonary physiology during pulmonary embolism. Chest 1992;101(Suppl 4):163–71S.

2. Malik AB, Johnson A. Role of humoral mediators in the pulmonary vascular response to pulmonary embolism. In: Weir EK, Reeves JT, eds. Pulmonary Vascular Physiology and Pathophysiology. Marcel Dekker: New York, 1989:445–68.

3. Sutton G, Hall R, Kerr I. Clinical course and late prognosis of treated subacute massive, acute minor, and chronic pulmonary thromboembolism. Br Heart J 1977;39:1135.

4. Rich S, Levitsky S, Brundage BH. Pulmonary hypertension from chronic pulmonary thromboembolism. Ann Intern Med 1988;108:425.

5. Moser KM, Daily PO, Peterson K, et al. Thromboendarterectomy for chronic, major vessel thromboembolic pulmonary hypertension: immediate and long-term results in 42 patients. Ann Intern Med 1987;107:560–5.

6. Nakayama Y, Sugimachi M, Nakanishi N, et al. Noninvasive differential diagnosis between chronic pulmonary thromboembolism and primary pulmonary hypertension by means of Doppler ultrasound measurement. J Am Coll Cardiol 1998;31:1367–71.

7. Eysmann SB, Palevsky HI, Reichek N, et al. Two-dimensional and Doppler echocardiographic and cardiac catheterization correlates of survival in primary pulmonary hypertension. Circulation 1989;80:353–60.

SECTION III

The Pulmonary Artery

31

Pulmonary stenosis

Martin St John Sutton MBBS

A 30-year-old man was noted to have a heart murmur after presenting to his family doctor complaining of fatigue. He had mild symptoms of dyspnea and palpitations but no syncope or chest pain. He had given up weight training at a gymnasium 5 days each week approximately one year earlier for unknown reasons.

On examination there was a prominent 'a' wave in the jugular venous pulse, normal heart rate, blood pressure and peripheral arterial pulse volume and contour. On auscultation he had a harsh ejection systolic murmur over the left upper chest and a single second heart sound consistent with pulmonary stenosis. Chest X-ray demonstrated a dilated main and branch pulmonary arteries. The ECG showed sinus rhythm, right axis deviation and mild right ventricular hypertrophy.

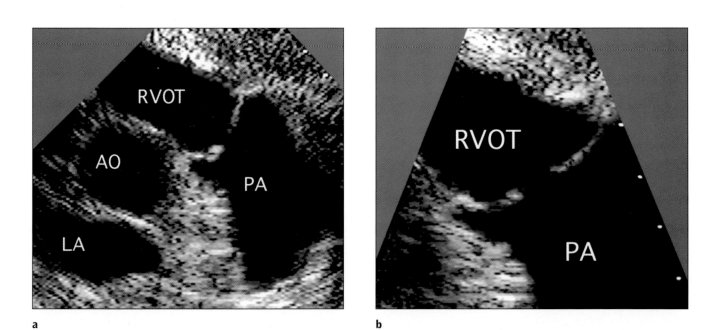

a
b

Figure 31.1
(a) The parasternal short axis at aortic valve level shows a mildly thickened pulmonary valve which domes in systole. The proximal pulmonary artery (PA) was enlarged owing to post-stenotic dilatation. The right ventricular outflow tract (RVOT) is mildly enlarged and the wall is mildly hypertrophied.
(b) Close-up view of the pulmonary valve from the parasternal position. The valve is thickened and domes in systole.

109

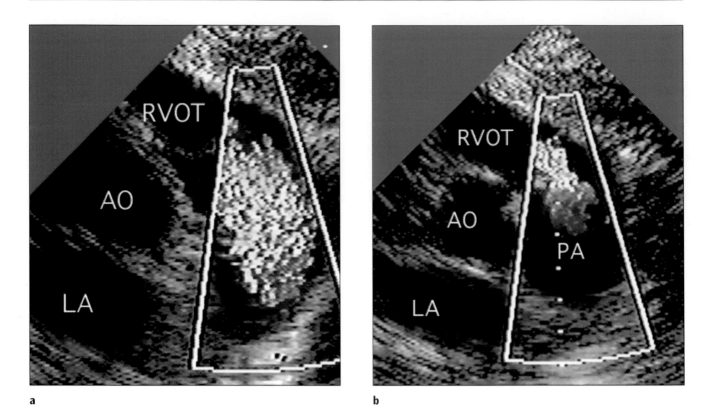

a   b

Figure 31.2

(a) Similar view to that in Figure 31.1 in systole. There is turbulent flow in the pulmonary artery which arises from the valve level. The jet has high velocity which is consistent with significant valvular stenosis.

(b) Similar view in diastole. A jet of pulmonary insufficiency arises at the level of the valve and extends a short way into the right ventricular outflow tract (RVOT). There is proximal flow convergence in the pulmonary artery (PA).

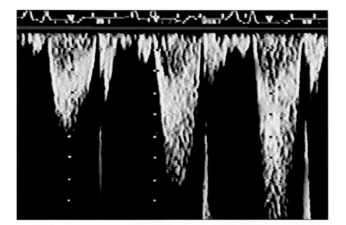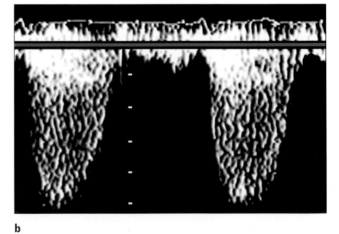

a   b

Figure 31.3

(a) Spectral display of pulsed-wave Doppler in the right ventricular outflow tract. During this tracing, the sample volume was advanced towards the pulmonary valve from the right ventricular outflow tract. The velocity increases as the sample volume is moved into the vena contracta, in which the blood flow accelerates through the valvular obstruction.

(b) Spectral display of continuous-wave Doppler across the pulmonary valve. The velocity profile peaks in mid-systole with a maximum velocity of 5.1 m/s indicating a peak gradient across the valve of 104 mmHg which is consistent with severe pulmonary stenosis. A double envelope is evident within the spectral envelope. The peak velocity in the right ventricular outflow tract is greater than 1 m/s.

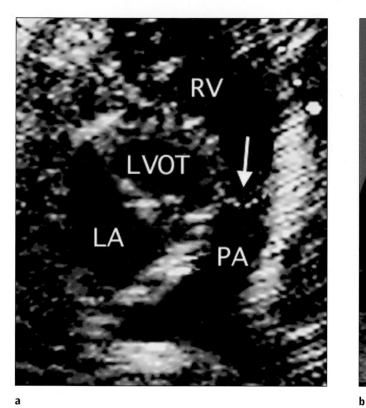
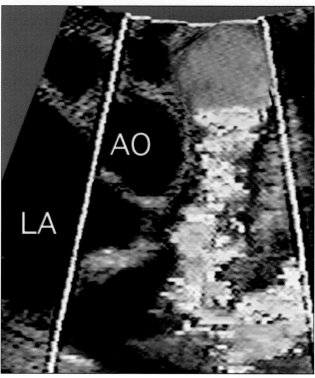

a   b

Figure 31.4
(a) Subcostal view of the pulmonary artery (PA) in long axis. The pulmonary valve (arrow) domes in diastole. The pulmonary artery and its branches are only mildly dilated in this view.
(b) The color flow Doppler signal indicates low velocity and laminar flow until the level of the pulmonary valve at which point the signal aliases. This indicates that the level of obstruction is the valve and helps to distinguish this entity from supra- or sub-valvar stenosis.

Discussion

The harsh ejection systolic murmur audible over the left upper chest and the single second heart sound together with the predominant 'a' wave in the jugular venous pulse all suggest pulmonary stenosis at valve level. The 'a' wave is the reflection of altered compliance of the hypertrophied right ventricle. The classic systolic doming of the thickened pulmonary valve and the post-stenotic dilatation of the pulmonary trunk are the two-dimensional echocardiographic stigmata of pulmonary valve stenosis. Doppler interrogation of the valve from the upper left parasternal region or in the subcostal view of the long axis of the pulmonary arterial trunk provides accurate quantitation of the severity of stenosis. Serial echocardiography is essential for evaluation of the stenosis, which may progress over years.[1]

Pulmonary stenosis with an intact ventricular septum is common in its mild form, but pulmonary stenosis is often associated with a ventricular septal defect, which should be definitively excluded. This patient was stable but had severe pulmonary stenosis. He underwent successful pulmonary valve replacement with a tissue valve, with resolution of his symptoms.

Reference

1. Rowland DG, Hammill WW, Allen HD, *et al*. Natural course of isolated pulmonary valve stenosis in infants and children utilizing Doppler echocardiography. Am J Cardiol 1997;79:344–9.

32

Massive pulmonary embolism

John Augoustides MD

A 45-year-old woman presented with recurrent shortness of breath and chest pain over 6 months. She had recently had blood-tinged sputum. She was known to suffer from chronic bronchitis on the basis of a 50-pack-year smoking history. She had no symptoms or signs of deep venous thrombosis. Her cardiovascular examination was significant for a precordial right ventricular heave and a loud P2 on auscultation, despite her hyperinflated lungs. Her EKG showed sinus rhythm with a dominant R-wave in lead V1 and her chest X-ray showed hyperinflation and a flattened diaphragm. An echocardiogram was ordered to evaluate her ventricular function and to grade her pulmonary hypertension.

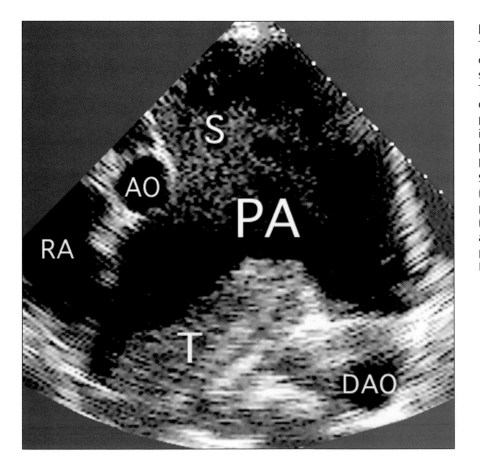

Figure 32.1
Transthoracic two-dimensional echocardiogram from the parasternal short-axis view at the base of the heart. The usual anatomy has been obliterated by the massively enlarged pulmonary artery (PA). Thrombus (T) is identified in the proximal right main branch. Both left and right main branches are severely dilated. Spontaneous echocardiographic contrast (S) or 'smoke' is identified in the proximal artery. The ascending aorta (AO) is of normal dimension but appears diminutive next to the pulmonary artery. RA, right atrium; DAO, descending thoracic aorta.

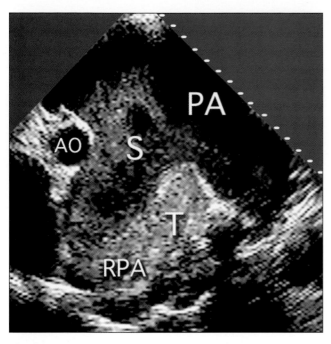

Figure 32.2

Transthoracic two-dimensional echocardiogram from the parasternal short-axis view at the base. Angulation of the transducer in a medial direction allows visualization of the right pulmonary artery (PA). The thrombus is again seen at the bifurcation and along the wall of the proximal right pulmonary artery. The spontaneous echocardiographic contrast (S) represents low-velocity flow.

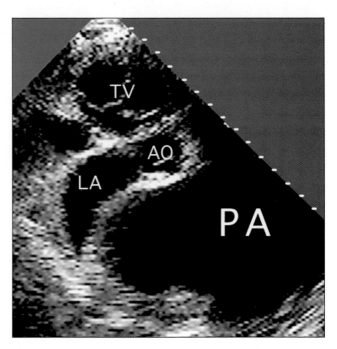

Figure 32.3

Transthoracic two-dimensional echocardiogram from an off-axis parasternal position at the base. The left atrium (LA) was so compressed by the massive pulmonary artery (PA) that it could be seen only in non-standard views. The left-sided chambers were otherwise impossible to visualize. The small left atrial size is due to severely reduced filling. The tricuspid valve (TV) is also seen in this image.

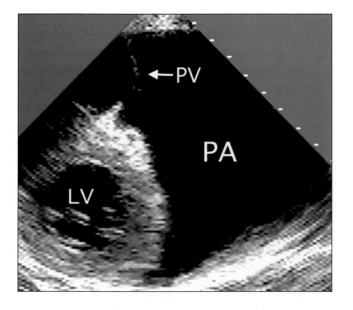

Figure 32.4

Transthoracic two-dimensional echocardiogram from the parasternal position. Another non-standard view demonstrates the underfilled left ventricle (LV), which measures approximately 3.8 cm in diameter in diastole. The pulmonary valve (PV) is displaced anteriorly.

Discussion

This woman presented with massive pulmonary thromboembolism. The source was not apparent on clinical assessment. The chronicity was suggested by her clinical history and the severely dilated pulmonary vasculature. The giant pulmonary artery dwarfed the aorta. In addition, the severity was suggested by the spontaneous echocardiographic contrast in the pulmonary artery, which is diagnostic of low velocity flow and probable major obstruction of the pulmonary vascular bed.

The distorted anatomy demands flexibility in the conduct of the echocardiographic examination as a search for appropriate non-standard views is undertaken. This massive pulmonary artery is at risk for aneurysm, rupture, dissection, and atrial compression, as in this case. The expected right heart echocardiographic findings would include right ventricular hypertrophy and dilatation, poor right ventricular function, pulmonary and tricuspid regurgitation. A patent foramen ovale, if present, could be the source of a significant right to left shunt.[1] The differential diagnosis of chronic thrombus in the pulmonary vascular bed is either primary or secondary.[2] Primary pulmonary thrombosis originates in the pulmonary vascular bed as governed by the triad of Virchow. Local blood flow may be sluggish, owing to severe pulmonary hypertension that is either primary or secondary. There may be a prothrombotic abnormality of the blood. The pulmonary arterial vessel wall may have intimal disruption from arteritis, e.g.

Takayasu's or dissection. Atheroma, however, is uncommon in the pulmonary vascular bed. Secondary pulmonary thrombosis results from extension of an embolus which commonly originates from the venous system of the lower extremity. Concomitant clinical evidence of deep venous thrombosis may be lacking. Lower extremity venous Doppler studies may be negative. Pelvic vein thrombosis may also be the source of large pulmonary emboli, mostly in women.

This differential is broad but significant with respect to therapeutic strategy. The etiology determines the therapeutic management. This patient had a negative workup for deep venous thrombosis, including a negative pelvic magnetic resonance image. She was diagnosed with idiopathic severe pulmonary hypertension. Her ultimate therapy would be bilateral lung transplantation, assuming adequate right ventricular function.

References

1. Kasper W, Meinertz, T, Henkel B, *et al*. Echocardiographic findings in patients with proved pulmonary embolism. Am Heart J 1986;112:1284–90.

2. Wittlich N, Erbel R, Eichler A, *et al*. Detection of central pulmonary artery thromboemboli by transesophageal echocardiography in patients with severe pulmonary embolism. J Am Soc Echocardiogr 1992;5:515–24.

33

Endocarditis with pericardial effusion

Jorge R Kizer MD
Susan E Wiegers MD

A 33-year-old man presented to the hospital with fever and pleuritic chest pain. He had a history of intravenous drug use. He had tested negative for HIV 6 months previously and his past medical history was otherwise unremarkable. Three days prior to this admission he had developed fevers with rigors. On the day of admission he had experienced sharp chest pain exacerbated by deep breaths and relieved by leaning forward.

The patient was an ill-appearing, cachectic man with a temperature of 103.4°F, a blood pressure of 95/40 mmHg and a heart rate of 114 bpm. Room air oxygen saturation was 93%. Breath sounds were decreased bibasilarly. The heart sounds were diminished but a II/VI systolic ejection murmur was audible at the right upper sternal border. A soft three-component pericardial friction rub was present. There were track marks in both upper extremities consistent with intravenous drug use. Laboratory examination was remarkable for marked leukocytosis with a left shift. Chest X-ray demonstrated small bilateral pleural effusions and atelectasis. Four out of four blood cultures grew *Staphlylococcus aureus* within 24 hours. Vancomycin and gentamicin were started in the emergency room before the blood culture results were available. However, he deteriorated rapidly with hypotension despite volume resuscitation and required pressor support. An echocardiogram was performed in the medical intensive care unit.

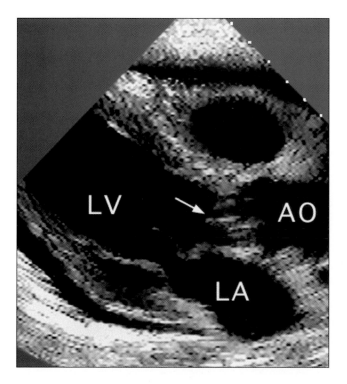

Figure 33.1
Parasternal long-axis view in diastole. The aortic valve is markedly abnormal and is diffusely thickened. A vegetation (arrow) prolapses into the left ventricular outflow tract. It is attached to the ventricular surface of the aortic valve. However, the entire valve is abnormal. There is a circumferential echo-free space surrounding the heart which represents pericardial effusion. LV, left ventricle; LA, left atrium; AO, aorta.

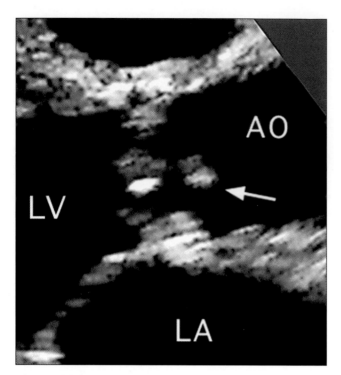

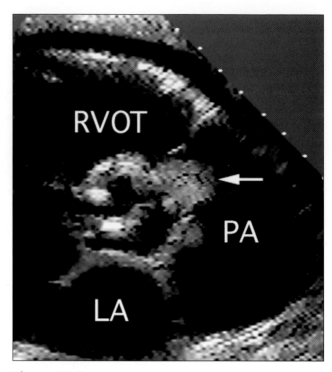

Figure 33.2
Close-up image from the parasternal long-axis view of the aortic valve in diastole. The 1 cm vegetation (arrow) is imaged on the aortic side (AO) of the aortic valve. It was highly mobile in real time, demonstrating high-frequency, chaotic motion. The walls of the aortic root are noted to be more than 5 mm in thickness. This sign is highly suggestive of aortic root abscess.

Figure 33.3
Parasternal short-axis view at the level of the base of the heart in diastole. The aortic valve (AO) is again seen to be markedly thickened along all three cusps. A mass (arrow) associated with the aortic root near the left coronary cusp projects into the pulmonary artery (PA). This represents an aortic root abscess with extension into the pulmonary artery. The mass is distal to the level of the pulmonary valve, which is imaged between the right ventricular outflow tract (RVOT) and the pulmonary artery. The posterior wall of the aortic root is also markedly thickened and contains echodensities which are highly suggestive of abscess. In this view, the pericardial effusion is seen anterior to the right ventricular outflow tract.

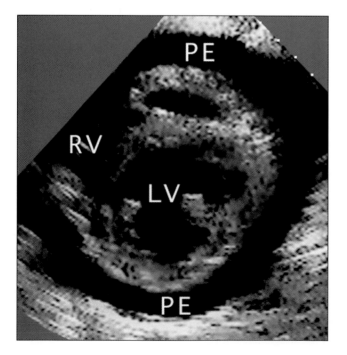

Figure 33.4
Parasternal short-axis view at the level of the papillary muscles. The circumferential nature of the pericardial effusion (PE) is apparent. It is moderate in size, being more than 1 cm in width. However, there were no echocardiographic signs of tamponade. On Doppler examination there was no evidence of respirophasic variation of tricuspid or mitral in-flow velocities. There was no right ventricular or right atrial collapse. It was not felt that the pericardial effusion in and of itself was contributing to the patient's hemodynamic instability.

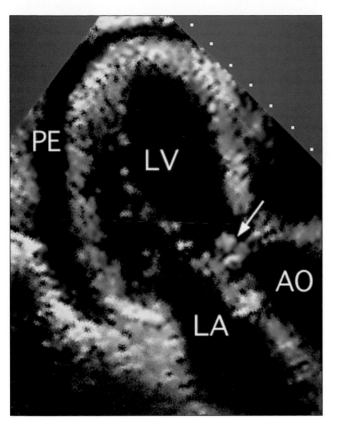

Figure 33.5
Apical long-axis view in diastole. Once again the vegetations (arrow) attached to the aortic valve are seen to project into the left ventricular outflow tract. The extension of the pericardial effusion (PE) around the apex is demonstrated. Note that the mitral valve appears to be normal with no evidence of vegetations. On color Doppler flow imaging there was moderate aortic regurgitation, which is not shown in these images.

Discussion

Annular abscesses more commonly involve the aortic root than the mitral valve ring. Clues to the diagnosis of abscess include recent onset of valvular regurgitation, high-level atrioventricular block, short duration of symptoms with rapid deterioration, a virulent pathogen, namely *Staphylococcus aureus*, and the presence of pericarditis, as in this patient.[1] However, clinical criteria and transthoracic echocardiography are much less sensitive for the diagnosis than transesophageal studies.[1,2]

Thickening of the aortic root to more than 2 mm and the presence of a pericardial effusion on transthoracic study should raise concern regarding the presence of an abscess.

Pericardial effusion in the setting of sub-acute, infective endocarditis is often not infectious in origin and is postulated to result from immunological mechanisms affecting the pericardium. However, in the setting of acute bacterial endocarditis, the presence of a pericardial effusion is commonly associated with valve ring abscess. Bacterial pericarditis may occur by extension from the valve ring abscess or myocardial abscess, rupture of a mycotic aneurysm caused by coronary embolization of infected material, or by simultaneous hematogenous seeding of the pericardium at the time of the original bacteremia.[3] This patient had a complicated aortic valve ring abscess that extended into the pulmonary artery. While an annular abscess may rupture into the right atrium, right ventricle or left atrium, extension into the pulmonary artery is less common, owing to separation of the fibrous skeletons of the great vessels. Emergency surgery was contemplated which would have consisted of reconstruction of the aortic valve annulus and placement of an allograft prosthesis. An allograft is highly preferable in this situation, as it is thought to be more resistant to reinfection.[4] This patient would have required repair of the pulmonary artery as well. Unfortunately, he suffered a pulseless electrical activity arrest on the morning after admission. Permission for autopsy was refused by the family. His fulminant course reflects the high mortality of this complication of endocarditis and underscores the importance of prompt recognition and surgical treatment.

References

1. Blumberg E, Karalis D, Chandrasekaran K, *et al.* Endocarditis-associated paravalvular abscesses. Do clinical parameters predict the presence of abscess? Chest 1995;107:898–903.

2. Afridi I, Apostolidou M, Saad R, *et al.* Pseudoaneurysms of the mitral-aortic intervalvular fibrosa: dynamic characterization using transesophageal echocardiographic and Doppler techniques. J Am Coll Cardiol 1995;25:137–45.

3. Wiegers SE, Plehn JF, Rajail-Khorasani A, *et al.* Purulent pericarditis and ventricular pseudoaneurysm in an intravenous drug abuser. Am Heart J 1988;116:1635–7.

4. Dossche KM, Defauw JJ, Ernst SM, *et al.* Allograft aortic root replacement in prosthetic aortic valve endocarditis: a review of 32 patients. Ann Thorac Surg 1997;63:1644–9.

34

Pulmonary embolism

Elizabeth A Tarka MD

A 67-year-old man presented to the emergency department complaining of acute dyspnea and sharp pleuritic chest pain. He had a history of severe chronic obstructive pulmonary disease and had recently returned from a 10-hour car trip. The physical examination revealed an obese male in moderate respiratory distress. His pulse was 130 bpm, blood pressure 100/65 mmHg, respiratory rate 28 and room air oxygen saturation 92%. The breath sounds were decreased at the right base with dullness to percussion. His cardiac examination revealed a tachycardic rhythm without audible murmurs or gallops. His right lower extremity was edematous. An electrocardiogram, chest X-ray, arterial blood gas and transthoracic echocardiogram were performed in the evaluation of this patient's symptoms.

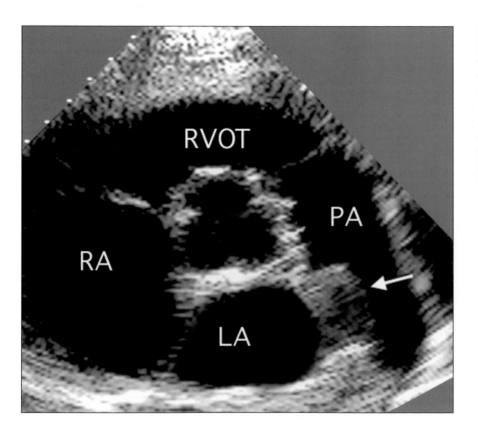

Figure 34.1
Parasternal short-axis view at the aortic valve level. There is a mass (arrow) visualized at the bifurcation of the main pulmonary artery (PA) which extends into the right pulmonary artery. The right atrium (RA) is dilated and the interatrial septum bows into the left atrium (LA) consistent with elevated right atrial pressure. RVOT, right ventricular outflow tract.

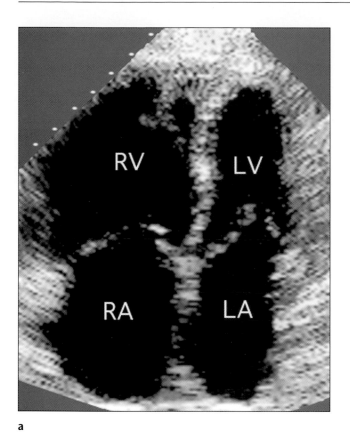

a

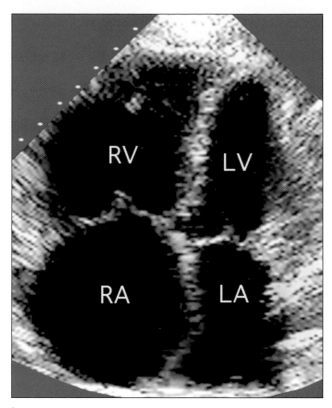

b

Figure 34.2

(a) Apical four-chamber view in diastole. The right ventricle (RV) is severely dilated, as is the right atrium (RA). Owing to right ventricular failure, the left ventricle (LV) is markedly underfilled and appears abnormally small. There is evidence of right ventricular hypertrophy with a hypertrophied moderator band seen in this and other apical images.

(b) Apical four-chamber view in systole. The right ventricular systolic function is profoundly decreased, with little change in the total area of the right ventricle between systole and diastole (compared to (a)). The right atrium is more dilated in this systolic frame compared to the diastolic frame, which suggests severe tricuspid regurgitation. The bowing of the interatrial septum into the left atrium is well seen in this image. This is due to the right atrial hypertension. The lateral wall of the left ventricle thickens normally but the septal motion is paradoxical.

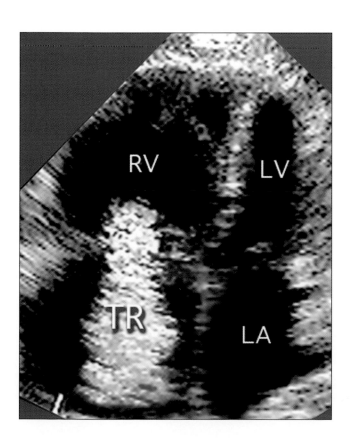

Figure 34.3

Apical four-chamber view in systole with color Doppler flow imaging. A turbulent jet of severe tricuspid regurgitation (TR) extends into the right atrium. The diameter of the jet at its origin at the level of the tricuspid valve is wide. The diameter of a regurgitant jet at the vena contracta correlates with the severity of the regurgitation.

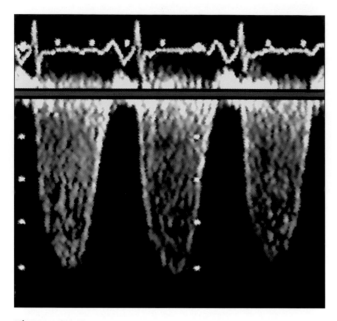

Figure 34.4
Spectral display of continuous-wave Doppler signals across the tricuspid valve from the apical position. The high-velocity systolic jet of tricuspid regurgitation is displayed below the baseline. The tricuspid regurgitation jet illustrated here has a velocity of 4 m/s which corresponds to an estimated systolic difference between the right ventricle and atrium of 64 mmHg as calculated by the modified Bernoulli equation. In the setting of a dilated right atrium, the right atrial pressure is assumed to be 15 mmHg, resulting in a peak pulmonary artery systolic pressure estimate of 79 mmHg.

Discussion

Echocardiography is a rapid, non-invasive strategy to aid in the diagnosis and therapeutic plan of acute pulmonary embolism. While direct visualization of the thrombus is confirmatory, this is usually not possible on a transthoracic study. However, parasternal short-axis and long-axis views of the pulmonary artery should always be attempted. The parasternal long-axis view of the pulmonary artery visualizes only the proximal pulmonary artery, but may demonstrate the presence of a proximal thrombus. From the standard parasternal long-axis position, the transducer is moved superiorly one intercostal space and angled anteriorly. Anterior and superior angulation of the transducer will bring the bifurcation into view. In addition, slight clockwise rotation of the transducer (5–10°) is helpful. The subcostal short axis may also demonstrate the bifurcation of the pulmonary artery in patients with a good subcostal window. The velocity of the tricuspid regurgitant jet should be measured in every possible view. Most tricuspid regurgitant jets are central

and the highest velocity is usually recorded from the apical four-chamber view.

Well accepted echocardiographic features supporting the diagnosis of pulmonary embolism exist. In acute right ventricular pressure overload states, the right ventricle is dilated and hypokinetic.[1] Flattening and abnormal movement of the interventricular septum toward the left ventricle secondary to ventricular interdependence results in a profound decrease in left ventricular preload.[2]

In patients without any underlying cardiac or pulmonary disease, a non-hypertrophied right ventricle is incapable of acutely generating a significantly elevated systolic pressure. In general, the normal right ventricle cannot generate a mean pulmonary artery pressure greater than 40 mmHg.[3] This corresponds to a maximum peak pulmonary artery systolic pressure of approximately 55 mmHg. The absence of right ventricular hypertrophy in a patient with signs of right ventricular pressure overload is evidence of an acute increase in pulmonary artery pressure. In this patient, the pulmonary artery systolic pressure was estimated at 79 mmHg by the modified Bernoulli equation using the tricuspid regurgitant jet velocity of 4 m/s and an assumed right atrial pressure of 15 mmHg. The patient's underlying chronic obstructive pulmonary disease had resulted in mild pulmonary hypertension, for which the right ventricular hypertrophy was a compensation. This ventricle was then able to generate a greater than normal systolic pressure in the setting of a superimposed acute insult from a large pulmonary embolism. Although not well visualized in these images, right ventricular hypertrophy is seen in the setting of chronic pulmonary hypertension. Subacute pulmonary embolism may also present with the echocardiographic findings in this case. Right ventricular hypertrophy and a tricuspid regurgitation velocity greater than 3.7 m/s are consistent with the diagnosis.[4] However, the presence of paradoxical septal motion and the clinical setting identified an acute pulmonary embolism superimposed on chronic pulmonary hypertension.

As suspected by the clinical history, this patient had an acute pulmonary embolus. While the right ventricle was able to generate a higher peak systolic pressure than usual, right ventricular failure had ensued, owing to the complete obstruction of the right pulmonary artery. In this case, the transthoracic study confirmed the diagnosis of pulmonary embolism and demonstrated severe right ventricular dysfunction. Therefore, the patient received intravenous tissue plasminogen activator. Echocardiographic diagnosis of right ventricular dilatation and hypokinesis have been proposed as indications for thrombolytic therapy even in hemodynamically stable patients.[5] A repeat transthoracic echocardiogram the following day revealed an estimated pulmonary artery systolic pressure (PASP) of 50 mmHg with improvement in the right ventricular function. The patient was discharged 6 days later on chronic anticoagulation.

References

1. Kasper W, Meinertz T, Hendel B, *et al.* Echocardiographic findings in patients with proved pulmonary embolism. Am Heart J 1986;112:1284–90.

2. Jardin R, Dubourg O, Gureret P, *et al.* Quantitative two-dimensional echocardiography in massive pulmonary embolism: Emphasis on ventricular interdependence and leftward septal displacement. J Am Coll Cardiol 1987;10:1201–6.

3. Come P. Echocardiographic recognition of pulmonary arterial disease and determination of its cause. Am J Med 1988;84:384–94.

4. Kasper W, Geibel A, Tiede N, *et al.* Distinguishing between acute and subacute massive pulmonary embolism by conventional and Doppler echocardiography. Br Heart J 1993;70:352–6.

5. Konstantinides S, Geibel A, Olschewski M, *et al.* Association between thrombolytic treatment and the prognosis of hemodynamically stable patients with major pulmonary embolism. Circulation 1997;96:882–8.

35

Thrombus associated with a pulmonary artery catheter

Susan E Wiegers MD

A 47-year-old man had a several-year history of dilated cardiomyopathy with progressive symptoms. He had been listed for a heart transplant and maintained in the hospital on chronic ionotropic infusion. Over the course of several days his condition deteriorated further and he was transferred to the intensive care unit in cardiogenic shock. A Swan–Ganz catheter was placed and the patient was aggressively treated. After 2 days, he remained critically ill and was taken to the operating room, where a left ventricular assist device was placed. A transesophageal study was performed in the operating room to assist in evaluation of right heart function. An incidental finding is illustrated below.

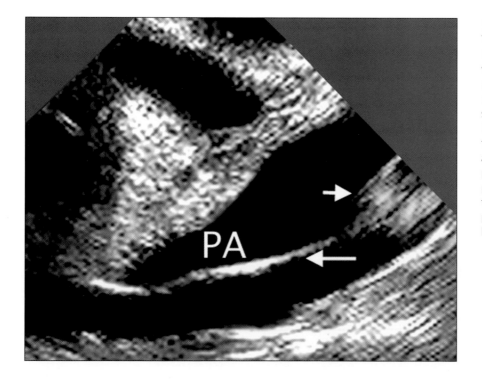

Figure 35.1
Transesophageal image in the longitudinal plane of the right ventricular outflow tract and the pulmonary artery (PA). Note that the pulmonary artery is the most anterior structure of the heart at this level and is thus farthest from the transesophageal probe. The pulmonary artery catheter (long arrow) is noted passing from the outflow tract into the pulmonary artery. A mass is attached to the catheter (short arrow) in the main pulmonary artery before the bifurcation.

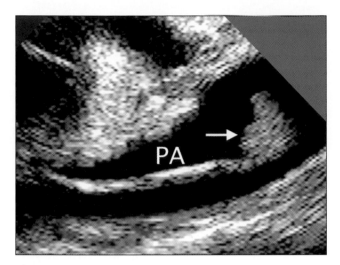

Figure 35.2
Similar transesophageal view of the thrombus (arrow) at a later part of the cardiac cycle. The clot was highly mobile, as evidenced by its changing position within the main pulmonary artery.

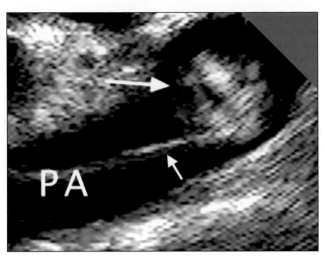

Figure 35.3
Magnified image of the thrombus with rotation of the probe to reveal the maximum size of the thrombus. The clot does not occlude the main pulmonary artery but is larger in diameter than either of the main branch pulmonary arteries, partially occluding the right pulmonary artery.

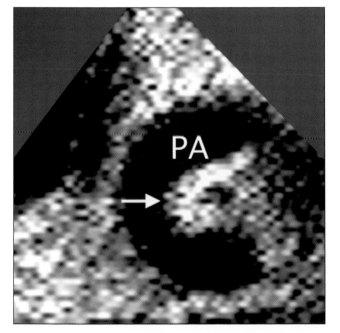

Figure 35.4
Short-axis view of the right pulmonary artery (PA) demonstrating the thrombus attached to the catheter (arrow), which is echodense compared to the thrombus.

Discussion

Thrombus formation on pulmonary artery catheters undoubtedly occurs far more often than is clinically recognized. Embolization of this large thrombus would have led to the death of this patient. The portion of the thrombus attached to the catheter in the main pulmonary artery was highly mobile, making embolization more likely. As far as could be determined in this seriously ill patient, he had not sustained a significant pulmonary embolus prior to the time of the transesophageal echocardiogram in the operating room. Cardiogenic shock with a very low flow state presumably predisposed him to thrombus formation. Percutaneous removal of the catheter is not recommended when such a large and extensive thrombus is identified. The clot was removed surgically prior to the removal of the Swan–Ganz catheter. Catheter formation is common on central lines[1] and has been reported on ventricular pacemakers with resultant embolization.[2,3] Thrombi associated with pulmonary artery catheters are much less commonly detected.

The patient was stabilized on a left ventricular assist device without mechanical support of the right ventricle. He underwent successful cardiac transplantation several months later.

References

1. Podolsky L, Manginas A, Jacobs L, *et al.* Superior vena caval thrombosis detected by transesophageal echocardiography. J Am Soc Echocardiogr 1991;4:189–93.

2. Porath A, Avnum L, Hirsch M, *et al.* Right atrial thrombus and recurrent pulmonary emboli secondary to permanent cardiac pacing—a case report and short review of literature. Angiology 1987;38:627–30.

3. Bastianon V, Menichelli A, Colloridi V, *et al.* Ventricular thrombosis during permanent endocardial pacing in a pediatric patient with hemorrheological disorders. Pacing Clin Electrophysiol 1985;8:164–9.

36

Pulmonary artery dissection

Gene Chang MD

A 43-year-old Caucasian man had end-stage pulmonary disease secondary to primary pulmonary hypertension. A giant pulmonary artery aneurysm with a chronic dissection had been diagnosed in the past. He was referred for lung transplantation. The patient was felt to be an acceptable transplant candidate and underwent successful bilateral sequential lung transplantation and complete reconstruction and replacement of the main pulmonary artery and the right and left pulmonary arteries when a suitable organ became available. A 24 mm × 12 mm bifurcation hemashield graft was placed from the pulmonary valve to the distal pulmonary arteries. Preoperative transthoracic and representative intraoperative transesophageal echocardiogram images of the chronic pulmonary artery dissection and subsequent repair are depicted below.

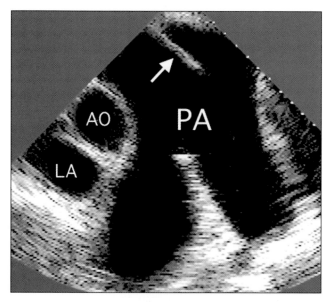

Figure 36.1
Transthoracic parasternal short-axis view at the level of the base of the heart. The normal architecture is distorted by the massively enlarged pulmonary artery (PA). The bifurcation of the main pulmonary artery and enlargement of the branch pulmonary arteries is well seen. A normal-sized aortic root is visualized to the left of the pulmonary artery. The left atrium (LA) is seen posteriorly. A flap is visible in the proximal main pulmonary artery (arrow) which runs towards the left main pulmonary artery but passes out of plane. It appears to end abruptly but this is an artifact, since the dissection flap spiraled into the left pulmonary artery.

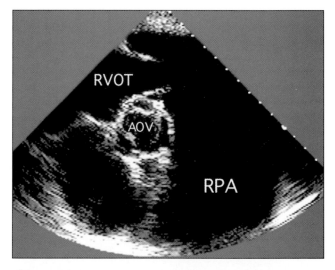

Figure 36.2
Transthoracic parasternal short-axis view at the level of the base of the heart. The transducer has been angled medially and superiorly from its position in the previous image. The left atrium is no longer visible and the right pulmonary artery (RPA) is imaged as it passes posteriorly to the aortic root towards the left of the screen (right side of the patient). It is markedly enlarged; the diameter is many times larger than the aortic root diameter. A normal aortic trileaflet valve is well seen. The pulmonary valve is open in this systolic frame and is positioned more anteriorly than its usual position. The leaflets cannot open fully to approximate the walls of the pulmonary artery, as they normally would, owing to the severe dilatation of that structure. The right ventricular outflow tract (RVOT) is also dilated.

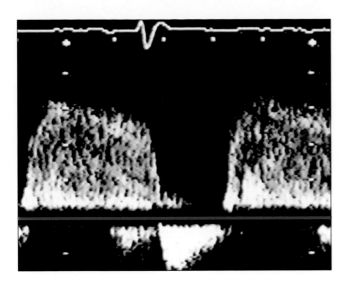

Figure 36.3
Spectral display of continuous-wave Doppler across the pulmonary valve taken from the parasternal position. In diastole, a high-velocity jet of pulmonary regurgitation is seen above the baseline. The peak velocity is 3.1 m/s (each calibration mark represents 1 m/s.) Therefore, the peak gradient between the pulmonary artery and the right ventricle at the onset of diastole is 38 mmHg. The true pulmonary artery diastolic pressure is this gradient plus the right ventricular diastolic pressure. The pulmonary artery diastolic pressure is therefore severely elevated. The systolic pulmonary artery pressure cannot be calculated from these values but only from the tricuspid regurgitation velocity, which is of course obtained in another view. The tricuspid regurgitation jet velocity was 4.8 m/s which predicts a peak pulmonary artery pressure of 107 mmHg, assuming a right atrial pressure of 15 mmHg.

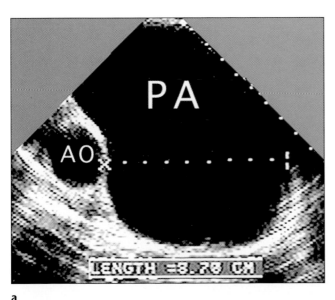

a

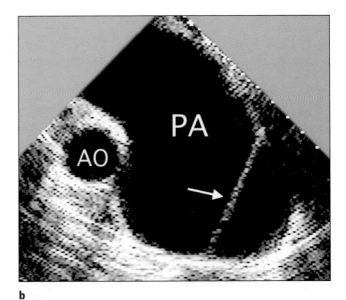

b

Figure 36.4
(a) Transesophageal echocardiogram from the high esophageal position in the transverse plane (imaging angle 0°). Although the image may superficially resemble Figure 36.1, they are taken from opposite directions. In the transesophageal images, the top of the image represents posterior structures. Therefore, the proximal pulmonary artery is imaged at the bottom of the screen and the level of the bifurcation of the pulmonary artery is seen at the top of the screen. The main pulmonary artery measures 8.7 cm, which is severely enlarged (normal < 2.5 cm). The normal-sized aorta is seen on the left of the screen.
(b) Transesophageal echocardiogram from the high esophageal position in the transverse plane (imaging angle 0°). The transducer has been withdrawn slightly and rotated to the left compared to the previous image. The dissection flap (arrow) is visible in the proximal portion of the main pulmonary artery running towards the left branch of the pulmonary artery, which goes off to the right of the screen and is not imaged. The right main pulmonary artery passes posteriorly to the ascending aorta (AO).

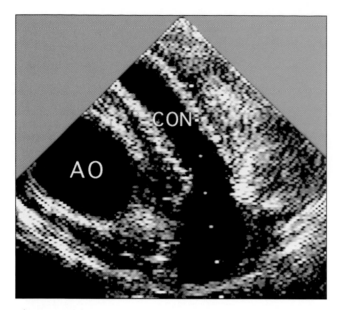

Figure 36.5
Post-pump transesophageal echocardiogram from the high esophageal position in the transverse plane (imaging angle 0°). The surgical conduit (CON), which has replaced the right main pulmonary artery, is clearly visible posterior to the aorta. The proximal pulmonary artery, at the bottom of the screen, is not well seen in this image but has also been replaced by a surgical conduit. The material of the conduit gives rise to a characteristic refraction pattern with multiple, short parallel lines. A mass consistent with surgical hematoma is noted posterior to the right pulmonary artery conduit.

Discussion

Primary pulmonary hypertension (PPH) is a disease characterized by sustained elevations of pulmonary pressure without a demonstrable cause, and defined in the National Institutes of Health (NIH) registry as a mean pulmonary artery pressure of ≥25 mmHg at rest or >30 mmHg with exercise.[1] The estimated incidence of PPH ranges from one to two cases/million people in the general population.[2] Dyspnea and fatigue represent the two major early symptoms reported in patients with PPH. However, the non-specific nature and subtlety of signs and symptoms at disease onset hinder early diagnosis. Typically, the mean time from the onset of symptoms to diagnosis is 2 years.[2] The pathogenesis typically involves pulmonary arteriolar medial hypertrophy, inflammation, vasoconstriction, and thrombosis in situ.[3] Chronic pulmonary arterial dissection, as noted in the above patient, is not typically noted with PPH, but has been described in the literature.[4]

Echocardiography is frequently performed early in the evaluation of patients with symptomatic dyspnea. The imaging modality can provide an estimate of pulmonary artery pressures, and may aid in the diagnosis of PPH by ruling out intrinsic myocardial, ischemic, valvular, or congenital heart disease. The diagnosis of PPH remains one of exclusion. Cardiac conditions which can cause pulmonary hypertension such as left ventricular failure and left-sided valve lesions must be excluded. Pulmonary function testing typically identifies mild abnormalities in lung function and progressive arterial hypoxemia with disease advancement.

Right heart catheterization, with or without exercise, confirms the diagnosis of PPH, and is instrumental in the initiation and monitoring of the response to therapy.[5] Nitric oxide, epoprostenol (prostacyclin), nitroprusside, and adenosine have all been used for acute assessment of pulmonary vasoreactivity. The most widely used medications for long-term therapy include calcium channel blockers nifedipine or diltiazem and intravenous epoprostenol.[1] Pulmonary artery pressure may also be estimated using the tricuspid regurgitation jet velocity via the modified Bernoulli equation. Although diagnosis of pulmonary hypertension is usually confirmed with pulmonary artery catheterization, response to therapy may be monitored by echocardiography. A direct evaluation of pulmonary vasoreactivity is imperative, since an initial response to vasodilator therapy has been shown accurately to identify patients likely to respond to long-term oral therapy. The pulmonary artery diastolic pressure may also be estimated, as demonstrated in Figure 36.3. In this case, the minimal value for the pulmonary artery diastolic pressure is 38 mmHg, which is considerably elevated.

This patient's markedly dilated pulmonary artery has displaced the other cardiac structures. Since the pulmonary valve and artery are the most anterior of the cardiac structures, transthoracic imaging is often more helpful than transesophageal imaging. With the transducer in the esophagus, the pulmonary artery is in the far field of the image. In this case, the dissection flap might initially be mistaken for one of the pulmonary valve leaflets. However, the pulmonary valve itself has been medially and anteriorly displaced by the pulmonary artery dilatation. The dissection flap sits in the usual position of the pulmonary valve as it spirals towards the left pulmonary artery and moves out of plane.

Unfortunately, PPH is a progressive disease with a poor prognosis and no known cure. The mean survival after diagnosis was 2.5 years for patients followed in the NIH registry, with a brighter prognosis for those patients responding to calcium channel blockers and/or epoprostenol treatment.[6] Lung transplantation, and combined heart–lung transplantation, represents a promising cure for PPH as no cases of recurrent PPH have been reported following transplantation. However, this treatment option remains restricted by the limited availability of organs. Additionally, the morbidity and mortality rates after lung transplantation are higher among patients with PPH than among those with other diagnoses. One-year survival rates after lung transplantation for PPH reportedly range from 65–70%.[7] Long-term survival is limited by the development of obliterative bronchiolitis, the major long-term complication of lung transplantation.

This patient developed recurrent severe pulmonary hypertension due to vascular graft stenosis and underwent successful pulmonary artery stent placements. He ultimately expired 3 years after successful transplantation, succumbing to progressive obliterative bronchiolitis.

References

1. Rick S, Dantzker DR, Ayres SM, et al. Primary pulmonary hypertension: a national prospective study. Ann Intern Med 1987;107:216–23.

2. Rubin, LJ. Current concepts: primary pulmonary hypertension. N Engl J Med 1997;336:111–17.

3. Rich, S. Clinical insights into the pathogenesis of primary pulmonary hypertension. Chest 1998;114:2375–415.

4. Masud S, Ishii T, Asuwa N, et al. Concurrent pulmonary arterial dissection and saccular aneurysm associated with primary pulmonary hypertension. Arch Pathol Lab Med 1996;120:309–12.

5. Groves BM, Badesch DB, Turkevitch D, et al. Correlation of acute prostacyclin response in primary (unexplained) pulmonary hypertension with efficacy of treatment with calcium channel blockers and survival. In: Hume JR, Reeves JT, Weir EK, eds. Ion Flux in Pulmonary Vascular Control, Plenum Press: New York, 1993:317–30.

6. D'Alonzo GE, Barst RJ, Ayres SM, et al. Survival in patients with primary pulmonary hypertension: results from a national prospective registry. Ann Intern Med 1991;115:343–9.

7. Hosenpud JD, Novick RJ, Bennet LE, et al. The Registry of the International Society for Heart and Lung Transplantation: thirteenth official report—1996. J Heart Lung Transplant 1996;15:655–74.

37

Acquired pulmonary stenosis after the Ross procedure

Susan E Wiegers MD

A 45-year-old man had undergone the Ross procedure 2 years earlier to correct aortic stenosis due to a calcified bicuspid valve. The procedure involved transfer of the native pulmonary valve to the aortic position and placement of a cryopreserved homograft in the pulmonary position. The surgical course had been uncomplicated.

Examination 2 years later revealed a loud ejection murmur at the left upper sternal border and a loud holosystolic murmur audible at the left and right lower sternal borders. Both murmurs increased with inspiration. The patient was asymptomatic, with a sedentary lifestyle.

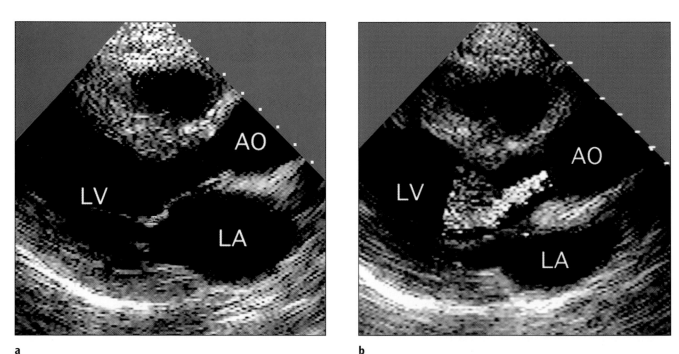

a   b

Figure 37.1
(a) Parasternal long-axis view in diastole. The left ventricular (LV) cavity size is normal and the walls are mildly hypertrophied. The left atrium (LA) is normal. The tip of the anterior leaflet of the mitral valve is mildly thickened. The aortic valve leaflets are not imaged. The aortic root (AO) is thickened which is consistent with surgical change.
(b) Color flow Doppler image in the same view. A high-velocity, turbulent jet arises from the aortic valve and extends into the left ventricular outflow tract. The ratio of the jet width at its origin to the left ventricular outflow tract diameter is less than 25% which indicated that the aortic regurgitation is mild. The regurgitant jet is central which excludes a paravalvular leak.

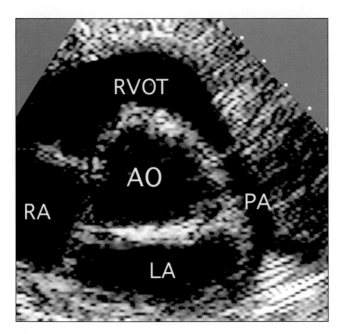

Figure 37.2
Parasternal short-axis view at the base of the heart. The discrepancy between the size of the aortic root (AO) and the pulmonary artery (PA) is clear. The pulmonary valve appears to be normal but is incompletely visualized. The bifurcation of the pulmonary artery is well demonstrated with the right main pulmonary artery passing posterior to the aortic root. The main pulmonary artery and the branches are small. The aortic root which contains the pulmonary autograft is mildly dilated, and thickening of the walls is again noted. The right ventricular outflow tract (RVOT) appears to be normal.

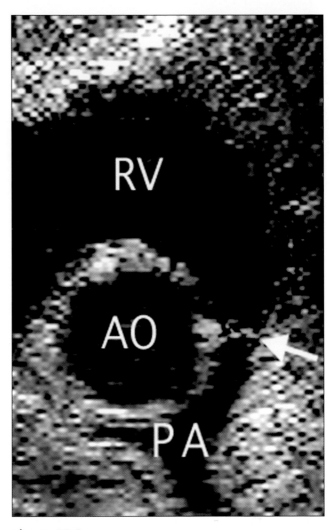

Figure 37.3
Subcostal short-axis view at the base of the heart. Again the discrepancy between the pulmonary artery and the aortic root size is demonstrated. The right ventricle appears to be mildly enlarged. However, right ventricular enlargement was not evident in the parasternal long- or short-axis views. Assessment of right ventricular size is problematic in the subcostal view, because of the off-axis imaging.

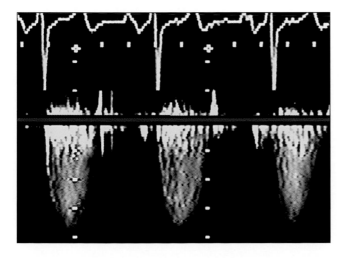

Figure 37.4
Spectral display of continuous wave Doppler across the pulmonary valve and the main pulmonary artery. The peak velocity is 3.7 m/s, predicting a peak gradient of 55 mmHg. The gradient is most likely to be a combination of valvular and supravalvular stenosis.

Discussion

The Ross procedure has been advocated as an alternative for the use of aortic homografts in patients requiring aortic valve replacement.[1] Transesophageal echocardiography is used intraoperatively to size the aortic root and to be sure that the pulmonary valve is of a comparable size. While the cross clamp and operative time are longer with the Ross procedure than with simple aortic valve homograft surgery, the perioperative morbidity and mortality have been similar.[2]

Aortic insufficiency has been reported to be mild in 10% of patients at one year in later studies where intraoperative echocardiography was standardly used to size the aortic root.[3] Trivial aortic regurgitation has been reported in a higher proportion of patients. The development of pulmonary stenosis in the cryopreserved homograft has been reported rarely. Supravalvular pulmonary stenosis, presumably at the suture line, has also occurred rarely.[4] This patient has not required intervention.

References

1. Gerosa G, Ross D, Brucke P, et al. Aortic valve replacement with pulmonary homografts. J Thorac Cardiovasc Surg 1994;107:424–37.

2. Santini F, Dyke C, Edwards S, et al. Pulmonary autograft versus homograft replacement of the aortic valve: a prospective randomized trial. J Thorac Cardiovasc Surg 1997;113:894–9; discussion 899–900.

3. David T, Omran A, Webb G, et al. Geometric mismatch of the aortic and pulmonary roots causes aortic insufficiency after the Ross procedure. J Thorac Cardiovasc Surg 1996;112:1231–7.

4. Lima V, Lazzam C, Benson L. Stenting for pulmonary artery stenosis following the Ross procedure. Catheterization Cardiovasc Diagn 1995;36:259–61.

38

Compression of the heart by anterior mediastinal mass

Susan E Wiegers MD

Dyspnea, cough and chest heaviness developed in a 45-year-old man with a history of Hodgkin's lymphoma treated 3 years previously with chemotherapy. The patient had had several episodes of syncope. He was admitted to the hospital where he was found to be hypotensive, tachypneic and tachycardic. A chest radiograph showed a very large anterior mediastinal mass and bilateral pleural effusions. An echocardiogram was performed to evaluate right heart function.

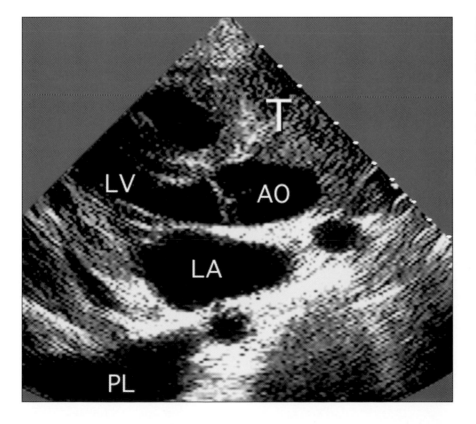

Figure 38.1
Parasternal long-axis view. The normal geometry of the heart is distorted by a large tumor mass (T) that appears to be compressing the ascending aorta (AO) and the right ventricular outflow tract. A small posterior pericardial effusion (PE) is present. A large left pleural effusion (PL) is separated from the pericardium by a dense mass that also represents a tumor.

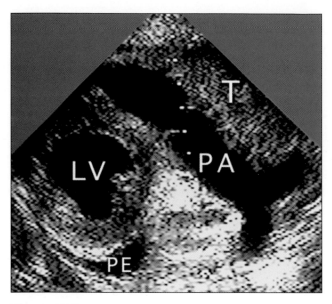

Figure 38.2
Parasternal long-axis view of the pulmonary artery (PA). The anterior mediastinal mass (T) extends to the level of the pulmonary artery and its bifurcation. There is an abnormal tissue density posterior to the pulmonary bifurcation which is also tumor. The left ventricle (LV) is imaged in short axis. Once again the small posterior pericardial effusion (PE) is visible.

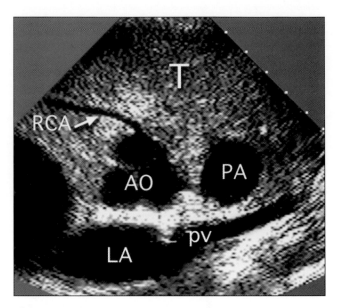

Figure 38.3
Parasternal short-axis view at the base of the heart. The mediastinal tumor has completely distorted the geometry and posteriorly displaced the pulmonary artery, which it encircles. The right coronary artery (RCA) is visible running through the tumor mass after its origin from the right coronary sinus of Valsalva. The caliber of the vessel is probably normal and there is no evidence of ostial compression. The left superior pulmonary vein (pv) is partially compressed by the mass.

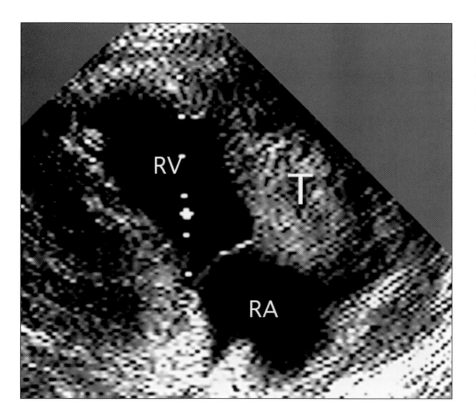

Figure 38.4
Parasternal long-axis right ventricular inflow view. The tumor (T) is seen anteriorly and compresses both the right ventricle (RV) and the right atrium (RA). In the distal right ventricle, it appears to be invading the wall of the ventricle.

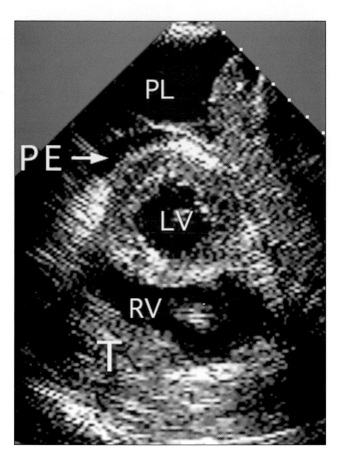

Figure 38.5
Posterior thoracic image. The large left pleural effusion allows imaging of the heart and mediastinal structures when the transducer is placed on the left posterior chest. The pleural effusion is adjacent to the transducer (top of the screen) and the right ventricle is in the far field of the image, anterior to the left ventricle. The left and right ventricles are shown in short axis and the tumor is once again imaged anterior to the right ventricle and lateral to the left ventricle. This view may occasionally be very helpful in imaging patients with poor anterior thoracic images due to surgery, bandages or chest tubes. A left pleural effusion is necessary for this image to be obtained.

Discussion

The patient's symptoms were due to compression of the anterior mediastinal structures by the large tumor mass that encased the heart and great vessels. Such a presentation is fortunately rare. The tumor mass was too large and intrinsically associated with vital cardiac structures to allow for surgical resection to correct the obstructive symptoms. The presence of the mass in the anterior mediastinum allowed infiltration of the paracardiac space with resultant outflow tract obstruction. Similar cases have been reported with invasion of the myocardium and intracardiac masses as well.[1] Primary lymphoma of the heart is a rare condition,[2] although metastatic involvement with extracardiac lymphoma is relatively common.

There was concern in this patient's case that treatment of the tumor with radiation or chemotherapy would lead to massive tumor necrosis with resultant swelling of the tumor and further compression of the cardiac structures. Owing to the patient's very poor condition, radiation therapy was undertaken. He had a transient improvement in his hemodynamics but subsequently deteriorated.

References

1. Halcox J. Non-surgical CHOP cures right ventricular outflow obstruction. Heart 1999;81:445–6.

2. Ceresoli G, Ferreri A, Bucci E, *et al*. Primary cardiac lymphoma in immunocompetent patients: diagnostic and therapeutic management. Cancer 1997;80:1497–506.

39

Pulmonary saddle embolism

Elizabeth A Tarka MD

A 76-year-old woman with rectal carcinoma successfully underwent an abdominal perineal resection. Two weeks later, she was admitted for acute dyspnea and fever. She reported several episodes of near syncope in the preceding days. On admission, her respiratory status rapidly deteriorated requiring intubation and transfer to the intensive care unit. She was hypotensive. Physical examination findings were notable for tachycardia, tachypnea, clear lungs, an accentuated second heart sound, and cyanosis. A transthoracic echocardiogram showed a dilated right ventricle and paradoxical interventricular septal motion. The remaining views were technically limited and a transesophageal echocardiogram was performed.

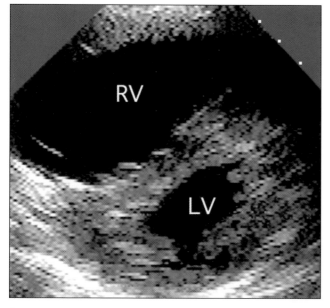

a

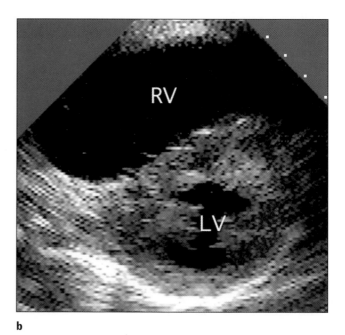

b

Figure 39.1
(a) Transthoracic parasternal short-axis echocardiogram of the left ventricle (LV) in diastole. The right ventricle (RV) is severely enlarged while the left ventricular cavity size is normal. There is marked flattening of the interventricular septum.
(b) Similar systolic image from the parasternal view. The interventricular septum has moved towards the right ventricle. Although it has thickened, the septum remains flattened in systole. This paradoxical septal motion is consistent with right ventricular volume and pressure overload. The fractional area change of the right ventricle is markedly decreased, indicating a severe decrease in right ventricular systolic function.

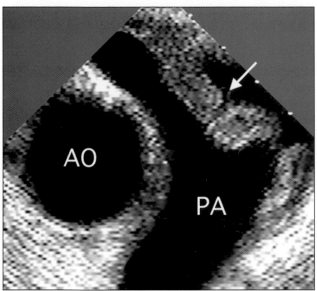

a

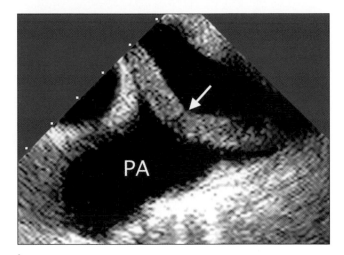

b

Figure 39.2

(a) Transesophageal echocardiogram from the high esophageal level in the transverse plane (imaging angle 0°). The proximal ascending aorta (AO), seen in short axis, is normal. The proximal pulmonary artery (PA) is at the bottom of the screen, since it is an anterior structure. The caliber of the vessel is normal and the bifurcation of the pulmonary artery is well seen. A portion of the right pulmonary artery is visualized as it passes posteriorly (at the top of the screen) to the aorta. The ostium of the left pulmonary artery is also seen, although the left pulmonary artery is always more difficult to visualize. A mobile mass (arrow), approximately 4 cm long, is seen in the right main pulmonary artery extending into the bifurcation. The head of the mass has prolapsed into the left main pulmonary artery. The saddle embolus is layered along the bifurcation of the pulmonary artery. Not only does it appear to be partially obstructing both the right and the left pulmonary arteries, it has a high risk for more distal embolization and pulmonary infarction.
(b) Several frames later in the same cardiac cycle, the thrombus (arrow) has moved within the pulmonary artery and appears to be occluding the bifurcation.
(c) Several frames later in the same cardiac cycle, the thrombus has now moved again and appears to be entering the left pulmonary artery.

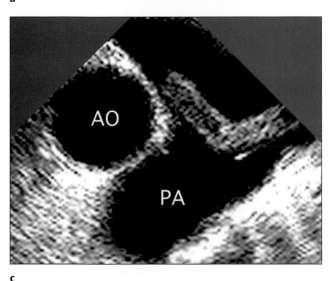

c

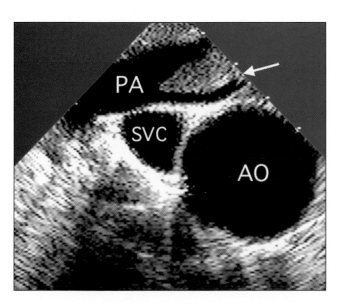

Figure 39.3

Transesophageal echocardiogram from the high esophageal level in the transverse plane (imaging angle 0°). The transesophageal probe has been withdrawn slightly and the entire probe rotated towards the right of the patient to visualize more of the right pulmonary artery (PA). The thrombus (arrow) extends well into the right main pulmonary artery and appears to partially occlude the vessel. SVC, superior vena cava.

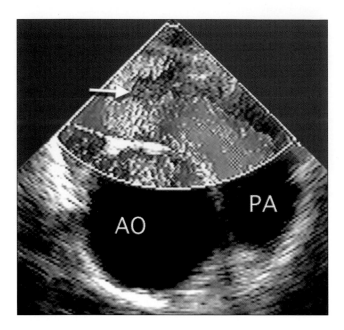

Figure 39.4
Similar transesophageal image to Figure 39.2 with color Doppler flow imaging. Once again the right main pulmonary artery is imaged posterior to the ascending aorta (AO). The saddle embolus (arrow) extends into the right main pulmonary artery. Laminar color Doppler flow is evident in the main pulmonary artery (PA) and the proximal right pulmonary artery. However, turbulent flow develops at the distal extent of the thrombus indicated by the arrow. The turbulent flow is due to partial obstruction of the vessel by the thrombus resulting in an increased velocity and disrupting the normal laminar flow in the vessel.

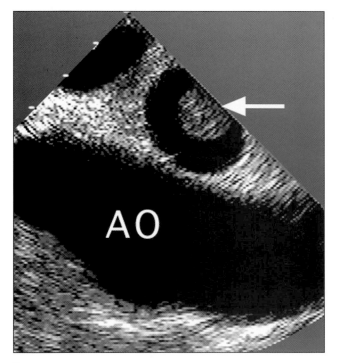

a

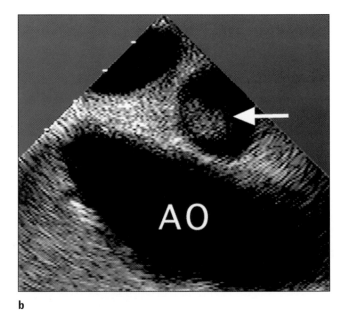

b

Figure 39.5
(a) Transesophageal echocardiogram from the high esophageal level in the longitudinal plane (imaging angle 90°). The right pulmonary artery is seen in short axis and contains a thrombus (arrow). The aorta (AO) is visualized in long axis.
(b) Several frames later in the same cardiac cycle, the thrombus (arrow) has moved within the pulmonary artery. In real time, the mass exhibited high-frequency chaotic motion.

Discussion

Confirming the diagnosis of pulmonary embolism in a critically ill patient is challenging. The standard diagnostic procedures such as ventilation-perfusion lung scans and pulmonary artery angiography are difficult to perform safely in a hemodynamically unstable patient. While there are characteristic findings on a transthoracic echocardiogram, the study is often technically limited in an intubated patient. The use of transesophageal echocardiography to detect thromboembolus in the pulmonary artery has been described.[1] The bifurcation of the main pulmonary artery and the course of the right pulmonary artery are easily visualized by this approach; however, the left branch is more difficult to image.

The confirmation of this life-threatening condition allows for the institution of prompt treatment. The administration of thrombolytic agents relieves the obstruction to pulmonary artery blood flow, thereby improving right ventricular function and reducing pulmonary artery resistance.[2] Anticoagulation to provide prophylaxis against additional thromboembolic events is administered as an adjunct to the thrombolytic agent.

Evaluation of the effect of lytic therapy can be monitored by transesophageal echocardiography.[3]

Because of this patient's recent surgery, she was not a candidate for thrombolytic therapy. Her rapid clinical deterioration prompted an emergency thromboendarterectomy in the operating room. The patient's hemodynamic and respiratory parameters dramatically improved. She was discharged on the tenth postoperative day on coumadin.

References

1. Nixdorff U, Erber R, Drexler M, *et al*. Detection of thromboembolus of the right pulmonary artery by transesophageal two-dimensional echocardiography. Am J Cardiol 1988;61:488–9.

2. Come P, Ducksoo K, Parker J, *et al*. Early reversal of right ventricular dysfunction in patients with acute pulmonary embolism after treatment with intravenous tissue plasminogen activator. J Am Coll Cardiol 1987;10:971–8.

3. Gelernt MD, Mogtader A, Hahn RT. Transesophageal echocardiography to diagnose and demonstrate resolution of an acute massive pulmonary embolus. Chest 1992;102:297–9.

40

Acquired supravalvular pulmonary stenosis

Martin St John Sutton MBBS
Susan E Wiegers MD

A 30-year-old asymptomatic woman 15 weeks into her first pregnancy was seen at her initial antenatal clinic visit at which time a clinical diagnosis of severe pulmonary hypertension was made. Doppler echocardiogram demonstrated a peak tricuspid regurgitant velocity of 4.5 m/s indicating a right atrial–right ventricular systolic gradient of 81 mmHg. She was referred for consideration of termination of pregnancy and tubal ligation on account of the high risk for maternal and fetal demise if the pregnancy was continued.

A detailed history and physical examination revealed a completely asymptomatic woman able to exercise in the gymnasium 5 days per week without exercise intolerance, chest pain, light headedness, syncope, or palpitations.

As an infant, she had presented with failure to thrive soon after birth. Her electrocardiogram showed septal Q waves and poor R wave progression across the anterior precordium. A chest X-ray revealed moderately severe cardiomegaly. She was treated with digitalis and diuretics for a diagnosis of congenital mitral regurgitation and severe left ventricular dysfunction. Progressive deterioration eventually led to cardiac catheterization which serendipitously demonstrated anomalous left coronary from pulmonary artery. She had corrective surgery with ligation of the origin of the left coronary artery from the pulmonary artery with construction of a side to side fistula between the coronary artery and the aortic root. After 10-year follow-up her left ventricular size and function had returned to normal and she was subsequently lost to follow-up.

On physical examination her jugular venous pressure was elevated by 20 cm with prominent 'v' waves. She had a right ventricular parasternal lift, a loud ejection systolic murmur with a thrill in the second left intercostal space and a holosystolic murmur in the fourth left intercostal space which varied with respiration. An electrocardiogram showed right axis deviation and right ventricular hypertrophy.

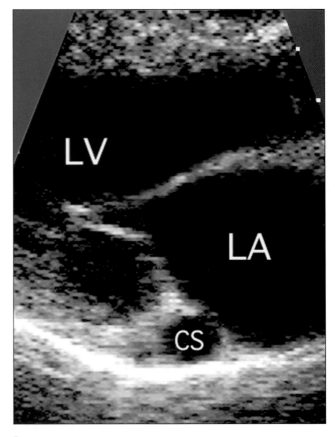

a

Figure 40.1
(a) Parasternal long-axis view with a close-up of the mitral valve, which is normal. The coronary sinus (CS) is dilated.

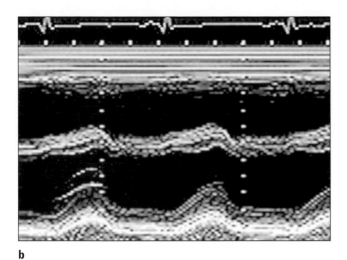

b

Figure 40.1

(b) M-mode echocardiogram from the parasternal position. The right ventricle is dilated and hypertrophied. The left ventricular systolic function is normal, but the interventricular septal motion is paradoxical.

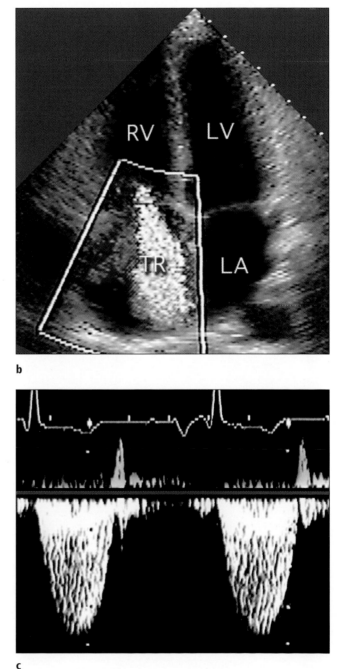

a

b

c

Figure 40.2

(a) Apical four-chamber view revealing a moderately enlarged and hypertrophied right ventricle that is apex-forming with mildly diminished function. The right atrium is mildly dilated.
(b) Similar systolic view with color Doppler flow imaging. There is moderately severe tricuspid regurgitation.
(c) Continuous-wave Doppler spectral display of tricuspid regurgitation. The peak velocity is 4.7 m/s (each calibration mark represents 1 m/s), indicating a right ventricular to right atrial gradient of 88 mmHg.

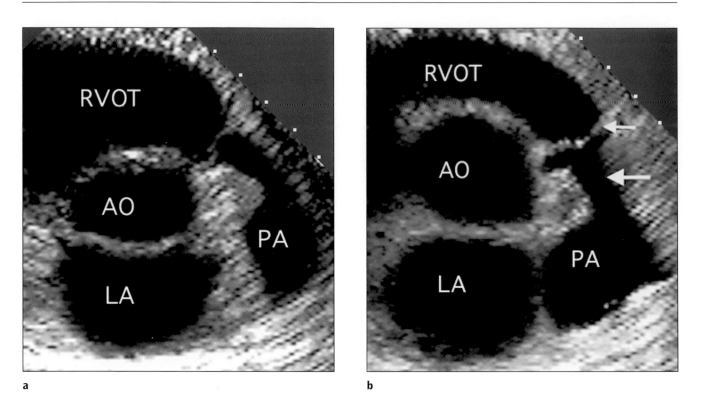

a

b

Figure 40.3
(a) Parasternal short axis view at the base of the heart. Approximately 1.5 cm distal to the pulmonary valve is a severe narrowing of the pulmonary artery.
(b) Close-up of the pulmonary artery confirming the severe narrowing of the proximal pulmonary artery and post stenotic dilatation. The pulmonary valve (small arrow) is mildly thickened and is closed in diastole. The supra-valvular obstruction (larger arrow) is visible in the proximal pulmonary artery. The obstruction appears to be caused by the baffle which was surgically created to direct aortic flow to the anomalous coronary artery.

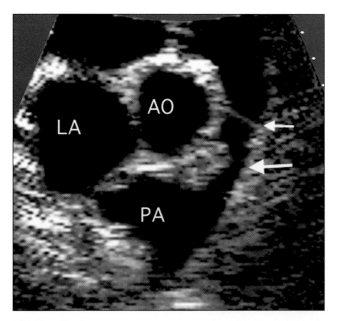

Figure 40.4
Short-axis view from the subcostal view demonstrating the normal pulmonary valve (small arrow) and the narrowed pulmonary artery (large arrow).

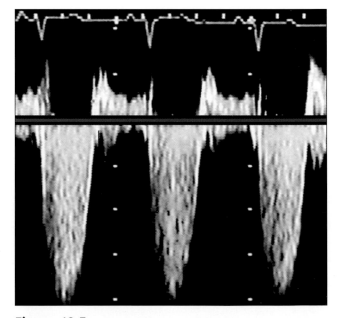

Figure 40.5
Continuous-wave Doppler spectral display across the pulmonary artery. The peak velocity is 4 m/s which predicts a peak gradient of 64 mmHg between the right ventricle and pulmonary artery.

Discussion

Two-dimensional echocardiography was rudimentary 30 years ago and not performed in this patient. Cardiomegaly, severe global left ventricular function and Q waves across the precordium in a newborn should suggest anomalous left coronary from the pulmonary artery. Echocardiography now allows for the non-invasive assessment of the proximal main pulmonary trunk and the proximal coronary arteries, which should be visualized and the direction of flow determined by color flow Doppler.[1] In the majority of newborns with this condition, the anomalous origin of the left coronary artery from the pulmonary trunk will be present with a single coronary artery arising from the right coronary sinus of Valsalva.[2] The treatment of this condition is early corrective surgery. When surgery is delayed in those who survive to 4–5 years, the likelihood of restitution of left ventricular function is seriously reduced, whereas left ventricular size and function can be expected to return to normal if corrective surgery is performed in the neonate. Late complications of early corrective surgery performed over two decades ago are dependent on the precise surgical procedure performed. In this patient, in whom surgery was performed 28 years before her current pregnancy, the construction of a side to side fistula with the aorta had established adequate left coronary flow to the myocardium, but the pulmonary artery was compromised and narrowed. As the patient grew, the pulmonary artery twisted along its long axis and became progressively distorted which partially obstructed flow in the main pulmonary trunk.

The diagnosis of pulmonary hypertension was difficult to reconcile with the harsh upper parasternal ejection systolic murmur, which suggested right-sided outflow tract obstruction. The pulmonary valve looked normal by echocardiography and the dilated right heart chambers and the high peak velocity of the tricuspid regurgitant jet suggested equivalent elevation of right ventricular and pulmonary artery pressures. Only visualization of the proximal main pulmonary artery allowed the correct diagnosis of severe suprapulmonary stenosis to be established. It is therefore critically important to examine both right heart chambers and the right-sided great artery (usually pulmonary artery) to exclude right-sided outflow tract obstruction. The gradient between the right ventricle and right atrium was 88 mmHg, while the gradient between the right ventricle and the pulmonary artery was 64 mmHg. Thus, the pressure in the pulmonary artery distal to the stenosis was 24 mmHg plus the right atrial pressure, which was estimated at 15 mmHg. The patient did not have severe pulmonary hypertension.

The patient was followed with serial monthly two-dimensional echocardiograms which showed no deterioration in right ventricular function and no change in the systolic gradient in her main pulmonary trunk. She completed an uneventful pregnancy, delivered a normal female baby vaginally at term and is to undergo elective patch enlargement of her main pulmonary artery. Balloon angioplasty is contraindicated because of the risk of compromising her left coronary artery flow via the fistula, which lies between the main pulmonary artery and the ascending aorta.

References

1. Takeshita S, Yamaguchi T, Kuwako K, *et al.* Anomalous origin of the left coronary artery from the pulmonary artery: direct assessment of anomalous and collateral coronary flow by pulsed Doppler echocardiography. Cathet Cardiovasc Diagn 1992;27:220–2.

2. Jureidini SB, Nouri S, Crawford CJ, *et al.* Reliability of echocardiography in the diagnosis of anomalous origin of the left coronary artery from the pulmonary trunk. Am Heart J 1991;122:61–8.

SECTION IV

The Left Atrium

41

Interatrial septal aneurysm

Jorge R Kizer MD
Susan E Wiegers MD

A 28-year-old woman developed the sudden onset of incoherent speech and right hemiplegia. She had no remarkable medical or surgical history. She had been taking oral contraceptives for many years. Her family history was unremarkable and she had no history of migraines or other neurological disorders.

On presentation to the emergency room her neurological examination was remarkable for a receptive aphasia and right hemiplegia. Computed tomography scan of the head revealed a left frontotemporal hypodensity consistent with an acute stroke. A thrombotic occlusion of the origin of the left middle cerebral artery was present on angiography. This patient was not a candidate for thrombolytic therapy because of a delay in presentation which exceeded 3 hours. Hospital workup for hypercoagulable states including pregnancy was negative. Lower extremity ultrasound Doppler examination was negative for deep venous thrombosis. She was managed with systemic anticoagulation and was discharged to a rehabilitation facility after a 10-day hospital stay. A transthoracic echocardiogram during her hospitalization was a poor-quality study. A transesophageal echocardiogram was performed to evaluate for a cardioembolic source.

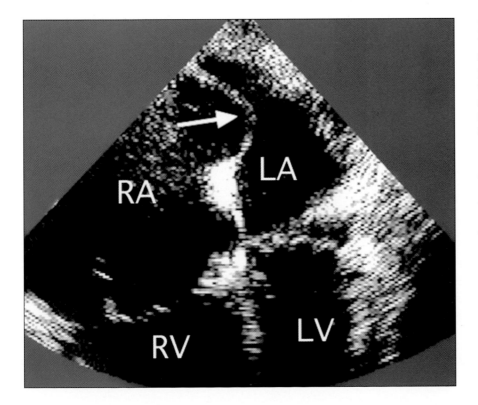

Figure 41.1
Transesophageal echocardiogram from the mid-esophageal level transverse plane (imaging angle 0°) of a modified four-chamber view. The interatrial septum (arrow) bulges into the left atrium. The base of the interatrial septal aneurysm measures over 1.5 cm. In addition, the depth of the aneurysm is also more than 1.5 cm. This is consistent with the diagnosis of interatrial septal aneurysm. Although the right atrium (RA) and right ventricle (RV) appear slightly enlarged in this view, this is due to the rightward angulation of the transducer.

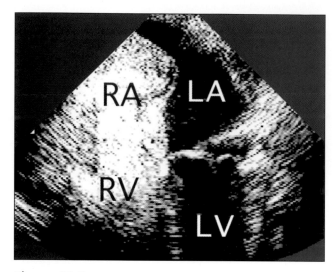

Figure 41.2
Transesophageal echocardiogram from a similar view after the intravenous injection of agitated saline. Ten milliliters of saline is agitated with 0.25 ml of air between 10-ml syringes connected by a three-way stopcock. After approximately five to 10 passes, the saline becomes cloudy. It is then injected into the vein and provides prompt opacification of the right side of the heart. These microbubbles are too large to cross the pulmonary circulation and are not normally seen in the left-sided heart chambers. In this view full opacification of the right atrium has been achieved. The bubbles have not yet crossed the tricuspid valve orifice into the right ventricle. The outline of the interatrial septal aneurysm is well delineated by the contrast. There is no definite evidence of microbubbles in the left atrium (LA) or left ventricle (LV).

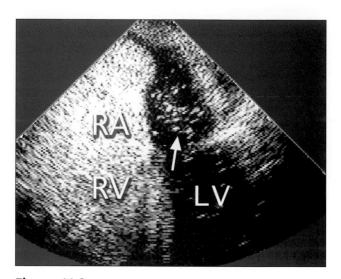

Figure 41.3
The patient performed a Valsalva maneuver with the next contrast injection. In this view, opacification of the right atrium and right ventricle by the microbubbles are well seen. After the release of the Valsalva maneuver the microbubbles are seen to have crossed the interatrial septum and are present in the left atrium (arrow). This finding is consistent with a patent foramen ovale which is associated with interatrial septal aneurysms.

Discussion

An interatrial septal aneurysm occurs when the interatrial septum underlying the area of the fossa ovalis is redundant and protrudes excessively into either atrial cavity.[1] While the degree of excursion required for classification has been arbitrary and variable in the literature, there is increasing consensus that a 15-mm displacement of a 15-mm base provides a criterion of high specificity.[2] Estimates on the prevalence of interatrial septal aneurysms in the general population have been as high as 1% in autopsy series[3] to 2.2% in a randomly selected cohort.[2] They are often considered incidental findings, although an association has been found with mitral valve prolapse.[4] Interatrial septal aneurysms may not be visible by transthoracic echocardiography. Because the interatrial septum is in the far field and is parallel to the ultrasound beam in the apical four chamber view, it may be difficult to delineate the anatomy of the interatrial septum. A highly mobile interatrial septal aneurysm may be mistaken for an atrial mass. Transesophageal echocar-

diography is often required to make the diagnosis. An interatrial septal aneurysm is associated with the presence of a patent foramen ovale, which may be diagnosed by color flow Doppler imaging or contrast injection.

Studies have demonstrated an association between interatrial septal aneurysm and stroke, particularly in young patients.[2] However, the risk of stroke conferred by this finding has not been prospectively evaluated. The prevalence of a coexisting communication either in the form of fenestrations of the interatrial septum or of a patent foramen ovale have ranged from 56 to 90%.[2,5] A possible stroke mechanism is paradoxical embolus through the interatrial communication. In addition, a thrombus may form in the cusp of the interatrial septal aneurysm with subsequent embolization. Studies have provided markedly different assessments of the importance of interatrial septal aneurysm in the risk of embolic cerebral vascular ischemic events.[6,7] The Lausanne stroke study showed a very low risk of recurrent stroke in patients with interatrial septal aneurysm as their only risk factor for cerebral embolic events.[6] In any case, it is very rare to see a thrombus within the interatrial septal aneurysm. In this patient it is possible that the combination of a hypercoagulable state conferred by oral contraceptives perhaps associated with either paradoxical embolus or thrombus formation within the interatrial septal aneurysm can be evoked to explain the embolic cardiovascular accident.

References

1. Belkin R, Kisslo J. Atrial septal aneurysm: Recognition and clinical relevance. Am Heart J 1990;120:948–57.

2. Agmon Y, Khanderia B, Meissner I, *et al.* Frequency of atrial septal aneurysms in patients with cerebral ischemic events. Circulation 1999;99:1942–4.

3. Silver M, Dorsey J. Aneurysms of the septum primum in adults. Arch Pathol Lab Med 1978;102:62–5.

4. Rahko P, Xu Q. Increased prevalence of atrial septal aneurysm in mitral valve prolapse. Am J Cardiol 1990;66:235–7.

5. Belkin R, Hurwitz B, Kisslo J. Atrial septal aneurysm: Association with cerebrovascular and peripheral embolic events. Stroke 1997;18:856–62.

6. Bogousslavsky J, Garazi S, Jeanrenaud X, *et al.* Stroke recurrence in patients with patent foramen ovale: the Lausanne Study. Lausanne Stroke with Paradoxical Embolism Study Group. Neurology 1996;46:1301–5.

7. IlerciL A, Meisner JS, Vijayaraman P, *et al.* Clinical significance of fossa ovalis membrane aneurysm in adults with cardioembolic cerebral ischemia. Am J Cardiol 1997;80:96–8.

42

Lipomatous hypertrophy of the interatrial septum

Susan E Wiegers MD

An elderly patient with a history of coronary artery disease and progressive aortic stenosis underwent combined coronary artery bypass grafting and aortic valve replacement. The patient had been experiencing exertional angina and dyspnea but had no history of arrhythmias or palpitations. Transesophageal echocardiography was performed during the procedure to monitor left ventricular function and the competency of the valve replacement.

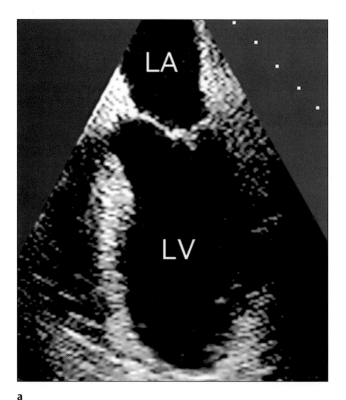

a

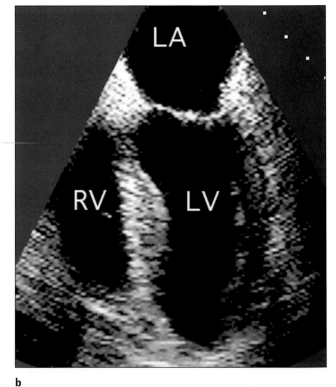

b

Figure 42.1
(a) Transesophageal four-chamber view from the mid-esophageal level in the transverse plane (imaging angle 0°). In this late diastolic frame the mitral valve has closed and the left atrium is slightly enlarged. The left ventricular cavity is enlarged. In this view the apex of the left ventricle is foreshortened as it typically is in transesophageal imaging.
(b) Similar transesophageal view in systole. Comparison of the endocardial borders with the diastolic frame indicates thickening of the lateral wall and proximal septum. The distal septum, however, maintains the deformation it exhibited in diastole and the wall appears thinned. The patient had sustained an anteroapical myocardial infarction in the past. The right ventricle is also mildly dilated in this systolic image consistent with decreased right ventricular function.

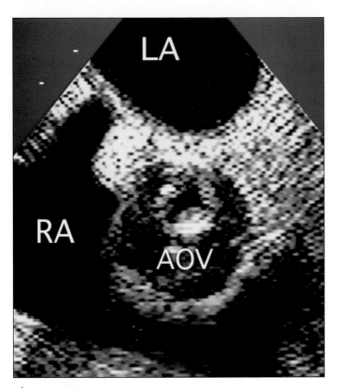

Figure 42.2
Transesophageal short-axis view of the aortic valve from the high esophageal level (imaging angle 40°). The valve (AOV) is heavily calcified and no definite orifice could be seen. The patient had senile calcific aortic stenosis on an anatomically normal tricuspid valve. However, the dense calcification has obscured the normal architecture and made delineation of the separate cusps impossible. Note the mass projecting from the interatrial septum into the right atrium.

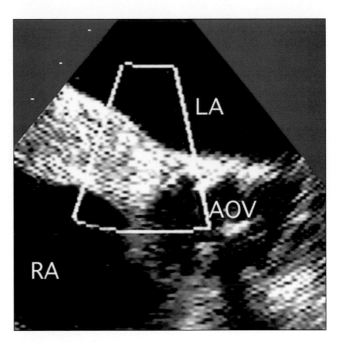

Figure 42.3
Close-up transesophageal view of the interatrial septum and aortic valve from the same transducer position as in Figure 42.2. The interatrial septum, identified between the left (LA) and right (RA) atria is thickened, measuring approximately 2 cm. The gain settings are high in this image but the septum appears echodense and refractile with a heterogeneous pattern that contains multiple septations surrounding very small, more echolucent areas. This appearance is consistent with adipose tissue.

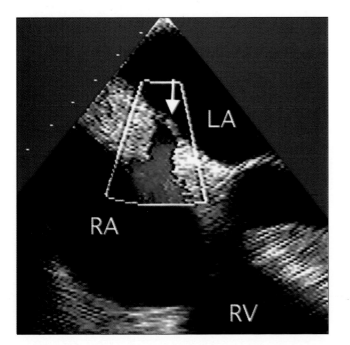

Figure 42.4
The nature of the interatrial septal thickening is diagnosed with further imaging of the septum. With the probe in the transverse plane (imaging angle 0°), the transducer is advanced slightly and rotated to the right. The entire interatrial septum is visualized. Two areas of marked thickening are present but the fossa ovalis (arrow) is spared and appears to be normal. Low-velocity flow is seen with the color flow Doppler imaging with no evidence of interatrial shunt flow. The process that involves the interatrial septum on either side of the fossa ovalis is identical, although the cephalad interatrial septum is somewhat thicker than the more proximal septum.

Discussion

The patient had calcific aortic stenosis and coronary artery disease which required surgical intervention. The transesophageal images demonstrated critical aortic obstruction and moderately decreased left ventricular function due to a previous myocardial infarction. An incidental finding on the transesophageal study was lipomatous hypertrophy of the interatrial septum. The classic pattern of distribution of the fatty infiltration, sparing the fossa ovalis, distinguishes this entity from other much rarer causes of interatrial septal thickening. Metastatic tumors may rarely involve the septum and amyloid heart disease may result in thickening of all of the atrial walls including the atrial septum.

On transthoracic imaging the sparing of the fossa ovalis leads to the typical 'dumb-bell' shape which is best appreciated in the four-chamber view or the subcostal view of the atrial septum. Visualization of this pattern is diagnostic of lipomatous hypertrophy and obviates the need for any further imaging. At times, massive lipomatous hypertrophy may obscure the area of the fossa, raising concern of a right atrial tumor. In this unusual instance, transesophageal echocardiography may be necessary to image the area of the fossa ovalis and demonstrate its freedom from infiltration. The lipomatous infiltration does not protrude into the left atrium and lipomatous hypertrophy is not a viable explanation for a left atrial mass.

Significant lipomatous hypertrophy of the atrial septum is defined as a thickening greater than 2 cm. Histological examination of surgically obtained specimens has revealed multivacuolated fat and atypical hypertrophied myocytes in many.[1] Lipomatous hypertrophy is associated with increasing age, body mass and the thickness of the adipose tissue in the atrioventricular groove.[2] The etiology of the entity and the exact nature of the lipomatous hypertrophy is not known. Lipomatous hypertrophy can be distinguished from a lipoma by the lack of a defined capsule. The condition is thought to be associated with atrial arrhythmias but this may be due to testing bias. The indications for surgery are very controversial and obstruction to flow is rarely present.[3] Nevertheless, surgical resection of massively thickened septa due to fatty infiltration has been reported. The surgery may require reconstruction of the septum and a portion of the atrial wall.[4,5] There is no evidence that surgical resection will reduce the incidence of atrial arrhythmias.

References

1. Burke A, Litovsky S, Virmani R. Lipomatous hypertrophy of the atrial septum presenting as a right atrial mass. Am J Surg Pathol 1996;20:678–85.

2. Shirani J, Roberts W. Clinical, electrocardiographic and morphologic features of massive fatty deposits ('lipomatous hypertrophy') in the atrial septum. J Am Coll Cardiol 1993;22:226–38.

3. Zeebregts C, Hensens A, Timmermans J, et al. Lipomatous hypertrophy of the interatrial septum: indication for surgery? Eur J Cardio-Thorac Surg 1997;11:785–7.

4. Oxron D, Edelist G, Goldman B, et al. Echocardiography and excision of lipomatous hypertrophy of the interatrial septum. Ann Thorac Surg 1999;67:852–4.

5. Alcocer J, Datz W, Hattler B. Surgical treatment of lipomatous hypertrophy of the interatrial septum. Ann Thorac Surg 1998;65:1784–6.

43

Impending paradoxical embolism

Elizabeth A Tarka MD

A 62-year-old woman with colon cancer presented to her primary care physician's office complaining of left hand clumsiness. She also reported episodes of slurred speech and right hand paresthesias. Each episode resolved completely within one hour of the onset of symptoms. Physical and neurological examinations were unremarkable. She was admitted to the hospital and computed tomography of the head was normal. Aspirin and heparin were started. Further evaluation included a normal carotid ultrasound examination. A transthoracic echocardiogram revealed a mobile biatrial mass and a transesophageal echocardiogram was performed. Owing to the nature of the right atrial mass, lower extremity venous duplex study was performed and revealed bilateral femoral deep venous thromboses.

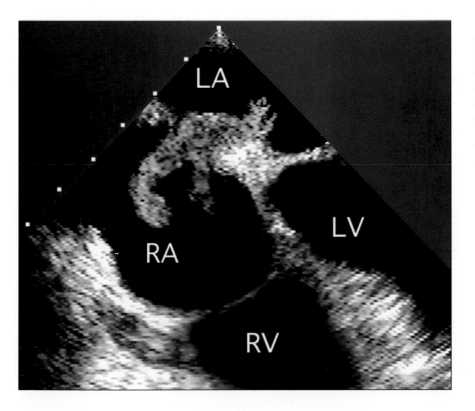

Figure 43.1
Transesophageal four-chamber view at the mid-esophageal level (imaging angle 0°). A mass is present in the right atrium (RA) and extends into the left atrium (LA). It appears to be one continuous structure that straddles the interatrial septum at the level of the fossa ovalis. In real time, both the right and left atrial masses were highly mobile.

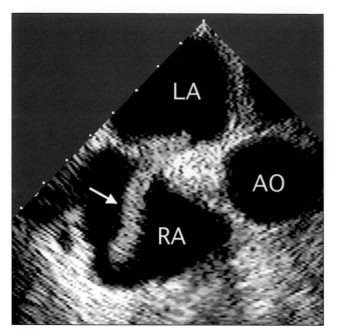

Figure 43.2
Transesophageal echocardiogram from the high esophageal level in the transverse plane (imaging angle 0°). The proximal ascending aorta (AO) in short axis is normal. The mass (arrow) is present in the right atrium (RA) and traverses the interatrial septum. The mass appeared discrete and did not originate from either vena cava.

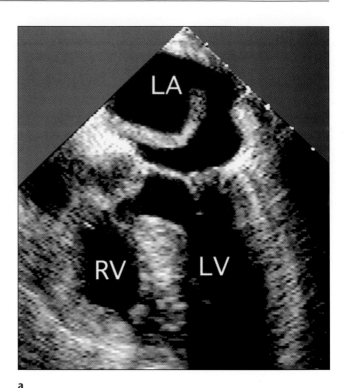

a

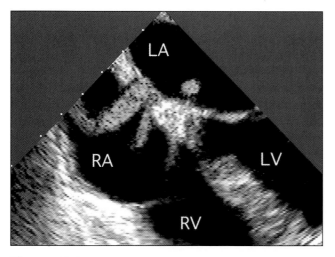

Figure 43.3
Transesophageal four-chamber view at the mid-esophageal level in the transverse plane (imaging angle 0°). During diastole, the mass is seen in the right atrium and is obviously attached to the interatrial septum. Also, visualized in the left atrium, is an echodensity which appears to be a separate mass. There was chaotic motion of the left atrial mass and the lobes of the right atrial mass.

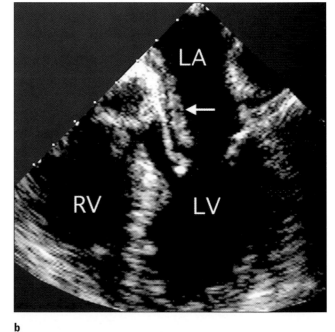

b

Figure 43.4
(a) Transesophageal echocardiogram at the mid-esophageal level with anteflexion. From this systolic image, it is clear that the left atrial mass seen in Figure 43.3 is actually one long structure that is attached to the interatrial septum. The left atrium (LA) and left ventricle (LV) are normal.
(b) During diastole, the mass (arrow) courses along the anterior leaflet of the mitral valve and prolapses across the valve orifice.

Discussion

Paradoxical embolism was first described by Connheim in 1877 and refers to the embolic entry of a venous thrombus into the systemic circulation through a right to left shunt.[1] In order for this to occur, an abnormal communication between the right and left circulations and a favorable pressure gradient promoting right to left shunting must be present. Before the advent of echocardiography, impending paradoxical embolism was diagnosed predominantly on postmortem examination. The main clinical clue is the presence of a pulmonary embolus in association with a systemic embolus. In 1985, the first case of echocardiographic identification of an impending paradoxical embolism was reported.[2] The development of non-invasive strategies using echocardiography to define interatrial communications have facilitated the diagnosis of paradoxical embolism. A recommended strategy in evaluating patients with an arterial embolism includes a transthoracic echocardiogram with contrast and provocative maneuvers. If the results are unrevealing, a contrast transesophageal echocardiogram should be performed if clinically indicated.[3]

Once the diagnosis of impending paradoxical embolism is made, systemic anticoagulation is the initial therapy to reduce future embolic events. Emergency intracardiac embolectomy with closure of a patent foramen ovale is recommended in all surgical candidates.[3] This patient had surgery and the thrombus was successfully removed. The patent foramen ovale was closed and the postoperative course was uneventful. She was anticoagulated and discharged on the fourth postoperative day.

References

1. Loscalzo J. Paradoxical embolism: clinical presentation, diagnostic strategies, and therapeutic options. Am Heart J 1986;112:141–5.

2. Nellesen U, Daniel WG, Matheis G. Impending paradoxical embolism from atrial thrombus: correct diagnosis by transesophageal echocardiography and prevention by surgery. J Am Coll Cardiol 1985;5:1002–4.

3. Meachem III RR, Headley A, Bronze M, *et al.* Impending paradoxical embolism. Arch Intern Med 1988;158:438–48.

44

Secundum atrial septal defect

Susan E Wiegers MD
Martin St John Sutton MBBS

A 37-year-old woman, 16 weeks pregnant, developed recurrent palpitations associated with near syncope. She went to the emergency room where an electrocardiogram revealed atrial fibrillation with a heart rate of 160 bpm, right bundle branch block, right axis deviation, and right ventricular hypertrophy. She had no history or symptoms of heart disease and no family history of congenital heart disease. A chest X-ray was recovered from 4 years previously taken following a motor vehicle accident and demonstrated mild cardiomegaly. She had recently noted exercise intolerance and mild dyspnea but had ascribed these symptoms to pregnancy. She was treated with intravenous digitalis and beta-adrenergic receptor blockers and reverted to sinus rhythm.

On examination she had an elevated jugular venous pressure with a 'v' wave, a parasternal lift, a widely split second heart sound with augmentation of the pulmonary component and a low-frequency diastolic murmur at the lower left sternal border. These clinical findings suggested an atrial septal defect with moderate pulmonary hypertension and tricuspid regurgitation. She was advised to consider termination of the pregnancy because of the presence of pulmonary hypertension and the associated risk to the fetus and herself. However, she decided to continue with the pregnancy but agreed to stop work and rest.

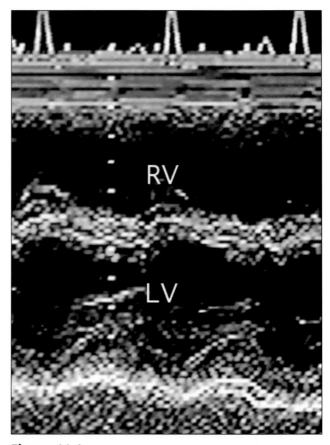

Figure 44.1
M-mode electrocardiogram from the parasternal position of the right ventricle and left ventricle at the level of the mitral valve chords. The left ventricle is normal in size with normal systolic function, as evidenced by the normal fractional shortening. The right ventricle, however, is dilated and the right ventricular free wall is hypertrophied.

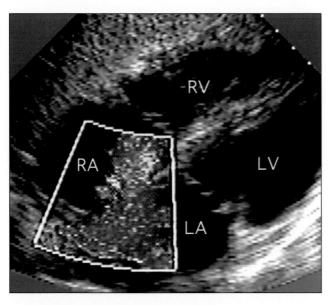

a

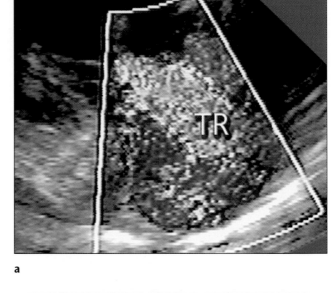

a

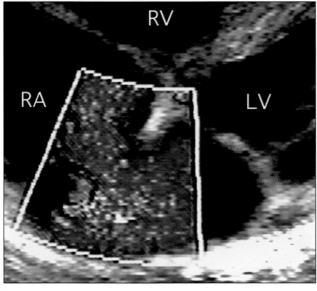

b

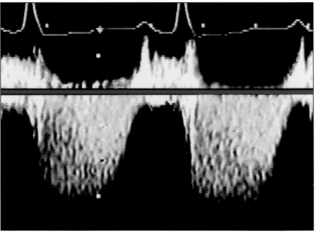

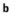

b

Figure 44.2
(a) Subcostal view of the four-chambers of the heart with color flow Doppler imaging. The right ventricle is dilated. The hypertrophy of the right ventricular free wall is not well seen in this image. A large color jet crosses the interatrial septum from the left atrium into the right atrium through an atrial septal defect. The defect is in the mid-septum in the region of the fossa ovalis which is diagnostic of a secundum atrial septal defect.
(b) Close-up image of the secundum defect. The color Doppler jet measures approximately 1.9 cm as it crosses the septum. This represents a large atrial septal defect with significant left to right shunt flow.

Figure 44.3
(a) Parasternal right ventricular inflow view with color flow Doppler imaging in systole. The right atrium and ventricle are dilated. A jet of moderate tricuspid regurgitation (TR) arises from the level of the tricuspid valve and fills a significant portion of the right atrium in this view. The tricuspid regurgitation jet is turbulent and of relatively high velocity.
(b) Spectral display of continuous-wave Doppler from the apical position across the tricuspid valve. The tricuspid regurgitation is the systolic signal below the baseline with a peak velocity of approximately 3 m/s. This predicts the gradient between the right atrium and the right ventricle of 36 mmHg using the modified Bernoulli equation. Assuming a right atrial pressure of 10 mmHg, the peak pulmonary artery systolic pressure is 46 mmHg, consistent with moderate pulmonary hypertension.

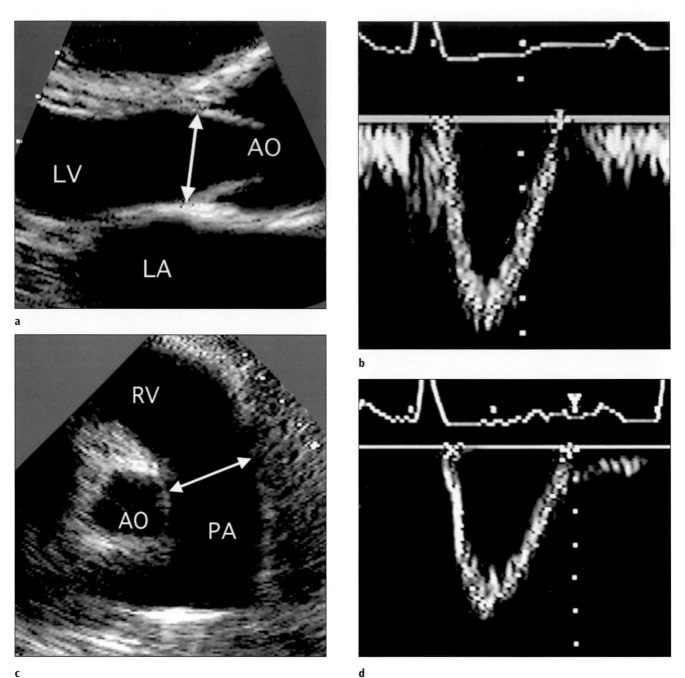

a

b

c

d

Figure 44.4

(a) Measurement of pulmonary flow to systemic flow ratio (Qp/Qs). Close-up of the left ventricular outflow tract from the parasternal long axis. The outflow tract diameter is measured immediately below the aortic valve leaflets and is rounded to the nearest millimeter. In this image the diameter of the outflow tract is 2.0 cm.

(b) Spectral display of pulsed-wave Doppler from the apical position in systole. The sample volume has been placed in the left ventricular outflow tract, immediately below the aortic valve leaflets. The velocity time integral (VTI) is the area under the curve of the spectral envelope and can be digitized on-line with most ultrasound systems. (Vertical calibration mark = 20 cm/s; horizontal calibration mark = 200 m/s) The VTI was 24 cm.

(c) Parasternal short-axis view at the level of the base of the heart. The pulmonary artery is enlarged. The diameter is measured 1 cm distal to the pulmonary valve leaflets, which are not well demonstrated in this image. The diameter measured 2.9 cm. The enlarged right main pulmonary artery branch passes posteriorly to the aortic root.

(d) Spectral display of pulsed-wave Doppler from the same transducer position as in Figure 44.4c. The sample volume has been placed at the same level in the pulmonary artery where the diameter was measured. The VTI was 33 cm. Note the scale is different from that in Figure 44.4b, although the calibration marks represent the same values.

Discussion

This patient had a large secundum atrial septal defect with a significant left to right shunt which had been present since birth. Atrial septal defects are the most common congenital abnormality seen in adults after bicuspid aortic valves. Even large atrial septal defects are generally well tolerated and asymptomatic into adulthood. Although the ratio of pulmonary flow to systemic flow can be very high, it is generally in the range of 2 : 1 to 5 : 1. The left to right shunt creates a 'useless circuit' of blood flow which traverses the atrial septal defect, the right atrium through the tricuspid valve to the right ventricle, through the pulmonary artery and the pulmonary circulation. The blood empties into the left atrium through the pulmonary veins and then crosses again to the right atrium. Eventually, the right atrium and ventricle dilate under the volume load. Mild pulmonary hypertension is common, although Eisenmenger's syndrome is relatively unusual.

Echocardiography is an extremely sensitive tool for the diagnosis of atrial septal defects.[1] Off-axis views of the interatrial septum from the apical windows or from the subcostal windows usually best image the septum. The direction of shunt flow can also be measured from these views. Because the left atrial pressure is higher throughout most of the cardiac cycle in a normal patient, the shunt flow is predominately left to right. Elevation of the right atrial pressure from severe tricuspid regurgitation or from pulmonary hypertension may result in bidirectional shunting or a complete reversal of flow with development of cyanosis (Eisenmenger's syndrome). However, this is distinctly unusual. A transient right to left flow can be seen during the respiratory cycle in normal patients.

Quantification of the left to right shunt may be accomplished in several ways using echocardiography. The usual approach is to apply the continuity equation to the left ventricular outflow tract and pulmonary arteries to calculate stroke volumes. The ratio of the pulmonary stroke volume to the systemic stroke volume gives the shunt ratio or Qp/Qs. In an anatomically normal heart, the right-sided stroke volume is equal to the left-sided stroke volume. However, with an atrial septal defect and left to right shunting, the pulmonary stroke volume will be higher than the stroke volume through the left ventricular outflow tract. The stroke volume is calculated by the formula:

$$SV = CSA \times VTI$$

where SV is the stroke volume, CSA is the cross-sectional area and VTI is the velocity time integral of the spectral Doppler envelope taken at the level in which the cross-sectional area is measured. The cross-sectional area of the left ventricular outflow tract and the pulmonary artery may be calculated, assuming the circular geometry, from the diameters measured in the transthoracic studies. In calculating the shunt ratio, after cancelling equal terms, the formula is:

$$QP/QS = (D_{PA})^2 \times VTI_{PA}/(D_{LVOT})^2 \times VTI_{LVOT}$$

where D_{PA} and D_{LVOT} are the respective diameters of the pulmonary artery and left ventricular outflow tract. Substituting in the values obtained in this patient, Qp/Qs = $(2.9)^2 \times 33/(2.0)^2 \times 24$ which is equal to 2.9 : 1. In other words, the flow through the pulmonary circuit is 2.9 times greater than the flow through the systemic circuit. This Doppler echocardiographic method has demonstrated excellent correlation with invasive measurements of shunt flow.[2]

Closure of atrial septal defects may be accomplished in adults with very low operative mortality and is generally recommended if the shunt ratio is greater than 2 : 1 or 2.5 : 1.[3-5] The patient had serial echocardiograms at monthly intervals during the third trimester of pregnancy and 3 months postpartum. Her pulmonary artery systolic pressure peaked at 60 mmHg before labor and delivery but decreased to 45–50 by 3 months postpartum. She had a laparoscopic tubal ligation and is undergoing elective surgical closure of her secundum atrial septal defect. This patient did not undergo catheterization or further testing prior to surgery.

References

1. Mehta RH, Helmcke F, Nanda NC, *et al*. Uses and limitations of transthoracic echocardiography in the assessment of atrial septal defect in the adult. Am J Cardiol 1991;67:288–94.

2. Dittmann H, Jacksch R, Voelker W, *et al*. Accuracy of Doppler echocardiography in quantification of left to right shunts in adult patients with atrial septal defect. J Am Coll Cardiol 1988;11:338–42.

3. Shibata Y, Abe T, Kuribayashi R, *et al*. Surgical treatment of isolated secundum atrial septal defect in patients more than 50 years old. Ann Thorac Surg 1996;62:1096–9.

4. Horvath KA, Burke RP, Collins JJ Jr, *et al*. Surgical treatment of adult atrial septal defect: early and long-term results. J Am Coll Cardiol 1992;20:1156–9.

5. Gatzoulis MA, Redington AN, Somerville J, *et al*. Should atrial septal defects in adults be closed? Ann Thorac Surg 1996;61:657–9.

45

Partial atrioventricular canal defect

Martin St John Sutton MBBS
Susan E Wiegers MD

A 40-year-old woman complained of increased dyspnea over a 6-month period so that she could no longer climb a flight of stairs or do her household chores without having to stop and rest. She had suffered from bronchial asthma since early childhood but her recent reduction in exercise tolerance was not associated with any bronchospasm. Four months before presentation, she suddenly developed rapid palpitations for which she went to her local emergency room. For the first time, she was found to be in atrial fibrillation. The chest X-ray showed an enlarged heart and increased pulmonary vascularity suggestive of an intracardiac shunt. She was treated with oral anticoagulants and digitalis and reverted to sinus rhythm but continued to have short paroxysms of atrial fibrillation.

Physical examination revealed an obese women with an oxygen saturation of 92% in room air without clubbing or cyanosis. She had an elevated jugular venous pressure with a prominent 'v' wave. Systolic blood pressure was normal and she was in atrial fibrillation. Her apical impulse was not located, on account of her body habitus, but there was a mild right ventricular lift indicative of right ventricular predominance. There was an apical pansystolic murmur of moderate mitral regurgitation and a softer pansystolic murmur at the lower sternal border. The pulmonary component of the second heart sound was loud, consistent with increased pulmonary artery systolic pressure. An electrocardiogram revealed sinus rhythm, left axis deviation, and right bundle branch block.

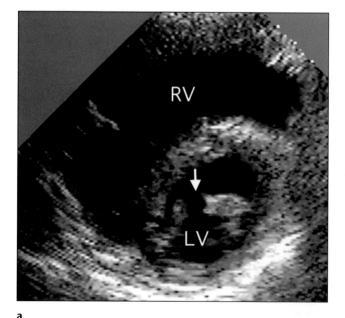

a

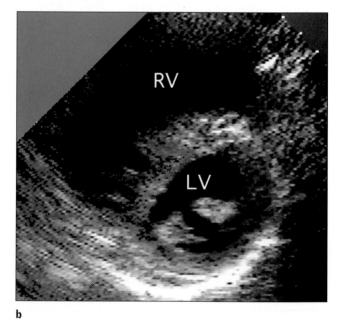

b

Figure 45.1
(a) Parasternal short-axis view at the level of the mitral valve leaflets in diastole. There is marked right ventricular hypertrophy and the right ventricle is enlarged. The interventricular septum is slightly flattened. There is a large cleft (arrow) in the anterior mitral valve leaflet. The anterior leaflet is thickened and the posterior leaflet is not well seen.
(b) Similar view in systole. The cleft in the anterior mitral valve leaflet is still visible. The interventricular septum remains flattened and the right ventricular systolic function is severely decreased.

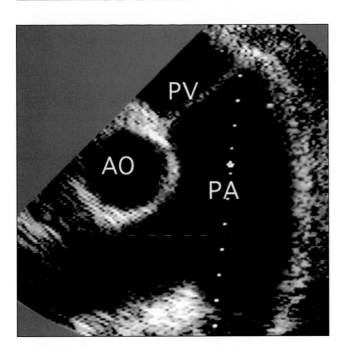

Figure 45.2
Parasternal short-axis view at the base of the heart. The pulmonary artery and its branches are seen in long axis. They are markedly dilated. The pulmonary valve (PV) appears anatomically normal, but there was moderate pulmonary regurgitation demonstrated by color flow Doppler (not shown).

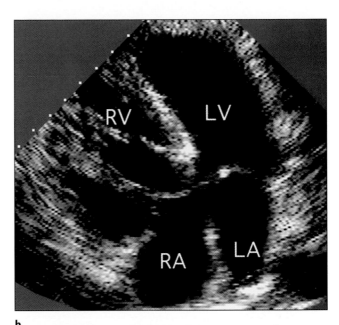
b

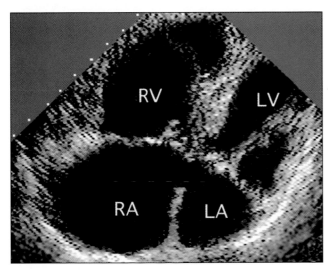
a

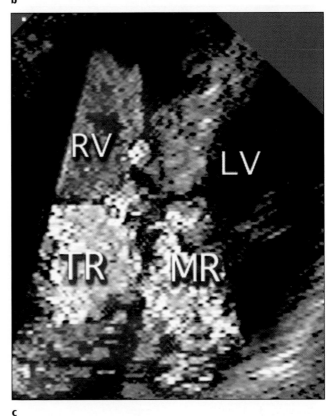
c

Figure 45.3
(a) A modified apical four-chamber view with the transducer placed medial to the true apex. The right heart chambers are enlarged and the right ventricle is hypertrophied. A defect of the primum interatrial septum is clearly visible. The mitral and tricuspid annuli are coplanar.
(b) A more standard apical four-chamber view. The transducer has been moved towards the patient's left and is now over the left ventricular apex. The septal leaflets of both the mitral and tricuspid valves are attached to the crest of the interventricular septum. The interventricular septum is intact and no ventricular septal defect is present.
(c) Similar view to that in (a), with color Doppler flow imaging showing moderate to severe mitral regurgitation (MR) and moderate tricuspid regurgitation (TR) in systole. Flow through the atrial septal defect is obscured by these two jets.

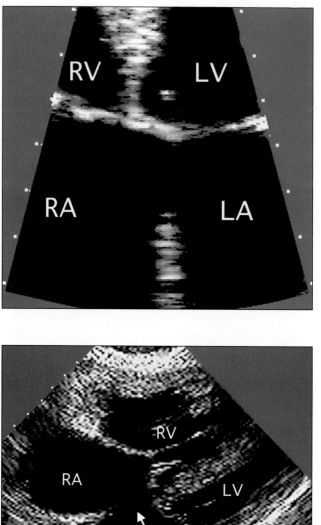

Figure 45.4
Close-up view of the crux of the heart from the apical four chamber view. The primum septum is absent, while the interventricular septum is intact. Both the mitral and the tricuspid valves arise at the same level from the interventricular septum.

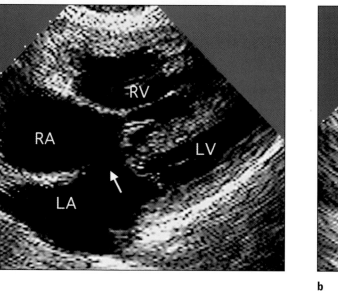

a

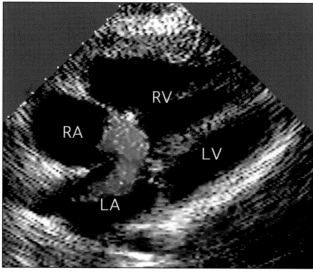

b

Figure 45.5
(a) Subcostal four chamber view in systole. The primum atrial septal defect (arrow) is at least 2 cm in diameter. The origin of the atrioventricular valves is again demonstrated.
(b) Similar view with color flow Doppler imaging. There is left to right flow across the atrial septal defect. Note the bowing of the interventricular septum into the left ventricle consistent with elevated right ventricular volume and pressure.

Discussion

This patient had previously undiagnosed congenital heart disease. The enlarged right heart chambers with the configuration of the ventricular septum indicated right ventricular pressure and volume overload and raised the question of an intracardiac shunt. The absence of the primum septum localized the level of the shunt, while color flow Doppler imaging determined the predominant direction of the shunt. Estimation of the right atrial–right ventricular pressure gradient enabled calculation of pulmonary artery systolic pressure. A cleft mitral valve is associated with partial and complete atrioventricular canal defects and must be looked for carefully in patients with this diagnosis. In addition, the interventricular septum must be interrogated to exclude a ventricular septal defect and establish the diagnosis as a partial rather than complete canal defect, as in this patient. The absence of the primum septum dictates that the septal leaflets of the two atrioventricular valves take origin from the ventricular septum at the same level.

Successful repair of this entity has been reported in adults who were previously undiagnosed.[1,2] Residual or recurrent mitral regurgitation is a significant long-term risk, and routine echocardiographic surveillance is recommended.[3] In patients who have undergone definitive repair in childhood, mitral valve abnormalities may cause symptoms in adulthood.

This patient underwent surgical repair, consisting of repair of the mitral valve cleft, and closure of the primum atrial septal defect. There was no residual mitral regurgitation on immediate postoperative transesophageal study.

The patient developed complete heart block in the immediate postoperative period, requiring pacemaker placement, but has recovered and returned to her usual activities.

References

1. Burke RP, Horvath K, Landzberg M, *et al*. Long-term follow-up after surgical repair of ostium primum atrial septal defects in adults. J Am Coll Cardiol 1996;27:696–9.

2. Abbruzzese PA, Napoleone A, Bini RM, *et al*. Late left atrioventricular valve insufficiency after repair of partial atrioventricular septal defects: anatomical and surgical determinants. Ann Thorac Surg 1990;49:111–14.

3. Barnett MG, Chopra PS, Young WP, Long-term follow-up of partial atrioventricular septal defect repair in adults. Chest 1988;94:321–4.

46

Sinus venosus atrial septal defect

Susan E Wiegers MD

A 40-year-old woman complained of palpitations, breathlessness and presyncope with vigorous exertion. She had not been aware of any cardiac problems but had not had access to regular medical care in her native country. On examination she had bilaterally clear lungs. There was a right ventricular heave. S1 was normal. The P2 component of S2 was loud and S2 was widely split and was fixed.

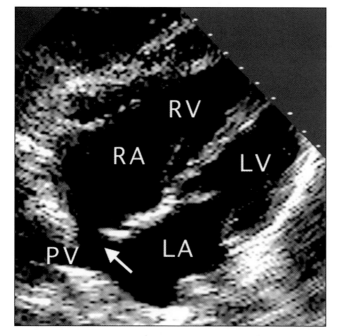

Figure 46.1
Subcostal view of the interatrial septum. The right atrium (RA) and right ventricle (RV) are dilated. The right ventricle is hypertrophied. A sinus venosus atrial septal defect (arrow) is seen in the interatrial septum. The defect measures over 1 cm in diameter in this view. The right inferior pulmonary vein (PV) inserts into the common area of the septal defect. The left atrium (LA) and left ventricle (LV) are of normal size.

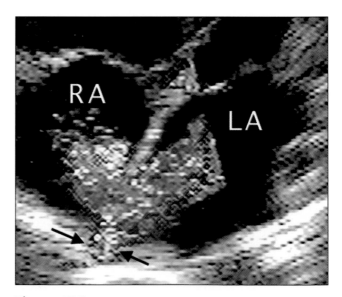

Figure 46.2
Close-up view of the distal interatrial septum with color flow Doppler imaging. The pulmonary venous inflow (arrows) from the right inferior vein is seen to enter both the left and the right atrium. The diagnosis of partial anomalous pulmonary venous return is confirmed by these images. The insertion of the inferior right vein is not imaged, but in this case was into the left atrium.

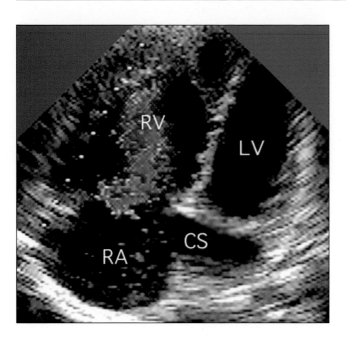

Figure 46.3
Off-axis apical view with posterior angulation of the transducer. The coronary sinus (CS) is imaged entering the right atrium. The coronary sinus is dilated, owing to the presence of a persistent left superior vena cava (not imaged) as well as elevated right-sided pressures. Pulmonary hypertension had developed in this patient due to the longstanding left to right shunt. Right-sided dilatation may occur in the setting of an interatrial shunt without pulmonary hypertension. However, coronary sinus dilatation would be expected only in the presence of elevated right atrial pressure.

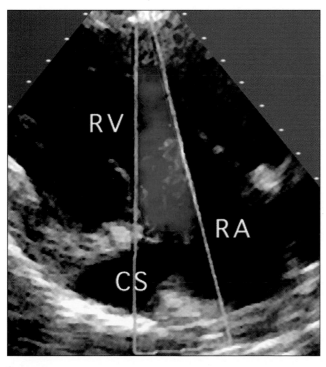

a

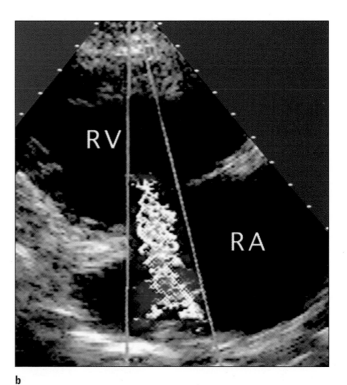

b

Figure 46.4
(a) Parasternal long-axis right ventricular inflow view with color Doppler imaging in diastole. The tricuspid valve leaflets are imaged in diastole with normal tricuspid valve inflow. The coronary sinus is seen entering the right atrium in the usual position but is once again seen to be severely dilated. Right atrial and ventricular dilatation are again appreciated.
(b) Systolic frame of the same view. A high-velocity turbulent jet of tricuspid regurgitation is seen arising from the level of the tricuspid valve and extending into the right atrium. The peak velocity of the jet was measured as 4.8 m/s (not shown), predicting a peak pulmonary artery pressure of 92 mmHg. Significant right ventricular dysfunction is appreciated from the comparison of the systolic and diastolic images.

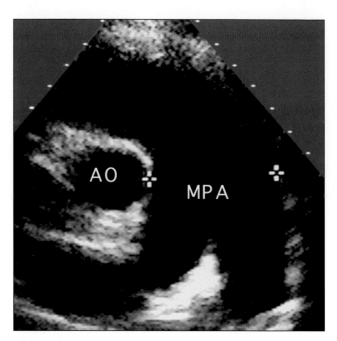

Figure 46.5
Parasternal short-axis view of the main pulmonary artery (MPA) and the proximal ascending aorta (AO). The pulmonary artery is normally the size of the aortic root. In this case it measures over 4.3 cm in diameter. The dilatation is due to the combined effects of the volume overload of the left to right shunt and ensuing pulmonary hypertension.

Discussion

Only 10% of atrial septal defects occur at the level of the sinus venosus. The embryology may differ from primum and secundum atrial septal defects. Some authorities believe this to be an abnormality of the superior vena caval insertion into the right atrium. Anomalous pulmonary venous return is associated only with this type of atrial septal defect. Some or all of the pulmonary veins may be displaced and insert into the superior or inferior vena cava. Even if the veins are in an anatomically normal position, the relationship between the defect and the venous insertion may allow passage of inflow to the right atrium. The size of the shunt flow from the left atrium to the right atrium depends on the size of the defect and the relative distensibility of the cardiac chambers.

Sinus venosus defects are the most commonly missed atrial septal defects because the lesion is in the far field of the image on transthoracic examination. Subcostal views are important in improving detection of the sinus venosus type of defect. Transesophageal echocardiography[1] and three-dimensional echocardiography[2] are also helpful. It is mandatory that all of the pulmonary veins be identified prior to surgical correction. The insertion of anomalous veins may be well outside the standard operative exposure. The short axis of the suprasternal notch view (see Chapter 25) may be very helpful in excluding partial anomalous pulmonary veins. Magnetic resonance imaging may be necessary to detect the veins in the thorax or abdominal cavity.

Persistent left superior vena cava is a generally benign lesion that occurs in isolation and in association with other congenital lesions. In the most common type, the right superior vena cava inserts normally into the right atrium. However, the fetal left superior vena cava does not involute but maintains its connection to the coronary sinus. The coronary sinus dilates, because of the increased flow. In this case the diagnosis of persistent left superior vena cava was confirmed by bilateral injection of agitated saline into the brachial veins. Injection in the right arm resulted in opacification of the right atrium with prompt appearance of contrast in the left atrium as well, owing to a small right to left shunt across the atrial septal defect. Injection of contrast into the left brachial vein resulted in the opacification of the coronary sinus prior to contrast appearing in the right or left atrium.

References

1. Pascoe RD, Oh JK, Warnes CA, *et al.* Diagnosis of sinus venosus atrial septal defect with transesophageal echocardiography. Circulation 1996;94:1049–55.

2. Lange A, Walayat M, Turnbull CM, *et al.* Assessment of atrial septal defect morphology by transthoracic three dimensional echocardiography using standard grey scale and Doppler myocardial imaging techniques: comparison with magnetic resonance imaging and intraoperative findings. Heart 1997;78:382–9.

47

Left atrial appendage thrombus

Susan E Wiegers MD

A 67-year-old man had sustained several myocardial infarctions. He had had documented episodes of paroxysmal atrial fibrillation but had not been anticoagulated, owing to chronic alcoholism. He presented with the acute onset of aphasia and left hemiparesis. His wife noted that he had complained of palpitations several days earlier but had seemed well until his neurological event. His cardiac examination was unremarkable. An electrocardiogram demonstrated normal sinus rhythm, inferior and septal Q waves. No hemorrhage was present on head computerized tomography scan. There was abrupt cut-off in the right middle cerebral artery on magnetic resonance angiogram which was felt to be consistent with a cardioembolic event. The transthoracic echocardiogram showed only decreased left ventricular systolic function and a dilated left atrium. A transesophageal echocardiogram was ordered to evaluate the source of the embolism.

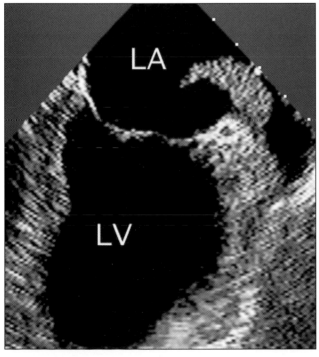

a

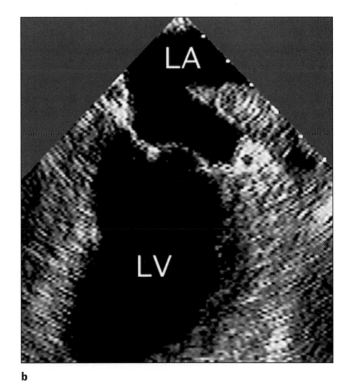

b

Figure 47.1
(a) Transesophageal echocardiogram from the mid-esophagus in the longitudinal plane (imaging angle 90°) in diastole. The left atrium (LA) is moderately dilated. A mobile mass (arrow) is seen to protrude into the left atrium from the atrial appendage, which is also dilated. The characteristics of this mass and its location are diagnostic of left atrial thrombus. The left ventricle (LV) is dilated.
(b) In systole, the mass has moved within the appendage, and the tip of the thrombus was highly mobile. Wall motion abnormalities of the inferior wall at the base (on the left of the screen) and the anterior wall at the base and mid-ventricular level (on the right of the screen) are evident in this systolic frame, representing the areas of his two previous infarctions.

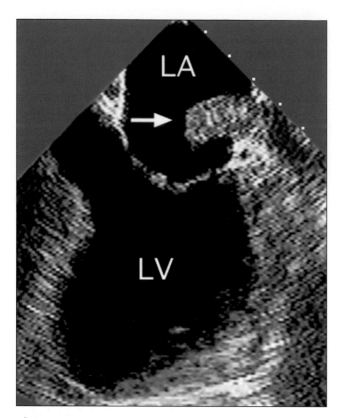

Figure 47.2
Transesophageal echocardiogram from the mid-esophagus in the transverse plane (imaging angle 0°) of a modified four-chamber view. The left atrial thrombus (arrow) is again seen to arise in the appendage and protrude into the left atrium (LA). The left ventricular outflow tract is visible between the anterior mitral valve leaflet and the left ventricular septum. Comparison of the postition of the thrombus in these two frames demonstrates that the thrombus was highly mobile.

Discussion

This patient with paroxysmal atrial fibrillation had a large left atrial thrombus that originated in the left atrial appendage but protruded into the left atrium. Although

recent technical advances in transthoracic echocardiography have allowed the visualization of the left atrium in more cases than previously, transesophageal echocardiography is still the definitive diagnostic test.[1] The differential diagnosis of this mass is limited, given the appearance of the mass and its location within the body of the appendage. The clinical setting was also highly consistent with atrial thrombus.

Atrial fibrillation increases the risk of cardiovascular accident by a factor of 5. The recurrence rate of stroke is extremely high, between 10 and 20% per year. The presence of left atrial appendage thrombus is associated with dense spontaneous contrast in the left atrium and decreased velocities in the appendage.[2] Appendage velocity can be measured most easily in the transesophageal study by placing the sample volume within the body of the appendage. In atrial fibrillation, there will be flow into and out of the appendage at irregular intervals. A low velocity probably reflects decreased atrial contractile function and must predispose to stagnation of blood within the appendage. A velocity of less than 0.3 m/s is associated with an increased risk of thrombus.[2]

This patient was anticoagulated with heparin followed by warfarin. He had several recurrent episodes of paroxysmal atrial fibrillation and was started on amiodarone for prophylaxis. It was thought, given his decreased left ventricular function present on echocardiography, that he would not tolerate procainamide or beta-blockers.

References

1. Omran H, Jung W, Rabahieh R, *et al.* Imaging of thrombi and assessment of left atrial appendage function: a prospective study comparing transthoracic and transesophageal echocardiography. Heart 1999;81:192–8.

2. Anonymous. Transesophageal echocardiographic correlates of thromboembolism in high-risk patients with nonvalvular atrial fibrillation. The Stroke Prevention in Atrial Fibrillation Investigators Committee on Echocardiography. Ann Intern Med 1998;128:639–47.

48

Left atrial myxoma

John Augoustides MD
Susan E Wiegers MD

A 65-year-old woman presented with fever and right-sided weakness. She also reported intermittent episodes of shortness of breath. She was otherwise well and reported no other neurological deficit. She had no peripheral stigmata of infective endocarditis. Her pulse was regular and a holodiastolic murmur was best heard at the cardiac apex and with radiation to the axilla. The rest of her cardiac examination was unremarkable. She had a right hemiplegia. Her laboratory studies were unremarkable and her electrocardiogram showed normal sinus rhythm. An echocardiogram was ordered to evaluate the murmur and to search for a cardiac source of embolus.

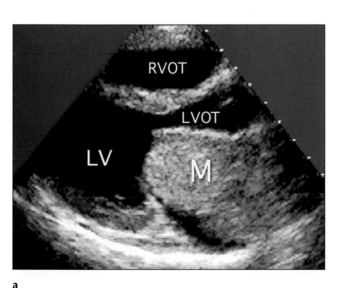

a

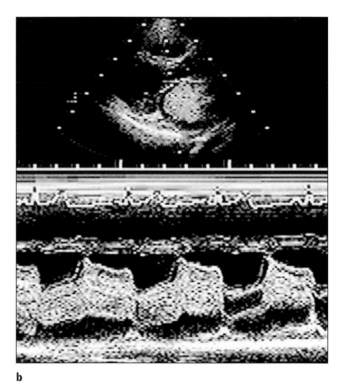

b

Figure 48.1
(a) Parasternal long-axis view in diastole. The left atrium is filled by a large mass (M) which appears to occlude the mitral valve orifice. The mass is heterogeneous and has a speckled pattern. It prolapsed into the mitral valve orifice in diastole and was slightly mobile within the left atrium. The left ventricular outflow tract (LVOT) appears slightly narrowed but there was no significant obstruction to outflow.
(b) M-mode echocardiogram from the parasternal position taken at the level of the mitral valve leaflets. The motion of the mitral valve is not normal and resembles that of mitral stenosis. However, the entire interleaflet area is filled by an echodensity that is consistent with an interatrial mass.

c

Figure 48.1

(c) Parasternal long-axis view in diastole with color Doppler flow imaging of mitral valve inflow. There is flow around the mass, but the turbulence of the jet is consistent with some degree of stenosis.

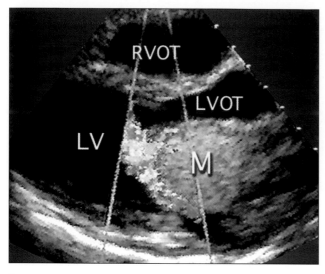

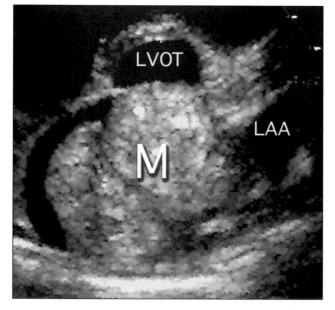

Figure 48.2

Off-axis parasternal short-axis view of the mass (M) which appears multilobulated with variations in the echodensity and demarcations within the mass itself. The attachment to the interatrial septum is not evident in this view although it was demonstrated in other views. The left atrial appendage (LAA) is enlarged, owing to the increased interatrial pressure. The off-axis angle has led to visualization of the left ventricular outflow tract (LVOT) rather than the aortic valve.

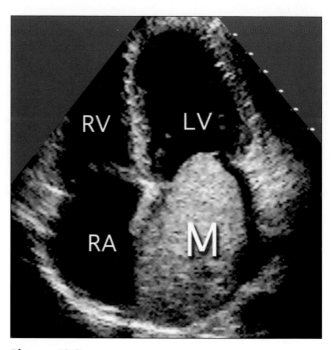

Figure 48.3

Apical four-chamber view of the mass (M) within the left atrium. The broad attachment to the interatrial septum can be appreciated in this view. However, for specific delineation of the origin of the mass, it is necessary to completely visualize the pulmonary veins and to exclude the origin of the mass from the pulmonary veins. Bronchogenic carcinomas may extend into the left atrium in some cases and simulate a myxoma. The right sided chambers are slightly dilated in this view due to the pulmonary hypertension which resulted from the functional mitral stenosis caused by the mass.

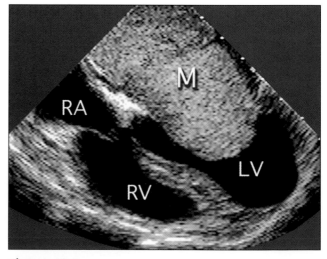

Figure 48.4

Transesophageal echocardiogram from the mid-esophageal level in the transverse plane (imaging angle 0°). The myxoma fills the left atrium and protrudes through the mitral valve in diastole into the left ventricular cavity. The mild dilatation of the right ventricle is again evident.

Discussion

The atrial myxoma was one of the first diagnoses made by M-mode echocardiography.[1] Myxomas account for approximately 40% of benign cardiac tumors with approximately 75% of these found in the left atrium. The transthoracic echocardiogram is diagnostic of atrial myxoma because of the appearance and behavior of the mass. The single mass is usually attached to the interatrial septum by a stalk. Only 6–8% of myxomas arise in the ventricles.

The consistency of a myxoma is gelatinous which can allow deformation throughout the cardiac cycle. Myxomas may be lobular but are rarely polypoid. Cystic echolucencies are characteristic and are detectable in about 25% of cases.[2] The size and mobility of a myxoma allows various degrees of prolapse through the mitral valve in diastole. The damage to the valve leaflet results from 'wrecking-ball' trauma rather than from any metastatic spread. Right atrial myxomas have also been reported to result in severe damage to the tricuspid valve by the same mechanism.[3] As myxomas increase in size to fill the left atrium, they cause progressive functional valvular stenosis with resultant pulmonary hypertension. Occasionally left atrial myxomas may also directly impede pulmonary venous inflow. Valvular regurgitation will vary from mild to severe. Tumor embolization has been reported to multiple organs and to the coronary arteries. Immediate surgical removal has been recommended, owing to the long-term potential for serious complications.[4] Reconstruction of the interatrial septum may be required if the attachment of the tumor is broad and sessile, rather than the more common stalk attachment.

Serial echocardiography is indicated in the long-term follow-up after surgery to detect recurrence, which may result from inadequate surgical resection or as part of a familial syndrome with a propensity to the development of myxomas. The familial syndrome is also associated with pigmented skin lesions and endocrine tumors.[5]

This patient's presentation is entirely explained by the left atrial myxoma. Tumor embolization accounted for her hemiplegia. The increasing degree of functional mitral stenosis caused exercise intolerance. She underwent cardiac surgery with removal of the tumor and bypass grafting of the right coronary artery which demonstrated an 80% lesion in the mid-vessel on preoperative coronary angiography.

References

1. Nomeir A. Watts L, Seagle R, et al. Intracardiac myxomas: twenty-year echocardiographic experience with review of the literature. J Am Soc Echocardiogr 1989;2:139–50.

2. Thier W, Schluter M, Krebber H. Cysts in left atrial myxomas identified by transesophageal cross-sectional echocardiography. Am J Cardiol 1983;51:1793–5.

3. Turlapati R, Jacobs L, Kotler M. Right atrial myxoma causing total destruction of the tricuspid valve leaflets. Am Heart J 1990;120:1227–31.

4. Reynen, K. Cardiac myxomas. N Engl J Med 1995;333:1610–17.

5. Vidaillet HJ, Seward J, Fyke FE, et al. Syndrome myxoma: a subset of patients with cardiac myxoma associated with pigmented skin lesions and peripheral and endocrine neoplasms. Br Heart J 1987;57:247–55.

49

Left atrial thrombus

Riti Patel MD

An elderly woman presented with multiple complaints, most notable for several episodes of severe presyncope. Three of these episodes had been associated with severe shortness of breath and had resolved when she lay down. She had had a St Jude's mechanical valve placed in the mitral position 6 years prior to presentation. There was no obvious cause for her symptoms found by history or physical examination, and subsequently the patient had a transthoracic echocardiogram to assess the valve function. The gradients across the prosthetic valve were normal. However, there was a suggestion of a left atrial abnormality. The images of the valve were technically limited and she underwent transesophageal echocardiography for further evaluation. Later, it was discovered that the patient had often been subtherapeutically anticoagulated.

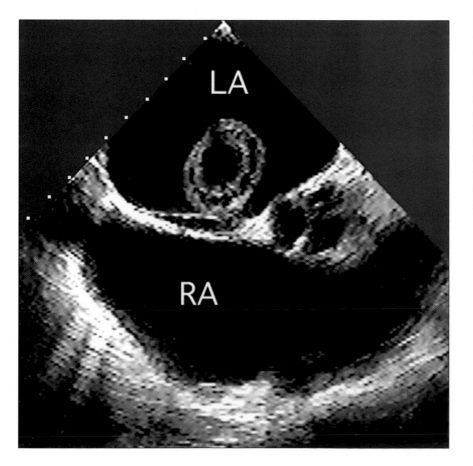

Figure 49.1
Transesophageal echocardiogram from the high esophageal level. There is biatrial enlargement. The aortic valve is imaged in short axis on the right of the image. There is a laminated round mass in the left atrium which measures 3 cm in diameter. The mass appears to have multiple layers surrounding a central area of lucency. Multiple frames fail to reveal a stalk or attachment to the left atrial wall. In fact, the mass moved freely around the left atrium.

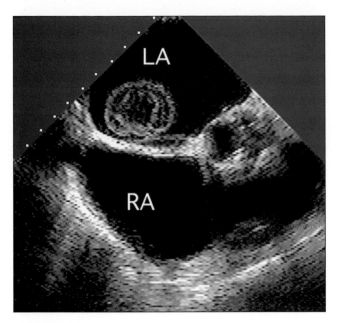

Figure 49.2
Similar view several frames later in the cardiac cycle. The mass rolled along the interatrial septum in a revolving motion with no evidence of attachment.

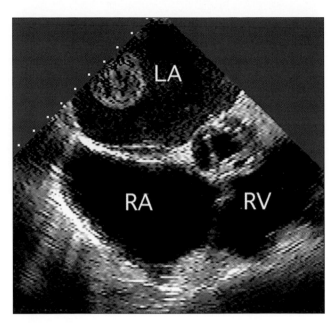

Figure 49.3
In this systolic frame, the mass is now in the center of the left atrial cavity where it continued to rotate slowly.

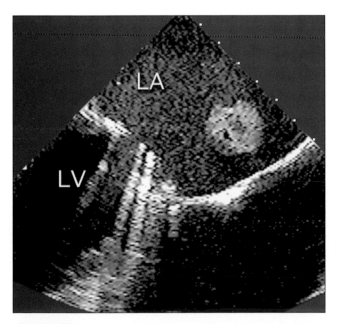

Figure 49.4
Image from the mid-esophagus in the longitudinal plane (imaging angle 90°). The mass is now near the anterior left atrial wall. The prosthetic valve is open in diastole and both leaflets are visualized. There is dense spontaneous echo contrast in the left atrium, which is consistent with low flow.

Images from the transesophageal echocardiogram show a circular, mobile mass consistent with thrombus. When compared to the orifice of the mechanical valve, the free floating thrombus is clearly large enough to occlude the mitral valve completely.

Discussion

A variety of conditions such as myocardial infarction, valvular disease, trauma, and arrhythmias place cardiovascular patients at risk for thrombus formation.[1] Often, underlying endocardial injury with subsequent platelet aggregation serve as the incipient events. In this case, subtherapeutic anticoagulation in the presence of a mechanical mitral valve certainly contributed to formation of the large left atrial thrombus in a dilated left atrium.[2]

A recent study by Leung et al. attempted to quantify the rate of stroke or other embolic events and identify risk factors for the development of these events in patients identified as having mobile and immobile left atrial thrombi by transesophageal echocardiography.[3] The study quantified the annual embolic event rate to be 10.4%. The presence of moderate or severe left ventricular dysfunction was found to be an independent predictor of death. History of thromboembolism, mobile thrombus, or thrombus with a maximum dimension of 1.5 cm or greater were found to be independent predictors of future embolic events. However, a major limitation of the study was that information on the levels of anticoagulation was unavailable.

This patient had an unusual thrombus in that it was not attached to the prosthetic valve, the sewing ring, the left atrial appendage, or the wall. Although pannus formation and thrombus may cause prosthetic valve obstruction,[4] this thrombus was not associated with the valve, although it was frequently seen to approach the orifice. It bounced around the left atrium, striking the walls and crossing the atrial cavity with a rolling motion. The laminated appearance suggested that it had been present for some time, perhaps enlarging during episodes of subtherapeutic anticoagulation. The patient was considered to be at risk for acute valvular obstruction by the thrombus, which was larger than the prosthetic valve orifice. It was thought that her presyncopal episodes might have been due to transient valvular obstruction by the thrombus.[5] In addition to embolic events, she was at increased risk for the develop-

ment of arrhythmias. As a result, this patient underwent successful surgical removal of the left atrial thrombus with resolution of her symptoms.

References

1. Mahy I, Al-Mohammad A, Cargill R. Left atrial thrombus as an early consequence of blunt trauma. Heart 1998;79:198–9.

2. Barbetseas J, Pitsavos C, Aggeli C, et al. Comparison of frequency of left atrial thrombus in patients with mechanical prosthetic cardiac valves and stroke versus transient ischemic attacks. Am J Cardiol 1997;80:526–8.

3. Leung D, Davidson P, Cranney G, Walsh W. Thromboembolic risks of left atrial thrombus detected by transesophageal echocardiogram. Am J Cardiol 1997;79:626–9.

4. Vitale N, Renzulli A, Agozzino L, et al. Obstruction of mechanical mitral prostheses: analysis of pathologic findings. Ann Thorac Surg 1997;63:1101–16.

5. Vitale M, Agnino A, Serena D, et al. Asymptomatic large left atrial thrombus. Texas Heart Inst J 1997;24:376–8.

50

Left atrial thrombus and spontaneous contrast

Susan E Wiegers MD

A 55-year-old woman with severe rheumatic mitral stenosis and chronic atrial fibrillation was to undergo mitral valve replacement. Her insurance company refused admission for anticoagulation with intravenous heparin prior to surgery. Oral anticoagulation with warfarin was discontinued 3 days prior to admission and she was admitted for a same-day surgical procedure. This transesophageal echocardiogram was performed in the operating room after the patient was anesthetized and intubated.

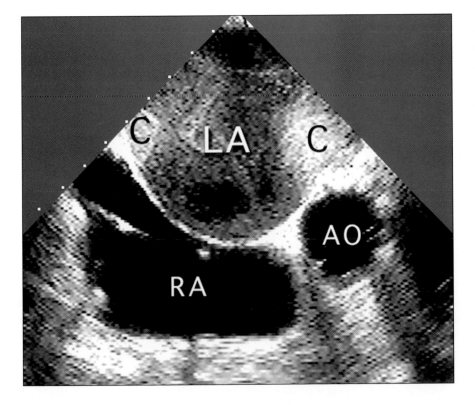

Figure 50.1
Transesophageal echocardiogram from the mid-esophageal level (imaging angle 0°) at the level of the aortic root (AO). The transducer has been rotated slightly to image the interatrial septum. The left atrium (LA) is severely enlarged, measuring over 7 cm in this view. Marked spontaneous echo contrast is evident within the left atrium. In real time this contrast swirled slowly. Comparison to the right atrium which had normal flows demonstrates a distinct difference. Two large thrombi (C) are evident within the left atrial cavity as sessile echodensities that did not move with the cardiac cycle and appeared to be attached to the wall. The interatrial septum is intact but bows towards the right, owing to the elevated left atrial pressure.

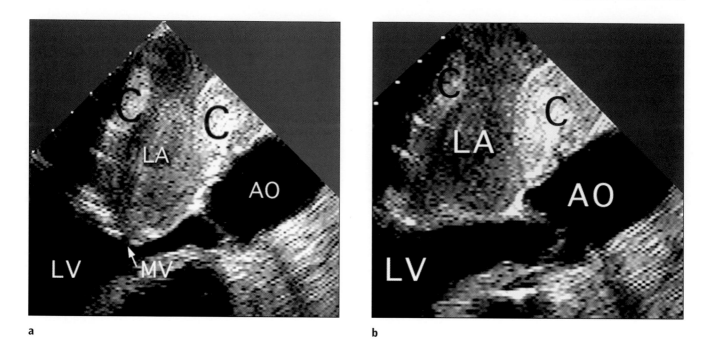

a

b

Figure 50.2

(a) Transesophageal echocardiogram from the mid-esophageal level in the longitudinal plane (imaging angle 90°). The left atrium (LA) is again seen to be severely enlarged and filled with spontaneous echo contrast and clot (C). The mitral valve (MV) is calcified and domes in diastole. The left ventricle is poorly seen in this view. The aortic valve appears to be thickened in this diastolic frame. (b) Similar transesophageal echocardiogram in systole. The mitral valve is again noted to be severely thickened and calcified. The aortic valve leaflet domes in systole, owing to rheumatic involvement and commissural thickening, which cannot be seen on this view. There is a significant difference in echodensity between the two thrombi in the left atrium. The more echobright thrombus appears to be calcified which is evidence of chronicity.

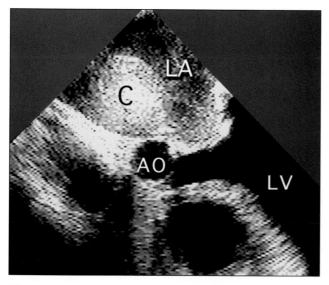

Figure 50.3

Transesophageal echocardiogram from the mid-esophageal level in the transverse plane (imaging angle 90°) in a modified four chamber view. The medial thrombus is the calcified one and measures over 3 cm in diameter.

Discussion

The patient had multiple risk factors for the development of left atrial thrombus including severe mitral stenosis, chronic atrial fibrillation, and an enlarged left atrium.[1] Transesophageal echocardiography is far more sensitive for the diagnosis than transthoracic imaging.[2] Left atrial thrombi most commonly form within the left atrial appendage. The echodensity may be similar to the atrial wall and surrounding tissue, making it difficult to distinguish thrombi from normal structures on transthoracic studies. Non-visualization of the left atrial appendage on a transthoracic study in a patient with a dilated left atrium due to mitral stenosis is associated with the presence of a thrombus within the left atrial appendage. Documentation is much more reliable via the transesophageal window where the difference between the thrombus and the surrounding structures is much more easily appreciated. Spontaneous echocardiographic contrast is an echocardiographic variable associated with the development of atrial thrombi.[3] Similarly, a decreased velocity of blood flow in the left atrial appendage (less than 0.4 m/s) is also associated with an increased risk of developing thrombi. This patient had critical mitral stenosis but very little mitral regurgitation. The presence of significant mitral regurgitation, even in the presence of chronic atrial fibrillation and an enlarged left atrium, decreases the risk of thrombus formation.[4]

This patient's thrombi were extensively calcified, attesting to their chronicity despite long-term oral anticoagulation at therapeutic levels. Although the thrombi appeared immobile, they protruded into the left atrial cavity and lined a portion of the interatrial septum. Their presence would have precluded percutaneous valvuloplasty if this had been a consideration. The surgical procedure involved placement of a St Jude's mitral valve and debridement of the left atrial thrombi. The patient was managed with intense anticoagulation postoperatively.

References

1. The Stroke Prevention in Atrial Fibrillation Investigators Committee on Echocardiography. Transesophageal echocardiographic correlates of thromboembolism in high-risk patients with atrial fibrillation. Ann Intern Med 1998;128:639–47.

2. Thomas MR, MonaghanMJ, Smyth DW, *et al*. Comparative value of transthoracic and transoesophageal echocardiography before balloon dilatation of the mitral valve. Br Heart J 1992;68:493–7.

3. Rittoo D, Sutherland G, Currie P, *et al*. A prospective study of left atrial spontaneous echo contrast and thrombus in 100 consecutive patients referred for balloon dilation of the mitral valve. J Am Soc Echocardiogr 1994;7:516–27.

4. Blackshear J, Pearce L, Asinger R, *et al*. Mitral regurgitation associated with reduced thromboembolic events in high-risk patients with non-rheumatic atrial fibrillation. Stroke Prevention in Atrial Fibrillation Investigators. Am J Cardiol 1993;72:840–3.

51

Cor triatriatum

Martin St John Sutton MBBS
Susan E Wiegers MD

A 47-year-old man had a heart murmur detected at a life insurance examination and was referred for evaluation. He was asymptomatic except for mild shortness of breath on moderate exertion which had progressed over the prior year. He had no risk factors for coronary heart disease but had a history of rheumatic fever at the age of seven years, at which time he was told he had a heart murmur. He had no family history of congenital heart disease.

On examination he looked fit and had no edema, a normal jugular venous pressure and normal peripheral pulses. He was in sinus rhythm and normotensive. His apical impulse was unremarkable. On auscultation there was a normal first and second heart sound without augmentation of pulmonary closure, and a systolic murmur at the apex which was consistent with a flow murmur. An electrocardiogram showed sinus rhythm with normal axis, intervals and morphology.

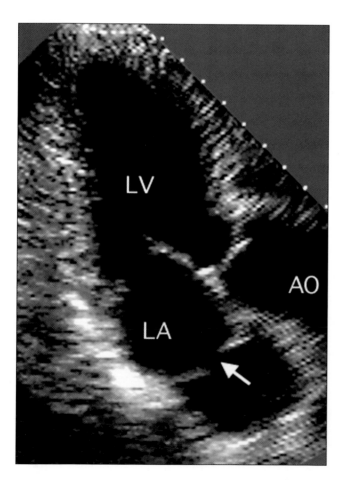

Figure 51.1
In the apical long-axis view of the left ventricle there is a membrane running across the atrium parallel to the mitral valve orifice, dividing the left atrium into two almost equal-sized chambers with a normal non-rheumatic mitral valve. The posterior chamber receives the pulmonary veins and the more apically placed chamber is contiguous with the atrial appendage.

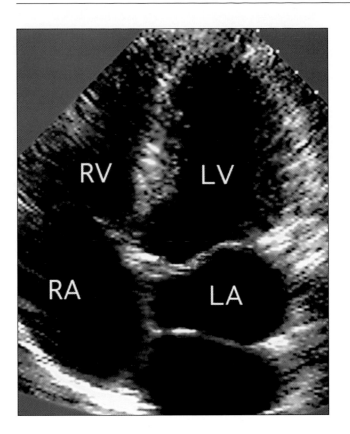

Figure 51.2
The apical four-chamber view shows that the left atrium is not dilated, making significant obstruction at the membrane level unlikely. The normal right atrial and ventricular sizes and absence of tricuspid regurgitation suggest low pulmonary artery systolic pressure. Importantly the posterior left atrial chamber receives the pulmonary veins, while the left atrial appendage drains into the chamber adjacent to the mitral valve.

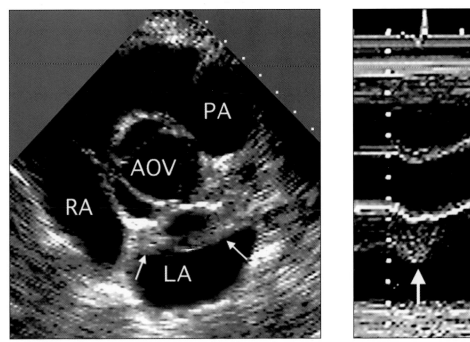

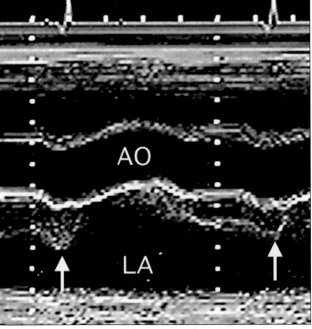

a

b

Figure 51.3
(a) Parasternal short-axis view demonstrating the membrane (arrows) in the left atrium.
(b) M-mode echocardiogram from the parasternal position. The right ventricular outflow tract is seen anteriorly. The aortic root is normal. The left atrium is only mildly enlarged. There is a structure (arrows) within the left atrium that represents the membrane.

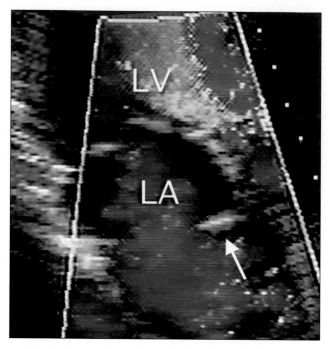

Figure 51.4
Color flow Doppler imaging in the long-axis view shows that the orifice in the membrane does not cause aliasing and indicates a low diastolic gradient across the membrane.

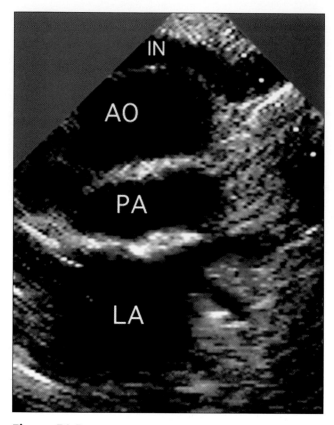

Figure 51.5
Suprasternal notch view with the transducer directed posteriorly to demonstrate the pulmonary veins entering the posterior portion of the left atrium. The innominate (IN) vein, seen in long axis, is the most superior structure in this view. The transverse aorta (AO) is demonstrated in short axis with the right pulmonary artery (PA) in long axis as it passes under the aortic arch. The left pulmonary veins (on the right of the screen) enter the left atrium normally. The right veins are not as well seen on this image.

Discussion

The diagnosis in this patient is cor triatriatum which is easily established unequivocally by two-dimensional echocardiography. Cor triatriatum is an uncommon congenital anomaly in which there is persistence of the common pulmonary vein, which receives the confluence of the pulmonary veins from both lungs. The membrane may be hemodynamically inconsequential, or may be severely obstructive and result in pulmonary venous and subsequently pulmonary arterial hypertension. The diagnosis is made by demonstrating that the pulmonary veins drain into the superior or posterior left atrial compartment and that the left atrial appendage drains into the anterior or inferior chamber. Early diagnosis is important because resection of this supramitral valve obstruction results in restitution of pulmonary artery pressures to normal.[1]

Membranes with multiple openings or large single openings are asymptomatic and cause no obstruction to flow, as in this patient. Cor triatriatum is occasionally found as an incidental finding in patients undergoing echocardiography or transesophageal study for other reasons.[2]

References

1. Tahernia AC, Ashcraft KW, Tutuska PJ. The diagnosis of cor triatriatum sinistrum in children: a continuing dilemma. South Med J 1999;92:218–22.

2. Jeong JW, Tei C, Chang KS, et al. A case of cor triatriatum in an eighty-year-old man: transesophageal echocardiographic observation of multiple defects. J Am Soc Echocardiogr 1997;10:185–8.

52

Bronchogenic carcinoma invading the left atrium

Victor A Ferrari MD

A 65-year-old smoker with no previous cardiac history presented with a 3-month history of chest pain, palpitations, dyspnea on exertion, and non-productive cough. She had noted an unintentional 45-pound weight loss over the past 6 months, and denied fever, chills, night sweats, or hemoptysis. She described a 50 pack-year smoking history, but had stopped smoking 15 years ago.

On physical examination, the jugular venous pressure was normal, with normal carotid pulse contours. The lung examination was notable for decreased air movement in the left upper lung field with bronchial breath sounds. On auscultation, she had a normal S$_1$, and a normally split S$_2$.

There was a grade I/VI systolic ejection murmur at the right upper sternal border with no diastolic murmur. The remainder of the examination was normal. Laboratory testing and electrocardiogram were normal. Chest X-ray demonstrated a large dense left upper lobe mass, measuring 14 × 10 cm, with no pleural effusion.

A transthoracic echocardiogram demonstrated normal left ventricular size with normal left ventricle function, and an ill-defined echodensity along the lateral left atrial border which could not be distinguished as an extra- or intracardiac structure. Transesophageal echocardiography was undertaken to better define this abnormality.

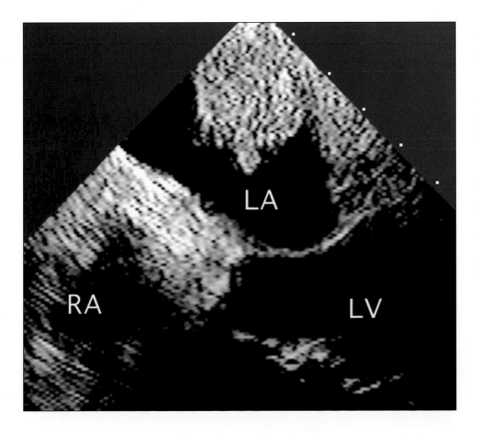

Figure 52.1
Transesophageal echocardiogram from the mid-esophagus in the transverse plane (imaging angle 0°). The close-up image of the left atrium (LA) from the four-chamber view demonstrates a left atrial mass. The left atrium, right atrium (RA), and left ventricle (LV) are identified. The tumor is large with a homogeneous appearance, and has two areas that were mobile in real time. The mass involves a majority of the left atrium, and extends along the lateral left atrium to the mitral annulus, but did not obstruct the mitral valve. The interatrial septum is thickened, owing to lipomatous hypertrophy and not from infiltration by the tumor.

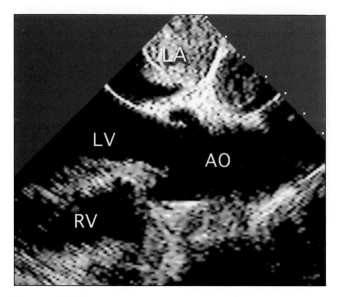

Figure 52.2
In the longitudinal plane (imaging angle 90°), the left atrium (LA) is seen posterior (top of the image) to the ascending aorta (AO), and the right ventricle (RV) is located anteriorly to the left ventricle (LV). The tumor occupies a significant portion of the left atrium, particularly at the superior aspect.

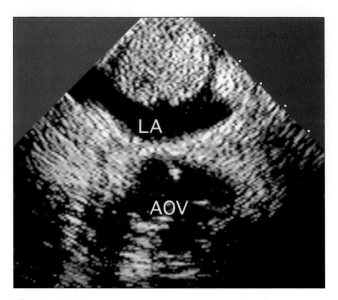

Figure 52.3
In the transverse plane at a location in the superior left atrium (LA) (imaging angle 30°), there is near complete obstruction of the left superior pulmonary vein by the tumor, with the majority of the upper left atrium occupied by the mass. The left inferior pulmonary vein was partially obstructed by the mass, but the right pulmonary veins were not involved. AOV, aortic valve.

Discussion

The differential diagnosis of cardiac masses includes thrombus, tumor and vegetations. Thrombi in the left atrium may be of several types, and are usually located along the walls (mural) or in the left atrial appendage. Mural thrombi usually occur in the setting of severe dilatation of the left atrium, which was not seen in this case. So-called 'tumor thrombus' can be seen in malignancies which have highly thrombotic properties, such as renal cell carcinoma, and can extend from the renal veins to the right atrium via the inferior vena cava. While a thrombus might be possible, owing to a lung malignancy in this patient, it is more common to see extension of the tumor itself into the left atrium via the pulmonary veins. Vegetations may be of bacterial, fungal, or murantic origin. It would be unusual to see a vegetation in this location within the heart, although fungal infections can produce large vegetations. The mitral valve was not involved by this process, making vegetation extremely unlikely. Tumors can be of primary cardiac origin or metastatic, and may be either benign or malignant. The most likely etiology of this patient's mass is a malignant tumor that is metastatic from a lung carcinoma.

Primary cardiac tumors are much less common than metastatic tumors to the heart. The incidence ranges from 0.0017% to 0.28% in autopsy series. Approximately 75% of cardiac tumors are benign. Of the malignant tumors, 75% are sarcomas, with the majority in adults being angiosarcomas and rhabdomyosarcomas. Symptoms can be quite non-specific in patients with left atrial tumors, with non-productive cough, paroxysmal nocturnal dyspnea, and dyspnea on exertion as common presenting complaints. The diagnosis of cardiac tumors has been significantly improved since the advent of non-invasive imaging techniques such as transthoracic and transesophageal echocardiography.[1–4] While differentiation of benign versus malignant tumors can be difficult from imaging techniques alone, several features may be helpful. Malignant tumors are more likely to be located along the atrial free wall or on the right side of the heart. They are more commonly associated with hemorrhagic pericardial effusions, local mediastinal invasion, rapid change in size, and extension into the pulmonary veins.

This patient had several of the characteristic symptoms and echocardiographic findings of a metastatic tumor invading the heart. She had a non-productive cough and weight loss, which, in a former smoker, are worrisome symptoms for a lung malignancy. Weight loss is an uncommon symptom in patients with primary cardiac malignancies. Metastatic tumors to the heart, particularly those that involve the atria, may cause atrial arrhythmias or symptoms consistent with pericarditis, including pericardial effusions. Dyspnea on exertion may be due to pulmonary vein obstruction by a tumor, a pericardial effusion with increased intrapericardial pressure, or hypoxemia secondary to altered ventilation/perfusion matching. The atrium is a common location to find metastatic tumors, and primary or secondary tumors of the heart may be present along the lateral walls. The complete occlusion of the pulmonary vein is a common finding in metastatic lung cancers. Since the pulmonary veins are in the far field in transthoracic studies, transesophageal echocardiography is frequently necessary to demonstrate the extension from the pulmonary veins into the left atrium.[5,6]

Although surgical resection of similar tumors has been reported,[7] the patient was found to have distal bony metastases. She received combination chemotherapy and radiation with some decrease in the size of the tumor.

References

1. Reeder GS, Khandheria BK, Seward JB, Tajik AJ. Transesophageal echocardiography and cardiac masses. Mayo Clin Proc 1991;66: 1101–9.

2. Salcedo EE, Cohen GI, White RD, Davison MB. Cardiac tumors: diagnosis and management. Curr Probl Cardiol 1992;17:73–137.

3. Lee TM, Chen MF, Liau CS, Lee YT. Role of transesophageal echocardiography in the management of metastatic tumors invading the left atrium. Cardiology 1997;88:214–17

4. Awad M, Dunn B, al Halees Z, et al. Intracardiac rhabdomyosarcoma: transesophageal echocardiographic findings and diagnosis. J Am Soc Echocardiogr 1992;5:199–202.

5. Lynch M, Balk MA, Lee RB, Martin RP. Role of transesophageal echocardiography in the management of patients with bronchogenic carcinoma invading the left atrium. Am J Cardiol 1995;76:1101–2.

6. Capdeville H, Hearn C, Rice T, et al. Left atrial metastasis of a large cell carcinoma of the lung in an asymptomatic patient: transesophageal echocardiographic evaluation. J Cardiothorac Vasc Anesth 1997;11:492–4.

7. Torre W, Rabago G, Barba J, et al. Combined surgical approach for sarcoma lung metastasis with atrial involvement. Thorac Cardiovasc Surg 1999;47:125–7.

SECTION V

The Mitral Valve

53

Mitral valve prolapse

Susan E Wiegers MD

A 70-year-old man had a long history of a systolic murmur. Two years previously his doctor had noted atrial fibrillation. The ventricular rate was controlled without therapy and he was not treated with any medications. His exercise tolerance deteriorated over several weeks and he presented to his doctor complaining of severe dyspnea on exertion, orthopnea and new pedal edema. The physical examination was notable for elevated jugular venous pressures, bibasilar rales in both lung fields and a 4/6 holosystolic murmur which was loudest at the apex. An echocardiogram was done to assess the patient's cardiac function. The diagnosis of flail mitral valve leaflet was made and the patient underwent mitral valve repair. Intraoperative transesophageal images are also shown.

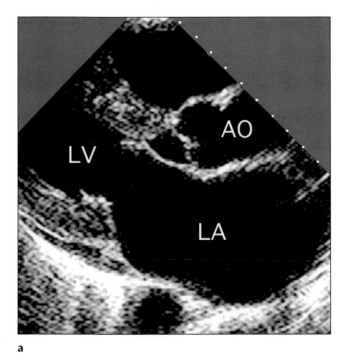

a

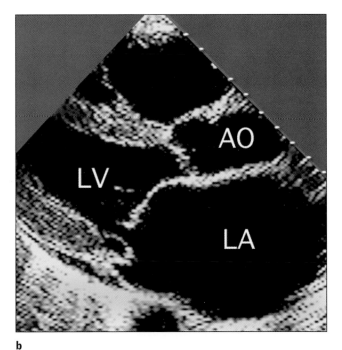

b

Figure 53.1
(a) Parasternal long-axis view in diastole. There is moderate concentric left ventricular hypertrophy with a normal chamber size. The left atrium (LA) is markedly dilated. The aortic valve and ascending aorta (AO) also appear to be normal. The mitral valve leaflets are slightly thickened at the tips. The posterior mitral leaflet is not as well seen as the anterior leaflet but does not appear to be abnormal in this view. (b) Similar parasternal long-axis view in late diastole; the aortic valve has not yet opened. The anterior mitral valve leaflet is in normal position. However, the body of the posterior mitral leaflet flails into the left atrium, pointing away from the left ventricle. A thin cord attached to the tip of the leaflet is seen doubling back towards the left ventricular cavity. Right ventricular enlargement is evident in this view.

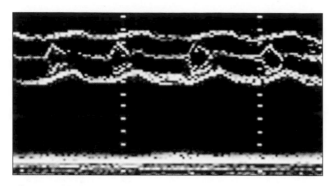

Figure 53.2

M-mode echocardiogram from the parasternal position at the level of the aortic valve. The left atrium is markedly dilated. The aortic valve demonstrates early closure. It opens relatively normally and the leaflets approximate the walls of the aortic root. However, the leaflets begin to close at the point of maximal excursion. This pattern of early closure is consistent with decreased stroke volume.

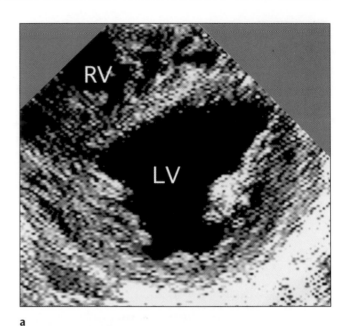

a

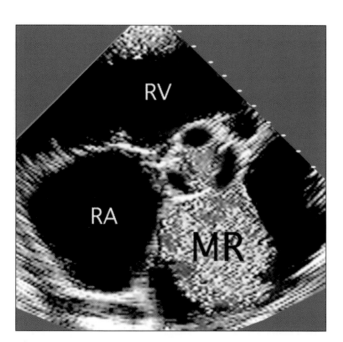

Figure 53.3

Parasternal short-axis view in systole at the level of the aortic valve. The partial opening of the aortic valve is demonstrated by the color jet that outlines the orifice of the aortic valve. It can be difficult to distinguish decreased opening due to a low stroke volume from decreased opening of the valve due to aortic stenosis, possibly from a rheumatic process. However, in the other views of the aortic valve in this patient, the leaflets are not thickened and do open fully in the very beginning of systole, which rules out aortic stenosis. The turbulent jet of mitral regurgitation (MR) filling the left atrium is well seen even in this view, which is perpendicular to the mitral regurgitation jet. The right atrium (RA) and right ventricle (RV) are both dilated.

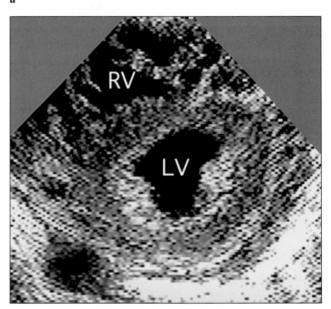

b

Figure 53.4

(a) Parasternal short-axis view of the left ventricular cavity in diastole. There is flattening of the interventricular septum. The view is slightly off-axis but the walls appear concentrically thickened with no evidence of scarring. In particular, the inferior wall appears to be normal. The papillary muscles are both imaged at this level and also appear to be anatomically normal. (b) Similar parasternal short-axis view in systole. Interventricular septal flattening persists in systole. This pattern is consistent with right ventricular volume and pressure overload. The fractional area change in the left ventricle (LV) indicates excellent systolic function, at least at this level, with no wall motion abnormalities. The right ventricle (RV), however, demonstrates a decreased change in area which is suggestive of right ventricular dysfunction. A trivial pericardial effusion is present, but is visible only in systole.

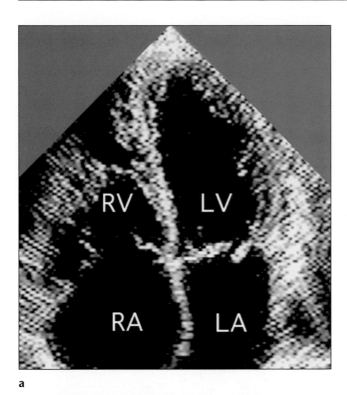

a

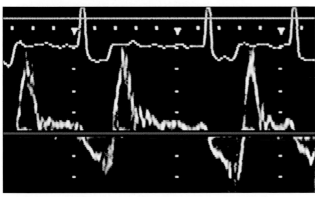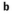

b

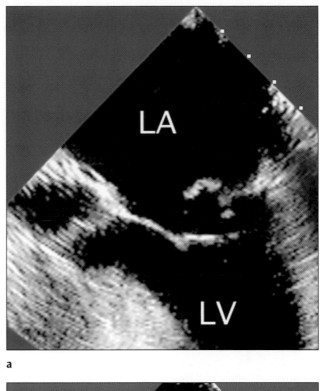

a

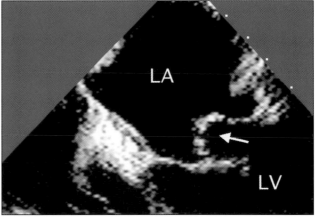

b

Figure 53.5

(a) Apical four-chamber view in systole. Once again, the posterior leaflet of the mitral valve flails into the left atrium (LA). The anterior leaflet appears to be in a normal position and would coapt with a normal posterior leaflet. Right ventricular cavity dilatation is well appreciated in this view. The right atrium (RA) is markedly dilated and the tricuspid valve leaflets fail to coapt, owing to annular dilatation rather than prolapse of the leaflets. (b) Spectral display of pulsed-wave Doppler with the sample volume in the right superior pulmonary vein taken from the apical position. There is systolic reversal of flow into the pulmonary vein. The flow is below the baseline or away from the transducer in systole, indicating blood flow from the left atrium into the pulmonary veins during systole. The filling of the left atrium, indicated by flow towards the transducer or above the baseline, occurs predominantly during early diastole.

Figure 53.6

(a) Intraoperative transesophageal echocardiogram from the mid-esophageal level in the transverse plane (imaging angle 0°). The posterior leaflet of the mitral valve flails into the left atrium and is seen well behind the anterior mitral leaflet. The left atrium is markedly enlarged. A portion of the left ventricular outflow tract and the aortic valve is seen on the left of the screen. (b) Intraoperative transesophageal echocardiogram from the transverse plane (imaging angle 0°) of the four-chamber view. This is a close-up of the mitral valve. In this systolic frame, a scallop of the posterior mitral valve leaflet (arrow) prolapses into the left atrium. The portion of the mitral valve which is flail is not visualized in this frame. There was torrential mitral regurgitation which is also not shown in this picture.

Discussion

The patient no doubt had had significant mitral regurgitation for some time, given the level of pulmonary hypertension and the left atrial dilatation. Although pulmonary hypertension is usually due to mitral stenosis or left ventricular dysfunction which develops as the result of severe chronic mitral regurgitation, it may occur with isolated severe mitral regurgitation and preserved left ventricular function.[1] Severe elevation of pulmonary pressures may be present in a minority of cases. The patient's hypertrophied and dilated right ventricle are the result of chronic pulmonary hypertension. Progressive tricuspid annular dilatation is the result of right ventricular remodelling secondary to the volume load. Consequently, tricuspid regurgitation may further increase and produce further annular dilatation. This patient had a tricuspid regurgitation jet velocity of 3.1 m/s. Applying the modified Bernoulli equation (pressure gradient = $4\,v^2$) where v is the velocity of the tricuspid regurgitation jet measured by continuous-wave Doppler, the pressure gradient between the right ventricle and the atrium is 38 mmHg. Assuming the right atrial pressure is 15 mmHg, the estimated peak pulmonary artery pressure is 53 mmHg. At this level of peak right ventricular systolic pressure, flattening of the interventricular septum in systole could be expected. Its presence in diastole represents elevated diastolic volume from significant tricuspid regurgitation.

The patient's acute decompensation was most probably due to chordal rupture and a sudden increase in the severity of mitral regurgitation. The left ventricle is mildly dilated, as demonstrated in the apical four-chamber view. However, the ventricle has not had time to adapt to the sudden increase in mitral regurgitation and the severe volume load. The flail portion of the posterior leaflet is evidence of acute severe mitral regurgitation, which is generally poorly tolerated. Reversal of flow in the pulmonary veins during systole is evidence of severe regurgitation but needs to be incorporated into assessment of all the characteristics of the mitral regurgitation. The pulmonary vein flow may be sampled from the apical position in a transthoracic study or from a high esophageal position in the transesophageal study. If the jet of mitral regurgitation is eccentric, it is important to sample the veins on the opposite side of the jet. Normally, most forward flow into the left atrium occurs in systole. Severe mitral regurgitation disturbs the usual filling pattern and most filling occurs in diastole. In the operating room, pulmonary vein flow reversal may be the best acute assessment of the improvement in severity of mitral regurgitation after mitral valve repair.[2]

Multiplane transesophageal echocardiography is an important tool in the operating room for evaluating the mechanism of mitral regurgitation and planning the operative strategy.[3] Transesophageal echocardiography in particular allows prediction of the surgical strategy and allows assessment of the surgical results.[4]

This patient was treated with diuresis and digoxin with minimal improvement. He underwent mitral valve repair with resection of the flail scallop and placement of an annuloplasty ring. A tricuspid annuloplasty ring was also placed. Immediate post-pump images demonstrated mild mitral regurgitation and moderate tricuspid regurgitation. The pulmonary artery pressure measured by pulmonary artery catheter dropped to 39 mmHg. The patient recovered from surgery and has returned to his usual activities.

References

1. Alexopoulos D, Lazzam C, Borrico S, et al. Isolated chronic mitral regurgitation with preserved systolic left ventricular function and severe pulmonary hypertension. J Am Coll Cardiol 1989;14:319–22.

2. Pieper EP, Hellemans IM, Hamer HP, et al. Value of systolic pulmonary venous flow reversal and color Doppler jet measurements assessed with transesophageal echocardiography in recognizing severe pure mitral regurgitation. Am J Cardiol 1996;78:444–50.

3. Stewart WJ, Griffin B, Thomas JD. Multiplane transesophageal echocardiographic evaluation of mitral valve disease. Am J Cardiac Imag 1995;9:121–8.

4. Hellemans IM, Pieper EG, Ravelli AC, et al. Prediction of surgical strategy in mitral valve regurgitation based on echocardiography.

54

Mixed rheumatic valve disease

Susan E Wiegers MD

A 26-year-old man was seen in the medical clinic complaining of shortness of breath when climbing stairs. He had immigrated from India several years previously and had no previous diagnosis of heart disease. Cardiac examination revealed a laterally displaced point of maximal impulse which was thought to be diffuse. S_1 was loud and S_2 normal. A loud systolic ejection murmur radiated to the carotids from the right upper sternal border. A loud holosystolic murmur and a soft diastolic rumble were audible at the apex. There was a blowing diastolic murmur at the left lower sternal border.

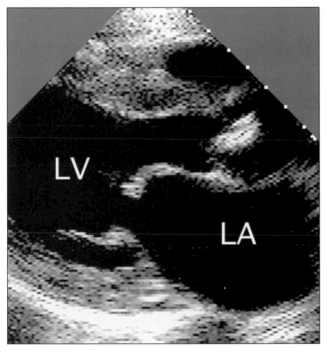

a

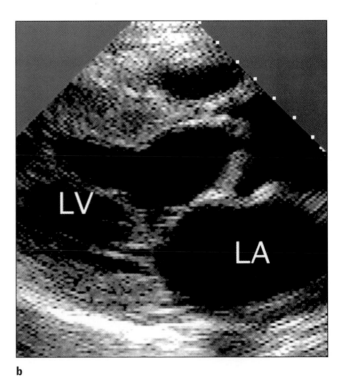

b

Figure 54.1
(a) Parasternal long-axis view demonstrating doming of the mitral valve in diastole. The mitral valve leaflets are thickened and the motion of the posterior leaflet is also restricted. It does not approximate the posterior wall of the left ventricle (LV) in this image, which is taken at the maximum opening of the valve. The attachment of thickened mitral valve chordae to the posterior leaflet is also visualized. The left ventricle is dilated and there is moderate hypertrophy. The left atrium (LA) is also dilated. The aortic valve is markedly thickened and calcified. The aortic annulus appears to be normal but the leaflets themselves are heavily calcified.
(b) Parasternal long-axis view in systole. The aortic valve is diffusely thickened and domes, owing to commissural fusion. The thickened subvalvular attachments to both mitral valve leaflets are clearly visible. The left ventricular systolic function is moderately decreased.

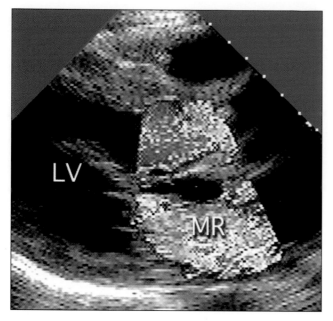

Figure 54.2

Parasternal long-axis view in systole with color flow Doppler imaging. The left atrium is filled with a turbulent jet of mitral regurgitation (MR) which appears severe in degree. The presence of significant aortic stenosis is evident by the abrupt development of high-velocity turbulent flow in the left ventricular outflow tract at the level of the aortic valve. The flow in the left ventricular outflow tract itself is laminar and of low-velocity. The left ventricular systolic function is again noted to be moderately decreased. In the setting of significant mitral regurgitation, this represents severe systolic dysfunction.

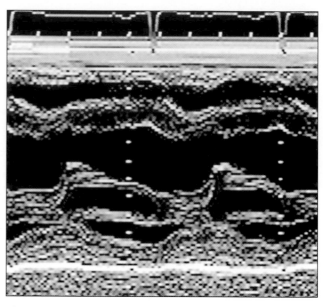

Figure 54.3

M-mode echocardiogram from the parasternal position at the level of the mitral valve leaflets. The mitral valve leaflets are thickened. The decreased E to F slope and the anterior motion of the posterior mitral valve leaflets in diastole are pathognomonic for rheumatic mitral stenosis.

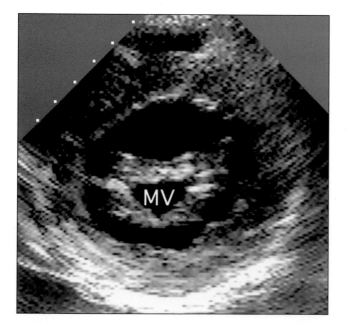

Figure 54.4

Parasternal short-axis view of the mitral valve orifice (MV) in diastole. The thickening and focal calcifications of both leaflets is evident. The leaflets are restricted from opening by commissural fusion at both the lateral and the medial commissures. This process results in the triangular shape of the orifice at the level of the commissures.

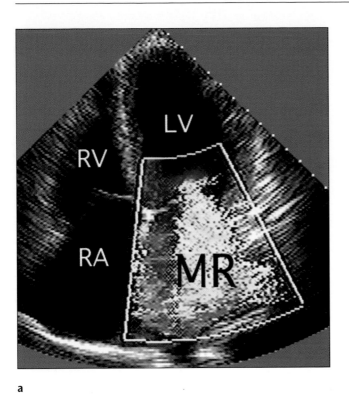

a

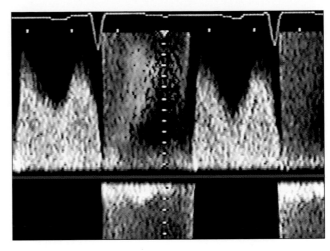

b

Figure 54.5

(a) Apical four-chamber view with color Doppler flow imaging across the mitral valve. In systole there is a turbulent jet of mitral regurgitation arising from the mitral valve plane and extending into the left atrium. The broad jet extends to the posterior wall of the left atrium consistent with severe mitral regurgitation. (b) Spectral display of pulsed-wave Doppler across the mitral valve from the apical position. Each vertical scale mark represents 20 cm/s. The peak mitral valve inflow velocity is 2.2 m/s which represents a peak gradient of 19 mmHg. The pressure half-time of the mitral valve E wave is prolonged and suggestive of mild mitral stenosis. In this case the transvalvular gradient results from the mild valvular obstruction and the high mitral inflow due to the severe mitral regurgitation.

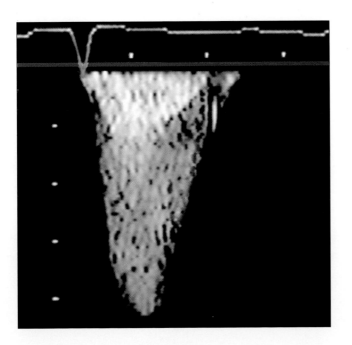

Figure 54.6

Spectral display of continuous-wave Doppler across the aortic valve from the aortic position. The peak and mean gradient across the valve are 71 and 49 mmHg which is consistent with severe aortic stenosis.

Discussion

Rheumatic heart disease continues to be a common cause of valvular heart disease, especially in developing countries where presentation with advanced disease at a young age is frequent. In this case, the aortic and mitral valves are both regurgitant and stenotic. Multivalvular involvement is common for rheumatic disease. The pathophysiological process involves thickening and fusion of the commissures. The orifice is narrowed by the commissural fusion, creating obstruction to flow. The thickening of the commissures disrupts the coaptation of the valve and creates regurgitation. The orifice of a severely affected valve can become fixed (the so-called 'fish-mouth' valve), resulting in significant regurgitation and stenosis.

This patient had mixed valvular disease and left ventricular dysfunction. The ventricular response to each of the valvular lesions differs. It is instructive to consider which of the hemodynamic loads has resulted in left ventricular dilatation and systolic dysfunction. At least moderate and possibly severe aortic stenosis is present. The aortic valve area calculation by continuity equation is 1.1 cm. However, there is detectable leaflet motion which is enough to exclude critical aortic stenosis.[1] The left ventricle responds to increasing degrees of outflow obstruction by hypertrophy of the walls with preservation of the ventricular cavity size and systolic function. Gender differences in the response to aortic stenosis have been reported.[2] However, in isolated aortic stenosis dilatation, to this degree, a fall in left ventricular ejection fraction would not be expected unless the patient had critical aortic stenosis and was in a state of significant hemodynamic compromise. The ventricular response to aortic regurgitation is dilatation with no change in relative wall thickness. Relative wall thickness compares the dimensions of the walls to the cavity radius:

Relative wall thickness = IVS + PWT/LVID
(normal range: 0.33–0.36)

where IVS and PWT are the dimensions of the interventricular septum and posterior wall, respectively, and LVID is the internal diameter of the left ventricle in diastole. This patient has eccentric hypertrophy with mild increase in relative wall thickness as well as a significant increase in the left ventricular dimensions. The overall left ventricular mass has therefore increased significantly.

The mitral valve is mildly stenotic. There is ample evidence on the echocardiographic study that severe obstruction is not present. First of all, the parasternal long-axis view demonstrates an opening of at least 1 cm in this plane. Therefore, the mitral valve area is likely to be greater than 1 cm². This estimate is confirmed in the parasternal short-axis view of the mitral orifice where the valve area may be planimetered. Secondly, the pressure half-time of the spectral envelope of the Doppler signal across the mitral valve is only mildly prolonged, which is suggestive of mild stenosis. In any case, the left ventricle is usually small and underfilled in mitral stenosis so it is unlikely that this valve lesion accounts for the left ventricular remodelling.

Severe mitral regurgitation is also present, owing to the rheumatic involvement of the valve. The mitral regurgitation may be exacerbated by annular dilatation but the original lesion was clearly rheumatic in nature. Assessment of the severity of mitral regurgitation depends on the relative size of the color Doppler jet compared to the left atrial area. Correlation with qualitative measures of mitral regurgitation obtained invasively is generally good, although eccentric jets may be difficult to assess.[3] Both the left atrium and the left ventricle dilate in the setting of chronic severe mitral regurgitation. Left atrial dimensions correlate best with the severity of the mitral regurgitation, although in this patient mitral stenosis no doubt contributed to the left atrial enlargement. The absence of left ventricular enlargement does not rule out severe mitral regurgitation.[4] Eventually, compensatory mechanisms to the increased volume load from the mitral regurgitation fail, and left ventricular failure ensues.

The patient responded to diuresis with a modest improvement in his symptoms. He underwent replacement of the mitral and aortic valves, which was complicated by the need for a permanent pacemaker and the development of atrial fibrillation.

References

1. Hoffman R, Flachskampf F, Hanrath P. Planimetry of orifice area in aortic stenosis using multiplane transesophageal echocardiography. J Am Coll Cardiol 1993;22:529–34.

2. Legget M, Kuusisto J, Healy N, et al. Gender differences in left ventricular function at rest and with exercise in asymptomatic aortic stenosis. Am Heart J 1996; 131:94–100.

3. Enriquez-Sarano M, Tajik AJ, Bailey KR, et al. Color flow imaging compared with quantitative Doppler assessment of severity of mitral regurgitation: influence of eccentricity of jet and mechanism of regurgitation [published erratum appears in J Am Coll Cardiol 1993;22:342]. J Am Coll Cardiol 1993;21:1211–19.

4. Burwash IG, Blackmore GL, Koilpillai CJ. Usefulness of left atrial and left ventricular chamber sizes as predictors of the severity of mitral regurgitation. Am J Cardiol 1992;70:774–9.

55

Mitral stenosis with large left atrial thrombus

Susan E Wiegers MD

An 85-year-old woman with a history of rheumatic heart disease presented with an acute embolic cardiovascular accident. The patient had refused surgery in the past despite severe dyspnea on exertion due to severe mitral stenosis and aortic stenosis. She had been in chronic atrial fibrillation for at least 8 years but had refused anticoagulation because of her concerns about medication side effects. She had recently agreed to treatment with subcutaneous heparin twice a day.

On physical examination the patient was an ill-appearing cachetic woman who was disoriented and hemiplegic. Her neck veins were distended to 9 cm above the right atrium. The point of maximal impulse was non-displaced. S_1 was loud. S_2 was normal. There was an opening stamp with a loud diastolic murmur heard at the apex. There was a very harsh systolic ejection murmur at the left upper sternal border. An echocardiogram was done to assess the patient's valvular disease and to rule out a cardiac source of embolism.

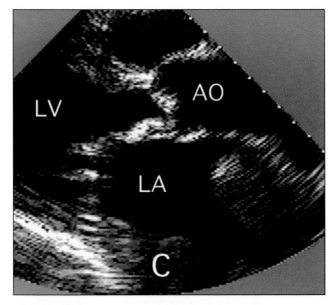

Figure 55.1
Parasternal long-axis view in diastole. The left atrium (LA) is severely dilated. A large homogeneous mass (C) lines the superior and posterior walls of the left atrium. A small opening in the thrombus at the insertion of the left superior pulmonary vein is seen. This laminated thrombus has reduced the effective volume of the left atrium. The mitral valve is calcified and thickened. It domes in diastole consistent with significant mitral stenosis. The left ventricle (LV) is of normal size. The aortic valve is markedly thickened in this diastolic image.

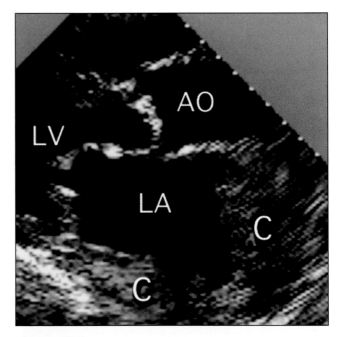

Figure 55.2
Lateral angulation of the transducer again in diastole demonstrates the extent of the clot (C) within the left atrium. Pulmonary venous inflow has kept a small channel in the inferior portion of the thrombus. This has prevented the development of pulmonary venous obstruction which would be a concern in this case. The thrombus otherwise appears to be adherent to the inferior and superior walls of the left atrium.

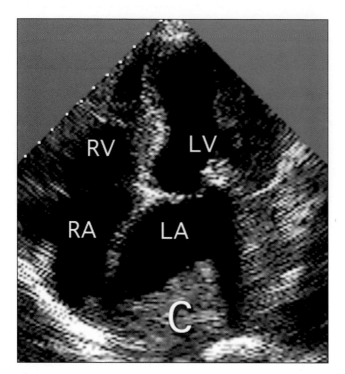

Figure 55.3

Apical four-chamber view demonstrating the large thrombus (C) within the left atrium (LA). The thrombus occupies nearly one-half of the area of the left atrium in this view and spans the area of insertion of the right and left superior pulmonary veins. The left atrium itself is markedly dilated, owing to the mitral stenosis and the longstanding atrial fibrillation. The right atrium (RA) is mildly dilated, as is the right ventricle (RV).

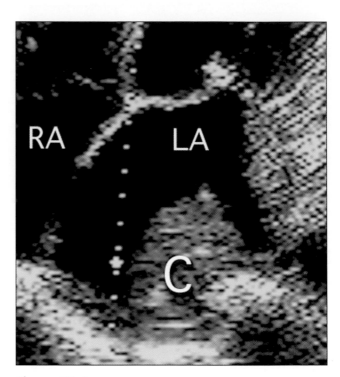

Figure 55.4

Close-up image of the left atrium and thrombus in systole from the previous apical four-chamber view. Once again the channels for pulmonary venous inflow both on the right and the left are visualized. The thrombus (C) protrudes into the left atrial cavity but was completely immobile.

Discussion

This elderly woman has severe mitral stenosis and moderate aortic stenosis. The left atrium is dilated, owing to the mitral valve obstruction as well as chronic atrial fibrillation. The mass within the left atrium appears to be a thrombus. The stasis of blood within the left atrium due to the mitral stenosis has led to the development of a laminated clot along the walls of the left atrium. Tumor is in the differential diagnosis of this mass. Most left atrial thrombi arise within the left atrial appendage, because this is the area with the most static flow within the left atrium. The location of the thrombus is unusual in this case but has probably developed over a long time period because of low velocity of blood flow from both the obstruction to mitral flow and atrial fibrillation. A tumor might have the same echogenic characteristics as this mass. However, the two most common tumors would be a myxoma or a metastatic neoplasm. Myxomas are usually attached to the interatrial septum and do not layer along the atrial walls. Metastatic left atrial masses are often bronchogenic carcinomas which arise from a pulmonary vein rather than

sparing the origins of the venous inflow. In this situation the flow from the pulmonary veins has prevented deposition of the thrombus within the pathway of flow and the clot has accumulated along the walls, where the stasis of blood flow is most pronounced.

Transthoracic echocardiography is not a sensitive diagnostic tool for the diagnosis of left atrial thrombus.[1] In this case, the thrombus was so large that it was easily visualized. However, left atrial thrombi are often restricted to the left atrial appendage where blood flow velocities may be low. Transesophageal echocardiography is often necessary for the diagnosis of left atrial thrombus. However, highly mobile thrombi or very large ones such as this may sometimes be visualized on transthoracic study. Newer transthoracic systems may be more sensitive for the diagnosis of left atrial clot. While percutaneous valvuloplasty would generally be contraindicated in patients with left atrial thrombus, successful procedures in emergency situations have been reported under transesophageal guidance.[2]

Transesophageal echocardiography was unnecessary in this patient and was not performed. The patient was eventually convinced of the inadequacy of her current anticoagulation regimen. She was treated with 1 week of intravenous heparin and anticoagulated with warfarin. The goal International Normalized Ratio (INR) was 2.5. She was discharged to a rehabilitation facility and after 6 months had not had a recurrent embolic event. Transthoracic echocardiogram demonstrated a decrease in the size of the left atrial thrombus but incomplete resolution.

References

1. Thomas MR, Monaghan MJ, Smyth DW, *et al*. Comparative value of transthoracic and transoesophageal echocardiography before balloon dilatation of the mitral valve. Br Heart J 1992;68:493–7.

2. Chirillo F, Ramondo A, Dan M, *et al*. Successful emergency percutaneous balloon mitral valvotomy in a patient with massive left atrial thrombosis: utility of transesophageal echocardiographic monitoring. Cardiology 1991;79:161–4.

56

Percutaneous balloon mitral valvuloplasty under transesophageal guidance

Bruce D Klugherz MD

A 28-year-old pregnant woman (G2P1) developed shortness of breath both on exertion and at rest during the second trimester. Her first pregnancy, two years earlier, had been complicated by similar but milder symptoms. She had not received a cardiovascular evaluation at that time. A transthoracic echocardiogram revealed moderate mitral stenosis with fusion of the commissures. The valve was neither calcified nor regurgitant. The patient had immigrated to Britain during this pregnancy and had no known history of rheumatic fever.

She became progressively more symptomatic over the next month and the decision to undertake a percutaneous balloon mitral valvuloplasty was made. To minimize the radiation exposure, the procedure was done with transesophageal guidance and pelvic shielding.

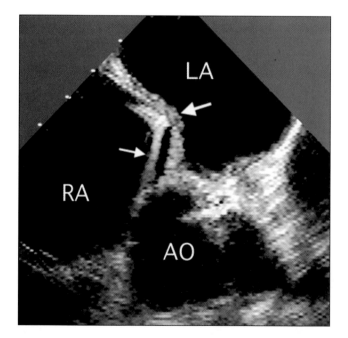

Figure 56.1
Transesophageal echocardiogram from the level of the midesophagus in the transverse plane (imaging angle 0°). This image is taken slightly above the aortic valve leaflets, imaging the aortic root (AO) in short axis. A Mullin's sheath has been advanced via the right femoral vein and positioned in the right atrium (RA). Within the sheath is a Brockenbrough transseptal needle. The entire apparatus is oriented towards the fossa ovalis, resulting in bulging of the interatrial septum towards the left atrium (LA). Upon confirmation of position, the interatrial septum is punctured by the Brockenbrough needle. In this image, the tip of the needle is abutting the interatrial septum. The point at which the needle will cross the plane of the interatrial septum is indicated by the large arrow. An artifact from the catheter (small arrow) extends along the ultrasound scan line from the catheter into the right atrium.

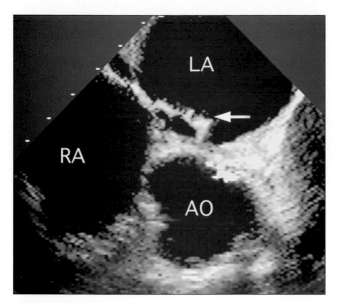

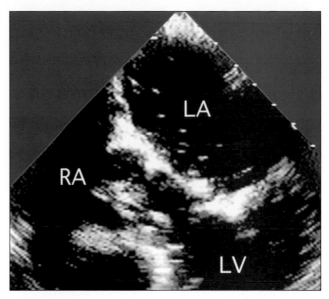

Figure 56.2
Transesophageal echocardiogram from a similar plane as in
Figure 56.1. A special guidewire of the Inoue balloon system
has passed through the trans-septal sheath and crossed the
interatrial septum. The distal loops of the guidewire are
visualized in the left atrium (arrow). The puncture site may be
enlarged with an Inoue dilator, and the Inoue balloon
catheter may then be advanced over the guidewire.

Figure 56.3
Transesophageal echocardiogram from the mid-esophageal
level of the modified four-chamber view in the transverse axis
(imaging angle 0°). The Inoue balloon catheter has been
advanced over the guidewire and is now evident in the left
atrium (LA). The mitral valve plane is visualized between the
left atrium and left ventricle (LV) but the leaflets are not well
seen in this image. Flushing of the catheter with saline has
resulted in a small amount of echocardiographic contrast in
the left atrium.

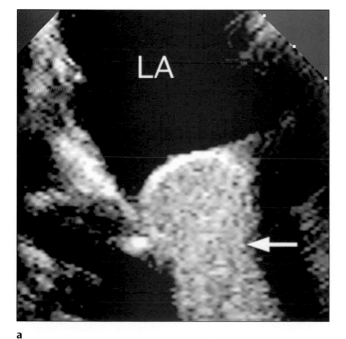

a   b

Figure 56.4
(a) Transesophageal echocardiogram from the mid-esophageal level of the modified four-chamber view in the transverse axis
(imaging angle 0°). The Inoue balloon has been properly positioned across the stenotic mitral valve and inflated. Waisting of the
balloon near its mid-section represents restriction by the stenotic mitral valve (arrow). AO, aorta; LA, left atrium.
(b) With the balloon fully expanded, a waist is no longer apparent (arrow), consistent with successful commissural rupture.

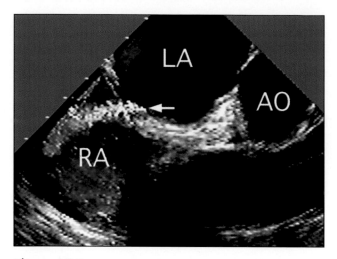

Figure 56.5
Transesophageal image from the mid-esophagus (imaging angle 90°). All of the valvuloplasty apparatus has been removed. There is no longer a catheter in the left atrium or right atrium. Color Doppler flow imaging identifies a small jet of turbulent left to right flow (arrow) across the interatrial septum indicating the presence of a residual iatrogenic atrial septal defect at the site of trans-septal puncture. Such defects are common, but rarely physiologically significant.

Discussion

Percutaneous mitral balloon valvuloplasty (PMBV) is now an established alternative to surgical mitral commissurotomy for the treatment of symptomatic mitral stenosis. The principle mechanism by which balloon inflation reduces the stenosis severity is by splitting of the fused commissures.[1] The Inoue balloon catheter technique, introduced in 1984 and approved for use in the United States in 1994, is favored in many institutions. It utilizes a low-profile, easily maneuverable catheter which is size-adjustable and self-positioning. Using the Inoue technique, an approximate 50% reduction in the trans-mitral gradient and a doubling of the mitral valve area are typically observed.[2] Results are best in the absence of significant leaflet thickening, immobility, and calcification, and with minimal subvalvular apparatus involvement.[3]

PMBV is ideally suited for pregnant patients with mitral stenosis who develop progressive symptoms as a result of the physiological increase in cardiac output and reduction in diastolic filling time which occurs with pregnancy. In a recent series of 44 patients, successful treatment was achieved in 100% of patients with all experiencing functional improvement.[4] Exposure of the fetus to scattered ionizing radiation is of obvious concern in such patients. Echocardiography is an essential tool in the assessment of patients undergoing PMBV. Both transthoracic and transesophageal echocardiography are routinely performed to screen patients for the procedure. Preprocedural transesophageal echocardiography is particularly valuable in identifying the presence of a left atrial thrombus, which if unnoticed can have grave consequences if the procedure is carried out. During the procedure, transesophageal echocardiography affords precise visualization of the interatrial septum and mitral apparatus, facilitating proper positioning of the trans-septal needle and balloon catheter, respectively. Immediate post-inflation assessment of the leaflet excursion, residual gradient and mitral regurgitation is also possible. It also reduces the use of ionizing radiation which should be kept to a minimum in all patients, but especially pregnant women. Transesophageal guidance has had little use as a total substitute for fluoroscopic guidance, but further research is ongoing to determine the safety of such a strategy.[5]

Residual atrial septal defects at the site of the trans-septal puncture may be seen in the majority of patients immediately after the procedure with the use of transesophageal echocardiography, the most sensitive technique for their detection. Intracardiac shunts may be detected by oximetry in a much smaller number, 25% of patients, immediately after the procedure. The shunts are rarely clinically significant and the majority close during short-term follow-up.

References

1. Kaplan J, Isner J, Karas R, *et al*. In vitro analysis of mechanisms of balloon valvuloplasty of stenotic mitral valves. Am J Cardiol 1987;59:318–23.

2. Herrmann H, Ramaswamy K, Isner J, *et al*. Factors influencing immediate results, complications, and short-term follow-up status after Inoue balloon mitral valvotomy: a North American multicenter study. Am Heart J 1992;124:160–66.

3. Abascal V, Wilkins G, O'Shea J, *et al*. Prediction of successful outcome in 130 patients undergoing percutaneous balloon mitral valvotomy. Circulation 1990;82:448–56.

4. Ben Farhat M, Gamra H, Betbout F, *et al*. Percutaneous balloon mitral commissurotomy during pregnancy. Heart 1997;77:564–7.

5. Kultursay H, Turkoglu C, Akin M, *et al*. Mitral balloon valvuloplasty with transesophageal echocardiography without using fluoroscopy. Cathet Cardiovasc Diagn 1992;27:317–21.

57

Ischemic mitral regurgitation

John Augoustides MD
Susan E Wiegers MD

A 75-year-old man presented to his family practitioner with increasing shortness of breath. He had recovered from a myocardial infarction 6 months previously. He denied any recent chest pain or palpitations. On physical examination his pulse was irregular and he had bibasilar rales. On cardiac examination, an apical systolic thrill was palpable, as well as an apical holosystolic murmur with radiation to the axilla. An office electrocardiogram revealed atrial fibrillation and left axis deviation. A transthoracic echocardiogram was ordered to evaluate left ventricular function and the new systolic murmur.

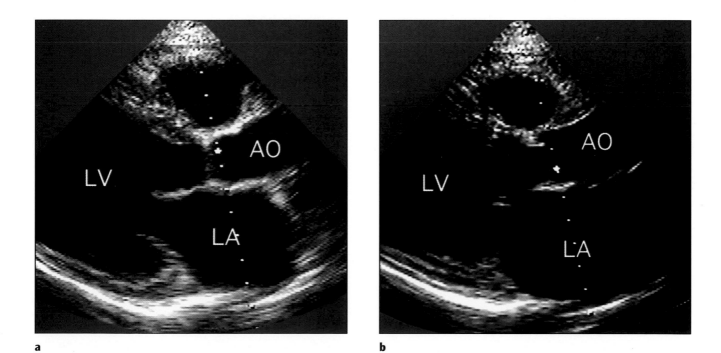

a   b

Figure 57.1
(a) Parasternal long-axis view in diastole. The left ventricle (LV) is severely dilated. The posterior wall is thinner than the interventricular septum. The left atrium (LA) is also moderately dilated. (b) Similar view in systole. Marked systolic expansion of the left atrium is suggestive of severe mitral regurgitation. The left ventricle remains enlarged. Comparison of the internal dimensions between systole and diastole indicate a severely decreased fractional shortening, indicative of decreased left ventricular function. Left ventricular dysfunction has resulted in a decreased stroke volume which fails to open the aortic valve fully, as demonstrated in this image.

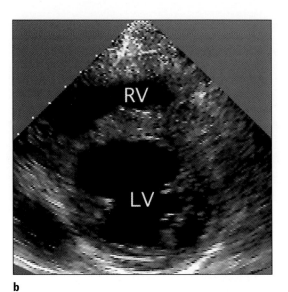

a

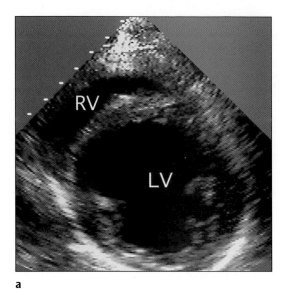

b

Figure 57.2

(a) Parasternal short-axis view in diastole. The left ventricle is again noted to be dilated. The inferior and the posterior walls are thinned and echodense compared to the septum and the anterior wall which is diagnostic of scar from an old myocardial infarction. (b) Parasternal short-axis view in systole. The inferior and posterior walls do not thicken to the same extent as the anterior wall. The posterior wall, in particular, exhibits severe hypokinesis.

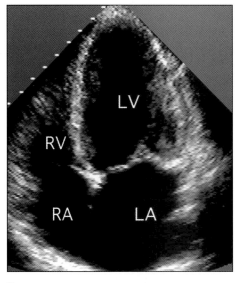

a

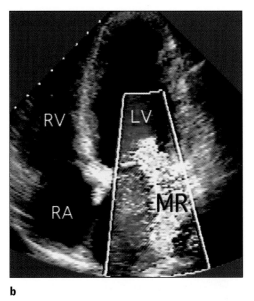

b

Figure 57.3

(a) Apical four-chamber view in early systole. The right ventricular (RV) systolic function appears to be normal. The right atrial (RA) size is also normal. Left ventricular (LV) systolic function is decreased and the chamber enlargement can be appreciated even in systole. The left atrium (LA) is moderately to severely enlarged. Incomplete closure of the mitral valve is present. The leaflets form a triangle at the coaptation point rather than lying horizontally. Incomplete closure of the mitral valve may result from annular dilatation or from papillary muscle dysfunction. There is dropout of the interatrial septum because the structure is parallel to the ultrasound beam in this view. Subsequent images demonstrate that there is no anatomic abnormality of the septum. (b) Similar view in a later systolic frame with color flow Doppler imaging. A torrential jet of mitral regurgitation (MR) fills a large portion of the left atrium and enters the pulmonary veins posteriorly. The jet actually rebounds off the posterior wall of the left atrium and circles the chamber. The aliased, high-velocity jet arises from the level of the mitral leaflet coaptation which is apically displaced, owing to the incomplete closure of the valve. The leaflets form a triangle with the apex pointing towards the left ventricular apex. The normal valve coapts in the plane of the annulus. Note that the interatrial septum has moved rightwards due to the increased left atrial pressure. It is no longer parallel to the ultrasound beam and is imaged in its entirety.

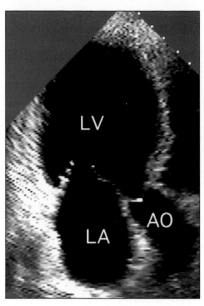

a

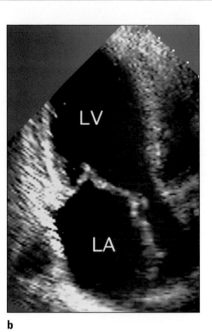

b

Figure 57.4

(a) Apical long-axis view of the mitral valve in diastole. The mitral leaflets appear to be normal although they are not fully opened in this image. The left ventricle is severely dilated. (b) Similar view in systole. The incomplete closure pattern of the mitral leaflet is again appreciated in this long-axis image. The posterior leaflet is fixed with little change in position between systole and diastole. A fixed leaflet may be caused by rheumatic heart disease but, in this case, the normal motion of the anterior leaflet rules out that possibility. In addition, the leaflets do not show thickening, which would invariably be present if rheumatic valvular disease were present. The posterior leaflet is tethered by the annular dilatation and the posterior papillary muscle dysfunction due to inferior infarction. The result is a relatively immobile posterior leaflet. The triangular closing of the mitral valve leaflets is clearly demonstrated.

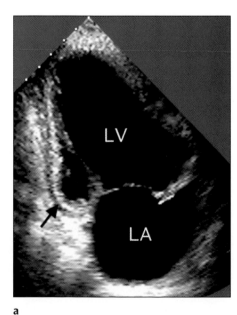

a

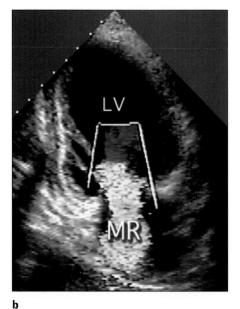

b

Figure 57.5

(a) Apical two-chamber view in systole. There is an aneurysm (arrow) of the inferior wall at the base of the ventricle which exhibits systolic bulging. The basilar inferior wall is echodense and thinned, evidence of a scar. The posterior mitral leaflet is fixed and tethered towards the left ventricle. The anterior mitral valve leaflet is able to assume a normal anatomic position but coaptation is incomplete, owing to the posterior leaflet dysfunction. (b) Similar systolic view with color Doppler flow imaging. The mitral regurgitation jet is eccentrically directed along the posterior wall of the left atrium by the over-riding anterior leaflet.

Discussion

This patient has severe chronic mitral regurgitation as evidenced by the dilated left atrium and left ventricle. Echocardiography is very sensitive for the diagnosis of mitral regurgitation. However, quantification of the severity has been more difficult, largely owing to the absence of a 'gold standard' for comparison. Invasive assessments are also qualitative measures. The most common technique in clinical practice is visually to compare the area of the mitral regurgitation jet to the area of the left atrium.[1] In this case, the mitral regurgitation fills the left atrium on color Doppler flow imaging which is diagnostic of severe regurgitation. An eccentric jet may impinge on the left atrial wall and cause the jet to spread out along the wall in the plane perpendicular to the imaging plane which may result in underestimation of the jet area.[2] It is reasonable to upgrade the severity of an eccentric jet by one grade because of this effect. Other methods for diagnosing severe mitral regurgitation include demonstrating reversal of systolic flow in the pulmonary veins.[3]

The anatomic mechanism of mitral regurgitation in this patient is understood by observing the function of the mitral leaflet at the level of the mitral annulus. Incomplete mitral leaflet coaptation is due to a fixed posterior leaflet and a dilated mitral annulus. The dilated annulus is due to cavity enlargement from ventricular remodelling as a gradual response to the volume load and to the infarction. The geometry of the annulus is further disrupted by the inferior aneurysm. The presence of the aneurysm also indicates an ischemic insult to the posterior papillary muscle. The distortion of the papillary muscle pulls the posterior leaflet into the ventricle and does not allow it to coapt correctly in systole. The mitral regurgitation jet is directed posteriorly. Mitral annular dilatation alone creates a centrally directed jet of mitral regurgitation. Asymmetric mitral leaflet motion allows leaflet over-ride and eccentric mitral regurgitation. The mitral regurgitation is severe, owing to the combined annular and leaflet pathology. The mitral regurgitation is eccentric, owing to the dominance of the fixed leaflet mechanism.

Although the patient was considered a relatively high-risk surgical candidate, he underwent coronary artery bypass grafting and mitral valve replacement. Had the dilated annulus been the sole cause of the regurgitation it might have been addressed with an annuloplasty ring. However, the presence of the inferior wall aneurysm and the papillary muscle dysfunction makes the success of a simple repair much less likely. The patient underwent placement of a mechanical bileaflet mitral valve. He was weaned from bypass on inotropic support and required ventilation in the intensive care unit for 2 days postoperatively. However, he had an uncomplicated course on transfer to the ward and was discharged to home on the 8th postoperative day on oral anticoagulants.

References

1. Bolger A, Eigler N, Maurer G. Quantifying valvular regurgitation. Limitations and inherent assumptions of Doppler techniques. Circulation 1988;78:1316–18.

2. Chen C, Thomas J, Anconina J, et al. Impact of impinging wall jet on color Doppler quantification of mitral regurgitation. Circulation 1991;84:712–20.

3. Klein A, Obarski T, Stewart W, et al. Transesophageal Doppler echocardiography of pulmonary venous flow: a new marker of mitral regurgitation severity. J Am Coll Cardiol 1991;18:518–26.

58

Acute papillary muscle rupture

Susan E Wiegers MD

A 65-year-old woman with a long history of tobacco use had sustained an uncomplicated inferior myocardial infarction 2 weeks previously. She had been doing well at home but had the sudden onset of sharp chest pain followed by severe dyspnea. She was brought to the emergency depart-

ment where she was found to be in pulmonary edema and required intubation. A new loud systolic murmur was heard at the apex and an echocardiogram was obtained. A transesophageal echocardiogram was performed immediately following the transthoracic study.

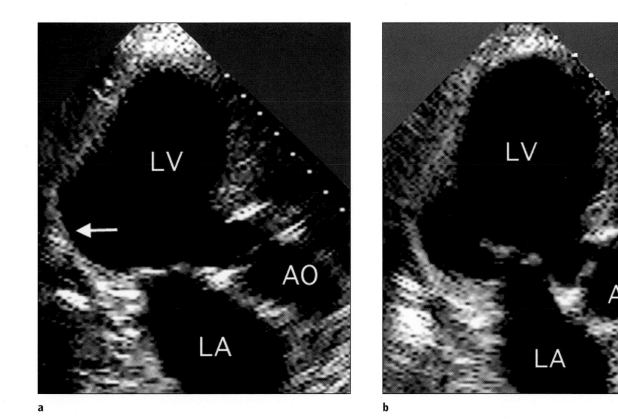

a   b

Figure 58.1
(a) Transthoracic apical long-axis view in early systole demonstrates dyskinesis (arrow) of the posterior wall at the base. The posterior wall bulges in systole and the myocardium is thinned. Since ventricular remodelling has already occurred the posterior wall motion abnormality is probably due to the previous infarction rather than an acute event. LV, left ventricle; LA, left atrium; AO, aorta. (b) Diastolic image in the same view. There is diastolic deformity of the posterior wall which confirms the presence of a posterior aneurysm. The tip of the posterior mitral valve leaflet appears markedly thickened, but this is difficult to appreciate in the still frame.

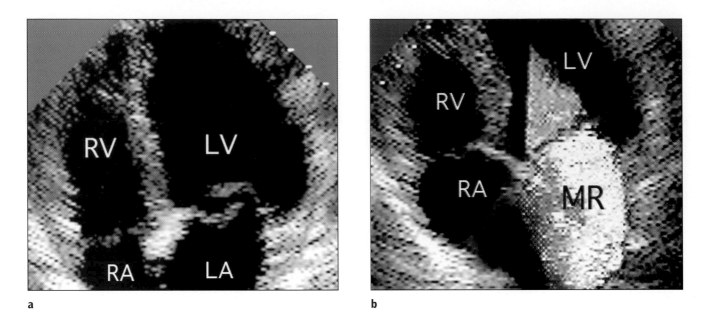

a   b

Figure 58.2

(a) Transthoracic apical four-chamber view in early diastole. The scale is different from that of the previous figure. The left ventricle is dilated and the lateral wall at the base is thinned. The posterior leaflet of the mitral valve (attached to the lateral annulus) is thickened at the tip. In real time, there appeared to be a large mass on the tip of this leaflet. (b) Systolic image in the same view with color flow Doppler imaging. A turbulent jet of torrential mitral regurgitation (MR) fills the left atrium. The interatrial septum bows into the right atrium (RA), owing to the increase in left atrial pressure. The lateral wall of the left ventricle (LV) is akinetic. The wall motion abnormality involves not only the posterior wall as seen in the previous figures, but the lateral wall as well. The left ventricular ejection fraction is moderately reduced. In the setting of severe mitral regurgitation, this apparent moderate reduction in ejection fraction may represent severe left ventricular dysfunction.

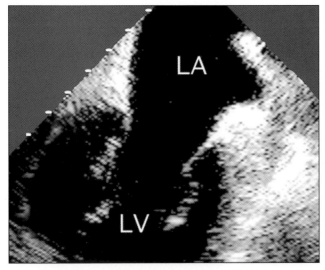
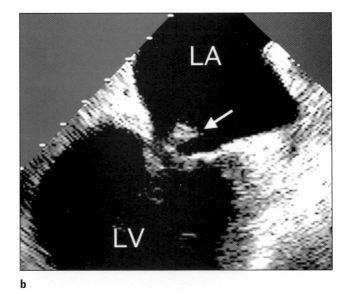

a   b

Figure 58.3

(a) Transesophageal diastolic image of the mitral valve leaflets from the mid-esophagus and imaging plane of approximately 70°. The mitral valve leaflets open normally. The left atrium (LA) is not enlarged, indicating the acute nature of the severe mitral regurgitation. The basilar posterior wall is seen on the left of the screen and a portion of the aneurysm is visualized, although not clearly. (b) In this systolic image from the same view, the head of the posterior medial papillary muscle (arrow) prolapses into the left atrium. It is attached to the posterior mitral valve leaflet. The ruptured papillary muscle tip can be recognized by its characteristic shape. The triangular shape of the ruptured portion of the papillary muscle is appreciated with the apex of the triangle closest to the leaflet and the base of the triangle projecting into the left atrium. The systolic deformation of the posterior wall is seen on the left of the screen.

Discussion

The large wall motion abnormality in this case is indicative of a posterolateral basilar aneurysm. Severe mitral regurgitation may result from annular dilatation or from papillary muscle dysfunction. However, in this case, the history of acute chest pain followed by hemodynamic collapse is suggestive of an acute event such as papillary muscle rupture. The transthoracic study ruled out the other cause of a loud systolic murmur after myocardial infarction which is ventricular septal defect. It is easily appreciated on the transthoracic images that the mitral valve is abnormal. However, the ruptured head of the papillary muscle was visible in this case only on transesophageal imaging. Transesophageal studies are more sensitive and specific for flail mitral valve leaflet.[1] The size and triangular shape of the papillary muscle head indicates that the rupture occurred in the body of the papillary muscle. Rupture may occur at the chordal level, the tip of the papillary muscle or in the body of the papillary muscle itself. Progressively more severe mitral regurgitation is associated with these lesions.

Rupture of the head of a papillary muscle results in acute torrential mitral regurgitation which is always poorly tolerated and often rapidly fatal. This patient was immediately taken to the catheterization laboratory for coronary angiogram followed by emergency mitral valve replacement with coronary artery bypass grafting. Her course was complicated by acute renal failure, but she survived.

Reference

1. Himelman RB, Kusumoto F, Oken K, et al. The flail mitral valve: echocardiographic findings by precordial and transesophageal imaging and Doppler color flow mapping. J Am Coll Cardiol 1991;17:272–9.

59

Systolic anterior motion of the mitral valve causing left ventricular outflow tract obstruction after mitral valve repair

Susan E Wiegers MD

A 57-year-old man underwent mitral valve repair for symptomatic mitral regurgitation. He had a long history of mitral valve prolapse due to a myxomatous valve. His symptoms had progressed over the course of the past 6 months. Preoperative evaluation showed no evidence of coronary disease and severe prolapse of a scallop of the posterior mitral valve leaflet. He was taken to the operating room and underwent resection of a scallop of the posterior mitral leaflet with annular plication and placement of an annuloplasty ring. He was markedly hypotensive when weaning from bypass despite triple pressor infusion.

Transesophageal echocardiography demonstrated left ventricular outflow tract obstruction secondary to severe systolic anterior motion of the mitral valve. In addition, there was severe residual mitral regurgitation. The hypotension responded only partially to weaning from the inotropic agents. A second bypass run was undertaken. The repair was taken down and the patient underwent sliding plasty with undercutting of P_1 and P_2 scallops. After the second bypass run, the patient was easily weaned from bypass. He did not require pressor agents to maintain his blood pressure and there was no residual mitral regurgitation.

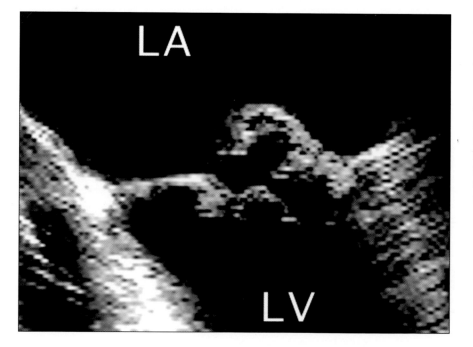

Figure 59.1
Transesophageal echocardiogram from the mid-esophageal level in the transverse plane (imaging angle 0°) prior to the surgical repair. This close-up of the mitral valve is taken from a four-chamber view in systole. A large scallop of the posterior leaflet of the mitral valve prolapses into the left atrium (LA). The leaflet is thickened and myxomatous. Left ventricular (LV) systolic function (not shown here) was normal.

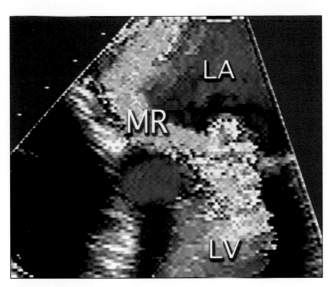
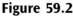

Figure 59.2

Similar transesophageal echocardiogram from the mid-esophageal level and the transverse plane (imaging angle 0°) with color flow Doppler imaging in systole. The prolapsing posterior leaflet directs the jet of mitral regurgitation (MR) medially along the interatrial septum. The left atrium (LA) is noted to be enlarged. Proximal acceleration of the jet can be appreciated on the left ventricular (LV) side of the mitral valve. This is a sign of severe mitral regurgitation.

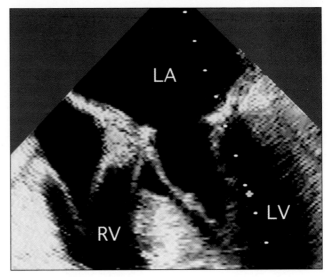

Figure 59.3

Intraoperative transesophageal echocardiogram taken after the first pump run. The transducer is in the mid-esophagus. The imaging plane is 0°. This four-chamber image demonstrates the mitral annuloplasty ring in place which appears as two echodense structures in the mitral annulus. Comparison with Figure 59.1 demonstrates that the mitral annulus has been significantly reduced in size.

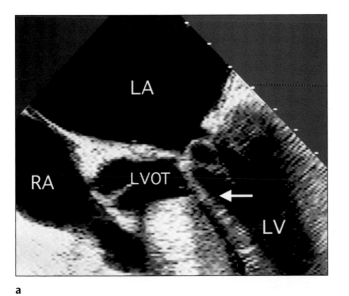

a

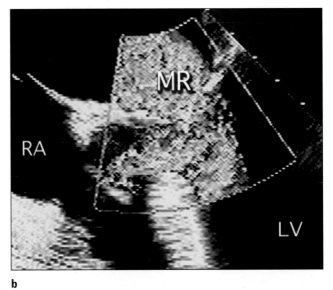

b

Figure 59.4

(a) Similar transesophageal image in a four-chamber view with the transducer withdrawn slightly compared to the level in Figure 59.3 allowing imaging of the left ventricular outflow tract (LVOT). This systolic image demonstrates marked systolic anterior motion of the anterior mitral valve leaflet (arrow) with obstruction of the left ventricular outflow tract. Again, it is noted that the left atrium is enlarged but the mitral valve annulus has been significantly reduced in size. The right atrium and right ventricle appear underfilled. The patient was on maximal inotropic support at this time. (b) Similar transesophageal echocardiogram with color flow Doppler imaging in systole. The jet of mitral regurgitation (MR) is central rather than eccentric as it had been previously. However, it is still severe in degree. There is a high-velocity turbulent jet in the left ventricular outflow tract that was caused by the systolic anterior motion of the mitral valve and the resultant dynamic obstruction. The systolic anterior motion of the mitral valve leaflet disrupts normal coaptation, resulting in significant mitral regurgitation.

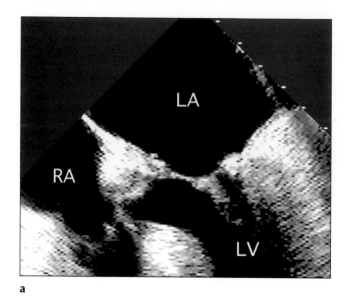
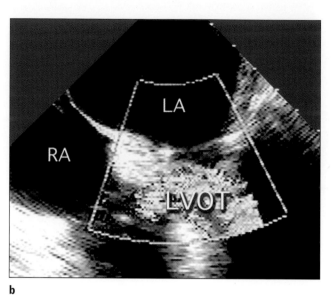

a   b

Figure 59.5

(a) Transesophageal echocardiogram from the mid-esophageal level after the second pump run. The patient is no longer on inotropic support. Systolic anterior motion of the mitral valve is no longer present and the left ventricular outflow tract is no longer obstructed in this systolic image. (b) Similar transesophageal echocardiogram with color flow Doppler imaging. There is no residual mitral regurgitation. The left ventricular ejection jet seen in the left ventricular outflow tract is no longer of high velocity or turbulent.

Discussion

This patient had classic mitral valve prolapse with a myxomatous valve and was an excellent candidate for mitral valve repair. Intraoperative transesophageal echocardiography is an important component in the strategy to assess the adequacy of repair and evaluate surgical complications.[1] Systolic anterior motion of the mitral valve has been reported after mitral valve repair both with a rigid annuloplasty ring and without a ring.[2] The presumed mechanism of the systolic anterior motion involves a distortion of the geometry of the anterior mitral valve leaflet in relation to the ejection jet of the left ventricle. The annuloplasty ring brings the posterior mitral annulus closer to the left ventricular outflow tract. A redundant anterior mitral valve leaflet may then be displaced into the ejection jet, subjecting it to the Venturi effect.[3] The left ventricular outflow tract obstruction may result in profound hypotension immediately following weaning from cardiopulmonary bypass. The use of inotropic agents may exacerbate the obstruction not only by increasing the velocity of the ventricular ejection which increases the Venturi effect, but also by causing a further decrease in the left ventricular volume which brings the anterior mitral valve leaflet into the outflow tract. Some patients respond promptly to discontinuation of inotropic agents, use of beta-blockade and volume infusion. However, patients with intractable hypotension will require a second pump run. A sliding plasty with undercutting of the scallops will usually eliminate the systolic anterior motion and subsequent outflow tract obstruction. If not, mitral valve replacement may be necessary.[4]

In addition to left ventricular outflow tract obstruction, systolic anterior motion of the mitral valve leaflet disrupts normal valvular coaptation and results in significant mitral regurgitation. This patient had worsened mitral regurgitation after the initial repair. Resolution of the systolic anterior motion eliminated the mitral regurgitation. Care should be taken in evaluating patients after mitral valve repair to carefully visualize the anterior mitral valve leaflet in systole and to assess the left ventricular outflow tract.[5] The apical four-chamber view in the standard transesophageal image may not image the left ventricular outflow tract. Retroflexion of the transducer at the mid-esophageal level will usually bring the outflow tract into view. In addition, transgastric images simulating the apical long-axis view can also be attempted. The presence of chordal systolic anterior motion is quite common after mitral valve repair[6] and is of no hemodynamic consequence. It should be carefully distinguished from valvular systolic anterior motion. Doppler interrogation of the outflow tract may also reveal high-velocity aliased flow consistent with dynamic outflow tract obstruction. A high level of suspicion is necessary when evaluating patients in the operating room after mitral valve repair to rule out these complications.

References

1. Stewart WJ, Griffin B, Thomas JD. Multiplane transesophageal echocardiographic evaluation of mitral valve disease. Am J Cardiac Imag 1995;9:121–8.

2. Eishi K, Kawazoe K, Kawashima Y. Systolic anterior motion of the mitral valve after mitral valve repair without a ring. Ann Thorac Surg 1993;55:1013–14.

3. Kreindel MS, Schiavone WA, Lever HM, *et al.* Systolic anterior motion of the mitral valve after Carpentier ring valvuloplasty for mitral valve prolapse. Am J Cardiol 1986;57:408–12.

4. Stewart WJ, Currie PJ, Salcedo EE, *et al.* Intraoperative Doppler color flow mapping for decision-making in valve repair for mitral regurgitation. Technique and results in 100 patients. Circulation 1990;81:556–66.

5. Freeman W, Schaff H, Khandheria B, *et al.* Intraoperative evaluation of mitral valve regurgitation and repair by transesophageal echocardiography: incidence and significance of systolic anterior motion. J Am Coll Cardiol 1992;20:599–609.

6. Cohen K, Norris L, Montemayor I, *et al.* Systolic anterior motion of the chordal apparatus after mitral ring insertion. Am Heart J 1992;124:666–70.

60

Systolic anterior motion of the mitral valve after mitral valve replacement

Susan E Wiegers MD

A 73-year-old man with a history of a myxomatous mitral valve developed progressive, severe shortness of breath. Evaluation demonstrated prolapse of the anterior mitral valve leaflet and severe mitral regurgitation. The patient underwent mitral valve replacement at another hospital. It was elected to place a bioprosthesis because of the patient's age and history of gastrointestinal bleeding. The

patient was discharged from the hospital on the seventh postoperative day and recovered normally. However, when he saw his cardiologist in follow-up 4 weeks later, he complained of continued dyspnea on exertion. The cardiologist noted a loud harsh systolic ejection murmur, loudest at the left lower sternal border, and an echocardiogram was obtained.

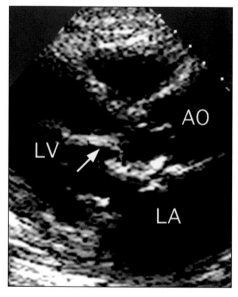

a

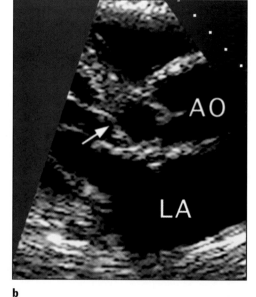

b

Figure 60.1
(a) Parasternal long-axis view in diastole. The left atrium (LA) is mildly enlarged. The stents of the bioprosthesis are echodense and project in a parallel fashion into the left ventricular cavity from the mitral valve annulus. The preserved native anterior mitral valve leaflet is observed also attached to the annulus extending down to the papillary muscle level which is just out of view. There is mild left ventricular hypertrophy and the left ventricular cavity appears normal in size at this level. The aortic root (AO) is normal and the aortic valve is closed in diastole. (b) Similar parasternal long-axis view in systole. The stents of the bioprosthesis are still visible. However, the native anterior mitral valve leaflet (arrow) demonstrates marked systolic anterior motion and is seen to obstruct the left ventricular outflow tract. Note that the stents of the bioprosthesis have not changed their orientation. The bioprosthetic leaflets themselves are not visualized in this transthoracic echocardiogram. The thin leaflets of the bioprosthesis are difficult to image in the acoustic shadow of the echodense stents. Owing to the outflow tract obstruction, the aortic valve leaflets are closed in this systolic frame.

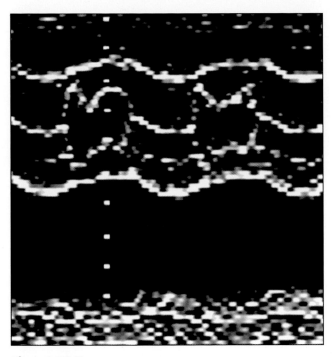

Figure 60.2
M-mode echocardiogram taken from the parasternal position of the aortic valve. Rather than the normal rectangular opening of the aortic valve, early closure of the aortic valve is demonstrated. The timing of the early closure of the aortic valve corresponds to the maximum gradient generated across the left ventricular outflow tract. This finding is characteristic of dynamic left ventricular outflow tract obstruction.

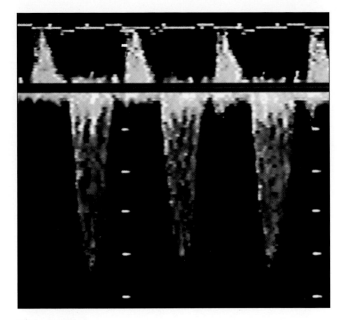

Figure 60.3
Spectral display of continuous-wave Doppler outflow velocity taken from the apical position across the left ventricular outflow tract. Each calibration mark represents 100 cm/s or 1 m/s. Thus the peak outflow velocity is over 4 m/s, predicting an outflow tract gradient of 64 mmHg. Although not well seen, the diastolic inflow into the left ventricle across the mitral valve also has increased velocity although the pressure half-time is normal. This is due to the fact that the bioprosthesis is mildly stenotic compared to a native valve.

Discussion

Preservation of the papillary muscles and chordal apparatus has become a standard surgical technique in mitral valve replacement. Preservation of these structures prevents the decline in left ventricular systolic function that is seen after mitral valve replacement in which the papillary muscles and chordal apparatus are removed.[1] The presence of the mitral valve tensor apparatus preserves the geometry of the ventricle. This may be why results of mitral valve repair are superior to mitral valve replacement in terms of postoperative left ventricular function.

This patient underwent the relatively unusual procedure of having a mitral valve bioprosthesis placed with preservation of the entire mitral valve structure including the mitral valve leaflets. As can be seen from the echocardiographic images, this presented no problem in diastole. However, by displacing the anterior mitral valve leaflet towards the interventricular septum, the leaflet was drawn into the left ventricular outflow tract by Venturi forces of the ejecting blood in systole. This created systolic anterior motion of the mitral valve leaflet with severe left ventricular outflow tract obstruction. The stent of the bioprosthetic valve holds the leaflet into the ejection jet, ensuring it will be forced into the left ventricular outflow tract in systole. The problem was exacerbated by the patient's normal left ventricular function and the geometry of his septum. Note the mild proximal bulging of the septum which is visualized in Figure 60.1. Left ventricular outflow tract obstruction by the native anterior mitral valve leaflet has been reported in this situation.[2,3] Not surprisingly, the practice of performing mitral valve replacement over unresected mitral leaflets is no longer generally accepted. Patients with small ventricular cavities and proximal systolic bulging may be particularly at risk for this complication. It is clear that ventricular dilatation might protect from this complication. Symptomatic systolic anterior motion of the mitral valve has also been reported after placement of an annuloplasty ring for mitral valve repair.

The patient failed to respond to beta-blockers and calcium channel blockers designed to decrease the force of left ventricular contraction. He was so symptomatic that he required repeat cardiac surgery in which the anterior mitral valve leaflet was removed. The bioprosthesis was left in place. Intraoperative transesophageal echocardiography confirmed resolution of the outflow tract obstruction and the patient has done well postoperatively.

References

1. David TE, Uden DE, Strauss HD. The importance of the mitral apparatus in left ventricular function after correction of mitral regurgitation. Circulation 1983;68:II76–82.

2. Bortolotti U, Milano A, Tursi V, *et al.* Fatal obstruction of the left ventricular outflow tract caused by low-profile bioprosthesis in the mitral position. Chest 1993; 103:1288–9.

3. Esper E, Ferdinand F, Aronson S, *et al.* Prosthetic mitral valve replacement: late complications after native valve preservation. Ann Thorac Surg 1997;63:541–3.

61

Marfan's syndrome

Susan E Wiegers MD

A-38-year old man was the tallest of his three brothers, who were all over 6 feet 3 inches. His habitus was notable for an asthenic build, long fingers and a mild pectus excavatum. He was well, but a murmur was noted by a family member who was a nursing student. Referral to an internist revealed no other significant data. The patient had no exercise limitation and had never experienced chest pain. He did not have a high arched palate or lens dislocation. There was no family history of sudden death or cardiovascular disease. A loud systolic murmur was noted across the entire precordium. Echocardiography was undertaken to evaluate the murmur.

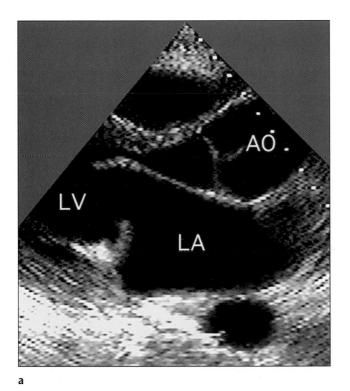
a

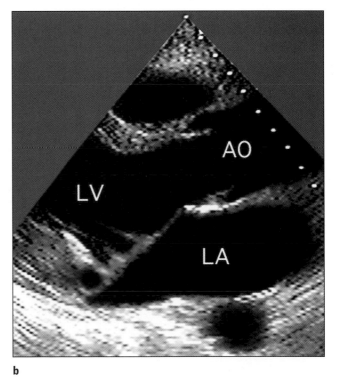
b

Figure 61.1
(a) Parasternal long-axis view in diastole. The mitral valve is markedly abnormal. The anterior mitral leaflet is thickened and myxomatous. The posterior leaflet is also noted to be thickened. The left ventricular cavity (LV) is dilated and measures approximately 6 cm. The left atrium (LA) is also enlarged. The aortic root and ascending aorta (AO) are enlarged, measuring approximately 4 cm. The descending thoracic aorta, which is seen posterior to the left atrium, is of normal caliber. (b) Parasternal long-axis view in systole. The markedly abnormal motion of the mitral valve is now evident. The myxomatous anterior leaflet appears to hinge at the annulus and billows into the left atrium. The posterior leaflet prolapses particularly at the annular attachment. *continued overleaf*

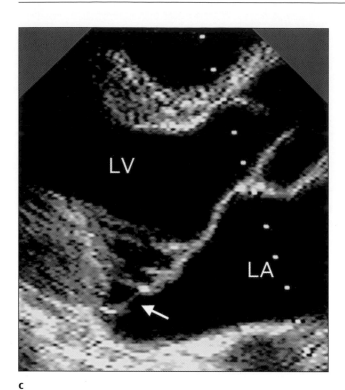

c

Figure 61.1 *continued*
(c) Close-up view of the mitral valve in systole. The arrow demonstrates the marked prolapse of the posterior leaflet of the mitral valve into the left atrium.

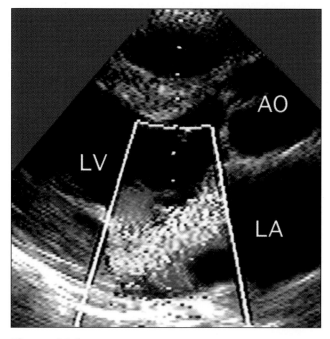

Figure 61.2
Parasternal long-axis view in systole with color flow Doppler imaging. A highly turbulent jet of mitral regurgitation fills the left atrium (LA). The jet originates at the posterior annulus, as evidenced by the PISA effect on the left ventricular side of the mitral valve at that site. The anteriorly directed jet courses up the long and myxomatous anterior leaflet towards the aortic root.

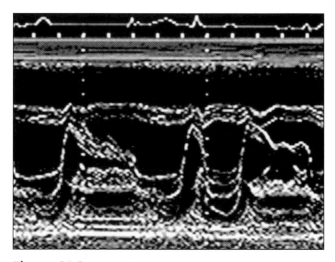

Figure 61.3
M-mode echocardiogram from the parasternal position of the mitral valve. Marked prolapse of the posterior mitral valve leaflet is demonstrated in systole. While two-dimensional echocardiography is far more sensitive and specific for the diagnosis of mitral valve prolapse, this classic M-mode finding is often present in patients with such severe prolapse. The thickening of the leaflets is also readily apparent.

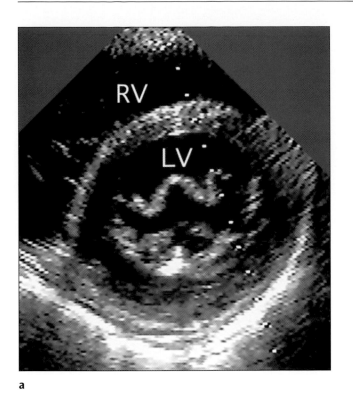

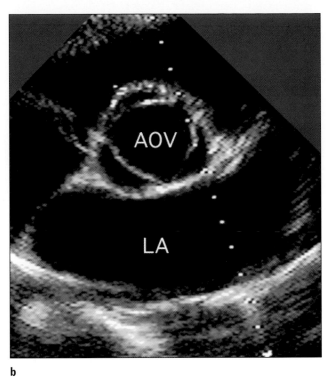

a   b

Figure 61.4
(a) Short-axis view from the parasternal position of the left ventricle in diastole at the level of the mitral valve leaflets. The mitral leaflets are noted to be thickened, myxomatous and highly redundant. The left ventricular cavity is dilated.
(b) Short-axis view from the parasternal position at the level of the base of the heart in systole. Left atrial (LA) enlargement is evident. The aortic valve (AOV) is normal but the root is dilated. The leaflets are not thickened and are anatomically normal.

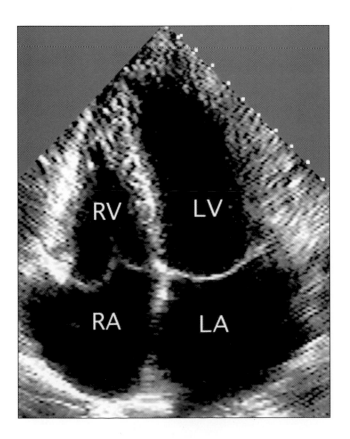

Figure 61.5
Apical four-chamber view in systole. The left ventricle is dilated and the left ventricular ejection fraction is slightly reduced. There is biatrial enlargement. The abnormally redundant anterior mitral valve leaflet is noted. There is also prolapse of the anterior leaflet of the tricuspid valve appreciated in this view.

Discussion

This patient had previously undiagnosed Marfan's syndrome. Now known to be caused by a defect in the fibrillin gene, it has long been diagnosed by clinical criteria.[1] The condition occurs in approximately 1 in 10 000 individuals and is inherited as an autosomal dominant syndrome with variable penetrance and expression; 20–40% of cases arise as spontaneous mutations.[2] Tall stature, arm span greater than total height, high arched palate, and arachnodactyly characterize the common physical findings. Cardiovascular complications include mitral valve prolapse which is often severe, aortic dilatation, and a propensity for aortic dissection.

This patient's echocardiographic findings were highly suspicious for Marfan's syndrome. Echocardiographers should be alert to the combination of marked myxomatous mitral valve abnormality in the setting of aortic annular dilatation. The mitral leaflets in this condition are elongated as well as myxomatous, and tend to billow into the left atrium in systole.[3] In this case, the prolapse of the posterior leaflet directed the regurgitant jet anteriorly towards the aortic root. The murmur was loudest at the left upper sternal border rather than the apex for this reason. The mitral regurgitation is usually progressive, owing to the valvular abnormality as well as the annular dilatation.

Serial echocardiographic follow-up is recommended to assess the mitral valve as well as the aorta. Progressive aortic root enlargement is an ominous sign and should precipitate surgical replacement of the aortic root and ascending aorta. A change in the aortic sinus dimension of more than 5% per year is predictive of aortic dissection or rupture.[4] In patients with Marfan's syndrome who present with acute chest pain, a high level of suspicion for the diagnosis or aortic dissection should be maintained. Transesophageal echocardiography is a rapid and reliable technique to diagnose dissection.[5]

The mitral regurgitation often results in the need for surgery as well. Mitral valve repair should not be attempted in patients with Marfan's syndrome because of the frequent need for reoperation. This patient demonstrated progressive enlargement of the left ventricle and a mild fall in the ejection fraction in serial studies. He has remained asymptomatic and has not yet undergone surgery.

References

1. Towbin J, Casey B, and Belmont J. Human genetics '99: the cardiovascular system. The molecular basis of vascular disorders. Am J Hum Genet 1999;64:678–84.
2. Tilstra D, Byers P. Molecular basis of hereditary disorders of connective tissue. Ann Rev Med 1994;45:149–63.
3. Pini R, Roman MJ, Kramer-Fox R, et al. Mitral valve dimensions and motion in Marfan patients with and without mitral valve prolapse. Comparison to primary mitral valve prolapse and normal subjects. Circulation 1989;80:915–24.
4. Legget M, Unger T, O'Sullivan C, et al. Aortic root complications in Marfan's syndrome: identification of a lower risk group. Heart 1996;75:389–95.
5. Simpson I, de Belder M, Treasure T, et al. Cardiovascular manifestations of Marfan's syndrome: improved evaluation by transoesophageal echocardiography. Br Heart J 1993; 69:104–8.

62

Thrombosis of a bioprosthetic mitral valve

Susan E Wiegers MD

A 42-year-old man had undergone mitral valve replacement for endocarditis secondary to intravenous drug use. A bioprosthetic mitral valve replacement had been placed, owing to the presence of active infection and a large annular abscess. The patient had been well for several years but not compliant with anticoagulation. He presented to the emergency room with a 1-week history of effort presyncope and progressive shortness of breath at rest. In the emergency room, he was in extremis, with evidence of a low perfusion state and pulmonary edema. Heart sounds were inaudible. A transthoracic echocardiogram demonstrated a large mass in the left atrium that was thought to be a thrombus. The patient was anticoagulated with intravenous heparin but deteriorated soon after presentation, requiring intubation. Transesophageal echocardiography was performed in the operating room, where the patient underwent emergency surgery.

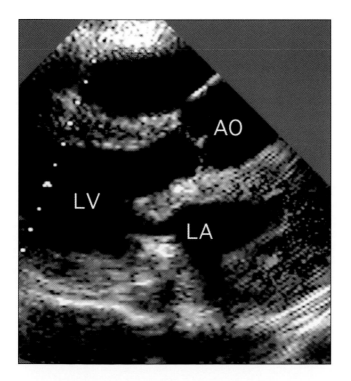

Figure 62.1
Parasternal long-axis view in diastole. The left atrium is filled with a homogeneous mass that involves the walls of the left atrium and leaves a small echolucent cavity. The stents of the bioprosthetic valve are echodense and project into the left ventricle but the valve leaflets are not imaged. The left ventricle is normal-sized, although the left atrium is enlarged. The aortic valve is normal.

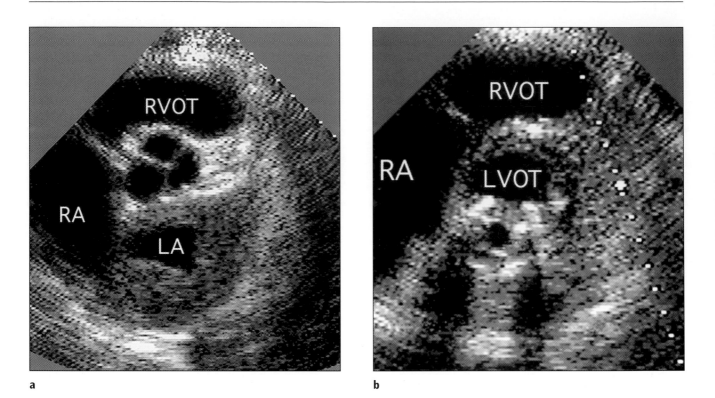

a   b

Figure 62.2

(a) Parasternal short-axis view at the level of the base of the heart in diastole. The aortic valve is tricuspid and appears normal. The thrombus fills the left atrium and extends into the left atrial appendage, which is seen on the right of the screen in the anterior portion of the left atrium.

(b) Parasternal short-axis view at the level of the mitral valve. The transducer has been angled inferiorly from the previous view to obtain this image. The three struts of the bioprosthetic valve are clearly demonstrated. The orifice appears to be narrowed by the left atrial thrombus, which appears to extend into the valve opening.

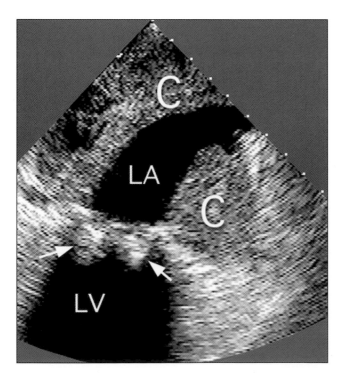

Figure 62.3

Transesophageal image from the mid-esophagus in the longitudinal view. The bioprosthetic mitral valve stents (arrows) project into the left ventricular cavity (LV). Although the stents are more echodense than the surrounding tissue, they are obscured by the large amount of thrombus which is present in the valve orifice. The left atrial cavity (LA) is narrowed by a large clot (C). To the right of the image, the thrombus obscures the left atrial appendage and projects into the left atrium proper. Laminated thrombus is also present along the interatrial septal side of the left atrium seen on the left of the image. No motion of the mitral valve leaflets was observed in real time.

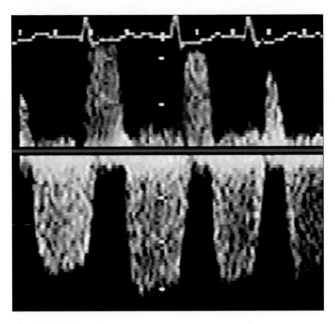

Figure 62.4
Spectral display of continuous-wave Doppler across the mitral valve. In the transesophageal approach, diastolic mitral inflow is seen as negative flow away from the transducer. The peak velocity of the mitral inflow is 3 m/s (calibration marks represents 100 cm/s or 1 m/s) which predicts a peak mitral valve gradient of 36 mmHg. The spectral envelope shows little change in the velocity during diastole which is consistent with a very long pressure half-time and critical mitral stenosis. An incomplete spectral envelope of mitral regurgitation is also noted.

Discussion

Owing to lack of compliance with anticoagulation and lack of long-term follow-up, this patient developed severe obstruction of his bioprosthetic valve several years after it was placed. The mass in the left atrium was laminated along the wall and homogeneous, making the thrombus the most likely diagnosis. Thrombosis of bioprosthetic mitral valves has been estimated to occur at a rate of less than 2% per patient-year, under optimal conditions.[1]

It is not always possible to obtain such excellent images of prosthetic mitral valves from the transthoracic approach. The stents of the valve are highly refractile and often cause enough shadowing to obscure the left atrium completely. In a critically ill patient with a mitral valve prosthesis, the echocardiographer should be ready to perform a transesophageal echocardiogram immediately if the transthoracic images do not yield a diagnosis. Transvalvular gradients can often be easily obtained from the apical transthoracic window and may demonstrate elevated velocities suggestive of valvular obstruction. Transvalvular gradients can also be obtained from the transesophageal windows. As opposed to the case with aortic gradients, it is generally quite easy to align the ultra-

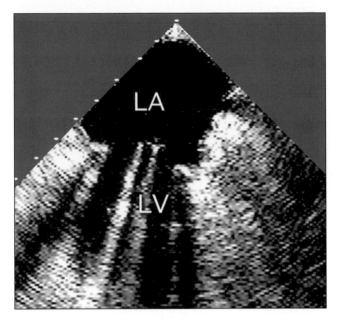

Figure 62.5
After the cardiopulmonary bypass and placement of a bileaflet mechanical valve. The diastolic view is similar to that of Figure 62.3. A St Jude's bileaflet valve is now present in the mitral position with normal opening of the leaflets in diastole. The left atrial clot has been surgically removed and the left atrial appendage has been ligated.

sound beam with the mitral inflow jet. In this patient, both approaches yielded essentially the same data.

Commonly pannus formation and rarely vegetation may also cause prosthetic valve obstruction.[2] In this case, the presence of the large left atrial mass excluded these two as etiologies of the patient's cardiogenic shock.

Thrombosis of the mitral valve in this patient was due to inadequate anticoagulation. The process was sub-acute but, when the obstruction reached a hemodynamically critical level, the patient developed cardiogenic shock. Thrombolytic therapy has been life saving in some patients with prosthetic valve thrombosis. However, in this patient the clot burden was too large and the patient too critically ill to attempt thrombolysis. Emergency mitral valve replacement was successful in this case.

References

1. Jamieson W, Munro A, Miyagishima R, et al. Carpentier-Edwards standard porcine bioprosthesis: clinical performance to seventeen years. Ann Thorac Surg 1995;60:999–1006.

2. Vitale N, Renzulli A, Agozzino L, et al. Obstruction of mechanical mitral prostheses: analysis of pathologic findings. Ann Thorac Surg 1997;63:1101–6.

63

Rheumatic mitral stenosis and severe pulmonary hypertension

Susan E Wiegers MD

A 60-year-old woman presented to the emergency room in rapid atrial fibrillation with profound shortness of breath. She had no history of cardiac problems and had never had rheumatic fever to her knowledge. Her youngest child was 25-years-old and all of her pregnancies had been uncomplicated. Cardiac evaluation in the emergency room revealed murmurs diagnostic of mitral stenosis, mitral regurgitation, and aortic stenosis and regurgitation. She was anticoagulated and cardioverted. Over the next 15 years she had progressive pulmonary hypertension documented by echocardiography but refused surgery. She was treated with diuretics, beta-blockers and digoxin.

Fifteen years after her initial presentation, she began to develop lower extremity edema which progressed to pitting of the abdominal wall. She had constant right upper quadrant pain, mild scleral icterus and severe shortness of breath. At her family's urging she finally presented to her cardiologist.

On physical examination she was mildly cachectic with a blood pressure of 100/60 mmHg. She was in atrial fibrillation at a rate of 60 bpm. Her cardiac impulse was not displaced but there was a right ventricular lift along the left sternal border. S_1 was soft, S_2 was single. There was a 3/6 holosystolic murmur at the apex and a 4/6 systolic ejection murmur at the right upper sternal border. A soft blowing diastolic murmur was audible at the lower sternal border and a loud diastolic rumble was also heard at the apex. The P_2 component was loud. There was a loud holosystolic murmur along the right lower sternal border which accentuated with inspiration. Echocardiography was performed to assess her valvular disease.

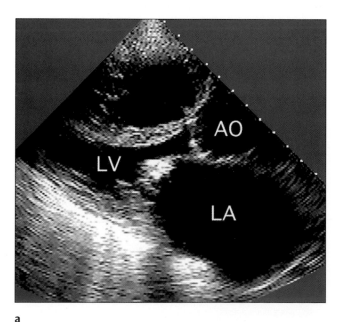

a

Figure 63.1

(a) Parasternal long-axis view in diastole. The left atrium (LA) is markedly enlarged. The mitral valve is severely calcified with the tips more affected than the body of the valve. The posterior leaflet is not visible, owing to the dense calcifications. This diastolic frame represents the maximum excursion of the valve, which was severely limited in its opening. The aortic valve is calcified and the ascending aorta (AO) is dilated although the root itself is not enlarged. The left ventricular cavity internal dimension (LV) is small, owing to the inversion of the curvature of the interventricular septum. The right ventricle is markedly enlarged. These findings are suggestive of severe pulmonary hypertension. The mitral valvular morphology is consistent with rheumatic disease.

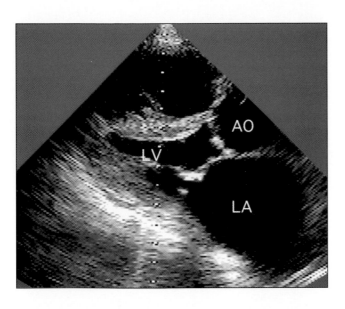

Figure 63.1

(b) Similar view in systole. The interventricular septum has moved towards the right ventricle. The systolic pressure in the left ventricle now exceeds right ventricular pressure, shifting the septum anteriorly. The septum still has an abnormal configuration with a slightly inverted radius of curvature, and the right ventricle is severely dilated. Comparison of the right ventricular area between systole and diastole reveals little change which is diagnostic of severe systolic dysfunction. Once again, dilatation of the left atrium and aorta is noted.

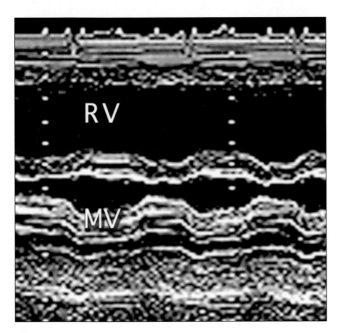

Figure 63.2

M-mode echocardiogram from the parasternal position at the level of the mitral valve leaflets. These findings are consistent with severe rheumatic disease. The right ventricle (RV), seen anterior to the left ventricle is severely dilated. Normally the right ventricular diastolic dimension should be less than two-thirds that of the left ventricular dimension. In this patient, the right ventricular dimension is larger than the left. In addition, the anterior wall of the right ventricle is severely hypertrophied (normal dimension is less than 5 mm). The interventricular septum is severely paradoxical and moves anteriorly in systole. The mitral valve leaflets are markedly thickened. Anterior motion of the posterior mitral valve leaflet in diastole is pathognomonic of mitral stenosis. The posterior wall is poorly seen in this view, owing to the sub-valvular thickening at the posterior annulus which is also evident in Figure 63.1a.

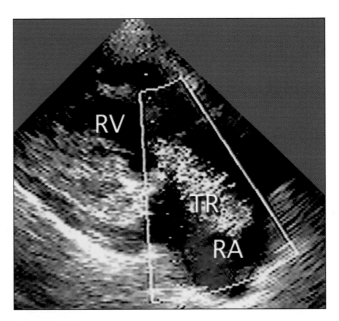

Figure 63.3

Right ventricular (RV) inflow view from the parasternal long-axis. The tricuspid leaflets are not well demonstrated here but open normally in diastole. There is a jet of moderate tricuspid regurgitation (TR) which arises at the level of the tricuspid valve leaflets and projects into the right atrium (RA). This high-velocity turbulent jet had a peak velocity of 4.2 m/s predicting a peak systolic gradient between the right venrtricle and right atrium of 71 mmHg. Assuming a right atrial mean pressure of 15 mmHg (no doubt an underestimate in this patient with signs of severe right-sided failure), the estimated peak pulmonary systolic pressure is 71 + 15 or 86 mmHg. Right ventricular hypertrophy is visualized in the anterior right ventricular free wall.

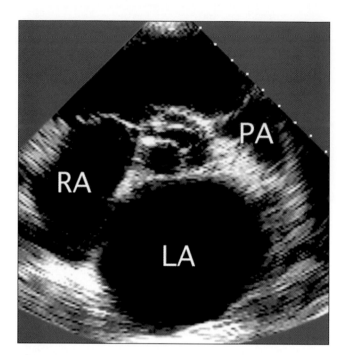

Figure 63.4
Parasternal short-axis view at the level of the base of the heart in systole. The left atrium (LA) is markedly dilated compared to the right atrium (RA) although the right atrium is itself also enlarged. Only the proximal pulmonary artery (PA) is visualized in this image. The aortic valve demonstrates thickening and calcification of the commissures with fusion between the non-coronary and left coronary cusps. Planimetry of the aortic valve area yielded a measurement of 1.1 cm².

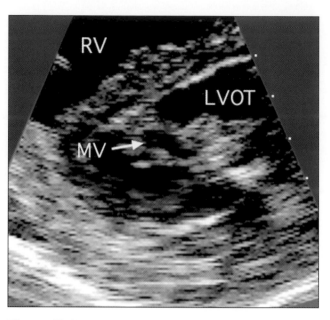

Figure 63.5
Off-axis image of the mitral orifice in a parasternal short-axis view. As is typical for rheumatic disease, sub-valvular thickening has distorted the mitral valve orifice so that it is no longer perpendicular to the parasternal long axis of the heart. This off-axis image was necessary to visualize the true mitral valve orifice (MV) which is very small measuring approximately 0.7 cm by 0.3 cm which yields a very small valve area if the orifice is assumed to be a rectangle (0.21 cm²). Planimetry of the valve orifice is made difficult by the heavy calcifications. LVOT, Left ventricular outflow tract; RV, right ventricle.

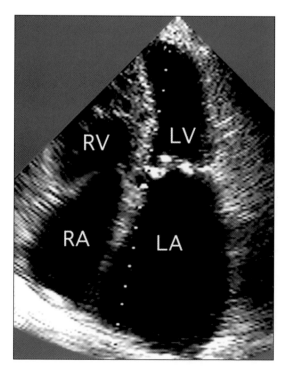

Figure 63.6
Apical four-chamber view in diastole. There is biatrial enlargement although the left atrium (LA) is considerably larger than the right atrium (RA). The left ventricular cavity (LV) is small and underfilled, while the right ventricle (RV) is severely enlarged. Bowing of the septum into the left ventricle is clearly demonstrated. The right ventricular diastolic pressure is greater than the left ventricular diastolic pressure, accounting for the shift. The mitral valve is severely calcified and practically immobile, as shown in this diastolic image.

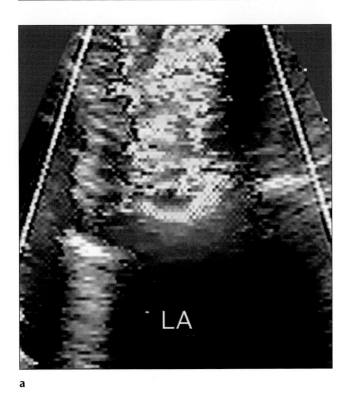

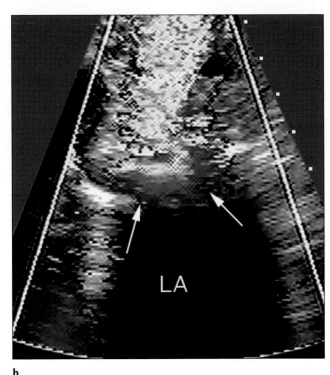

a

b

Figure 63.7

(a) Apical 4-chamber view in diastole with color Doppler flow imaging with a close-up view of the mitral valve. There is a turbulent jet, which arises at the level of the mitral valve and extends into the left ventricular cavity. This turbulent inflow is due to severe mitral stenosis. Note the PISA effect on the atrial side of the mitral valve. The proximal flow convergence is a sign of significant stenosis. It can also be used to calculate a mitral valve area (see Discussion).

(b) In using the proximal flow convergence method to calculate the mitral valve area, the distance between the initial color interface and the level of the first aliasing is measured. This represents the radius of a hemisphere upon whose surface the blood flow velocity is uniform and given by the Nyquist limit velocity.

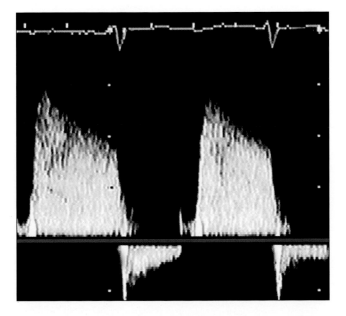

Figure 63.8

Spectral image of the continuous-wave Doppler across the mitral valve from the apical position. The peak velocity of the mitral valve inflow is 2.8 m/s, predicting a peak gradient of 31 mmHg. The pressure half-time of this slope is 198 s, which yields a mitral valve area estimate of 0.9 cm^2.

Discussion

This patient developed severe pulmonary hypertension and right-sided heart failure due to rheumatic mitral stenosis. This had been present for a number of years and was not treated surgically, at the patient's request. The development of cardiac cachexia and fixed supra-systemic pulmonary artery pressures is an ominous sign in end-stage rheumatic disease. Mitral valve replacement at this stage becomes a procedure with a very high morbidity and mortality. The patient also had symptoms of a low flow state which was the result of a fixed cardiac output from the severe mitral stenosis and the right-sided failure.

A variety of methods can be used to calculate the mitral valve area non-invasively. The planimetry of the valve orifice in this patient was limited by the dense calcifications, which made delimiting the edges of the orifice difficult. The pressure half-time method uses the formula:.

$$MVA = 220/\tau$$

where τ is the pressure half-time of the mitral inflow spectral pattern measured by continuous-wave Doppler. The formula was derived from clinical data by Hatle *et al.*[1]

A recently published application of the continuity principle uses proximal flow convergence to calculate the mitral valve area. The baseline of the color Doppler signal is adjusted by the sonographer so that the radius of the first alias of the color flow jet at the Nyquist limiting velocity is easily measured. Assuming circular geometry of the orifice, the mitral valve area is calculated as:

$$MVA = 2\pi R^2 \times V_{NYQUIST}/ V_{PEAK}$$

where MVA is the mitral valve area, R is the radius of the hemisphere as measured from the valve orifice to the level of the Nyquist limit, $V_{NYQUIST}$ is the velocity of the Nyquist limit and V_{PEAK} is the peak velocity through the mitral valve measured by continuous wave Doppler. In this case, the velocity at the Nyquist limit was set to be 0.35 m/s. The peak velocity across the valve measured by continuous wave Doppler was 2.8 m/s and the radius of the PISA hemisphere was 1 cm. Substitution of these values into the formula for the PISA method yields a calculated mitral valve area of 0.8 cm^2. This method correlates well with other invasive and non-invasive measurements of mitral valve area and can be easily applied with transesophageal echocardiography.[2,3]

The decision to operate on a patient with such severe pulmonary hypertension is a difficult one. It is likely that the near systemic pressures in this patient represent a level of fixed vascular disease that will not resolve with relief of the mitral valve stenosis. The patient had an echocardiographic score of 16 (out of 16) which predicts poor success and a high complication rate for a percutaneous procedure. A high echocardiographic score has also been shown to correlate with fixed pulmonary hypertension after intervention.[4] Nevertheless, successful surgical intervention has been undertaken even in elderly patients with severe pulmonary hypertension due to longstanding mitral stenosis.[5,6] On the basis of these published surgical results, the patient underwent mitral valve replacement with a mechanical prosthesis. She did not require coronary artery bypass grafting and an aortic valve was not placed, owing to the moderate degree of stenosis and the high morbidity associated with a double valve replacement in this patient. The pulmonary artery pressure fell to 40 mmHg systolic in the operating room, but subsequently increased to the range of 60 mmHg. The patient has done well after surgery and the signs of right heart failure have resolved.

References

1. Hatle L, Brubakk A, Tromsdal A, *et al.* Noninvasive assessment of pressure drop in mitral stenosis by Doppler echocardiography: application to diagnosis and evaluation of mitral valve disease. Br Heart J 1978;39:517–28.

2. Rodriguez L, Thomas J, Monterroso V, *et al.* Validation of the proximal flow convergence method: calculation of orifice area in patients with mitral stenosis. Circulation 1993;88:1157–65.

3. Deng Y.-B, Masayuki M, Xin-Fang W, *et al.* Estimation of mitral valve area in patients with mitral stenosis by the flow convergence method: selection of the aliasing velocity. J Am Coll Cardiol 1994;24:683–9.

4. Gamra H, Zhang H, Allen J, *et al.* Factors determining normalization of pulmonary vascular resistance following successful balloon mitral valvotomy. Am J Cardiol 1999;83:392–5.

5. Vincens J, Temizer D, Post J, *et al.* Long-term outcome of cardiac surgery in patients with mitral stenosis and severe pulmonary hypertension. Circulation 1995;92:II137–42.

6. Cesnjevar R, Feyrer R, Walther F, *et al.* High-risk mitral valve replacement in severe pulmonary hypertension—30 years experience. Eur J Cardio-Thorac Surg 1998;13:344–51.

64

Mitral valve endocarditis

Susan E Wiegers MD

A 42-year-old man had been admitted to the hospital with an acute abdomen. Surgical exploration revealed a perforated appendix. After surgery he received antibiotics for 2 weeks with a good response. He was discharged but noted pain at the site of an intravenous catheter. Over the course of the month he had fevers, occasional rigors and night sweats. He came back to the hospital after developing severe orthopnea which had rapidly appeared.

On examination he was dyspneic, febrile and tachycardic. The oxygen saturation was 89% on room air. The blood pressure was 100/60 mmHg and the pulse 125 bpm. There were rales in the basilar lung fields. A loud systolic murmur was audible and had not been noted on his previous admission. A transthoracic echocardiogram was performed after the patient was admitted to the coronary care unit. Based on the findings, a transesophageal echocardiogram was immediately performed.

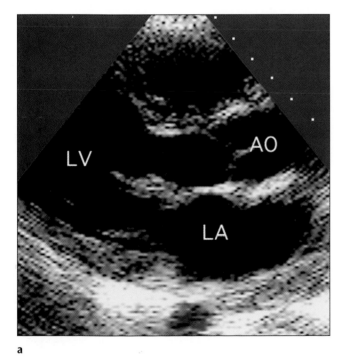

a

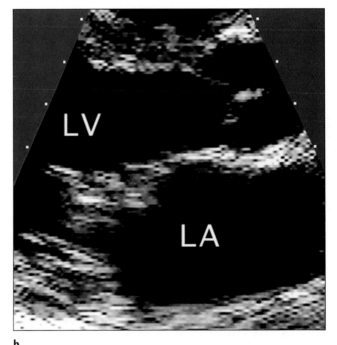

b

Figure 64.1
(a) Parasternal long-axis view in diastole from the transthoracic study. The left ventricle and atrium are of normal size. The anterior mitral valve leaflet is thickened and in this view appears myxomatous. The aortic valve is normal.
(b) Parasternal long-axis close-up view of the mitral valve in a later diastolic frame. It is now evident that the anterior mitral valve leaflet is markedly abnormal. The leaflet is over 1 cm thick and the appearance is highly suggestive of a large vegetation involving most of the leaflet. The posterior leaflet is not well visualized. *continued overleaf*

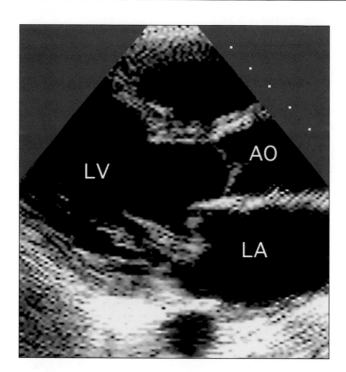

Figure 64.1 *continued*
(c) In early systole, the anterior leaflet prolapses into the left atrium. There is a hinge point in the leaflet close to the anterior annulus and the entire leaflet distal to this prolapses. This finding represents loss of structural support for the anterior leaflet and was associated with torrential mitral regurgitation.

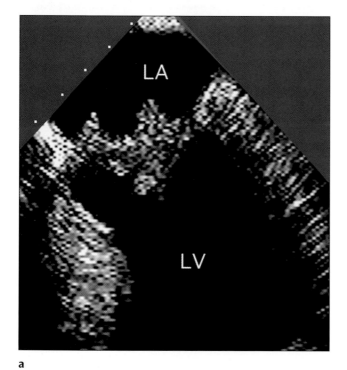

a

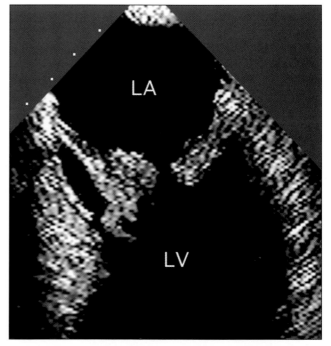

b

Figure 64.2
(a) Transesophageal echocardiogram from the transverse plane (imaging angle 0°). The mitral valve is imaged from the four-chamber view. There is a large mass which involves both the anterior and the posterior leaflets. The mass is multilobulated, fluffy in appearance and was mobile, with the individual lobulations displaying independent chaotic motion. The appearance was of a grape cluster attached to the valve. In this view, the vegetation appears to extend the length of the anterior leaflet to the annulus which is a risk factor for the presence of an annular abscess.
(b) In diastole, the vegetation clearly involves the posterior leaflet, which is thickened and abnormal. The vegetation on the anterior leaflet is broad based and involves primarily the atrial surface of the valve.

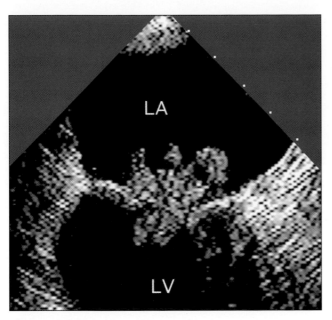

Figure 64.3

Transesophageal echocardiogram from the longitudinal plane (imaging angle 90°). The multiple lobulations on the valve are clearly visible. The annulus appears to be uninvolved.

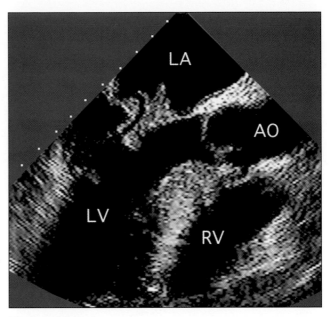

Figure 64.4

Transesophageal echocardiogram (imaging angle 135°). The aortic valve is normal and the anterior annulus of the mitral valve is intact. The vegetations extend down the chordae of the mitral valve.

Discussion

This patient had fulminant enterococcal endocarditis with acute severe mitral regurgitation that caused abrupt hemodynamic decompensation. Interestingly, the transthoracic images demonstrated a markedly abnormal valve with prolapse, but the nature of the abnormality was much more clearly demonstrated on the transesophageal echocardiogram. A high clinical suspicion is necessary to make the diagnosis of endocarditis in the setting of non-specific valvular abnormalities. It is standard practice in our laboratory to recommend transesophageal echocardiography to assess the valves if the clinical situation warrants this.[1] The criteria for the diagnosis of endocarditis have recently been revised to include echocardiographic findings.[2]

This patient underwent urgent valve replacement as he was not tolerating the acute severe mitral regurgitation and could not be stabilized medically. There was no evidence of abscess or involvement of the annulus at surgery and he was discharged on a 6-week course of intravenous antibiotics.

References

1. Bayer A, Bolger A, Taubert K, *et al*. Diagnosis and management of infective endocarditis and its complications. Circulation 1998;98:2936–48.

2. Durack D, Lukes A, Bright D. New criteria for diagnosis of infective endocarditis: utilization of specific echocardiographic findings. Duke Endocarditis Service. Am J Med 1994;96:200–9.

65

Mild mitral stenosis following percutaneous balloon mitral valvuloplasty

Susan E Wiegers MD

Bruce D Klugherz MD

A 28-year-old woman who had undergone percutaneous mitral valvuloplasty under transesophageal guidance during her last pregnancy came to the office for evaluation. Her symptoms had been relieved by the procedure and she was now feeling very well. She had delivered a healthy baby at 39 weeks' gestation with no complications. Her precordial examination was notable for a loud S_1 and a soft diastolic rumble following an opening snap. An echocardiogram was done to evaluate her rheumatic heart disease.

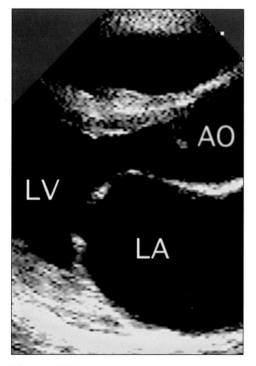

Figure 65.1
Parasternal long-axis view of the mitral valve in diastole. The left atrium (LA) is enlarged. The mitral valve leaflet tips are thickened and very slightly calcified. Both leaflets dome in diastole but are highly mobile and appear pliable. The aortic valve (AO) is mildly thickened but is not well visualized. The left ventricle (LV) is of normal size.

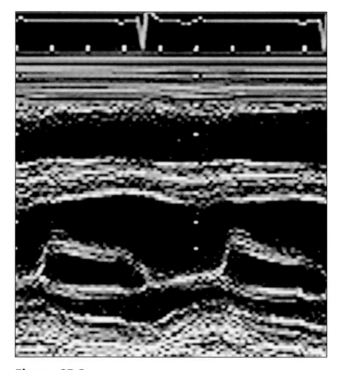

Figure 65.2
M-mode echocardiogram from the parasternal position of the mitral valve leaflets demonstrating the characteristic pattern of mitral stenosis. Both mitral valve leaflets are thickened and there is decreased excursion of the leaflets in diastole. The posterior leaflet appears more immobile than the anterior leaflet.

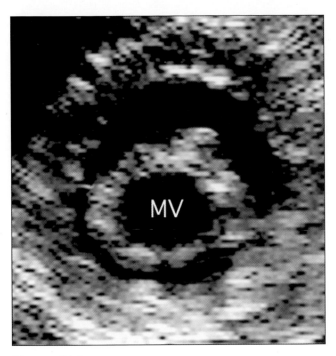

Figure 65.3
Parasternal short-axis view, a close up of the mitral valve (MV) orifice in diastole. This view is slightly off-axis to demonstrate the true mitral valve orifice. From this view the mitral valve area can easily be planimetered. The valve area by planimetry was 1.7 cm². The thickening of the anterior mitral valve leaflet is particularly evident. However the commissures have been disrupted by the mitral valvuloplasty with an excellent result.

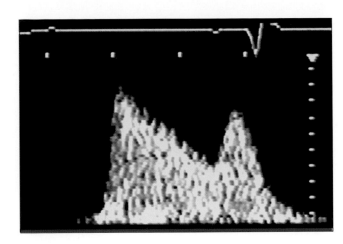

Figure 65.4
Spectral display of continuous-wave Doppler across the mitral valve in diastole with an apically positioned transducer. There is normal sinus rhythm as evidenced by the presence of both E and A waves in diastole. The peak velocity across the mitral valve is approximately 1.7 m/s. The pressure half-time is prolonged, consistent with mild mitral stenosis. The pressure half-time of the mitral inflow spectral display is 138 m/s. Using the pressure half-time formula (MVA = 220/τ, where τ is the pressure half-time), the valve area is estimated as 220/138 = 1.6 cm².

Discussion

An excellent result had been obtained previously with percutaneous valvuloplasty in this patient, whose mitral apparatus was ideally suited to the procedure. In the MGH echocardiographic scoring system of mitral stenosis, four anatomical characteristics of the valve are graded on a scale of 0 to 4, with 0 being normal and 4 being the most severely affected.[1] In this case, all four characteristics of leaflet mobility – leaflet thickening, leaflet calcification and subvalvular thickening and calcification – would be graded as a '1'. The total score would thus be 4. A low echo score correlates with a higher likelihood of successful results with the procedure.[2]

The highly mobile but stenotic mitral valve leaflet correlates with a loud S$_1$ on auscultation. In Figure 65.1, the parasternal long-axis view, the separation of the anterior and posterior mitral valve leaflets is approximately 1 cm. Since the medial–lateral (or horizontal) opening of a mitral valve is greater than the anteropos-

terior dimension, a 1-cm separation in the anterior–posterior axis predicts a mitral valve area greater than 1 cm². This examination was several months after the procedure which resulted in splitting of the commissures and increase in the valve area. Percutaneous mitral valvuloplasty usually results in an immediate increase in the mitral valve area with an average increase from 1 cm² to 2.2 cm². Improvement in functional class is immediate. Echocardiographic restenosis occurs in approximately 20% of patients.[3] The decision to treat her symptomatic mitral stenosis with percutaneous balloon valvuloplasty was appropriate since open commissurotomy carries a high risk of fetal wastage as a result of extracorporeal circulation, and closed mitral commissurotomy has been associated with an increased frequency of prematurity.[4]

Plainimetry of the mitral valve area is more reliable than the pressure half-time method immediately after valvuloplasty for evaluation of the true valvular orifice.[5] Planimetry of the valve in the short axis is operator-dependent, as care must be taken to image the smallest valve opening. Inappropriate location of the scanning plane more proximal to the annulus than the true orifice will give an erroneously large mitral valve area. The true mitral valve orifice is not likely to be parallel to the long axis of the left ventricle since the scarring process results in deformation of the subvalvular apparatus as well as fusion of the commissures. The valve area should be planimetered along the inner border of the orifice. In some patients, inadequate transthoracic images or inability to position the patient in the left lateral decubitus position will result in failure of this method. The pressure half-time method is less reliable immediately after valvuloplasty, owing to abrupt changes in the compliance of the left atrium after valvuloplasty which may change the relationship between pressure and the half-time. In addition, a residual interatrial connection with a left to right shunt will allow decompression of the left atrium into the right atrium as well as across the mitral valve. The decay of the pressure gradient will be more rapid and the pressure half-time shorter than in the absence of the left to right shunt. This will result in an overestimation of the valve area.[6]

References

1. Wilkins G, Weyman A, Abascal V, et al. Percutaneous balloon dilatation of the mitral valve: an analysis of echocardiographic variables related to outcome and the mechanism of dilatation. Br Heart J 1988;60:299–308.

2. Abascal VM, Wilkins GT, Choong CY, et al. Echocardiographic evaluation of mitral valve structure and function in patients followed for at least 6 months after percutaneous balloon mitral valvuloplasty. J Am Coll Cardiol 1988;12:606–15.

3. Desideri A, Vanderperren O, Serra A, et al. Long-term (9 to 33 months) echocardiographic follow-up after successful percutaneous mitral commissurotomy. Am J Cardiol 1992;69:1602–6.

4. Becker R. Intracardiac surgery in pregnant women. Ann Thorac Surg 1983;36:453–8.

5. Smith MD, Handshoe R, Handshoe S, et al. Comparative accuracy of two-dimensional echocardiography and Doppler pressure half-time methods in assessing severity of mitral stenosis in patients with and without prior commissurotomy. Circulation 1986;73:100–7.

6. Vasan R, Shrivastava S, Kumar M. Value and limitations of Doppler echocardiographic determination of mitral valve area in Lutembacher syndrome. J Am Coll Cardiol 1992;20:1362–70.

66

Prosthetic paravalvular leak

Victor A Ferrari MD

A 45-year-old man underwent an uncomplicated mitral valve replacement for severe bileaflet myxomatous disease and presented 1 month later with complaints of progressive exertional dyspnea, fatigue, and orthopnea. He denied fever, chills, sweats, or pain of any kind, and had no episodes of transient neurological deficits. His degree of anticoagulation had been excellent, with International normalized ratios (INRs) in the 3.2–3.6 range. On physical examination, he had a normal jugular venous pressure (JVP), and normal carotid pulse contours. The sternum was stable and pulmonary examination was normal. Crisp prosthetic heart sounds were present, and S_2 was normally split with a

prominent P_2. There was a grade II/VI blowing holosystolic murmur at the left lower sternal border and no diastolic murmur was appreciated. The remainder of the examination was normal. The electrocardiogram was unchanged from preoperatively. A transthoracic echocardiogram demonstrated normal left ventricular size with hyperdynamic left ventricular function, a moderately enlarged left atrium, and a suggestion of a jet of mitral regurgitation. Owing to artifact from the mechanical prosthesis, a paravalvular leak could not be excluded. Therefore, transesophageal echocardiography was performed for better assessment of the prosthetic valve function.

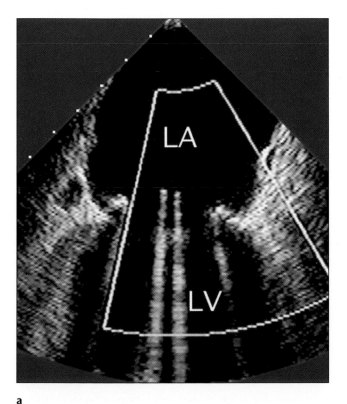

a

Figure 66.1

(a) Transesophageal echocardiogram from the mid-esophagus in the longitudinal plane (imaging angle 90°) demonstrating normal function of the St Jude's bileaflet valve in the mitral position. The left atrium (LA) and left ventricle (LV) are identified. In this plane, the posterior wall of the left ventricle is on the left, and the anterior wall to the right of the image. The typical echocardiographic signature of a normal St Jude's valve in diastole is demonstrated. The two vertical lines in the center of the valve plane (one for each leaflet of the valve) are fully open and almost parallel. There are no masses or other abnormalities in the valve orifice. Reverberation artifact from the highly refractile leaflets extends along the path of the ultrasound beam into the left ventricle. Incomplete opening of the leaflets or mobile echodensities affixed to the valve would raise the question of prosthetic valve endocarditis or subacute thrombosis of the valve. The left atrium is moderately enlarged.

continued overleaf

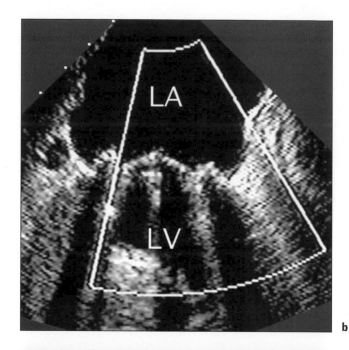

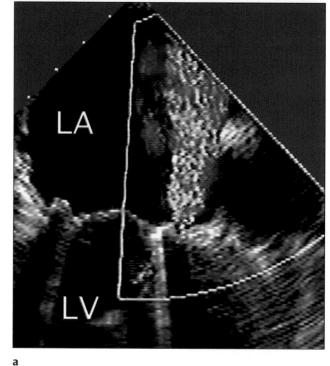

a

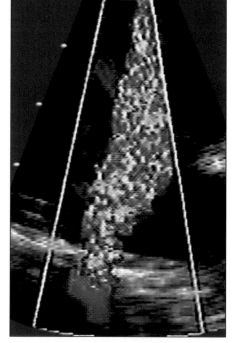

b

b

Figure 66.1 *continued*
(b) Similar view in systole, showing normal systolic closure of the leaflets with both mechanical leaflets at the valve plane. The normal angle between the leaflets at closure is approximately 120°. Note that the artifact from the metallic components of the valve is projected away from the transducer (top of image), permitting excellent visualization of the left atrium and the prosthesis. The valve appears to be well seated without evidence of obvious dehiscence or excessive mobility of the valve ring.

Figure 66.2
(a) Transesophageal echocardiogram from the mid-esophagus in the longitudinal plane (imaging angle 90°) with color flow Doppler imaging in a close-up view of the mitral valve prosthesis in systole. A large paravalvular leak (mosaic color pattern) is present along the anterior aspect of the sewing ring. Note that the area surrounding the leak appears normal without evidence of vegetations or mobile suture material. The normal closing jets of a St Jude valve are not imaged. However, from this and the subsequent image, it is clear that the mitral regurgitation is arising from the valve sewing ring, rather than through the prosthetic valve orifice. This is the distinction between paravalvular and valvular regurgitation.
(b) Close-up view of the systolic color Doppler jet representing the paravalvular leak. Rotation of the transducer has brought the largest dimension of the leak at its origin into view. The size of the color jet is approximately 5 mm at the origin of the paravalvular leak which is consistent with significant regurgitation. There is flow convergence on the ventricular side of the mitral valve at the site of the paravalvular leak. Calculation of an effective regurgitant orifice would be possible using the PISA equation.

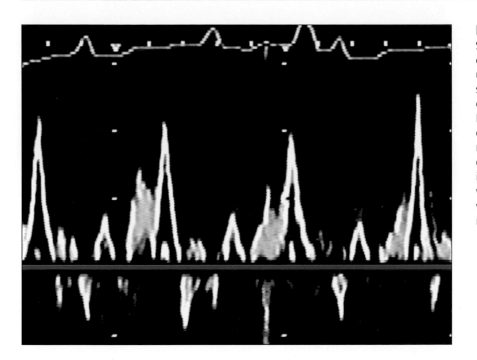

Figure 66.3
Spectral display of pulsed-wave Doppler evaluation of inflow from the left upper pulmonary vein demonstrates systolic blunting of inflow but no evidence of systolic flow reversal. Normally, the maximal left atrial filling occurs in systole. In this patient, the maximal filling clearly occurs in diastole but there is no reflux of blood into the pulmonary veins in systole which, in a simplified classification, would indicate a paravalvular leak of moderate degree.

Discussion

Paravalvular leaks can occur early (within 3 to 6 months following surgery) or late postoperatively. Early leaks are generally due to technical problems at surgery or due to dehiscence of sutures at the sewing ring. However, prosthetic valve endocarditis can occur at any time and should be excluded when a leak is detected. A larger percentage of cases of late paravalvular leak are due to endocarditis, which may be occult or sub-acute at presentation. If the leak is of moderate size or larger, it is generally recommended to repair the defect, provided the patient is a surgical candidate.

This patient presented with a symptom complex typical for an early significant periprosthetic valve leak. While the majority of patients will have a murmur on examination, up to 20% of patients will have no detectable abnormality on auscultation.[1] Signs of congestive heart failure are not universally present, and the patient may have symptoms only with exertion. The general assessment of prosthetic mitral valve function is usually satisfactory using transthoracic echocardiography; however, questions of paravalvular leaks or endocarditis require the improved visualization provided by transesophageal echocardiography.[2,3] Our patient presented with no symptoms of bacterial endocarditis nor poor anticoagulation which might raise the question of a valvular leak due to incomplete leaflet closure from an obstructing vegetation or thrombus.

Transesophageal echocardiography can discriminate a valvular from a paravalvular leak better than can transthoracic echocardiography. Owing to reverberation artifact from the leaflets and shadowing artifact from the sewing ring, mitral regurgitation jets may be obscured or altered so as to be nearly undetectable on transthoracic studies.[1,3] However, transthoracic Doppler interrogation of the mitral valve prosthesis may demonstrate an abnormally high transvalvular pressure gradient in the setting of a normal pressure half-time, which is a clue to the presence of significant mitral regurgitation. The standard criteria for grading the severity of mitral regurgitation in the case of central valvular leaks remains valid for prostheses. The three-dimensional area of the regurgitant color Doppler jet is assessed in several views and an overall jet volume is determined. In a mild paravalvular leak, the jet volume is less than 20% of the left atrial area, a moderate leak is 20–40% of the atrial area, and a severe leak encompasses more than 40% of the left atrial area, or causes systolic reversal of flow in the pulmonary veins. However, despite being a convenient index, pulmonary vein systolic flow reversal is not specific for the degree of mitral regurgitation. In addition, systolic flow reversal can be missed if only one pulmonary vein is sampled; therefore, recommendations state that at least two pulmonary veins be sampled during the examination. Unfortunately, pulmonary vein flow reversal is load dependent, with considerable overlap between groups of different regurgitation severity, and can also be seen in disorders such as constrictive pericarditis, restrictive or dilated cardiomyopathies, or certain arrhythmias. Eccentric paravalvular jets are frequently more difficult to quantify. Some authors have suggested a simplified approach for assessing mitral regurgitation using transesophageal echocardiography, whereby a jet is considered mild if it does not reach the mid-left atrium, moderate if it extends beyond the mid-left atrium but does not enter the pulmonary veins or left atrial appendage, and severe beyond these limits. Many severe central or eccentric jets will cause systolic flow reversal in the pulmonary veins.[4,5] While this is a simpler method, it is subject to some of the same problems with systolic pulmonary vein reversal outlined above.

Significant dehiscence causing instability or rocking of the prosthesis indicates an urgent situation that requires immediate attention. Catastrophic valve failure may occur under these conditions and repair should not be delayed if indicated.

References

1. Chen Y, Kan M, Chen J, *et al.* Detection of prosthetic mitral valve leak: a comparative study using transesophageal echocardiography, transthoracic echocardiography, and auscultation. J Clin Ultrasound 1990;18:557–61.

2. Alam M, Serwin JB, Rosman HS, *et al.* Transesophageal color flow Doppler and echocardiographic features of normal and regurgitant St. Jude medical prostheses in the mitral valve position. Am J Cardiol 1990;66:871–2.

3. Meloni L, Aru GM, Abbruzzese PA, *et al.* Localization of mitral periprosthetic leaks by transesophageal echocardiography. Am J Cardiol 1992;69:276–9.

4. Khanderia BK, Seward JB, Oh JK, *et al.* Value and limitations of transesophageal echocardiography in assessment of mitral valve prostheses. Circulation 1991;83:1956–68.

5. Hsiung M, Ku C, Wei J, *et al.* Transesophageal color Doppler flow imaging in the evaluation of prosthetic heart valves. Echocardiography 1992;9:583–8.

67

Mitral annular calcification

Susan E Wiegers MD

A 39-year-old man had been on dialysis for 4 years. He had a history of severe hypertension since his early twenties which had been largely untreated, owing to his lack of medical insurance. The patient was brought to the emergency room by his family after being found on the floor of his room, unable to rise, with hemiparesis. He was aphasic as well. Contrast computerized tomography scan of the head demonstrated an ischemic cardiovascular accident with no evidence of hemorrhage. This study was obtained while the patient was hospitalized.

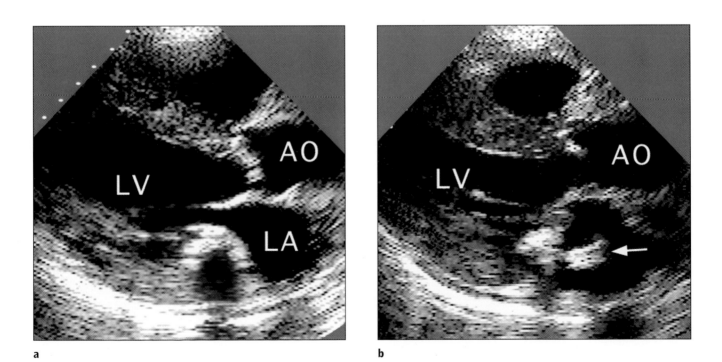

a   b

Figure 67.1
(a) Parasternal long-axis view in late diastole. There is dense mitral annular calcification of the posterior annulus. The left atrium (LA) is of normal size. However, there is a mass involving the mitral annulus that appears to extend into the left atrium. The left ventricle (LV) is hypertrophied but not dilated. The aortic valve also appears to be calcified.
(b) Similar systolic view. A portion of the mitral annular calcification projects into the left atrium (arrow). The aortic valve is calcified but is seen to open with systole.

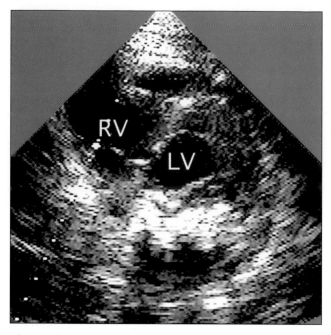

Figure 67.2
Parasternal short-axis view of the left ventricle at the level of
the mitral valve leaflets. The valvular architecture is obscured
by the dense posterior annular calcification, which is over
2 cm thick.

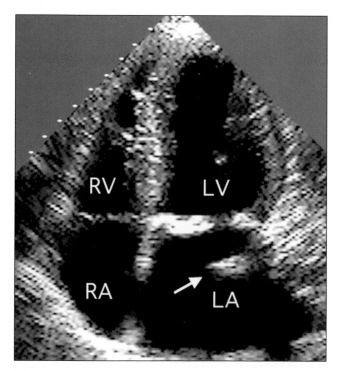

Figure 67.4
Apical four-chamber view in systole which again outlines the
dense calcification of the entire mitral annulus. The annular
calcification projecting into the left atrium (arrow) is seen in
this view as well. The right atrium and ventricle are noted to
be of normal size and the right ventricular systolic function is
normal.

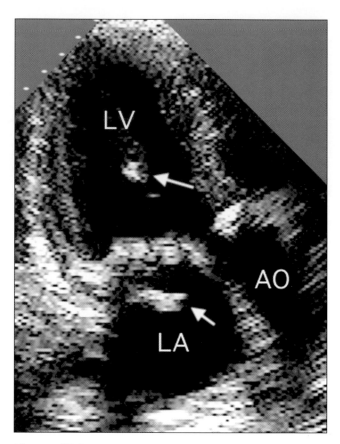

Figure 67.3
Apical long-axis view, demonstrating the thickening and
calcification of the mitral annulus that extends onto a portion
of the mitral valve leaflets. The projecting portion of the
annular calcification is clearly seen (short arrow). Calcification
of the tip of the posterior medial papillary muscle is also
noted (long arrow).

Discussion

Mitral annular calcification preferentially affects the
posterior annulus and is best visualized as an echodense
mass in the atrioventricular groove. In the parasternal
long axis, the mitral annular calcification may be seen at
the base of the posterior leaflet, while in the parasternal
short axis, it will appear as a bar in the most basilar
portion of the inferior wall. Exuberant mitral annular
calcification may project into the left atrium or into the
left ventricle. In real time, the calcified left atrial mass was
seen to be completely immobile, ruling out a calcified
mitral leaflet or vegetation. Occasionally a portion of the
mass may be mobile; this may represent associated thrombus.

Calcification of the mitral annulus is common in the
elderly. In patients over the age of 60, it was noted in 37%
of women and 15% of men in the Framingham study.[1] The

presence of mitral annular calcification and its extent were risk factors for the development of ischemic stroke in this population.[2] Mitral annular calcification may be a marker of a related cerebrovascular risk factor. Others have postulated that the mitral annular calcification is the nidus for formation of thrombi which embolize to the cerebral vessels, but this mechanism remains highly speculative.

Mitral annular calcification may extend into the valve leaflets creating stenosis or regurgitation.[3,4] Dense posterior mitral annular calcification may restrict the motion of the basal posterior wall and cause a wall motion abnormality unrelated to the presence of coronary disease. Calcification of both the mitral and the aortic annuli are more common in hemodialysis patients and is apparently related to abnormalities in calcium and phosphate metabolism.[5] Beside mechanical problems and cerebrovascular events, mitral annular calcification is associated with the development of conduction abnormalities requiring pacemaker therapy and carries a worse cardiovascular prognosis than in age-matched controls.[6]

References

1. Savage D, Garrison R, Castelli W, *et al*. Prevalence of annular calcium and its correlates in a general population based sample (Framingham Study). Am J Cardiol 1983;51:1375–8.

2. Benjamin EJ, Plehn JF, D'Agostino RB, *et al*. Mitral annular calcification and the risk of stroke in an elderly cohort. N Engl J Med 1992;327:374–9.

3. Labovitz AJ, Nelson JG, Windhorst DM, *et al*. Frequency of mitral valve dysfunction from mitral annular calcium as detected by Doppler echocardiography. Am J Cardiol 1985;55:133–7.

4. Aronow WS. Mitral annular calcification: significant and worth acting upon. Geriatrics 1991;46:73–5, 79–80, 85–6.

5. Maher ER, Young G, Smyth-Walsh B, *et al*. Aortic and mitral valve calcification in patients with end-stage renal disease. Lancet 1987;2:875–7.

6. Nair CK, Thomson W, Ryschon K, *et al*. Long-term follow-up of patients with echocardiographically detected mitral annular calcium and comparison with age- and sex-matched control subjects. Am J Cardiol 1989;63:465–70.

68

Hypertrophic cardiomyopathy and infective endocarditis

Riti Patel MD

A 49-year-old man with a history of alcohol abuse and hypertrophic cardiomyopathy presented with altered mental status, fever, and neck stiffness. He was found to have pneumococcal meningitis and was treated with antibiotics. Cardiac auscultation revealed a grade 4/6 holosystolic apical murmur. Progressive congestive heart failure and hypotension ensued, and the intensity of the murmur increased. A transthoracic echocardiogram was performed and revealed asymmetric septal hypertrophy, a mitral valve vegetation, severe mitral regurgitation, moderate aortic insufficiency, and normal left ventricular function. A transesophageal echocardiogram was performed.

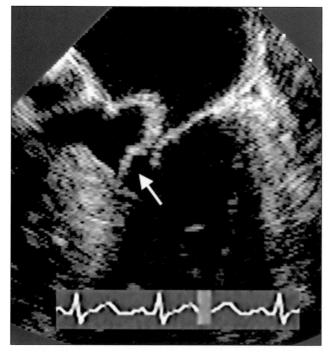

Figure 68.1
Transesophageal echocardiogram from the mid-esophageal position in the transverse plane (imaging angle 0°) in systole. There is systolic anterior motion of the mitral valve (arrow). The anterior leaflet, which appears thickened in this view, contacts the septum. The interventricular septum is hypertrophied compared to the lateral wall. The gradient progressively increases during systole as the cavity size of the left ventricle decreases, and the flow velocity and degree of obstruction increase.

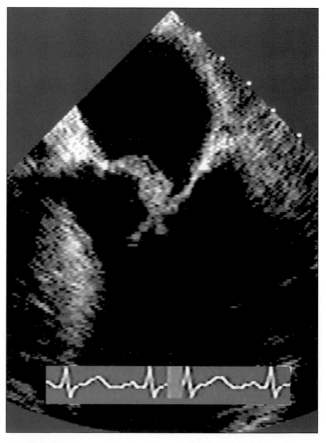

Figure 68.2
Similar view in an earlier systolic frame. The mitral valve is focally thickened in the mid-portion of the leaflet. The posterior leaflet appears entirely normal.

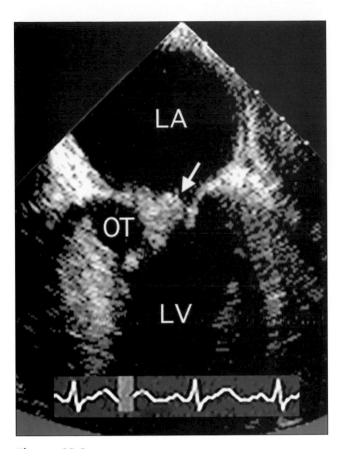

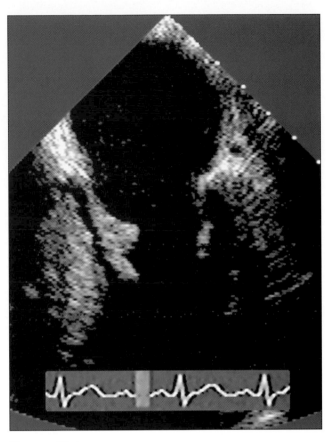

Figure 68.3
The transducer has been withdrawn, compared to the previous images, in this systolic frame. The mass attached to the mid-leaflet (arrow) is broad based and measures over 1 cm at the widest dimension. The focal nature of the lesion and its appearance are consistent with vegetation.

Figure 68.4
Diastolic frame from the four-chamber view. The vegetation is seen involving a large portion of the mitral leaflet. However, the annulus and the posterior leaflet are entirely normal.

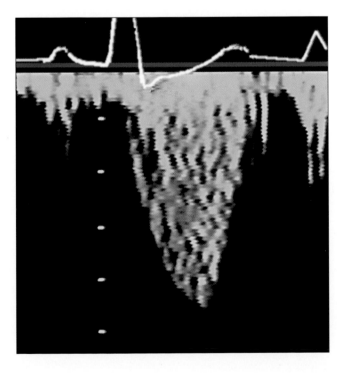

Figure 68.5
Spectral display of continuous-wave Doppler from the transthoracic echocardiogram across the left ventricular outflow tract (each calibration mark represents 1 m/s.) A late peaking systolic signal reaches over 4 m/s, predicting a peak outflow tract gradient of 80 mmHg.

Discussion

Infective endocarditis is a recognized complication of hypertrophic cardiomyopathy.[1,2] However, endocarditis in hypertrophic cardiomyopathy is seen predominantly in patients with left ventricular outflow tract obstruction, and is more common in those with both obstruction and a markedly dilated left atrium. Systolic anterior motion of the valve disrupts coaptation during systole and causes mitral regurgitation, also a predisposing factor for the development of endocarditis. In addition, there is a greater incidence of mitral valve abnormalities in the hypertrophic cardiomyopathy population, particularly leaflet prolongation and anomalous insertion of the papillary muscles into the mitral leaflets.[3,4] Currently, the American Heart Association recommends antibiotic prophylaxis for all patients with hypertrophic cardiomyopathy, regardless of whether obstruction is present or not.[5]

In this patient, images from the transesophageal echocardiogram clearly demonstrated a vegetation measuring approximately 1 cm × 5 mm on the atrial aspect of the anterior mitral leaflet. There was associated moderate mitral regurgitation. Ultimately, progression of sepsis and valvular disease resulted in his hemodynamic deterioration. Multi-organ failure precluded immediate surgery. Despite aggressive treatment with antibiotics, diuretics, and angiotensin converting enzyme inhibition, the patient developed worsening congestive heart failure and expired.

References

1. Allessandri N, Pannarale G, del Monte G, et al. Hypertrophic obstructive cardiomyopathy and infective endocarditis: a report of seven cases and a review of the literature. Eur Heart J 1990;11:1041–8.

2. Spirito P, Rapezzi C, Bellone P, et al. Infective endocarditis in hypertrophic cardiomyopathy: prevalence, incidence, and indications for antibiotic prophylaxis. Circulation 1999;99:2132–7.

3. Klues H, Roberts W, Maron B. Anomalous insertion of papillary muscle directly into anterior mitral leaflet in hypertrophic cardiomyopathy. Circulation 1991;84:1188–97.

4. Akihiko O, Masaya K, Mitsuhiro H, et al. HOCM with abnormalities of the mitral valve complex. J Heart Valve Dis 1997;6:60–2.

5. Dajani A, Taubert K, Wilson W, et al. Prevention of bacterial endocarditis. Recommendations by the American Heart Association. J Am Med Assoc 1997;272:1794–801.

69

Double orifice mitral valve

Martin St John Sutton MBBS
Susan E Wiegers MD

A 27-year-old woman complained of spontaneous rapid palpitations with which she developed atypical left submammary chest discomfort lasting for up to 40 min. There were no identifiable triggers for her palpitations except stressful situations. She recalled that her palpitations had been present since grade school, occurring every 2 to 3 years, but over the prior 6 to 9 months they had increased in frequency and duration.. Her only past medical history was of anorexia nervosa in adolescence; since then her body weight had been consistently above 115 lbs.

Previous investigations had included 48-hour ambulatory monitoring, which showed sinus tachycardia only, and a two-dimensional echocardiogram, which had reportedly demonstrated myxomatous mitral valve leaflets with systolic prolapse and mild mitral regurgitation. In view of her unremitting symptoms with beta-adrenergic receptor blockers and side effects from calcium channel antagonists, she sought a second opinion.

On examination she was asthenic, had a resting heart rate of 102 bpm in regular rhythm with no abnormal cardiac findings except for a soft apical pansystolic murmur radiating to the axilla consistent with mild mitral regurgitation. Clinical stigmata of hyperthyroidism were present and the diagnosis was confirmed biochemically. Electrocardiography demonstrated sinus tachycardia with non-specific ST and T wave changes inferiorly. An echocardiogram was performed to assess the history of an abnormal mitral valve.

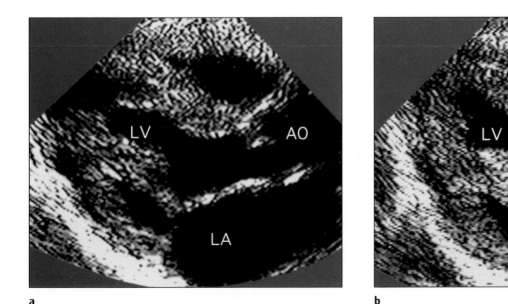

a   b

Figure 69.1
(a) Parasternal long-axis view in diastole. The mitral valve leaflets are abnormal and appear to be thickened. The papillary muscles demonstrate an abnormal attachment to the mitral valve leaflets. The left atrium is mildly enlarged and the left ventricular cavity is normal in size.
(b) Similar view in systole. The subvalvular apparatus assumes a mass-like appearance due to redundancy and myxomatous changes. The leaflets and the sub-valvular apparatus were excessively mobile.

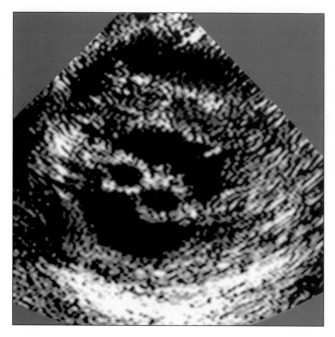

Figure 69.2
Parasternal short-axis view at the level of the mitral valve. There is duplication of the mitral valve orifice, resulting in two equal-sized circular orifices.

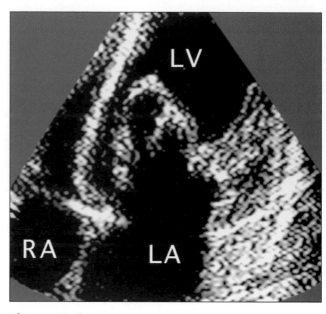

Figure 69.3
Close-up view of the mitral valve apparatus from the apical four-chamber view. The marked redundancy, especially of the anterior leaflet, and the abnormal insertions of the papillary muscles are evident in this diastolic frame. Doppler interrogation (not shown here) demonstrated mild mitral regurgitation and no evidence of mitral stenosis or dynamic outflow tract obstruction.

Discussion

This patient's symptoms were due to hyperthyroidism. However, echocardiography demonstrated a rare congenital anomaly of the mitral valve.[1] Careful inspection of the mitral valve in the parasternal long axis revealed marked redundancy of the subvalvular tissue, resembling a cleft mitral valve, as occurs in endocardial cushion anomalies. Several anomalies may produce a double-orifice mitral valve and most occur in association with partial or complete endocardial cushion defects.[2] There may be a complete division of the orifice by a fibrous band between the anterior and posterior leaflets. Four papillary muscles may be present with anomalous attachment to the central portion of the anterior mitral valve leaflet.[3,4] If the two individual mitral orifices are not in the same plane in the parasternal short axis, the bridging tissue can simulate a cleft.

Associated congenital lesions were excluded in this patient. Endocardial cushion defect is not present, as the apical four-chamber view clearly demonstrates that the septal leaflets of the mitral and tricuspid valves are not co-planar. The tricuspid valve inserts into the septum more apically than the mitral valve and the absence of defects in the primum or ventricular septa excludes a partial or complete atrioventricular canal defect. Duplication of the mitral valve orifice is uncommonly an isolated finding.

References

1. Mendelson M, Cole P, St John Sutton M, Double mitral valve orifice and primary pulmonary hypertension. Int J Cardiol 1989;22:261–4.

2. Trowitzsch E, Bano-Rodrigo A, Burger BM, et al. Two-dimensional echocardiographic findings in double orifice mitral valve. J Am Coll Cardiol 1985;6:383–7.

3. Ciampani N, Vecchiola D, Silenzi C, et al. The tensor apparatus in double-orifice mitral valve: interpretation of echocardiographic findings. J Am Soc Echocardiogr 1997;10:869–73.

4. Mao JT, Tang J, Li Y, et al. Double-orifice mitral valve with multiple papillary muscles—a report of two patients. Angiology 1999;50:771–5.

SECTION VI

The Left Ventricle

70

Post-infarction ventricular septal defect

Susan E Wiegers MD

A 62-year-old woman with rheumatoid arthritis had a long history of steroid use to control her disease. Four weeks prior to her current admission she had sustained a large anterior myocardial infarction which was complicated by atrial fibrillation and congestive heart failure. She had not received thrombolytic therapy, owing to delayed presentation to the emergency ward. No post-myocardial risk assessment was undertaken because the patient was felt by her treating physicians to be too frail. She was discharged on a calcium channel blocker to treat her hypertension and a lipid-lowering agent. One week after discharge she developed orthopnea and dyspnea on exertion which had not been present before her infarction. On the day of admission, her visiting nurse found her to be in more significant congestive heart failure and to be tachycardic. She was brought to her doctor's office where a loud systolic murmur was noted. She was in moderate congestive heart failure. She was admitted to the coronary care unit and an echocardiogram was performed.

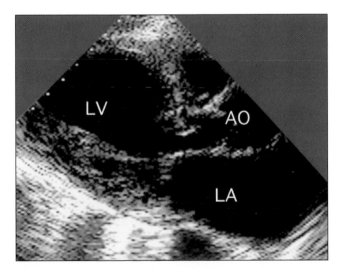

Figure 70.1
Parasternal long-axis view in systole. The left atrium (LA) is moderately dilated. The left ventricle (LV) is also significantly dilated. The proximal septum appears to contract but is akinetic beyond that. In fact, comparison to the diastolic view demonstrates systolic bulging in the distal septum consistent with aneurysm formation. The ascending aorta (AO) is normal. The interventricular septum in this image appears to have a normal texture.

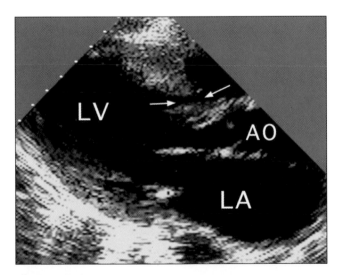

Figure 70.2
Similar parasternal long-axis view in diastole. Discontinuity in the mid-anterior interventricular septum (arrows) is noted. This ventricular septal defect is at the junction between the contracting and non-contractile myocardium of the septum. In this view, the ventricular septal defect appears to be approximately 3 mm wide. The anterior mitral valve leaflet is mildly thickened and mitral annular calcification is noted in the posterior annulus. The left atrium and left ventricle are again noted to be enlarged.

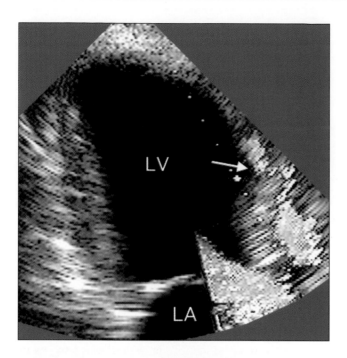

Figure 70.3
Apical long-axis view with color flow Doppler imaging in systole. The interventricular septum is on the right of the image. The turbulent high-velocity jet through the septal defect is identified by the arrow. The ventricular septal defect channel follows a seripiginous course through the interventricular septum as can be seen by the color flow.

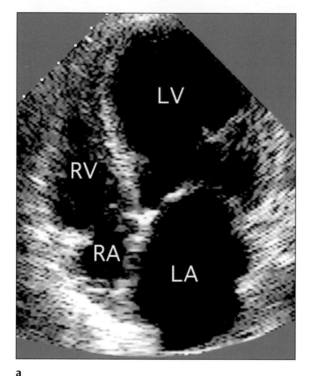

a

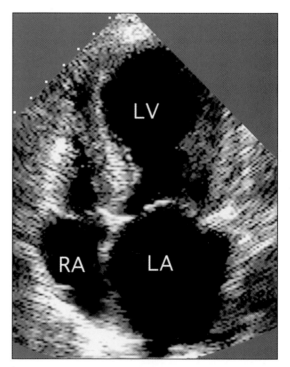

b

Figure 70.4
(a) Apical four-chamber view in diastole. The left atrium (LA) and left ventricle (LV) are markedly enlarged. The apex is dilated, consistent with aneurysm formation. The ventricular septal defect is not seen in this image. The right ventricular cavity is mildly dilated. Compared to the area of the left ventricular cavity, the right ventricle does not appear to be enlarged. However, the left ventricle is severely dilated and judging the size of the right ventricle by comparison to the left ventricle may lead to erroneous conclusions unless the left ventricular dilatation is kept in mind.
(b) Comparison of the left ventricular walls in systole demonstrates that the lateral wall thickens normally, as does the proximal interventricular septum. However, the septum at the mid-ventricular level is akinetic and the distal septum and apex bulge in systole which is diagnostic of an aneurysm. Note that, although the right ventricle was mildly dilated in the diastolic frame, the systolic function is hyperdynamic.

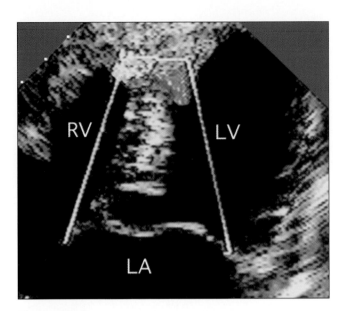

Figure 70.5
Slightly off-axis apical four-chamber view with color flow
Doppler imaging in a close-up of the interventricular septum.
The high-velocity turbulent jet through the ventricular septal
defect is seen towards the top of the screen. The red flow on
the left ventricular side of the defect indicates that the initial
course of the channel is towards the transducer at the apex.

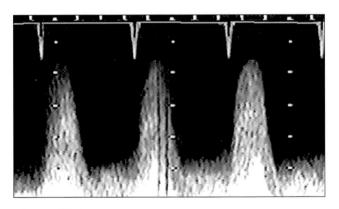

Figure 70.6
Spectral display of continuous wave Doppler from the
parasternal position across the ventricular septal defect. In
systole, a high-velocity jet from the left ventricle to the right
ventricle is identified. The peak velocity is 4.2 m/s consistent
with a gradient between the right ventricle and the left
ventricle of 71 mmHg (calibration marks represent 1 m/s).

Discussion

Two life-threatening complications of myocardial infarction may present in the first weeks after the event and be
heralded by the development of a new, loud systolic
murmur and the development of heart failure. Acute

mitral regurgitation due to papillary muscle rupture and
acute ventricular septal defect may be extremely difficult
to distinguish clinically, especially in the critically ill
patient. Emergency echocardiography is essential in differ-
entiating the two syndromes. Transthoracic images are
often adequate for diagnosis of both acute mitral regurgitation and ventricular septal defect. However, transesophageal images will be necessary if the cause of the
murmur and hypotension cannot be distinguished on the
transthoracic study.

Elderly patients, particularly those on steroids and
perhaps women, are more likely to sustain acute free-wall
rupture and interventricular septal rupture after infarction. There has been some suggestion that the use of
thrombolytic agents has contributed to an increased
incidence of these complications, although this remains
controversial.[1] Ventricular septal rupture is equally
common after anterior and inferior myocardial infarctions.[2] Infarct expansion and extensive myocardial
thinning may lead to intolerable wall stress, particularly at
areas with marked distortions in normal geometry, as in
this patient.[3] The average time to development of a
ventricular septal defect is approximately 5 days and the
defect may range from very small to a 1-cm hole in the
septum.[4] The ventricular septal defect may take a winding
course through the necrotic myocardium, leading to an
exit into the right ventricle far displaced from the left
ventricular site of the defect. Color flow within the interventricular septum, or high-velocity, turbulent flow in the
right ventricular apex may provide echocardiographic
clues to the diagnosis. The hemodynamic consequences of
the defect depend on the degree of shunt flow, residual
right ventricular function and response to the volume
overload as well as to the extent of coronary artery
obstruction. In this patient, the right ventricular function
was hyperdynamic and the gradient between the left and
right ventricle was high, indicating that the defect was
restrictive, at least on presentation. The modified
Bernoulli equation (pressure gradient $= 4v^2$, where v is the
velocity of the ventricular septal defect jet measured by
continuous-wave Doppler) can be used to calculate the
pressure difference between the two ventricles. In this
patient, the velocity of the ventricular septal defect jet was
4.2 m/s which, when substituted into the equation, yields
a 71-mmHg gradient between the ventricles. The systolic
blood pressure by cuff was 110 mmHg. Therefore, the
peak systolic pressure in the right ventricle, and by extrapolation the peak pulmonary artery systolic pressure is
obtained by subtracting the gradient between the ventricles from the cuff pressure. In this patient, the peak
pulmonary artery pressure can be estimated as 39 mmHg.

In the critically ill patient, stabilization with intra-aortic
balloon counterpulsation should be attempted, but deterioration in the hemodynamic status frequently demands
emergency surgery. Transesophageal echocardiography is

essential in the course of the operative repair. The distortion of the left ventricular geometry induced by the repair may lead to the development of mitral regurgitation, which should be addressed in the operating room. The right ventricular systolic function is an important determinant of the outcome of the surgery. The tissue which contains the ventricular septal defect is usually highly necrotic with little tensile strength, and residual shunts are not uncommon. Echocardiographic imaging will help determine the size of any residual shunt flow and aid in the decision to return to the operating room. It is no longer the practice to delay surgery, as the interim mortality was unacceptable. Rather, intervention should be undertaken as soon as possible using one of the recently described techniques.

This patient deteriorated hemodynamically over the course of 12 hours. An intra-aortic balloon was placed and she was taken to the operating room. An extensive ventricular septal defect was repaired using a bovine pericardial patch to exclude the infarcted septum from the left ventricular cavity.[5] Saphenous vein grafts were placed to the right coronary artery and a large obtuse marginal. The patient did well with the exception of a surgical infection of the venous harvest site. She was discharged on the 18th postoperative day.

References

1. Kinn JW, O'Neill WW, Benzuly KH, *et al*. Primary angioplasty reduces risk of myocardial rupture compared to thrombolysis for acute myocardial infarction. Cathet Cardiovasc Diagn 1997;42:151–7.

2. Mann JM, Roberts WC. Cardiac morphologic observations after operative closure of acquired ventricular septal defect during acute myocardial infarction: analysis of 16 necropsy patients. Am J Cardiol 1987;60:981–7.

3. Jugdutt BI, Michorowski BL. Role of infarct expansion in rupture of the ventricular septum after acute myocardial infarction: a two-dimensional echocardiographic study. Clin Cardiol 1987;10:641–52.

4. Di Summa M, Actis Dato GM, Centofanti P, *et al*. Ventricular septal rupture after a myocardial infarction: clinical features and long term survival. J Cardiovasc Surg 1997;38:589–93.

5. David TE. Operative management of postinfarction ventricular septal defect. Semin Thorac Cardiovasc Surg 1995;7:208–13.

71

Bullet in the heart

Susan E Wiegers MD

A 45-year-old woman was brought to the emergency room receiving basic life support after being shot in the chest during an altercation inside her home. She was intubated in the emergency room, and bilateral chest tubes were placed which drained a large amount of frank blood on the right. She initially required massive volume resuscitation but stabilized in the first several hours and was transferred to the trauma intensive care unit. She had severe damage to the right lung requiring a high inspired oxygen saturation. She remained hypotensive while receiving intravenous pressor agents and an echocardiogram was obtained to assess cardiac function. A transesophageal study was performed to confirm the finding of the transthoracic study.

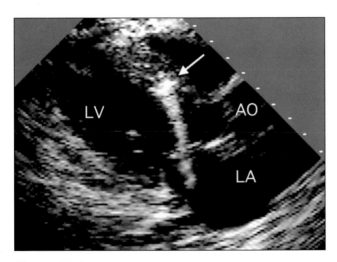

Figure 71.1
Transthoracic parasternal long-axis view in diastole. The view was obtained one intercostal space lower than the standard transducer position, because of bandages. The cardiac chambers appear to be normal in size, although the left atrium (LA) may be slightly dilated. The left ventricle (LV) appears to be normal. A highly refractile object (arrow) is visible in the interventricular septum. It is echodense and creates a reverberation artifact behind it which extends to the level of the left atrium. This density is a bullet fragment which appeared to be lodged within the septum and did not move relative to the cardiac structures. The valves appear normal although the imaging is limited. The pericardium is not well seen but there is a suggestion of consolidated material within the posterior pericardial space which would be expected to be thrombus.

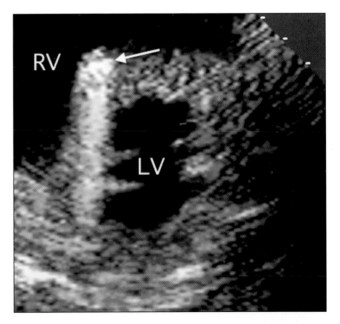

Figure 71.2
Transthoracic parasternal short-axis view at the level of the papillary muscles. This close-up image of the interventricular septum demonstrates that the bullet has lodged in the right ventricular side of the septum. It does not appear to be on the left ventricular side of the septum, as was suggested by the long-axis views, but seems to be more superficially located within the right ventricular (RV) endocardium. There is no evidence of ventricular septal defect or of damage to the valvular structures. A reverberation artifact is again seen posterior to the bullet in the line of the ultrasound beam. The left ventricular function was mildly decreased.

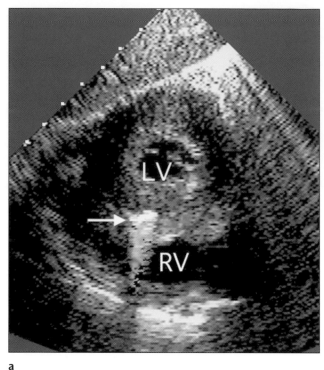

a

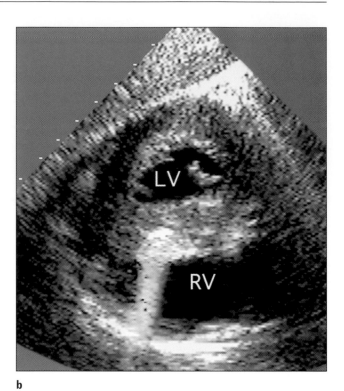

b

Figure 71.3

(a) The transesophageal study was performed several hours later, as the patient deteriorated hemodynamically. A transgastric image from the transesophageal echocardiogram study demonstrates the left (LV) and right (RV) ventricles in short-axis from the transverse plane (imaging angle 0°). The bullet fragment is once again seen in the right ventricular side of the interventricular septum with the reverberation artifact now extending into the right ventricle.

(b) Diastolic image from the same view. The left ventricular cavity is small and underfilled. The interventricular septum flattens, owing to right ventricular volume overload. The myocardium surrounding the bullet did appear to be thicker than the posterior wall and more refractile. However, it thickened normally in systole. Thus, it is unlikely that there was a significant hematoma surrounding the bullet fragment. The right ventricular area does not change significantly between the systolic and diastolic frames. The right ventricular failure was due to the acutely elevated pulmonary pressures from the lung injury. In addition, the patient may have had a more focal injury to the right ventricular wall due to the bullet. No significant pericardial effusion is seen on this study.

Discussion

Echocardiography is indispensable in the emergency room for evaluation of the trauma patient who is hypotensive. Immediate echocardiography may be related to improved survival since it allows rapid and accurate diagnosis of tamponade, hypovolemia and injury to the heart and great vessels.[1] Transthoracic echocardiography may be limited in patients with chest trauma either because of the placement of chest tubes and bandages in standard transthoracic transducer positions or because of the introduction of air into the mediastinum which limits ultrasound wave propagation into the chest. In this case the bullet passed through the right lung, causing severe mechanical and heat trauma. However, the right ventricular free wall

appears to have been penetrated without resulting in a significant pericardial effusion or tamponade. The absence of a pericardial effusion does not rule out significant cardiac trauma and a complete study should always be attempted.[2] Although embolization of bullet fragments to the heart has been reported,[3] the presence of the bullet within the interventricular septum made this unlikely.

In this patient the transthoracic study demonstrated that the bullet was embedded in the septum. The metal bullet is extremely echodense and results in a high-intensity signal returning to the transducer. The echocardiographic machine is unable to localize the artifact past the first interface which creates a type of reverberation artifact extending posteriorly along the direction of the ultrasound beam. This reverberation artifact makes the assessment of the surrounding septum difficult. An interventricular septal defect could not be excluded. Transesophageal echocardiography may be more reliable in diagnosing the presence and precise location of retained bullet fragments.[4] The possibility of esophageal trauma should be considered in any patient with penetrating mediastinal injuries. In the absence of an upper gastrointestinal bleed, however, the need for immediate transesophageal assessment usually precludes a detailed evaluation of the esophagus. The transesophageal study allowed the bullet fragment to be more precisely localized. It was seen to be on the right ventricular side of the septum and in no danger of eroding into the left ventricle. The bullet fragment also moved with the septum and appeared unlikely to embolize. Embolization of cardiac retained bullet fragments has been reported.[5] Given the stable location of the bullet fragment, as well as the patient's severe pulmonary injuries, no further treatment was undertaken. The patient eventually was weaned from mechanical ventilation. A follow-up echocardiogram taken 1 month later showed no change in the location of the bullet fragment, although the right ventricular function was improved compared to the previous study.

References

1. Plummer D, Brunette D, Asinger R, *et al*. Emergency department echocardiography improves outcome in penetrating cardiac injury. Ann Emerg Med 1992;21:709–12.

2. Hassett A, Moran J, Sabiston DC, *et al*. Utility of echocardiography in the management of patients with penetrating missile wounds of the heart. J Am Coll Cardiol 1986;7:1151–6.

3. Grewal KS, Sintek CF, Jorgensen MB. Bullet embolism to the heart. Am Heart J 1997;133:468–70.

4. Hashimi MW, Jenkins DR, McGwier BW, *et al*. Comparative efficacy of transthoracic and transesophageal echocardiography in detection of an intracardiac bullet fragment. Chest 1994;106:299–300.

5. Bilsker MS, Bauerlein EJ, Kamerman ML. Bullet embolus from the heart to the right subclavian artery after gunshot wound to the right chest. Am Heart J 1996;132:1093–4.

72

Ventricular mass after lung transplant

Susan E Wiegers MD

A 35-year-old woman with end-stage cystic fibrosis underwent orthotopic lung transplantation one year prior to this admission. She had done well on her routine immunosuppression regimen until approximately 2 weeks prior to the current admission, when she developed cough, low grade fevers and hemoptysis. Her clinical status rapidly deteriorated, precipitating admission to the hospital, where she required intubation and mechanical ventilation. The chest X-ray revealed extensive diffuse patchy infiltrates in both lungs. Bronchoscopic washings yielded hyphae consistent with fungal infection. The patient became septic and required multiple pressors to sustain her blood pressure. She remained extremely hypotensive despite full resuscitative efforts. An echocardiogram was ordered to evaluate the cause of hypotension in this critically ill patient.

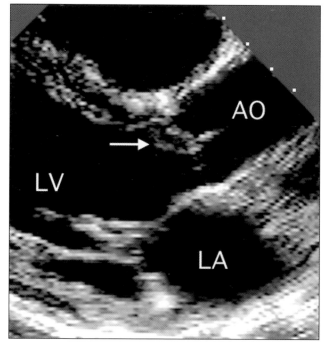

Figure 72.1
Parasternal long-axis view in late diastole. The left ventricle (LV) is of normal dimension as is the left atrium (LA) and the ascending aorta (AO). The mitral valve leaflets themselves appear to be normal. However, the chordal apparatus appears to be thickened. The most striking finding is a small hypoechoic mass (arrow) in the left ventricular outflow tract which may be associated with the right coronary cusp of the aortic valve.

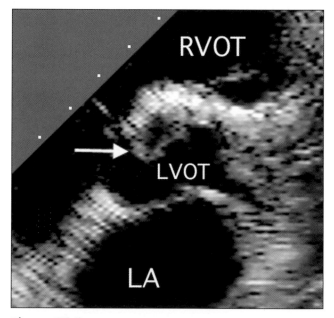

Figure 72.2
Parasternal short-axis view at the level of the left ventricular outflow tract (LVOT) just below the level of the aortic valve leaflets. A mass with a central clearing (arrow) is visualized attached to the septum in the anterior portion of the outflow tract. The mass has an unusual cystic appearance and attachment site which does not resemble the usual appearance of a subaortic membrane.

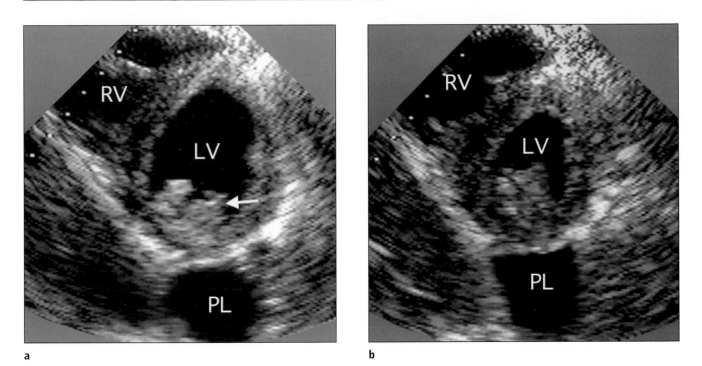

a   b

Figure 72.3

(a) Parasternal short-axis view from the transthoracic study at the level of the left ventricular papillary muscles. A left pleural effusion (PL) is demonstrated posterior to the left ventricle. The right ventricular cavity (RV) is mildly enlarged. The view is slightly off axis; however, a marked abnormality in the posterior wall of the left ventricle is demonstrated (arrow). This abnormality is in the region of the normal position of the posterior medial papillary muscle. The echodensity of this mass is different from that of the surrounding myocardium. The mass appears to project through the endocardium into the myocardium. There is no clear delineation from the surrounding tissue and the normal papillary muscle structure is not demonstrated.

(b)   Similar parasternal view in systole. The left ventricular systolic function is normal. There is mild flattening of the interventricular septum between the right ventricle and left ventricle consistent with right ventricular pressure overload. Once again the mass projects into the left ventricular cavity and the normal structure of the papillary muscle is not seen. This view is slightly more caudal than that of (a). The mass appears to extend towards the apex of the left ventricle.

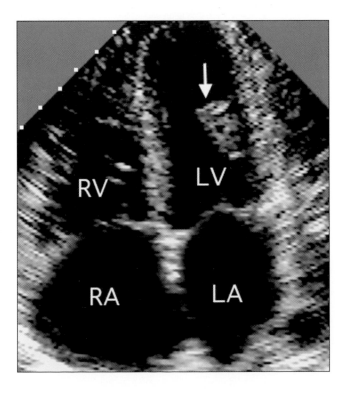

Figure 72.4

Apical four-chamber view, demonstrating the mass attached to the myocardium and projecting into the left ventricular cavity (arrow). The mass is near the normal position of a papillary muscle but its echodensity and position within the left ventricular cavity are extremely abnormal. Note that the left ventricular anatomy is otherwise normal. The right ventricle is mildly hypertrophied and the right atrium (RA) is enlarged.

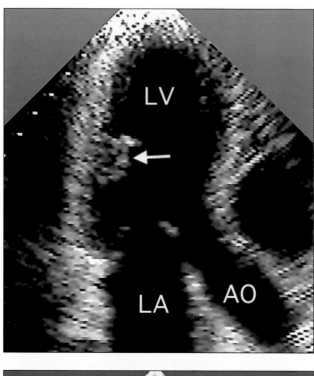

Figure 72.5
Apical long-axis view of the left ventricular mass (arrow). While the mass appears to occupy the normal position of the posterior medial papillary muscle, its orientation is extremely abnormal for a papillary muscle. The echodensity is different from that of the surrounding myocardium and the process appears to invade the posterior wall of the left ventricle.

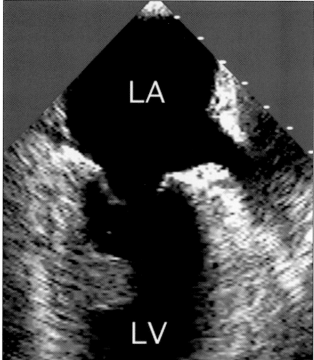

a

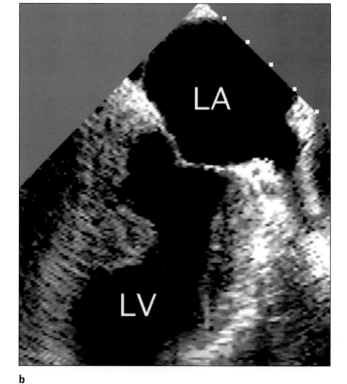

b

Figure 72.6
(a) Transesophageal echocardiogram from the mid-esophageal level in the longitudinal plane (imaging angle 90°). This two-chamber view demonstrates the mass more clearly than in the transthoracic images. The left atrium appears mildly enlarged and the left atrial appendage is well seen on the right of the screen. The mitral valve leaflets appear to be normal although they are not completely visualized in this projection. The left ventricular mass is clearly not a papillary muscle. The entire border of this mass contained very small, finger-like projections that were highly mobile in real time.
(b) Similar transesophageal view in systole. The mass did not contract with systole but appeared to be firmly attached to the left ventricular endocardium. In real time the motion of the mass clearly distinguished it from a papillary muscle.

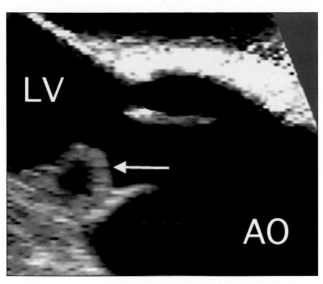

Figure 72.7
Transesophageal echocardiographic image from the mid-esophagus in the longitudinal plane (imaging angle 135°). The aortic valve leaflets are shown to be partially open in systole. The aortic root (AO) is imaged slightly off axis and was normal on complete inspection. The cystic mass (arrow) is seen to be attached to the septum. This mass had an area of central clearing and was not attached to the right coronary cusp of the aortic valve, although it is in close proximity.

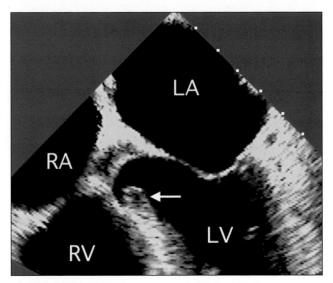
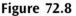

Figure 72.8
Transesophageal image from the mid-esophagus in the transverse plane (imaging angle 0°) of a modified four-chamber view. The endocardium of the interventricular septum appears to be thickened. Once again the cystic mass (arrow) is seen projecting into the left ventricular outflow tract. In this view it is clearly not attached to the aortic valve leaflets.

Discussion

The transthoracic echocardiogram was performed to evaluate a cause for hypotension in this patient. Left ventricular function was normal. In a septic patient, the decreased afterload may result in hyperdynamic left ventricular function.[1] Myocardial depression may also occur, resulting in ejection fractions in the normal range despite severely reduced systemic vascular resistance or decreased systolic function. In this case, the dilatation and mild decrease in right ventricular function were consistent with the acute pulmonary process that resulted in an increase in the pulmonary vascular resistance. Therefore, the most likely cause for the patient's hypotension was septic shock, as there was no echocardiographic evidence of cardiac failure.

An incidental finding on the transthoracic echocardiogram was the abnormal mass, initially thought to be an anomalous papillary muscle. However, the abnormality in the left ventricular outflow tract raised the question of a diffuse endocardial process. Furthermore, a transesophageal echocardiogram was undertaken to further delineate the abnormality. The transesophageal echocardiogram demonstrated an infiltrative process which had replaced the papillary muscle and was invading the myocardium below the papillary muscle insertion. A bacterial process is most unlikely to exhibit these findings, particularly in the absence of valvular lesions. Fungal myocarditis has been reported in immunocompromised

hosts with a very poor prognosis.[2–4] It is nevertheless very rare in the non-perioperative period.[5] Although cardiac tumors may have simulated the echocardiographic findings, the positive sputum Gram stain and the patient's septic state were all suggestive of a fungal process.

The patient was aggressively treated with maximum ionotropic support and antifungal agents but expired 2 days after the echocardiogram. Postmortem examination revealed aspergillus infection of the myocardium, endocardium, and lung. No other evidence of disseminated infection was found.

References

1. Jardin F, Brun-Ney D, Auvert B, *et al*. Sepsis-related cardiogenic shock. Crit Care Med 1990;18:1055–60.

2. Schwartz D. Aspergillus pancarditis following bone marrow transplantation for chronic myelogenous leukemia. Chest 1989;95:1338–9.

3. Hofman P, Gari-Toussaint M, Bernard E, *et al*. Fungal myocarditis in acquired immunodeficiency syndrome. Arch Maladie Coeur Vaisseaux 1992;85:203–8.

4. Rouby Y, Combourieu E, Perrier-Gros-Claude J, *et al*. A case of Aspergillus myocarditis associated with septic shock. J Infect 1998;37:295–7.

5. Sergi C, Weitz J, Hofmann W, *et al*. Aspergillus endocarditis, myocarditis and pericarditis complicating necrotizing fasciitis. Case report and subject review. Virchows Arch 1996;429:177–80.

73

Anomalous papillary muscle masquerading as a tumor

Martin St John Sutton MBBS

A 32-year-old woman complained of sudden onset of recurrent palpitations lasting for up to 2 hours, associated with lightheadedness and nausea. She also noticed while training for a marathon that her heart rate would suddenly increase by 30–40 bpm and take longer to return to normal after she had stopped running. She could not identify any triggers for her rapid heart rate and excluding caffeine from her diet had no impact on the frequency of her palpitations. She had had no previous heart disease, had no risk factors for coronary artery disease and no family history of congenital heart disease. Electrocardiography showed minor T wave inversion in the anterior precordial leads. A chest X-ray showed a normal cardiac silhouette and clear lung fields. An exercise stress test was entirely normal at high work load on a Bruce protocol. An echocardiogram was reported to show a 2 × 1.5 cm 'tumor' invading the myocardium in the anterior septum and left ventricular outflow tract and a transesophageal echocardiogram was said to be confirmatory. She was transferred for surgery.

On examination, she was normotensive and in regular rhythm without ectopic activity. Peripheral arterial pulses were present and equal bilaterally. The jugular venous pressure and apical impulse were normal. On auscultation there was a normal first heart sound and a normally splitting second heart sound and no ejection systolic murmur to suggest left ventricular outflow tract obstruction. Review of the electrocardiogram showed repolarization abnormalities in the anteroseptal region at rest which did not change with exercise; the chest X-ray was normal. A transthoracic echocardiogram was repeated.

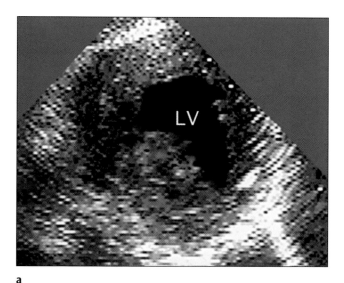

a

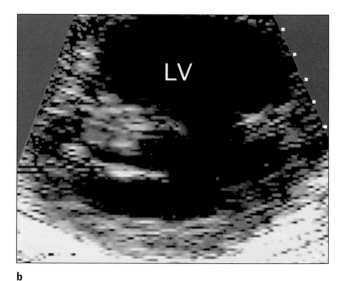

b

Figure 73.1
(a) Parasternal short-axis view at the mid-ventricular level. The 'mass' appears to be associated with the inferior wall and the septum at the apex. An important feature to note is that the acoustic property or signature of the lesion is similar if not identical to that of the myocardium.
(b) Close-up of the mass at the level of the mitral valve chords. The mass extends to this level although it is considerably smaller.

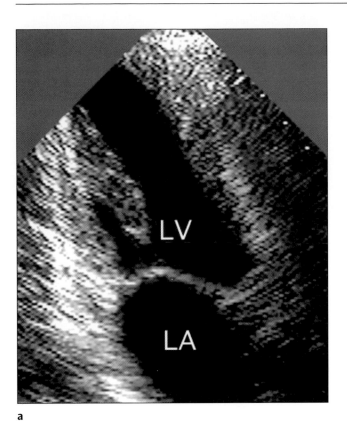

a

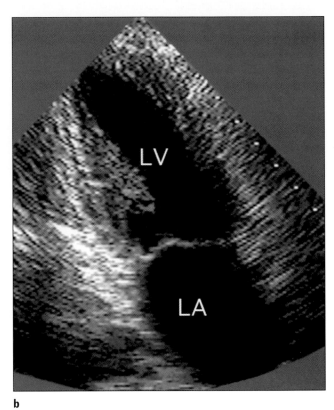

b

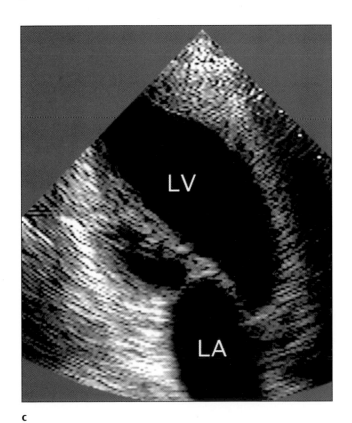

c

Figure 73.2

(a) Apical long-axis view demonstrating no evidence of the mass, but only a large posteromedial papillary muscle which is apically displaced. The mitral valve was competent.

(b) Apical two-chamber view demonstrating that the papillary muscle is present at the level seen in the short-axis view.

(c) Off-axis angulation allows the lesion to be reconstructed. The papillary muscle is abnormally large, is broad based, and has abnormal attachments to the anterior mitral leaflet. The tip of the muscle appears to insert directly onto the valve leaflets rather than via chordal attachments.

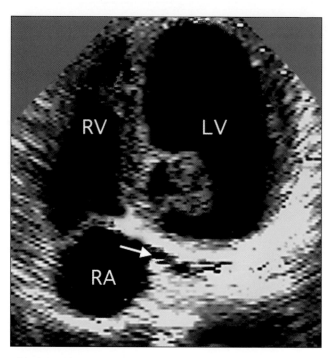

Figure 73.3
Off-axis apical four-chamber view. The transducer has been angled posteriorly as evidenced by demonstration of the coronary sinus (arrow) in the posterior atrioventricular groove. The anomalous papillary muscle attaches to the posterior septum at two levels but the body of the muscle is shown in short-axis.

Discussion

The erroneous diagnosis of tumor was made without sufficient attention being paid to two fundamental echocardiographic principles. First, whenever a mass is suspected, it is of paramount importance to attempt to reconstruct the lesion from orthogonal views to be certain that it is not an artifact. This reconstruction is often suboptimal if only the routine views/imaging planes are obtained. As in this patient the most useful diagnostic images were off-axis images that allowed the mass to be entirely visualized. Second, the acoustic properties of intracardiac masses provide information as to their composition. In this patient the acoustic appearance of the mass was indistinguishable from that of the myocardium, indicating that its composition was similar. Adherence to these two simple echocardiographic principles enabled this unusually located mass to be recognized as an ectopically placed papillary muscle. The electrocardiographic repolarization abnormalities in the anteroseptal leads, which initially caused concern, were congruent with the location of the 'tumor' reflecting the repolarization of this large ectopically located papillary muscle myocardium. The combination of off-axis parasternal and apical echocardiographic images allowed the complete papillary muscle to be traced from its septal origin to the mitral chords.

74

Pseudoaneurysm

Susan E Wiegers MD

A 78-year-old woman sustained an uncomplicated inferior myocardial infarction. An echocardiogram prior to discharge demonstrated mild thinning of the inferior wall and mild mitral regurgitation. She was subsequently well for over 2 years but had two transient ischemic attacks characterized by brief periods of aphasia and right hemiplegia. After the second episode, she presented to her primary care physician for evaluation. An echocardiogram was ordered as part of her workup. She had not experienced any chest pain since her myocardial infarction and had minimal dyspnea on exertion. Her physical examination was remarkable only for an S_4 on cardiac auscultation.

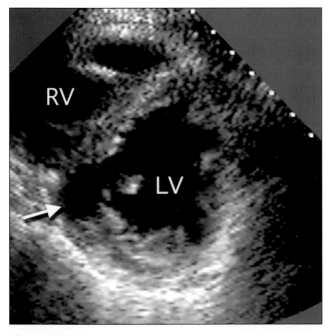

Figure 74.1
Parasternal short-axis view of the left ventricle at the level of the papillary muscles. The left ventricular cavity is of normal size. However, there is an outpouching of the inferior wall adjacent to the posteromedial papillary muscle. This outpouching (arrow) represents a well-developed pseudoaneurysm. The right ventricle is mildly dilated. The remainder of the left ventricle appears normal.

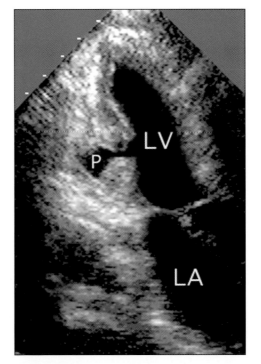

Figure 74.2
Apical long-axis view demonstrating the abrupt break in the inferoposterior wall endocardium just proximal to the posterior papillary muscle. The pseudoaneurysm (P) is well seen. The pseudoaneurysm cavity appears smaller than in the previous figure because it is irregularly shaped rather than spherical and symmetrical. The endocardium of the remainder of the left ventricular walls appear to be normal. The left atrium (LA) is mildly enlarged.

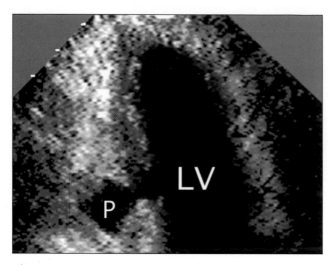

Figure 74.3
Close-up image of the pseudoaneurysm in the apical two-chamber view. The neck of the pseudoaneurysm is seen in the inferior wall. The walls of the pseudoaneurysm are not well delineated and in fact were lined with thrombus. The discontinuity in the inferior wall is clearly seen.

Discussion

Rupture of the myocardium into the pericardial space after a myocardial infarction usually results in sudden death due to cardiac tamponade. However, previous obliteration of the potential pericardial space by inflammation and scarring due to Dressler's syndrome, recurrent pericardial infections, or previous cardiac surgery may allow the rupture to be contained within a pocket of the pericardial space. The result is a pseudoaneurysm. This can be distinguished from a true aneurysm on the basis of the components of the wall of the chamber. The wall of a true aneurysm is lined with scar tissue and remnants of myocardial fibers, while the pseudoaneurysm's walls are lined by pericardium. Coronary arteries are present in the walls of a true aneurysm but never in a pseudoaneurysm. It is clear from Figure 74.1 that, had the patient's myocardial rupture been in a slightly different location, she would have presented with a ventricular septal defect rather than a pseudoaneurysm. The discontinuity in the myocardium is very close to the insertion of the interventricular septum. Rupture at this point would have been into the right ventricular cavity rather than the pericardial space.

Echocardiography usually allows for differentiation between true and false aneurysms. A pseudoaneurysm has a narrow neck at a site of abrupt discontinuity of the endocardium. The body of the chamber is usually greater than the dimension of the neck.[1] In contrast, the neck of a true aneurysm is typically as wide as the body. Cavity expansion is more pronounced with pseudoaneurysms and high-velocity diastolic flow out of the neck of the pseudoaneurysm into the left ventricular cavity is characteristic of a pseudoaneurysm but is not found with true aneurysms. The contour of the adjacent endocardium is also helpful. The abrupt discontinuity seen in this patient is never present in true aneurysms, where a gradual transition to the thinner walls of the aneurysm is characteristic. Occasionally, the differentiation cannot be made by even transesophageal echocardiography but other imaging modalities are not necessarily superior in this case. Confusion may result with paracardiac structures as well as true aneurysms. Atypical ventricular thrombi may appear to have central cavities and mimic the appearance of a pseudoaneurysm.[2]

The pseudoaneurysm may expand over time and cause multiple mechanical complications, even if it does not rupture. Distortion of the mitral valve and papillary muscle apparatus may result in mitral regurgitation.[3] The pseudoaneurysm cavity expands in systole and can compress other cardiac structures including the left atrium, coronary arteries, and the branch pulmonary arteries.[4] Owing to the risk of rupture over time, resection of pseudoaneurysms has been routinely recommended. Posteriorly located pseudoaneurysms are technically more challenging to repair, owing to difficulties in exposure and surgical access. Recently, it has been recommended that small stable pseudoaneurysms are better left untreated. This patient has a very small pseudoaneurysm that is not particularly expansile and may best be left unoperated. The development of pain, which is often chronic and radiates to the back for posterior pseudoaneurysms, congestive heart failure or demonstration of progressive expansion of the cavity are indications for urgent surgery. Thromboembolic complications are not infrequent. The risk of chronic anticoagulation in a patient with a pseudoaneurysm with an undefined risk of rupture should be seriously considered prior to proceeding.

This patient refused surgery and was anticoagulated with warfarin. An echocardiogram 8 months later showed no change in the size of the pseudoaneurysm cavity and she has been clinically stable.

References

1. Saner H, Asinger R, Daniel J, et al. Two-dimensional echocardiographic identification of left ventricular pseudoaneurysm. Am Heart J 1986;112:977–85.

2. Badano L, Piazza R, Bisignani G, et al. A large left ventricular thrombus evolving towards canalization and mimicking a left ventricular pseudoaneurysm: an echocardiographic study. J Am Soc Echocardiogr 1993;6:446–8.

3. Ezzat M, Abdelmeguid I, Leclerc D, et al. Left ventricular pseudoaneurysm associated with mitral regurgitation. Ann Thorac Surg 1992;53:504–6.

4. Cocina E, Rosas G, Ruiz F, et al. Left ventricular pseudoaneurysm: a cause of unilateral pulmonary edema by compressing the left pulmonary artery. Am Heart J 1996;132:1306–7.

75

Traumatic ventricular septal defect and mitral valve perforation

Susan E Wiegers MD

A 45-year-old man became suicidal while acutely intoxicated. After surviving a single vehicle accident he stabbed himself in the chest with a hunting knife. He was brought to the emergency room hypotensive and unresponsive. Emergency thoracotomy demonstrated hemopericardium, tamponade and a right ventricular laceration. The right ventricular wall was repaired and the patient was stabilized hemodynamically. He was easily extubated and transferred out of the intensive care unit. On the second postoperative day, the cardiology consultant heard a loud systolic murmur that had not been recorded on previous examinations. A transthoracic echocardiogram was performed.

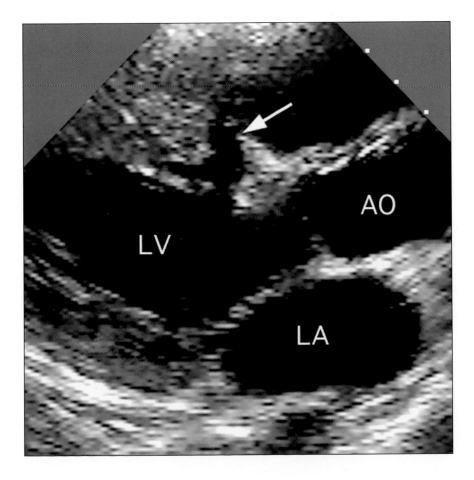

Figure 75.1
Parasternal long-axis view in systole. The left ventricle (LV), left atrium (LA), and aorta (AO) are of normal size. A large hole (arrow) is seen in the interventricular septum consistent with traumatic ventricular septal defect. The appearance is not one of a congenital ventricle septal defect. The defect is located in the proximal muscular septum and is quite large. However, the edges appear ragged. In addition, such a large congenital ventricle septal defect would have been clinically evident since childhood.

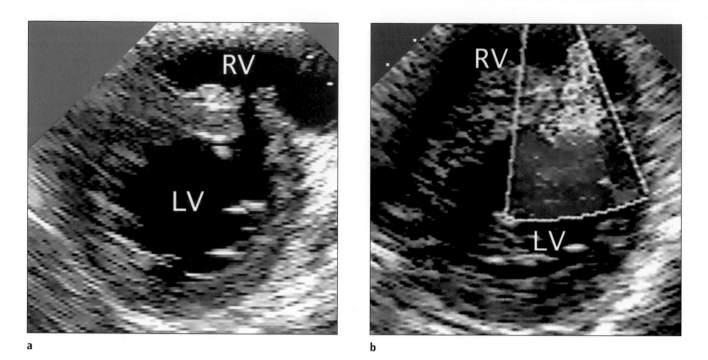

a   b

Figure 75.2

(a) Parasternal short-axis view. The ventricular septal defect is again demonstrated in the interventricular septum between the left (LV) and right ventricles (RV). There is a small mass in the left ventricle medial to the defect. This mass was highly mobile in real time. It represents a partially severed piece of septal myocardium that was attached by a short stalk of myocardium.

(b) Color Doppler flow imaging in the same parasternal view in systole. A wide high-velocity turbulent jet crosses the ventricular septal defect from the left to the right ventricle. The width of the color jet is approximately 1 cm which is a good estimate for the size of the ventricular septal defect (calibration marks are visible on the upper left-hand side of the image).

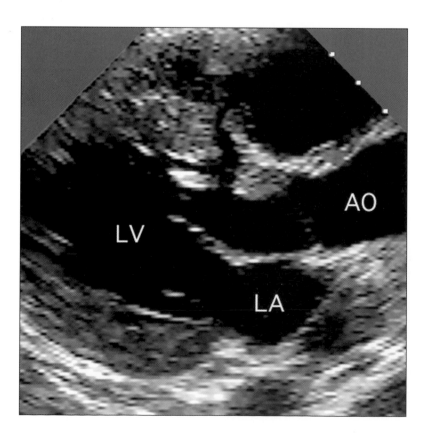

Figure 75.3

Parasternal long-axis view in diastole. This image is similar to Figure 75.1. However, in this diastolic image an odd angulation of the anterior mitral valve leaflet is seen. This motion, in which the distal leaflet moves at a different angle from that of the proximal leaflet around a hinge point, is highly suggestive of perforation. The hinge point is directly posterior to the ventricular septal defect which was itself directly posterior to the site of the right ventricular laceration (not shown here). Thus, the point of the knife passed through the right ventricular free wall, interventricular septum, and mitral valve, creating multiple defects.

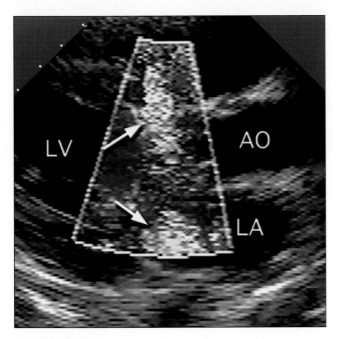

Figure 75.4
Color Doppler flow imaging of the parasternal long-axis view in systole. Perforation of the anterior leaflet of the mitral valve is confirmed by the presence of a turbulent jet of mitral regurgitation which originates at mid-leaflet (lower arrow). Again, the alignment of the ventricular septal defect and the mitral leaflet defect can be appreciated. The coronary sinus lies directly in the path of the knife blade but careful imaging did not reveal any abnormality of the coronary sinus.

Discussion

Patients with stab wounds to the chest who are unstable should undergo immediate surgical exploration.[1] Transesophageal echocardiography may be helpful in the operating room. Patients who are evaluated with immediate echocardiography may do better than patients in whom the test is delayed. This is because the echocardiogram allows for the immediate diagnosis of serious cardiac injuries and directs the approach to their treatment.[2] However, transthoracic echocardiography may not be sensitive enough for the diagnosis of cardiac injury in unstable patients.[3] A normal transthoracic study does not rule out significant cardiac problems and the presence of even a small pericardial effusion on the study makes surgical exploration mandatory. Furthermore, transthoracic studies may be of poor quality in up to 20% of patients with penetrating chest trauma.[4] Therefore, transesophageal echocardiography is felt to be a better test in the evaluation of patients with chest trauma. Transesophageal echocardiography has been found to be safe and highly accurate in this situation.[5]

Appropriate management of stab wounds to the heart involves repair of the right ventricular lacerations and stabilization of the patient. Prolonged cardiopulmonary bypass would be required for intracardiac repair of lesions and is to be avoided if possible, owing to patient instability and concern regarding the sterility of thoracotomies initiated in the emergency room. Echocardiography can be used intraoperatively if the patient fails to stabilize or postoperatively to evaluate any other abnormalities. This patient did not have a perioperative transesophageal echocardiogram and was doing well in the surgical intensive care unit when a loud murmur was noted. Traumatic ventricular septal defects have been reported after penetrating chest wounds.[6] Late sequelae of chest stab wounds may be detected in up to 25% of patients.[7]

References

1. Asensio JA, Stewart BM, Murray J, *et al*. Penetrating cardiac injuries. Surg Clin North Am 1996;76:685–724.

2. Plummer D, Brunette D, Asinger R, *et al*. Emergency department echocardiography improves outcome in penetrating cardiac injury. Ann Emerg Med 1992;21:709–12.

3. Meyer DM, Jessen ME, Grayburn PA. Use of echocardiography to detect occult cardiac injury after penetrating thoracic trauma: a prospective study. J Trauma 1995;39:902–7; discussion 907–9.

4. Johnson SB, Kearney PA, Smith MD. Echocardiography in the evaluation of thoracic trauma. Surg Clin North Am 1995;75:193–205.

5. Mollod M, Felner JM. Transesophageal echocardiography in the evaluation of cardiothoracic trauma. Am Heart J 1996;132:841–9.

6. Olsovsky MR, Topaz O, DiSciascio G, *et al*. Acute traumatic ventricular septal rupture. Am Heart J 1996;131:1039–41.

7. Demetriades D, Charalambides C, Sareli P, *et al*. Late sequelae of penetrating cardiac injuries. Br J Surg 1990;77:813–14.

76

Coronary fistula and traumatic ventricular septal defect

Susan E Wiegers MD

The patient in Chapter 75 was returned to the operating room 2 weeks after his initial injury where he underwent primary closure of the ventricular septal defect and single stitch repair of the mitral valve perforation. The traumatic ventricular septal defect was in close proximity to the left anterior descending artery which sustained trauma during the repair resulting in an anteroseptal wall motion abnormality postoperatively. Transesophageal echocardiography was performed in the operating room to guide the surgery.

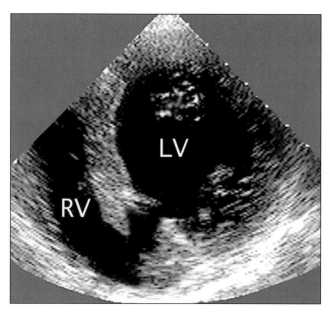

a

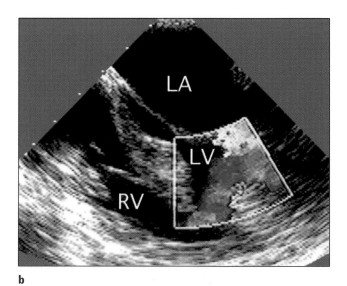

b

Figure 76.1

(a) Transesophageal echocardiogram from the transgastric view in the transverse plane (imaging angle 0°) at the level of the mitral chordae. There is a large ventricular septal defect measuring over 1 cm in diameter noted between the right ventricle (RV) and the left ventricle (LV). The right ventricle is mildly enlarged.

(b) Transesophageal image from the mid-esophageal level in a modified four-chamber view in the transverse plane (imaging angle 0°) with color flow Doppler imaging. There is a left to right shunt noted across the ventricular septal defect. The cropping of the color sector in this image has eliminated the high velocity turbulent jet on the right ventricular side of the ventricular septal defect.

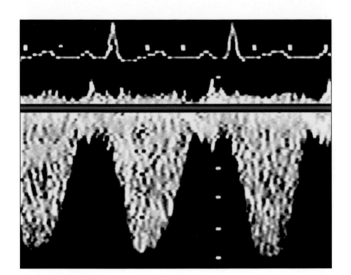

Figure 76.2
Spectral display of continuous-wave Doppler across the ventricular septal defect from the mid-esophageal level in the transverse imaging plane. In systole, there is a left to right jet of 5 m/s across the defect predicting a left ventricular to right ventricular gradient of over 100 mmHg. While this patient had not yet decompensated, his right ventricle was enlarged and was mildly hypokinetic, owing to the significant volume overload.

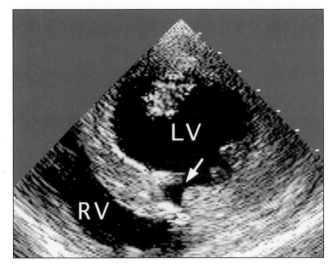

Figure 76.3
Transgastric echocardiogram from the transverse plane (imaging angle 0°) after the surgical repair immediately after weaning from cardiopulmonary bypass. A surgical patch is noted closing the ventricular septal defect (arrow). This was approached from the right ventricular side to avoid an incision into the left ventricular myocardium. The right ventricular size is slightly decreased compared to that in Figure 76.1a. The septum was severely hypokinetic after the repair.

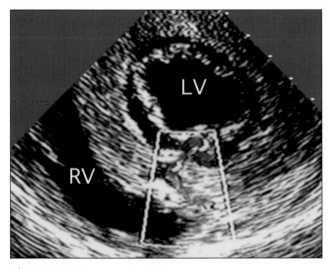

Figure 76.4
Transgastric image from the transverse plane (imaging angle 0°) with color Doppler flow imaging. There is no residual left to right shunt flow. However, a coronary artery within the interventricular septum empties into the blind pouch of the repaired ventricular septal defect. This represents a coronary artery fistula to the ventricular septal defect which was not appreciated prior to the repair. The large color jet of the ventricular septal defect flow obscured the smaller color Doppler jet of the coronary artery fistula in the images prior to the repair. The vessel was a large branch of the left anterior descending artery which was intramyocardial and had been lacerated during the stab wound. This had resulted in severe septal hypokinesis.

Discussion

The case is discussed in detail in the previous chapter (75). The transesophageal echocardiogram revealed additional information in the perioperative period that was not detected on the transthoracic study, despite excellent images. Owing to the fact that the septum had been hypokinetic for 2 weeks prior to the surgery, the coronary artery fistula was not considered to be a result of the current surgery. In addition, the demonstrated shunt was small, thus no further intervention was undertaken. The patient has continued to be stable from a cardiovascular standpoint with a residual ejection fraction of 45%.

Transesophageal echocardiography has been increasingly recognized as an invaluable tool in the management of patients with penetrating chest trauma, both on presentation and in the operating room.[1,2]

References

1. Porembka DT, Johnson DJD, Hoit BD, *et al.* Penetrating cardiac trauma: a perioperative role for transesophageal echocardiography. Anesth Analg 1993;77:1275–7.

2. Skoularigis J, Essop MR, Sareli P. Usefulness of transesophageal echocardiography in the early diagnosis of penetrating stab wounds to the heart. Am J Cardiol 1994;73:407–9.

77

Ventricular septal defect after a myocardial infarction

Susan E Wiegers MD

A 70-year-old man had been in excellent health until he sustained an acute anterior myocardial infarction. He had attributed his chest pain to gastroenteritis until 3 days after the initial episode when he had recurrence of the chest pain, followed by increasing dyspnea and weakness. On presentation to the emergency room he was in cardiogenic shock and was intubated. A loud systolic murmur was heard across the precordium. An electrocardiogram demonstrated Q waves in V3–V5 and persistent ST elevation. He was transferred by helicopter to a tertiary care center. A transthoracic echocardiogram was too technically limited to provide clinically useful information. A transesophageal echocardiogram was performed within 30 min of his arrival.

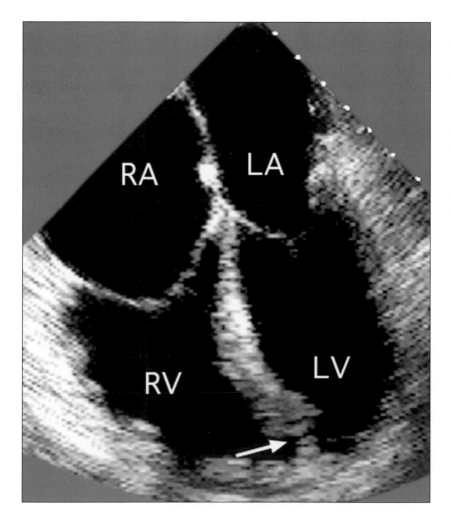

Figure 77.1
Transesophageal echocardiogram from the mid-esophageal level of the four-chamber view. The image is in the transverse plane (imaging angle 0°). The right atrium (RA) and right ventricle (RV) are severely dilated and the right ventricular function is severely decreased. The left ventricular ejection fraction appears to be normal but the septum and the apex do not thicken. The other walls were hyperdynamic. There is a defect in the distal septum (arrow) which appears to be a discontinuity in the endocardium.

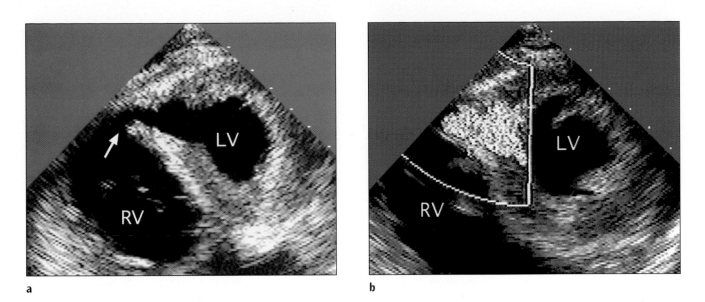

a   b

Figure 77.2
(a) Transgastric view of the short-axis at the level of the left (LV) and right ventricular (RV) apex. The image is again in the transverse plane (imaging angle 0°). There is a ventricular septal defect (arrow) with the septum prolapsing into the right ventricular apex in this systolic frame. The left ventricular apex is moderately dilated and severely hypokinetic in real time. The right ventricular apex is severely dilated and was akinetic. The ventricular septal defect measures over 1 cm on the left ventricular side.
(b) Transgastric view of the short-axis again in the transverse plane with color flow Doppler imaging. The probe has been withdrawn slightly compared with the previous image. The anterolateral papillary muscle is evident at the bottom right of the image. There is a large turbulent jet from the left ventricle to the right ventricle through the ventricular septal defect. The diameter of the color flow jet measures approximately 2 cm at its maximum width.

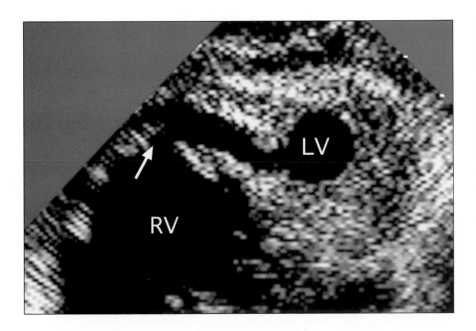

Figure 77.3
Similar view to that in Figure 77.2 except that the image is more apical. The ventricular septal defect is seen to extend to the very tip of the left ventricular cavity (arrow). A piece of the interventricular septum flails into the right ventricle in systole. There is a small posterior pericardial effusion at this level. The apex of the left ventricle was necrotic and it is likely that there was seepage of blood through the apex into the pericardial space. The rupture of the myocardium had occurred between the ventricles rather than between the left ventricle and the pericardial space.

Discussion

Transesophageal echocardiography was instrumental in the diagnosis of the cause of cardiogenic shock in this patient. Transthoracic images are often inadequate for diagnosis in patients who have been intubated and in those who cannot be adequately positioned for the examination. Transesophageal imaging is a rapidly available alternative which provides better image quality in the critically ill patient and allows for the diagnosis of the complications of myocardial infarction.[1]

This patient had a large apical ventricular septal defect due to rupture of an extensive portion of the interventricular septum at the apex. The hole in the septum was so large that a necrotic piece of the septum flailed into the right ventricular cavity in systole. The massive shunt flow through this very large defect overwhelmed the right ventricle, resulting in severe dilatation and systolic failure. Right ventricular akinesis is a poor prognostic sign in the acute setting. Survival after development of an acute ventricular septal defect depends on many factors, particularly the degree of the shunt flow, the presence of coronary artery disease in the non-infarcted territories, and the baseline left and right ventricular systolic function. Ventricular septal rupture is as common after inferior infarctions as anterior sites. However, the prognosis appears to be worse with inferior infarctions perhaps, owing to the association with right ventricular infarction and dysfunction which further limits the right ventricle's ability to handle the sudden volume load.[2] In addition, ventricular septal defects associated with inferior wall infarctions tend to occur towards the base of the heart, rather than the apex, making surgical access more difficult.

The transesophageal study in this patient demonstrated the extent of the defect which was large and suggested involvement of the apex itself in the necrotic process. Although pericardial effusions can be seen in patients with myocardial infarction, their presence may be a sign of impending rupture into the pericardial space. The flail portion of the septum was unlikely to hold sutures to allow for repair with a Dacron patch. Newer surgical techniques have allowed repair without suturing of necrotic myocardium.[3] This patient was taken as an emergency to the operating room. The initial repair of the ventricular septal defect appeared intact by transesophageal echocardiography but, as the patient was weaned from bypass, a small tear appeared in the apical myocardium which began to ooze profusely. On a second pump run, the apex was buttressed by a patch and the patient survived the surgery. The postoperative ejection fraction was approximately 30%. The right ventricular function was only mildly decreased. The patient was discharged to a rehabilitation facility on the 14th postoperative day.

References

1. Reeder GS. Identification and treatment of complications of myocardial infarction. Mayo Clin Proc 1995;70:880–4.

2. Anderson D, Adams S, Bhat A, et al. Post-infarction ventricular septal defect: the importance of site of infarction and cardiogenic shock on outcome. Eur J Cardio-Thorac Surg 1989;3:554–7.

3. Cooley D. Repair of postinfarction ventricular septal defect. J Cardiac Surg 1994;9:427–9.

78

Left ventricular pseudoaneurysm

Susan E Wiegers MD

A 40-year-old patient with mild cerebral palsy developed progressive shortness of breath over several months. Treatment with asthma medications was unsuccessful. After developing pedal edema and orthopnea, he underwent further evaluation. An electrocardiogram demonstrated evidence of a remote inferior myocardial infarction. A chest X-ray revealed a markedly enlarged cardiac silhouette. There was a totally occluded proximal right coronary artery on angiogram with non-critical left disease. Echocardiogram and ventriculogram revealed a large outpouching of the inferior wall with mildly reduced global function. These transesophageal images were obtained in the operating room.

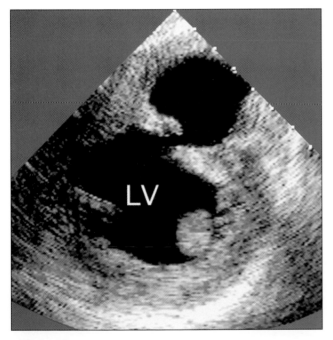

Figure 78.1
Transgastric echocardiogram in the transverse plane of the left ventricle (LV) in short-axis. The anterior wall is at the bottom of the screen. The anterolateral papillary muscle is visualized on the right of the screen within the left ventricular cavity. There is an abrupt discontinuity of the endocardium of the posterior wall with a large pseudoaneurysm behind the ruptured wall. The wall of the cavity appears to be lined with thrombus.

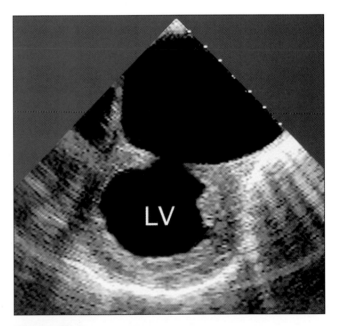

Figure 78.2
Rotation of the probe images the entire cavity of the pseudoaneurysm which was much larger than the left ventricle itself. The portion of the wall of the pseudoaneurysm imaged on the left of the screen is markedly thinned. The cavity of the pseudoaneurysm expanded in systole, while the left ventricular function appeared to be vigorous rather than expressing inferoposterior hypokinesis.

Discussion

A variety of echocardiographic criteria can be used to distinguish false aneurysms or pseudoaneurysms from true aneurysms of the left ventricular wall. While both are complications of transmural myocardial infarction, a true aneurysm results from the remodelling process. Infarct expansion can result in diastolic deformation of the infarcted segment with dyskinesis in systole. The neck of a true aneurysm is generally larger than the body of the aneurysm. A pseudoaneurysm is caused by contained rupture of the infarcted segment. Tamponade and death result if the rupture is not limited by pericardial adhesions. Pseudoaneurysms may not occur immediately after myocardial infarction but are a later event, occurring days or weeks after the infarction. The wall of the pseudoaneurysm is composed only of the visceral pericardium and thrombus. On echocardiogram, the neck of a pseudoaneurysm is narrower than the body and discontinuity in the endocardium can often be identified.[1,2]

Both aneurysms and pseudoaneurysms may be lined with thrombus and may exhibit systolic expansion. However, only a pseudoaneurysm will have high-velocity flow into the neck of the outpouching in systole and reverse the direction in diastole. Differentiation is clinically important since only pseudoaneurysms have a risk of late rupture. Both can cause congestive heart failure and be the source of thrombus formation with subsequent embolization.

Pseudoaneurysms may present as large paracardiac structures. The connection to the left ventricular cavity may not always be obvious. While pseudoaneurysm associated with myocardial infarctions may be seen adjacent to areas of wall motion abnormalities, those associated with surgical procedures or trauma may have more unusual connections that are difficult to identify. A posterior pseudoaneurysm after mitral valve replacement may be particularly difficult to image and diagnose.[3,4] At times transesophageal echocardiography may be necessary to delineate the connection between the pseudoaneurysm cavity and the left ventricular cavity.[5] Omniplane imaging may be helpful in evaluating the neck of the pseudoaneurysm and the connection to the left ventricle. The relationship of the neck to the mitral valve apparatus and papillary muscles may also be best assessed by transesophageal echocardiography. During the surgical procedure, transesophageal echocardiography is mandatory, as it will allow assessment of ventricular function and valvular competence after repair.

This patient tolerated the surgical repair and was left with a moderately decreased ejection fraction.

References

1. Mackenzie J, Lemole G. Pseudoaneurysm of the left ventricle. Texas Heart Inst J 1994;21:296–301.

2. Sorrell V, Callaway M, Zwischenberger J, et al. Left ventricular pseudoaneurysm. J Thorac Imaging 1994;9:258–9.

3. Sakai K, Nakamura K, Ishizuka N, et al. Echocardiographic findings and clinical features of left ventricular pseudoaneurysm after mitral valve replacement. Am Heart J 1992;124:975–82.

4. Chan R, Lubicz S, Oliver L, et al. Left ventricular false aneurysm complication mitral valve repair. Ann Thorac Surg 1993;56:175–6.

5. Stoddard, M., P. Dawkins, R. Longaker, et al. Transesophageal echocardiography in the detection of left ventricular pseudoaneurysm. Am Heart J 1993;124:534–9.

79

Biventricular aneurysm

Craig H Scott MD

A 69-year-old male patient with a history of a distal left anterior descending coronary artery territory infarction in the remote past, diabetes and end-stage renal disease underwent total left hip replacement surgery. On the third postoperative day, he became short of breath and complained of chest discomfort. An electrocardiogram showed inferior ST segment elevation, with evidence of right ventricular involvement in lead RV3. Cardiac catheterization demonstrated mid-vessel thrombosis of a large dominant right coronary artery. Angioplasty successfully re-established flow, but the patient had persistent ST segment elevation and developed Q waves in the inferior leads. He recovered and was sent home. Six weeks later, he presented to the emergency room with shortness of breath. A ventilation/perfusion scan was consistent with pulmonary embolus. An echocardiogram was performed to assess cardiac function.

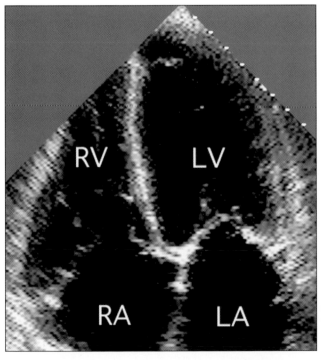

a

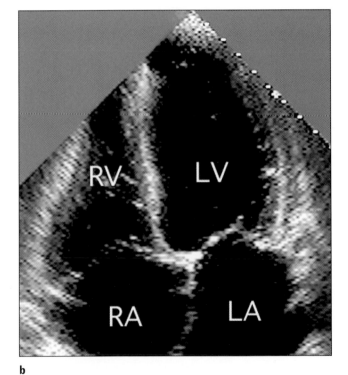

b

Figure 79.1
(a) Apical four-chamber view in diastole. All the cardiac chambers are moderately to severely enlarged. The distal septum demonstrates diastolic deformity which is consistent with left ventricular apical aneurysm.
(b) Similar systolic view. Comparison with the diastolic view demonstrates expansion of the left ventricular apex. The right ventricular free wall is also hypokinetic at the apex, which is more evident in subsequent images. A prominent moderator band is present running from the right ventricular free wall to the interventricular septum.

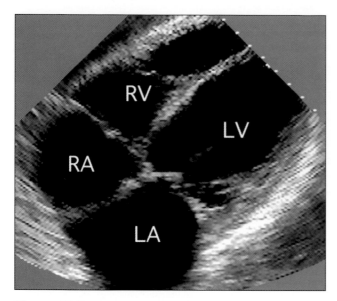

Figure 79.2
Subcostal four-chamber view in systole. The mid-right
ventricular free wall moves in normally during systole.
However, the apex is severely hypokinetic and the diameter
of the apex is wider than the mid-cavity. This regional wall
motion abnormality is due to infarction of the right
ventricular apex.

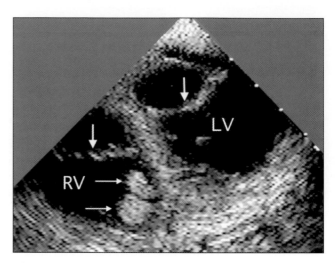

Figure 79.4
Off-axis parasternal short-axis image of the right and left
ventricular apices. There is a false chord (downward pointing
arrows) in the left (LV) and right ventricular (RV) apices. The
multiple thrombi (rightward pointing arrows) are again
evident in the right ventricular apex.

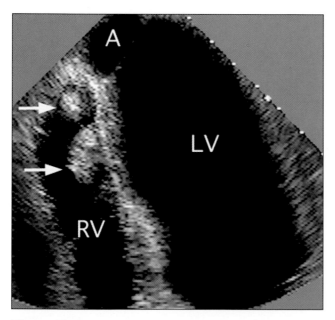

Figure 79.3
Off-axis apical four-chamber view of the left and right
ventricular apex. There is an aneurysm (A) of the left ventricle
(LV) at the apex. The walls of the aneurysm are thinned and
the diastolic deformation is evident. In systole, marked
dyskinesis resulted in further enlargement of the aneurysmal
segment. The right ventricular (RV) apex contains multiple
echodensities (arrows) attached to the interventricular septum.
These represent multiple apical thrombi. In real time, several
of the thrombi were highly mobile.

Discussion

Differentiation of an aneurysm, which involves all layers
of the ventricular wall, from a pseudoaneurysm, which
represents a contained rupture of the wall into the
pericardium, can be challenging. The distinction is important because therapy and prognosis differ. Pseudoaneurysms have a higher frequency of expansion and
rupture, thus requiring early surgical closure. A pseudoaneurysm often forms a neck or cylindrical channel
through the wall, whereas aneurysms tend to have more
smooth transitions from normal to fibrotic segments.[1]
However, a true aneurysm may appear to have a neck if
the ultrasound beam cuts obliquely through the walls of
the ventricle. The ultrasound beam is not infinitely thin.
If the aneurysm is relatively small, on the order of twice
the beam thickness which is approximately 1 cm, then the
edges of the beam will artifactually create the appearance
of a neck by projecting the left ventricular wall at the
junction of the aneurysm into its mouth. Overall, the
presence of a ventricular aneurysm is a poor prognostic
sign, independent of ejection fraction.[2]

Right ventricular infarction is present in half the
patients presenting with inferior infarction, typically in
patients with transmural infarctions of the inferioposte-
rior wall and/or the posterior septum.[3] Thrombi may
form in the akinetic segments of the right ventricle, probably by the same mechanisms as a left ventricular
aneurysm thrombus forms: stagnant blood flow and

abnormal endocardium.[4] The greatest risk in a right ventricular thrombus as a result of infarction without abnormal right to left shunting is pulmonary embolus. The long-term prognosis of this infrequently recognized complication of acute infarction is unknown, but treatment with anticoagulation is warranted in appropriate patients.

The differential diagnosis of a right ventricular mass includes normal structures, such as the moderator band and the papillary muscles from the tricuspid valve. Patients who have had prosthetic valves surgically implanted may have remnant papillary muscles and chordae tendinae that mimic a mass. Thrombus is uncommon, but may be seen especially in areas of hypokinesis. Endomyocardial fibrosis can result in a right ventricular apical mass, as well as subvalvular masses on the ventricular side of the tricuspid valve near the valve ring; however, these masses are rarely mobile. Both primary and metastatic tumors may involve the right ventricle but rarely as intraventricular mobile masses.

The patient was anticoagulated with resolution of his symptoms. The right ventricular thrombi decreased in size but were still present on a follow-up echocardiogram.

References

1. Hamilton K, Ellenbogen K, Lowe JE, *et al*. Ultrasound diagnosis of pseudoaneurysm and contiguous ventricular septal defect complicating inferior myocardial infarction. J Am Coll Cardiol 1985;6:1160–63.

2. Meizlish J, Berger HJ, Plankey RT, *et al*. Functional left ventricular aneurysm formation following acute anterior transmural myocardial infarction: incidence, natural history and prognostic implications. N Engl J Med 1984;311:1001–6.

3. Kinch JW, Ryan TJ. Right ventricular infarction. N Engl J Med 1994;330:1211–17.

4. Stowers SA, Leiboff RH, Wasserman AG. *et al*. Right ventricular thrombus formation in association with acute myocardial infarction: diagnosis by 2-dimensional echocardiography. Am J Cardiol 1983;52:912–13.

SECTION VII

Cardiomyopathies

80

Idiopathic hypertrophic sub-aortic stenosis

Susan E Wiegers MD

A 41-year-old woman with a history of diabetes mellitus developed progressive exercise intolerance over several months. She had led a predominantly sedentary life for many years but had recently experienced presyncope when putting away groceries. On physical examination, her blood pressure was 150/74 mmHg. She had a loud, harsh systolic ejection murmur over the precordium which increased with the release phase of the Valsalva maneuver.

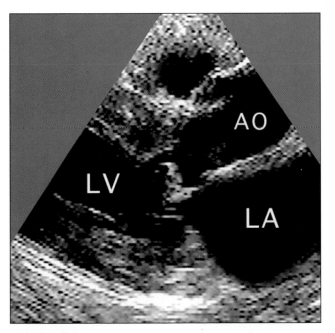

Figure 80.1
Parasternal long-axis view in systole demonstrating systolic anterior motion of the mitral valve. There is a sharp bend in the anterior mitral valve leaflet which is seen in the outflow tract in close proximity to the septum. There is hypertrophy of both the posterior wall and the septum. However, the septum is more than 1.3 times thicker than the posterior wall which is diagnostic of asymmetric septal hypertrophy. The left atrium (LA) is enlarged. The thickened aortic valve leaflets can be seen open in systole within the aortic root (AO). LV, left ventricle.

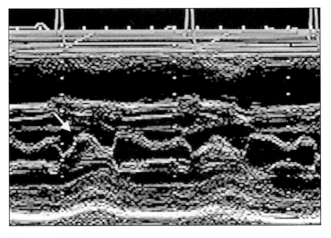

Figure 80.2
M-mode echocardiogram from the parasternal long-axis position demonstrating systolic anterior motion of the mitral valve (arrow). The anterior leaflet moves towards the septum during systole as identified by the QRS complex at the top of the screen.

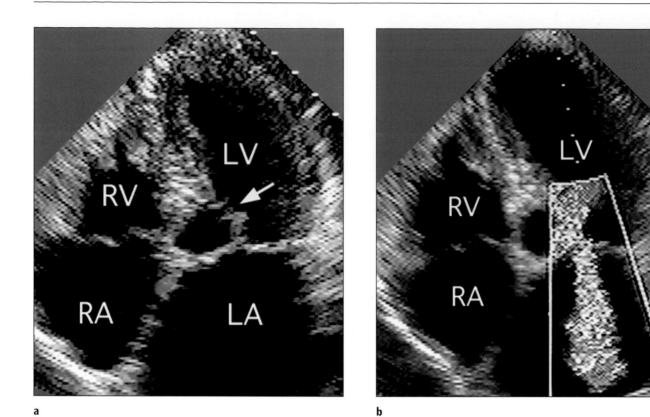

a

b

Figure 80.3
(a) Apical four-chamber view in systole. Both the concentric hypertrophy and the proximal septal bulging are well appreciated. The left atrium (LA) is markedly enlarged while the left ventricular (LV) cavity size is small. The mitral valve moves into the left ventricular outflow tract (arrow) and contacts the septum. The right atrium (RA) appears to be normal but the right ventricle (RV) is also hypertrophied.
(b) Apical four-chamber view with color Doppler flow imaging in systole. The color signal obscures the visualization of the systolic anterior motion. However, the turbulence in the left ventricular outflow tract begins at the level of the systolic anterior motion as demonstrated in (a). Note also the turbulent jet of moderately severe mitral regurgitation in the left atrium.

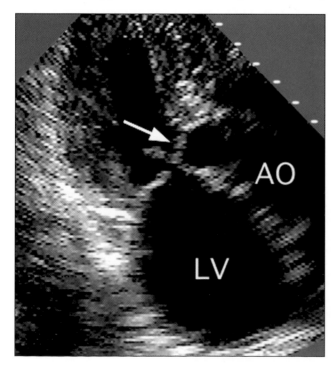

Figure 80.4
Apical long-axis view in systole again showing the anterior mitral valve leaflet in the left ventricular outflow tract (arrow). The contact with the septal bulge is particularly well seen. The posterior leaflet appears more restricted and the gap in the coaptation point is appreciated. This is the mechanism for the substantial mitral regurgitation in this case.

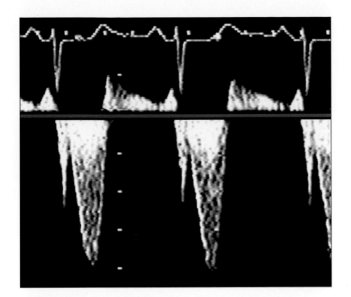

Figure 80.5
Continuous-wave Doppler spectral signal across the left ventricular outflow tract. The peak velocity is somewhat delayed, although the pattern is not the classic 'dagger' shape that is often seen with this entity. The peak velocity is approximately 4 m/s which predicts a peak systolic gradient of 64 mmHg.

Discussion

A number of genetic mutations have been associated with the clinical disease of idiopathic hypertrophic sub-aortic stenosis. The clinical presentation of this entity varies as does the prognosis, perhaps in part based on the under lying genetic abnormality. Many patterns of ventricular hypertrophy have been identified, although most commonly the interventricular septum is predominantly hypertrophied with the free wall less hypertrophied but involved.[1] In some studies the degree of hypertrophy did not correlate with symptoms, but the opposite has been found in other registries.

The timing of the systolic motion of the mitral valve leaflets correlates with the onset and the peak of the left ventricular outflow gradient.[2] However, the mechanism of systolic anterior motion has been a subject of debate and it appears to have several different etiologies. In patients with abnormal mitral valve leaflets characterized by elongation of the anterior leaflet, a sharp bend in the anterior leaflet at mid-valve level directs it into the outflow tract.[3] The result is localized contact of the leaflet with the septum. Our patient exhibits this pattern of systolic anterior motion. Other patients have anteriorly displaced papillary muscles and narrowed outflow tracts which result in broader contact of the anterior leaflet with the septum. No difference in resting gradients has been observed between these two types of patterns. Approximately 10%

of patients are thought to have sub-aortic obstruction based on the presence of an anomalous papillary muscle which inserts directly into the mitral leaflets with no chordae.[4] It is important to rule out this cause of obstruction in idiopathic hypertrophic sub-aortic stenosis (IHSS), since septal myomectomy would be unlikely to result in relief of the obstruction in such a case.

Restriction of the motion of the posterior leaflet of the mitral valve in relation to the more flexible and elongated anterior leaflet leads to failure of coaptation and resultant mitral regurgitation in systole. Those patients with elongated and flexible posterior leaflets have less mitral regurgitation when systolic anterior motion develops.[5] Mitral valve prolapse may also occur in the presence of severe systolic anterior motion. Right ventricular hypertrophy is common in patients with hypertrophic subaortic stenosis and may be more common in patients with severe symptoms.[6,7]

This patient responded to treatment with beta-blockers and disopyramide. Atrioventricular sequential pacemakers have been used in some patients to change the activation sequence of the interventricular septum and interrupt the outflow tract obstruction. Myomectomy has also been undertaken in severely symptomatic patients to decrease the degree of outflow tract obstruction.

References

1. Klues H, Schiffers A, Maron B. Phenotypic spectrum and patterns of left ventricular hypertrophy in hypertrophic cardiomyopathy: morphologic observations and significance as assessed by two-dimensional echocardiography in 600 patients. J Am Coll Cardiol 1995; 6:1699–708.

2. Lin C, ChenK, Lin M, et al. The relationship between systolic anterior motion of the mitral valve and the left ventricular outflow tract Doppler in hypertrophic cardiomyopathy. Am Heart J 1991;122:1671–82.

3. Klues H, Roberts W, Maron B. Morphological determinants of echocardiographic patterns of mitral valve systolic anterior motion in obstructive hypertrophic cardiomyopathy. Circulation 1993;87:1570–9.

4. Klues H, Roberts W, Maron B. Anomalous insertion of papillary muscle directly into anterior mitral leaflet in hypertrophic cardiomyopathy. Circulation 1991;84:1188–97.

5. Schwammenthal E, Nakatani S, He S, et al. Mechanism of mitral regurgitation in hypertrophic cardiomyopathy: mismatch of posterior to anterior leaflet length and mobility. Circulation 1998;98:856–65.

6. Suzuki J, Sakamoto T, Takenaka K, et al. Assessment of the thickness of the right ventricular free wall by magnetic resonance imaging in patients with hypertrophic cardiomyopathy. Br Heart J 1988;60:440–5.

7. McKenna W, Kleinebenne A, Nihoyannopoulos P, et al. Echocardiographic measurement of right ventricular wall thickness in hypertrophic cardiomyopathy: relation to clinical and prognostic features. J Am Coll Cardiol 1988;11:351–8.

81

Diastolic dysfunction

Martin G Keane MD

A 60-year-old woman with a history of hypertension presented with a complaint of progressive dyspnea over the past 2 years. She had never used tobacco and had no prior history of pulmonary disease. Physical examination demonstrated a prominent apical cardiac impulse with mild lateral displacement. The resting blood pressure was

160/94 mmHg. There was a I/VI systolic ejection murmur heard at the left sternal border, and an S$_4$ gallop was appreciated. The remainder of the examination was normal. An echocardiogram was performed to evaluate left ventricular function.

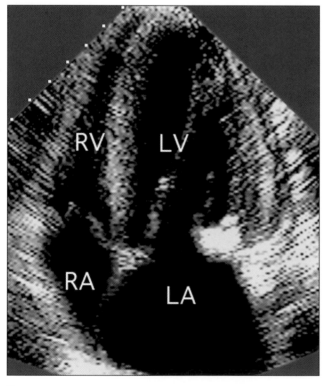

a

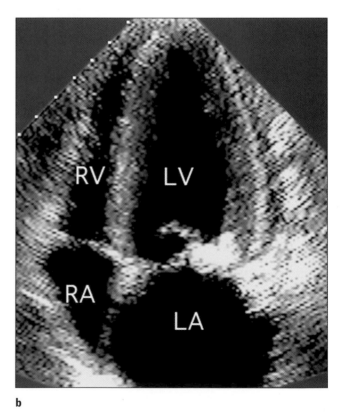

b

Figure 81.1
(a) Apical four-chamber view in diastole. The left ventricular (LV) cavity is normal in size, but there is moderate left ventricular hypertrophy. The left atrium (LA) is moderately dilated. The mitral valve is mildly thickened, and there is moderate mitral annular calcification most dense in the lateral annulus.
(b) Apical four-chamber view in systole. During systole, systolic anterior motion of the mitral valve chords is seen. There is no asymmetric septal hypertrophy present and the mitral apparatus does not approach the septum. Color Doppler interrogation of the mitral valve revealed moderate mitral regurgitation (not shown).

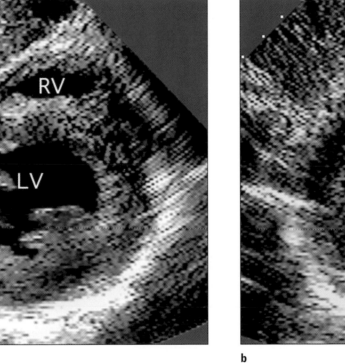

Figure 81.2
Spectral display of pulsed Doppler flow velocity across the mitral valve. There is a diminutive E-wave (early diastolic filling), with a more prominent A-wave (atrial kick). This pattern is consistent with abnormal diastolic relaxation and diastolic dysfunction.

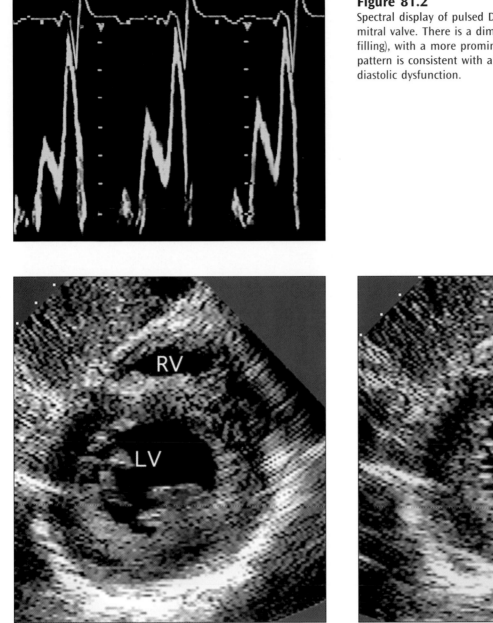

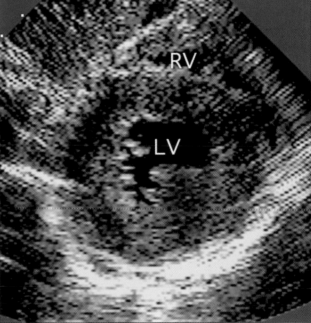

a   b

Figure 81.3
(a) Subcostal short-axis view of the left ventricle in diastole. The moderate hypertrophic thickening of the left ventricular walls is better appreciated in this diastolic frame. The ventricular walls measure 1.4 cm. The hypertrophy is concentric, with uniform thickness of the interventricular septum as compared with the other walls. The papillary muscles are also hypertrophied. Right ventricular hypertrophy is also present, as the wall measures over 5 mm.
(b) Subcostal view in systole. The systolic function is normal.

Discussion

Left ventricular hypertrophy represents an initially adaptive response, preserving optimal ventricular performance in the presence of pressure or volume overload. In the later stages of hypertrophy, enhanced interstitial collagen deposition, diminished capillary density, and abnormal myofibrillar function can result in overt systolic left heart failure. Abnormalities of diastolic filling are associated with the changes of ventricular hypertrophy, often predating or coexisting with systolic left ventricular failure. Left ventricular diastolic filling is determined by the complex interaction of many factors, including atrial and ventricular compliance, ventricular relaxation, atrial systolic function, ventricular interaction, and pericardial constraint.[1] Changes in any of these parameters can lead to abnormal diastolic function. Hypertrophy of the walls and associated ultrastructural changes augment intrinsic myocardial stiffness, and shift the passive filling of the ventricle to a steeper portion of the left ventricular diastolic pressure–volume relationship. In addition, metabolic abnormalities of the hypertrophic myocardium compromise the active relaxation of the ventricle.

Pulsed Doppler assessment of left ventricular inflow is the most commonly used echocardiographic technique to assess diastolic function. The simplest model of the overall diastolic filling process can be represented as an early phase and a late (or atrial) phase. Early diastolic flow is detected by the E velocity on pulsed Doppler interrogation. Changes in the atrioventricular driving forces, including atrial pressure at the time the atrioventricular valve opens, early diastolic ventricular pressure, and the active relaxation of the ventricle, affect the peak E velocity and its rate of decline (deceleration slope or time).[1] The velocity and duration of the subsequent A-wave is determined by the volume remaining in the atrium, atrial contractile function, and ventricular compliance. These velocity envelopes are also affected by age, preload, and heart rate.[1] The peak E-wave velocity in a normal adult varies within the range of 0.6–1.0 m/s, with a deceleration time of approximately 200 m/s.[2] Normally, most ventricular filling occurs in early diastole. Therefore, the A wave is typically of lower velocity.

With moderate degrees of hypertrophy, active relaxation of the ventricle becomes abnormal, with a smaller proportion of filling during the early phase occurring over a longer period of time. The E-wave velocity declines and the deceleration time is prolonged. A larger residual volume at atrial contraction results in high A-wave velocity, with reversal of the velocity ratio between E and A waves. This pattern has become most commonly identified with diastolic dysfunction, and is demonstrated by the present case study. With more significant hypertrophy, there is more consequential deterioration in the passive compliance characteristics of the ventricular chamber. This results in elevation of overall diastolic pressure, as well as a more rapid increase in chamber pressure with volume inflow. Therefore, severe

diastolic dysfunction may be characterized by a high E-wave velocity with a short deceleration time (< 150 m/s), as the pressure between atrium and ventricle equilibrates rapidly. The amount of flow during atrial systole is accordingly reduced, with a diminutive A wave. This pattern is classically associated with restrictive disease, including severe hypertrophy, infiltrative cardiomyopathies, and end-stage dilated cardiomyopathy. At intermediate stages of hypertrophic disease, there may be normalization of the filling pattern, as the E-wave peak velocity gradually increases and the deceleration time decreases.

Additional methods that allow more detailed analysis of diastolic function include assessment of pulmonary venous flow on either transesophageal or transthoracic echocardiography,[3] color M-mode and tissue Doppler.[4] Although not typically utilized in daily clinical practice, these newer techniques augment traditional pulsed Doppler analysis, and may enhance assessment of global and regional diastolic function.

Systolic anterior motion of the mitral valve is typically in the constellation of echocardiographic findings of hypertrophic obstructive cardiomyopathy. Varying degrees of systolic anterior motion, often chordal, can occur in other patients owing to the Venturi forces within the hypertrophic or hyperdynamic ventricle, as in this case. The patient's symptoms were due to diastolic dysfunction which caused elevated left atrial pressures, especially during exercise induced tachycardia. She was treated with an aggressive antihypertensive regimen.

References

1. Nishimura RA, Tajik AJ. Evaluation of diastolic filling of left ventricle in health and disease: Doppler echocardiography is the clinician's Rosetta Stone. J Am Coll Cardiol 1997;30:8–18.

2. Cohen GI, Pietrolungo JF, Thomas JD, Klein AL. A practical guide to assessment of ventricular diastolic function using Doppler echocardiography. J Am Coll Cardiol 1996;27:1753–60.

3. Keucherer HF, Kusumoto F, Muhiudeen IA, et al. Pulmonary venous flow patterns by transesophageal pulsed Doppler echocardiography: relation to parameters of left ventricular systolic and diastolic function. Am Heart J 1991;122:1683–93.

4. Garcia MJ, Thomas JD, Klein AJ. New Doppler echocardiographic applications for the study of diastolic function. J Am Coll Cardiol 1998;32:865–75

82

Dilated cardiomyopathy—Batista repair

Gene Chang MD

A 26-year-old man known to have severe idiopathic dilated cardiomyopathy, moderate to severe mitral regurgitation, moderate pulmonary hypertension (pulmonary artery pressure of 48/30 mmHg), and polysubstance abuse presented to an outside hospital with increasing shortness of breath, orthopnea and weakness. He did not improve on dual inotropic therapy. The patient was not an appropriate cardiac transplant candidate, because of continued substance abuse, but was referred for further evaluation and therapeutic intervention. A partial left ventriculectomy (Batista repair) and reimplantation of the anterior papillary muscle were undertaken. Immediate postoperative transesophageal echocardiography revealed a marked reduction in left ventricular end-diastolic dimensions (8.5 cm to 6.5 cm), improvement in left ventricular function (10% to 20%), and significant reduction in observed mitral regurgitation (3+ to 1+). Postoperatively, the patient required an intra-aortic balloon pump and inotropic support as well as intravenous antibiotics for a coagulase-negative staphylococcal line infection. The patient was ultimately discharged from the hospital on postoperative day 27 in stable condition.

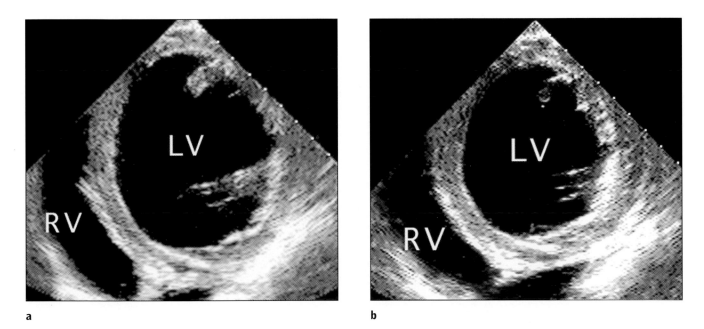

a   b

Figure 82.1
(a) Preoperative transgastric echocardiogram in the transverse plane (imaging angle 0°) of the left ventricle (LV) at the mid-ventricular level. In diastole, the left ventricle diameter is 8.5 cm. The right ventricle (RV) is also seen in short-axis and is severely enlarged.
(b) Comparison of the ventricular dimensions in this systolic frame demonstrates severely decreased biventricular function. The end-systolic diameter is > 6.5 cm and the estimated ejection fraction is 10%. The dilated ventricle, normal wall thickness and severely decreased ejection fraction are all consistent with the diagnosis of dilated cardiomyopathy.

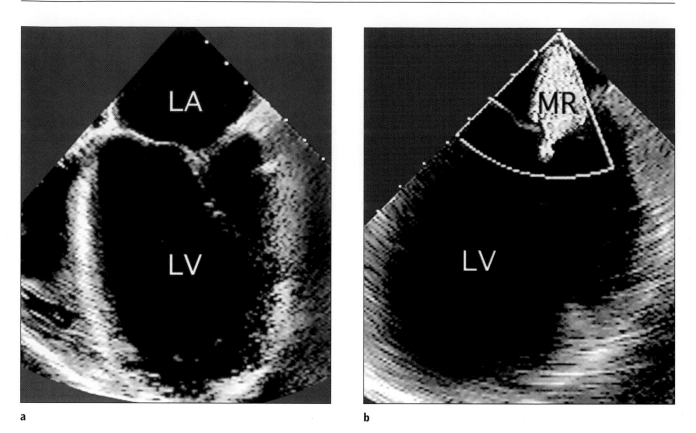

a   b

Figure 82.2

(a) Preoperative transesophageal echocardiogram in the transverse plane (imaging angle 0°) of the four-chamber view in systole. The left ventricle (LV) is severely dilated. Progressive ventricular remodelling has produced a ventricle with a globular shape. The transverse axis approaches the dimension of the long axis. The left atrium (LA) is only partially imaged but the mitral valve annulus is markedly dilated.

(b) Similar transesophageal echocardiogram with color flow Doppler imaging in systole. Moderate to severe mitral regurgitation (MR) arises as a central jet, which is consistent with functional regurgitation often seen in patients with dilated cardiomyopathy. The mechanism is thought to be failure of the leaflets to coapt properly due to the annular dilatation. Note that the mitral regurgitation arises well on the ventricular side of the mitral annulus which is due to incomplete closure of the mitral valve.

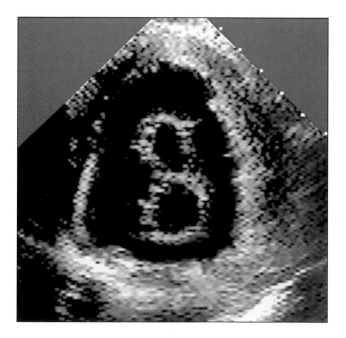

Figure 82.3

Postoperative transgastric echocardiogram in the transverse plane (imaging angle 0°) of the left ventricle at the level of the mitral valve leaflets in diastole. A partial left ventriculectomy has been performed with mitral valve repair via the Alfieri technique, yielding the characteristic 'figure of eight' appearance (see below). Following the surgical remodeling procedure, the left ventricle is significantly reduced in diameter, measuring 6.5 cm at end-diastole.

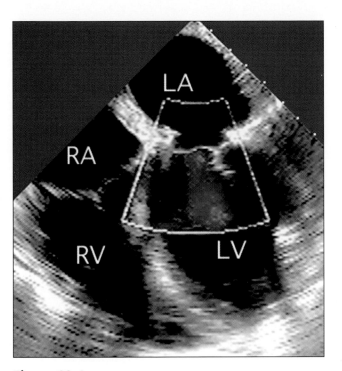

Figure 82.4
Postoperative transesophageal echocardiogram in the transverse plane (imaging angle 0°) with color flow Doppler imaging. The four-chamber view is imaged in systole similar to the preoperative Figure 82.2, in which the scale is the same. The left ventricular dimension has been significantly reduced. An annuloplasty ring is evident in the left atrium (LA) and no mitral regurgitation is evident. The base of the anterior papillary muscle has been reattached to the apical-lateral wall following the resection of a portion of the posterolateral wall. It is seen on the right of the image along the left ventricular lateral wall.

Discussion

Congestive heart failure has become one of the leading public health issues in cardiovascular medicine. The Framingham study reported a 12% increase per year in the incidence of congestive heart failure associated with an approximately 33% mortality rate within 2 years of diagnosis.[1] While cardiac transplantation has emerged as an effective therapy for patients with end-stage heart failure, its widespread application is thwarted by a limited supply of donors. This imbalance has provided the impetus for the development of other effective therapeutic modalities.

Partial left ventriculectomy, also known as heart reduction surgery or the Batista operation, has become popular as potential surgical therapy for end-stage dilated cardiomyopathy. First pioneered by the Brazilian surgeon Randas Batista in humans in 1994, it is based on the concept that a dilated ventricle with severe dysfunction would become more efficient with a reduction in size and a restoration of a more normal mass–diameter relationship.[2] The procedure involves a triangular wedge resection of the posterolateral wall of the left ventricle, beginning at the apex and extending to the atrioventricular groove. One or more marginal or posterolateral coronary artery branches may be excised with the resection. The resultant change in the geometry and juxtaposition of the papillary muscles of the mitral valve necessitates a valve repair to ensure competency. Typically, the central portion of the free edges of the anterior and posterior leaflets are sutured together into a double-orifice mitral valve (Alfieri technique). This yields a characteristic 'figure of eight' appearance on echocardiography in the short-axis view (Figure 82.3). The left ventriculotomy is then closed with bovine pericardium. The overall result is a surgically remodeled, smaller left ventricular cavity. Laplace's Law relating wall stress to the diameter of the chamber would predict a decrease in wall stress due to the surgery. Based on his initial 300 cases, Batista reported an encouraging 60% 2-year survival rate.[3]

The largest published single-center experience in the USA with the surgery has been at the Cleveland Clinic.[4] Fifty-seven consecutive patients (54 awaiting cardiac transplantation, 95% with idiopathic dilated cardiomyopathy) with a mean age of 53 years undergoing partial left ventriculectomy and mitral valve repair were prospectively studied. All patients had a left ventricular end-diastolic diameter of > 7 cm and were in New York Heart Association (NYHA) class III or IV, similar to the patient depicted above. Measurements made 3 months after the procedure demonstrated significant improvements in mean ejection fraction (14.4% ± 7.7% to 23.3% ± 10.7%), left ventricular end diastolic diameter (8.4 ± 1.1 cm to 6.3 ± 0.9 cm) and NYHA class (3.6 ± 0.5 to 2.2 ± 0.9) from preoperative baseline ($P < 0.001$). In addition, while 40% of patients were dependent on inotropic therapy preoperatively, no patients required inotropic support at 3 months after the procedure. Actuarial survival was reported to be 82% at 1 year. Unfortunately, left ventricular assist device support was required as rescue therapy in 17% of patients and in-hospital mortality was 3.5%. Actuarial freedom from procedure failure, defined as death or transplant relisting, was only 58% at 1 year.

Partial left ventriculectomy is emerging as a potential surgical treatment option for the population with end-stage heart failure given the favorable reported outcomes in initial studies. However, these results remain less than ideal and caution is advised as significant early morbidity and mortality have been noted with this surgery. Further investigation is needed, with better patient selection and operator experience, to improve outcomes.

References

1. Kannel WB, Belanger AJ. Epidemiology of heart failure. Am Heart J 1991;121:951–7.

2. Batista RJV, Santos JLV, Takeshita N, *et al*. Partial left ventriculectomy to improve left ventricular dysfunction in end-stage heart disease. J Cardiac Surg 1996;11:96–7.

3. Starling RC, Young JB. Surgical therapy for dilated cardiomyopathy. Cardiol Clin 1998;16:727–37.

4. McCarthy JF, McCarthy PM, Starling RC, *et al*. Partial left ventriculectomy and mitral valve repair for end-stage congestive heart failure. Eur J Cardiothorac Surg 1998;13:337–43.

83

HIV-associated cardiomyopathy

Robert H Li MD

A 32-year-old man with advanced AIDS (CD4 count of 130 cells/mm^3) presented with 3–4 weeks of progressive exertional dyspnea and lower extremity edema. The patient complained of dyspnea with recumbency, occasionally awakening him at night. He had a history of recurrent opportunistic infections including multiple episodes of pneumonia. He did not have a productive cough, fevers, or chills on presentation.

On physical examination, the patient was cachectic and in mild respiratory distress at rest. The temperature was 99°F, blood pressure 98/60 mmHg, and the pulse 86 bpm. Lung examination revealed rales at the bases bilaterally with dullness at the right base. The heart rhythm was regular, the point of maximal impulse diffuse and displaced laterally, and a third heart sound was present. There was a II/VI holosystolic murmur at the cardiac apex that radiated to the axilla. The jugular venous distention was 11 cm. There was no hepatosplenomegaly or ascites, but there was 1–2+ non-tender pitting edema of the lower extremities extending to the knee. A chest radiograph revealed increased interstitial markings bilaterally, a small left pleural effusion and an enlarged cardiac silhouette. An echocardiogram was performed to assess left ventricular function.

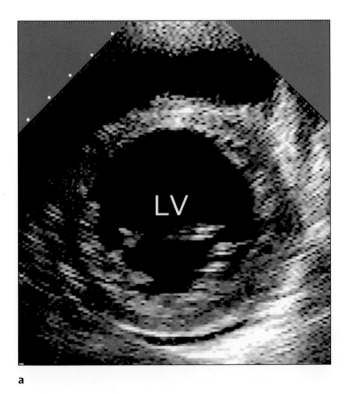

a

Figure 83.1

(a) Parasternal short-axis view in diastole at the level of the papillary muscles. The left ventricle (LV) is dilated. The pattern of left ventricular enlargement is consistent with eccentric hypertrophy in that the wall thickness is not increased while the left ventricular cavity dimension has increased significantly. The right ventricle appears enlarged in this view. The anteroposterior dimension of the right ventricular cavity measures over 2 cm. Right ventricular enlargement may be difficult to assess in the parasternal short-axis and the cavity size should be further evaluated in the apical or subcostal views. There is a small pericardial effusion posterior to the left ventricle.

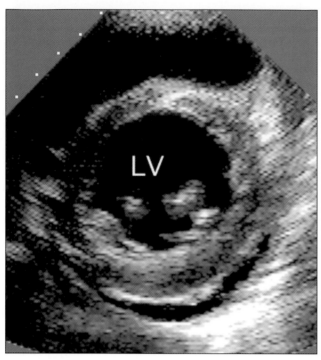

b

Figure 83.1
(b) Similar parasternal short-axis view in systole. Comparison of the fractional area change of the left ventricular cavity reveals severely decreased left ventricular systolic function. In addition, the right ventricular cavity size has also changed little in this systolic frame. The posterior pericardial effusion is seen more clearly, owing to the anterior motion of the posterior left ventricular wall.

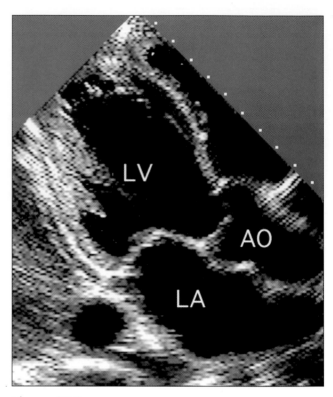

Figure 83.2
Apical three-chamber view of the left ventricle in diastole. The left ventricular cavity (LV) is again seen to be dilated and globular in this diastolic frame. The posterior medial papillary muscle is double-headed and can be seen attached to the posterior wall. The location, chordal attachments to the mitral valve, and the motion of the papillary muscle distinguish it from a thrombus. The left atrium (LA) is also enlarged. The ascending aorta (AO) is of normal size.

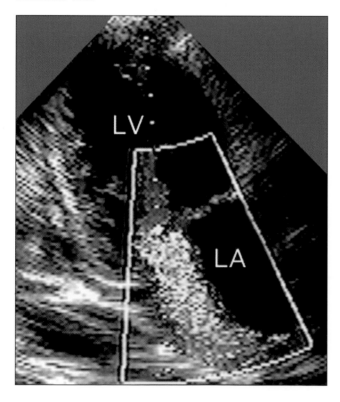

Figure 83.3
Apical two-chamber view in systole with color flow Doppler interrogation of the left atrium (LA) The severely decreased left ventricular (LV) function is confirmed in this view. A large jet of mitral regurgitation extends into the left atrium arising at the level of the mitral valve. The jet of mitral regurgitation reaches the back wall of the left atrium and was moderate to severe in degree. In the setting of severe mitral regurgitation, the left ventricular function should be hyperdynamic. Therefore, left ventricular systolic function may be even more profoundly decreased than is appreciated by the apparent fractional area change.

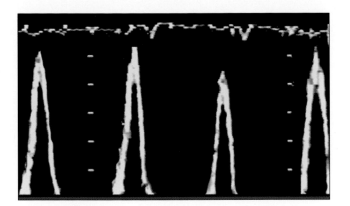

Figure 83.4
Spectral display of pulsed-wave Doppler from the apical position. The sample volume has been placed at the mitral valve leaflet tips. There is no early filling wave despite the presence of normal sinus rhythm. The E and A waves have fused, owing to tachycardia. The deceleration slope of the inflow wave is much shorter than 150 ms. This is consistent with severe restrictive physiology. A restrictive inflow pattern carries a very poor prognosis in the setting of systolic left ventricular failure. Note the mild respiratory variation in the inflow velocities which is due to pericardial constraint of the dilated ventricles.

Discussion

Assessment of left ventricular systolic function must be confirmed in orthogonal views such as the parasternal short-axis and the apical four-chamber view. The fractional area change in the parasternal short-axis view is often greater than that in the four-chamber view in patients with normal left ventricular function. This patient had global hypokinesis of a dilated left ventricle which was well seen in multiple views. The quality of the images is enhanced by the presence of the small circumferential pericardial effusion.

Although pulmonary infections are the leading cause of dyspnea in HIV patients, primary cardiac disease must also be considered in the differential diagnosis. Symptoms due to heart disease in HIV patients are frequently erroneously attributed to other organ systems. Cardiac abnormalities in patients with HIV infection are frequent, involving both the pericardium and the myocardium.[1,2] Pericardial effusions have been reported in up to 40% of patients with HIV infection on screening echocardiography and appear to occur with increasing incidence as the CD4 count declines.[3] The effusions are generally small to moderate in size and sterile, and rarely cause symptoms. The minority of patients have associated clinical evidence of pericarditis. The pericardium and myocardium can also be involved in neoplastic diseases common to HIV-infected patients, such as Kaposi's sarcoma or non-Hodgkin's lymphoma, usually

in the setting of widespread neoplastic disease. Echocardiography may reveal nodular or focal thickening of the pericardium due to tumor deposits, but diffuse involvement has also been reported.

Myocardial dysfunction with dilated cardiomyopathy is an important manifestation of AIDS-related cardiac disease. The prevalence of left ventricular dysfunction has been estimated to be 10–40% in patients with advanced AIDS.[4] Although it was previously thought that most patients were asymptomatic, recent data suggest that symptoms due to cardiomyopathy may be under-recognized. A large study following patients with early HIV disease (asymptomatic, CD4 count 400 cells/m^3) reported an annual incidence of 1.5% of dilated cardiomyopathy (defined as an ejection fraction of less than 45% and a left ventricular end-diastolic volume index of > 80 ml/m^2).[5] The majority of patients who developed cardiomyopathy had CD4 counts of less than 400 cells/mm^3, and all of the patients had symptomatic heart failure. Diagnosis is best made with two-dimensional echocardiography; endomyocardial biopsy is not likely to identify a treatable cause. Treatment is with standard therapy for dilated cardiomyopathy (angiotensin converting enzyme inhibitors, diuretics, anticoagulation, and digoxin). Unfortunately, the prognosis is extremely poor, with a mean survival in one study of 101 days compared with 472 days in those patients without dilated cardiomyopathy.

The etiology of the myocardial dysfunction is not well understood but is probably secondary to myocarditis caused by infectious agents such as coxsackie B virus, cytomegalovirus, Epstein–Barr virus, toxoplasma, and possibly HIV itself. Numerous immunological phenomena have also been implicated.[5] Cardiomyopathy can occasionally be caused by medications used to treat HIV-related complications, such as doxorubicin or alfa-interferon, both used for the treatment of Kaposi's sarcoma. Co-morbidities such as cocaine and ethanol abuse, infective endocarditis associated with injection-drug use, and nutritional deficiencies may also play a contributing role.

A previous echocardiogram of the patient performed 1 year earlier for evaluation of a murmur had been completely normal. This patient developed progressive left ventricular dysfunction in concert with his decline in CD4 counts. The diagnosis of the severe decrease of left ventricular function was important in this patient as it allowed directed therapy that improved his respiratory distress and avoided invasive evaluation for atypical pneumonia.

References

1. Anderson D, Virmani R. Emerging patterns of heart disease in human immunodeficiency virus infection. Hum Pathol 1990;21:253–9.

2. Currie PF, Jacob AJ, Foreman AR, *et al.* Heart muscle disease related to HIV infection: prognostic implications. Br Med J 1994;1605–7.

3. Heidenreich PA, Eisenberg MJ, LL K, *et al.* Pericardial effusion in AIDS: incidence and survival. Circulation 1995;3229–34.

4. Herskowitz A, Vlahov D, Willoughby S, *et al.* Prevalence and incidence of left ventricular dysfunction in patients with human immunodeficiency virus infection. Am J Cardiol 1993;71:955–8.

5. Barbaro G, DiLorenzo G, Grisorio B, *et al.* Incidence of dilated cardiomyopathy and detection of HIV in myocardial cells of HIV-positive patients: Gruppo Italiano per lo Studio Cardiologico dei Pazienti Affetti da AIDS. N Engl J Med 1998;1093–9.

84

Radiation-induced heart disease

Robert H Li MD
Susan E Wiegers MD

The patient was a 40-year-old man who had developed increasing dyspnea and exertional chest pain over the past few months. He had received mantle radiation in his adolescent years for lymphoma and had not received recent medical follow-up. He recalled an episode of aphasia and left arm weakness several months earlier which had lasted for an hour. He had not sought medical attention until he was unable to catch his breath. He admitted to worsening orthopnea and exertional presyncope over the past few months.

Physical examination revealed a thin man in mild respiratory distress. The blood pressure was 104/56 mmHg, the pulse was 100 bpm, and the respiratory rate was 18 breaths/min. The lungs had bibasilar rales with end-expiratory wheezes. Cardiac examination revealed a diffuse, hypokinetic PMI, a III/VI systolic ejection murmur along the left sternal border, and a soft diastolic murmur. A third heart sound was present. The jugular venous pressure was approximately 12 cmH$_2$O. The carotid pulse had a diminished and slowed upstroke. The abdomen was mildly distended with an enlarged, tender liver. There was 2+ pitting edema of the lower extremities. A chest radiograph revealed an enlarged cardiac silhouette and slightly increased interstitial markings throughout.

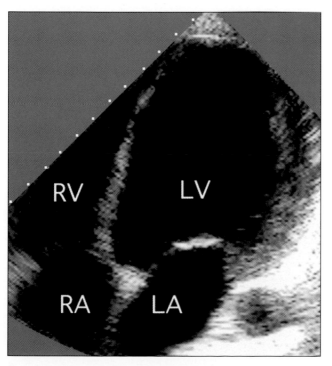

a

Figure 84.1

(a) Apical four-chamber view in diastole. The left ventricle is globular and severely enlarged. The left atrium and right atrium appear proportionate to the left ventricle and at first glance may strike the interpreter as being of normal size. They are in fact both significantly enlarged, as is the right ventricle. The mitral valve is thickened and calcified in this early diastolic frame.

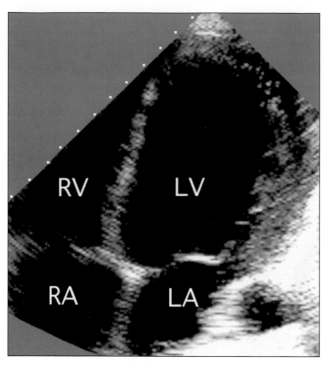

b

Figure 84.1

(b) Similar apical four-chamber view in systole. There is little change in the area of the left ventricle or right ventricle which signifies profoundly decreased function. In real time, the left ventricular ejection fraction was visually estimated at 10%. The lateral wall does appear to thicken slightly when compared to the diastolic image, but there is no real change in the interventricular septal thickness. The apex is not well imaged but gives the impression of a slight inward motion.

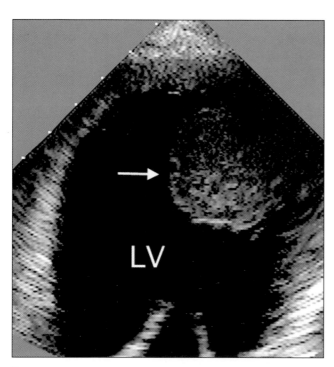

a

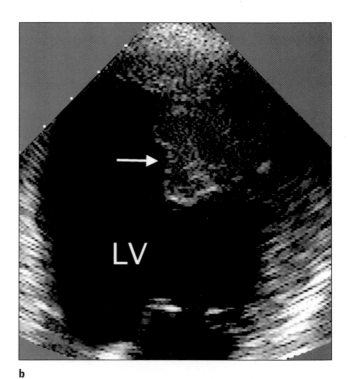

b

Figure 84.2

(a) Close-up image of the apex from the apical two-chamber view. This image is slightly off axis and the left ventricular cavity is foreshortened. There is a large echodensity attached to the distal anterior wall (arrow). This thrombus measured approximately 3 cm by 3.5 cm and was highly mobile on the real-time images.

(b) The protruding thrombus was mobile throughout the cardiac cycle. Comparison of the contour of the thrombus adjacent to the marking arrow demonstrates that another portion of the thrombus has rotated into view in this later image, demonstrating the marked mobility of the thrombus.

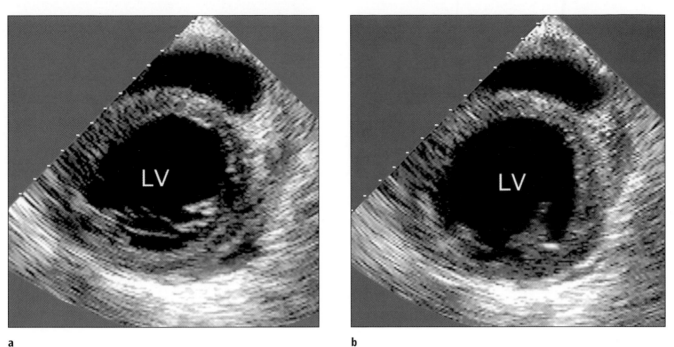

a   b

Figure 84.3

(a) Parasternal short-axis view of the left ventricle at the level of the mitral valve leaflets. Again, the severe dilatation of the ventricle is obvious. There is a small posterior pericardial effusion imaged posterior to the lateral wall.

(b) Similar view with the transducer angled more towards the apex of the heart resulting in a short-axis view at the level of the papillary muscles. There is a large mass in the region of the lateral papillary muscle which was a portion of the thrombus. The ventricular dilatation has distorted the usual position of the papillary muscles.

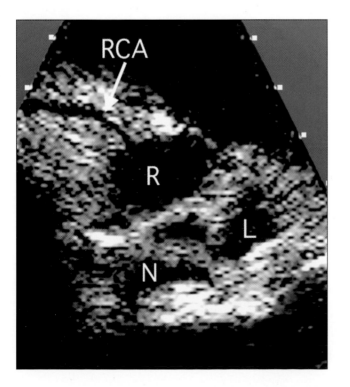

Figure 84.4

The thickened and calcified aortic valve commissures have partially fused, resulting in a 'fish-mouth' appearance of the aortic valve. The right (R), left (L) and non-coronary (N) cusps of the aortic valve are thickened and fixed. The resultant orifice is also fixed and thus severely stenotic and moderately regurgitant. Thickening of the aortic root due to fibrosis associated with the radiation therapy has led to marked narrowing of the right coronary artery (RCA).

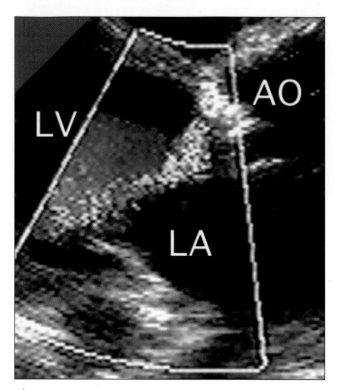

Figure 84.5
Parasternal long-axis view of the aortic valve with color flow
Doppler imaging in diastole. The fixed leaflets fail to coapt
and result in mild to moderate aortic regurgitation, which is
seen as a turbulent jet arising from the thickened and
calcified aortic valve leaflets.

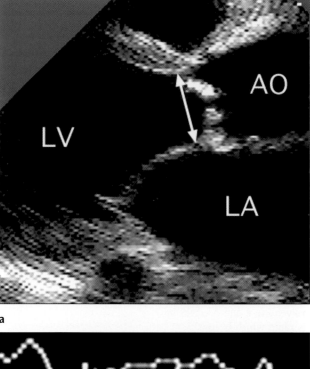

a

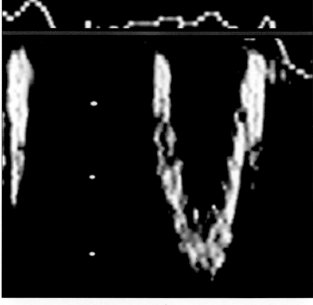

b

Figure 84.6
(a) Parasternal long-axis view of the left ventricular outflow
tract in systole. The outflow tract diameter is measured on-
line immediately below the valve leaflets. It should be
measured only in this view. The measurement is 2.3 cm,
which is larger than the normal 2.0 cm in an adult but in this
case consistent with the ventricular dilatation and
longstanding aortic regurgitation.
(b) Spectral display of pulsed-wave Doppler from the apical
five-chamber view. The sample volume has been placed in
the left ventricular outflow tract just below the aortic leaflets.
The velocity–time integral can be measured on line and in
this case was 14 cm.
(c) Spectral display of continuous-wave Doppler from the right
parasternal position. The peak velocity across the valve was
lower from the apical position because the ejection jet across
the aortic valve was eccentric. The measurements were also
taken from the right sternal edge and the suprasternal notch.
The peak velocity here is 3.2 m/s and the velocity–time
integral is 73 cm.

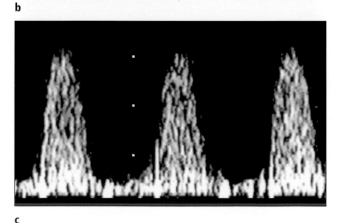

c

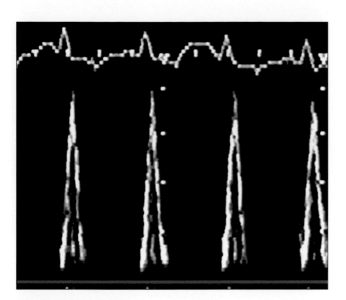

Figure 84.7
Spectral display of pulsed-wave Doppler across the mitral valve. The E and A waves have fused. The deceleration slope is rapid which is consistent with restrictive cardiomyopathy.

Discussion

The patient had advanced cardiomyopathy due to severe coronary artery disease associated with his previous radiation therapy. The diffuse narrowing of the coronary arteries is characteristic of this injury and makes bypass grafting impossible. The moderate aortic regurgitation and the severe stenosis may have also contributed to the left ventricular dysfunction. Fibrosis of the myocardium itself may also occur as a late sequela of radiation therapy.

Calculation of the aortic valve area relies on accurate velocities measured by Doppler echocardiography and by appropriate measurement of the left ventricular outflow area. Since the diameter of the left ventricular outflow tract is squared in the formula, any error in this measurement will propagate a substantial error in the final calculation. The continuity equation gives the aortic valve area as:

$$CSA_{AV} = \pi(D_{LVOT}/2)^2 \times VTI_{LVOT}/ VTI_{AV}$$

where CSA_{AV} is the aortic valve area, D_{LVOT} is the diameter of the left ventricular outflow tract, VTI_{LVOT} is the velocity–time integral of the pulsed-wave spectral Doppler pattern in the left ventricular outflow tract, and VTI_{AV} is the velocity-time integral across the aortic valve measured by continuous-wave Doppler. In this case, substitution into the equation yields:

$$AVA = 3.14(2.3/2)^2 \times 14/73 = 0.8 \text{ cm}^2$$

Planimetry of the valve from Figure 84.4 yielded a similar result. The continuity equation correlates well with invasively obtained data and may preclude the need for catheterization prior to operation in selected patients.[1] In this patient with profoundly decreased left ventricular function, a transaortic velocity of 3 m/s is indicative of severe stenosis. The peak gradient of only 36 mmHg is due to the cardiac failure and low flow across the valve. The continuity equation is essential in judging the severity of aortic stenosis in this case, as reliance on the peak and mean gradients alone will significantly underestimate the stenosis.

Left ventricular thrombus formation occurs primarily in three settings: recent transmural myocardial infarction, dilated cardiomyopathy, and left ventricular aneurysm. Two-dimensional echocardiography is the modality of choice for the detection of left ventricular thrombus, with both a high sensitivity (77–95%) and a high specificity (88–95%). The echocardiographic appearance of ventricular mural thrombus can vary from small to large, single to multiple, sessile to pedunculated, and fixed to mobile. In this patient, the thrombus was not seen until off-axis views were obtained. While the standard views may survey a normal apex, this patient's apex was too dilated to be completely imaged in the usual views. Close-up imaging (or zoom focusing) allows further evaluation. The differential diagnosis of the mass includes tumors as well as thrombus. The association with profoundly decreased left ventricular systolic function and the marked mobility of the mass favor thrombus as the diagnosis. It is very rare to see a thrombus overlying an area of normally contracting myocardium and this should raise the suspicion for alternative diagnoses.

Left ventricular thrombi are commonly seen after acute myocardial infarction. They were reported in 25–50% of patients with acute anterior infarctions in older series. Ten per cent of those patients experienced cerebral emboli.[2] More recent echocardiographic data in patients treated with thrombolytics and aggressive anticoagulation in the acute setting have demonstrated a decreased incidence in patients with anterior infarcts.[3] Ventricular thrombi are rarely (4%) seen after inferior infarcts. Thrombi are most commonly detected during the first week after an anterior myocardial infarction and generally occur in the ventricular apex. The thrombus usually develops over a region of myocardium that is akinetic, dyskinetic, or aneurysmal. Thrombi are less likely to regresses in patients with persistent left ventricular dilatation or worsening apical wall motion abnormality 3 months after infarction.[4] When a chronic left ventricular aneurysm is present, thrombus may be detected in up to 50% of patients. In comparison to patients with recent myocardial infarction and thrombus, systemic embolization occurs less frequently in patients with ventricular aneurysms. Higher-risk patients are those with thrombi that are mobile or protrude into the ventricular cavity, or are associated with ejection fractions of less than 35%.[5]

Dilated cardiomyopathy is the third setting in which left ventricular thrombi may be frequently seen. Postmortem studies have revealed thrombi in 60–75% of these patients. Thrombi tend to remain unchanged without anticoagulation, and decrease in size in patients receiving systemic anticoagulation.[6] The rate of systemic embolization in patients with cardiomyopathy has been estimated to be 4–5% per year, and is likely to be higher in patients with demonstrated left ventricular thrombus.

This patient had end-stage cardiomyopathy due to coronary disease and radiation damage and was not a candidate for revascularization or valve replacement. The right heart failure evident on his echocardiogram was due to the longstanding left ventricular dysfunction and possibly intrinsic pathology. He was anticoagulated with systemic heparin and stabilized with inotropic support. Serial echocardiograms demonstrated a decrease in the size of the thrombus, although it remained mobile. He underwent orthotopic heart transplantation 3 months after admission.

References

1. Roger VL, Tajik AJ, Reeder GS, *et al.* Effect of Doppler echocardiography on utilization of hemodynamic cardiac catheterization in the preoperative evaluation of aortic stenosis. Mayo Clin Proc 1996;71:141–9.

2. Fuster V, Halperin J, Chesebro J, *et al.* Left ventricular thrombi and cerebral embolism. N Engl J Med 1989;320:392–5.

3. Greaves SC, Zhi G, Lee RT, *et al.* Incidence and natural history of left ventricular thrombus following anterior wall acute myocardial infarction. Am J Cardiol 1997;80:442–8.

4. Kupper AJ, Verheugt FW, Peels CH, *et al.* Left ventricular thrombus incidence and behavior studied by serial two-dimensional echocardiography in acute anterior myocardial infarction: left ventricular wall motion, systemic embolism and oral anticoagulation. J Am Coll Cardiol 1989;13:1514–20.

5. Jugdutt B, Sivaram C, *et al.* Prospective two-dimensional echocardiographic evaluation of left ventricular thrombus and embolism after acute myocardial infarction. J Am Coll Cardiol 1989;13:554–64.

6. Stratton J, Nemanich J, Johannessen K, *et al.* Fate of the left ventricular thrombi in patients with remote myocardial infarction or idiopathic cardiomyopathy. Circulation 1988;78:1388–93.

85

Endomyocardial fibrosis

Susan E Wiegers MD
Lilian P Joventino MD

A 35-year-old man began noticing pedal edema, abdominal distension and exertional dyspnea. The symptoms progressed over the course of several months until he could no longer work. He presented to his physician and was found to have a markedly elevated peripheral eosinophil count. Physical examination revealed marked jugular venous distension with prominent 'a' and 'v' waves, ascites and severe pitting edema to the abdominal wall. Laboratory examination was also notable for mild renal insufficiency. A chest X-ray demonstrated mild congestive heart failure and a moderately enlarged cardiac silhouette. An echocardiogram was ordered to evaluate the patient's cardiac function.

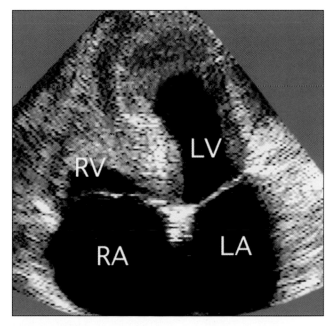

Figure 85.1
Apical four-chamber view in systole. Left ventricular (LV) and right ventricular (RV) cavities are fringed by large masses filling the apices of both ventricles. The right ventricular cavity is two-thirds filled and the left ventricular cavity approximately one-third filled. Both the left atrium (LA) and the right atrium (RA) are enlarged.

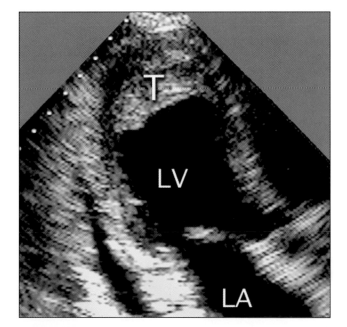

Figure 85.2
Apical long-axis view in diastole. The mass (T) is again noted to be filling the left ventricular (LV) apex. The mass itself is echodense and did not contract in real time. However, the overall left ventricular systolic function was normal and the myocardium at the apex contracted normally. The mitral valve is mildly thickened and the aortic valve is poorly seen. There is a small circumferential pericardial effusion which is seen in this and other frames.

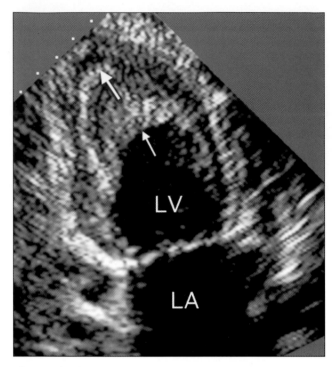

Figure 85.3
Apical two-chamber view of the left ventricle in systole. The larger arrow marks the left ventricular apical endocardium. The smaller arrow marks the limits of the mass filling the left ventricular cavity. Immediately adjacent to the small arrow is a very echobright area which is consistent with calcification within the mass.

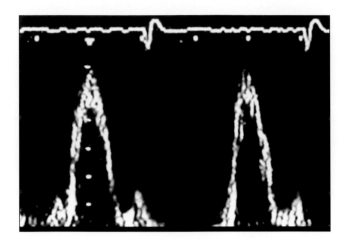

Figure 85.4
Spectral display of pulsed wave Doppler ultrasound from the apical position. The sample volume has been placed at the tips of the mitral valve leaflets. In diastole, a high-velocity E-wave demonstrates a very short deceleration time, which is the time for the signal to go from the peak velocity to the baseline. Each horizontal marking represents 200 ms. It is clear that the deceleration from the peak of the E-wave to the baseline is less than 150 ms. The A-wave is almost not detectable. This spectral Doppler pattern is consistent with restrictive physiology. The masses filling the left ventricle are non-distensible, resulting in the Doppler inflow pattern.

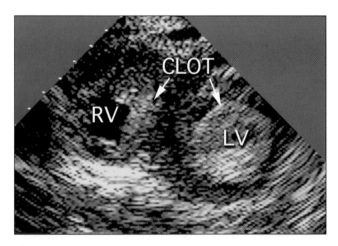

Figure 85.5
Parasternal short-axis view at the left level of the ventricular apices. Both left ventricular (LV) and right ventricular (RV) apices are dilated. However, the left ventricular apex cavity is completely filled by a mass (arrow), the right ventricular apex is partially filled by a similar mass (arrow). The pericardial effusion is once again seen anteriorly. In real time it was appreciated that these masses were non-distensible and did not contract, although there was motion of the myocardium.

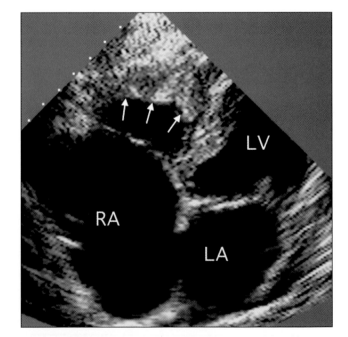

Figure 85.6
Off-axis apical four-chamber view from a medial position of the right ventricle and right atrium (RA). The right ventricular cavity is almost completely replaced by the mass (arrows) which fills the cavity and extends almost to the level of the tricuspid valve. The restriction to inflow has resulted in the marked right atrial enlargement.

Discussion

This patient had endomyocardial fibrosis associated with Loeffler's endocarditis. Two forms of hypereosinophilic syndrome can lead to obliterative myocardial fibrosis. The first is tropical eosinophilic endomyocardial fibrosis and the second is the non-tropical variant associated with idiopathic hypereosinophilic syndrome.[1] The eosinophils are abnormal cells which are toxic to the underlying myocardium, resulting in severe endocardial thickening, which can lead to obliteration of the ventricular cavities. The endocardial deposits consist of thrombotic and fibrotic material which may calcify. The myocardial systolic function is usually not affected but profound diastolic dysfunction results in severe symptoms of cardiac failure. Either or both ventricles may be affected. The echocardiographic pattern is characteristic, with the ventricular apices being more affected than the other portions of both ventricles. The echodense material is non-contractile but is distinguished from thrombus formation associated with apical aneurysm and Chaga's disease by the relatively normal motion of the underlying endocardium.[2] Calcification within the mass is common, and was seen in this patient.[3] Other conditions associated with endomyocardial fibrosis include schistosomiasis and Behçet's disease.[4]

Diastolic dysfunction results from the reduction in ventricular volume as well as the non-distensible nature of the material filling the ventricles. The restrictive Doppler pattern is characterized by a tall E-wave with a rapid deceleration time, and is evidence of advanced disease.[5] A dip and plateau are seen with invasive hemodynamic assessment and correlate with the Doppler pattern. Biatrial enlargement is also the rule, and was present in this patient.

The prognosis of endomyocardial fibrosis is poor, with most patients dying from progressive heart failure. Severe fixed pulmonary hypertension from recurrent pulmonary emboli has also been reported with the syndrome.[6] Pulmonary hypertension may result from chronically elevated pulmonary venous pressures due to the diastolic filling restriction. Surgical resection of the thrombotic material has been successfully undertaken in selected patients and appears to improve survival compared to historical controls. The decortication procedure may result in the need for mitral or tricuspid valve replacement during the procedure.[7] The atrioventricular valves may also be directly involved with the process, again necessitating valve replacement. Complete heart block, precipitated by the surgical decortication, may result in the need for a permanent pacemaker. Symptomatic relief with the surgery is generally good, and patients experience an improvement in exercise tolerance along with a demonstrable decrease in diastolic pressures and an increase in cardiac output.[8] Recurrence of the condition after surgery has been reported but is not present in the majority of patients.

References

1. Shabetai R. Restrictive, obliterative and infiltrative cardiomyopathies. In: Alexander R, Schlant R, Fuster V, eds. *Hurst's The Heart*, McGraw-Hill: New York, 1998:2085–6.

2. Acquatella H, Schiller N, Puigbo J, *et al*. Value of two-dimensional echocardiography in endomyocardial disease with and without eosinophilia. A clinical and pathologic study. Circulation 1983;67:1219–26.

3. Vijayaraghavan G, Balakrishnan M, Sadanandan S, *et al*. Pattern of cardiac calcification in tropical endomyocardial fibrosis. Heart Vessels 1990;Suppl 5:4–7.

4. Huong D, Wechsler B, Papo T, *et al*. Endomyocardial fibrosis in Behçet's disease. Ann Rheum Dis 1997;56:205–8.

5. Appleton CP, Hatle LK, Popp RL. Demonstration of restrictive ventricular physiology by Doppler echocardiography. J Am Coll Cardiol 1988;11:757–68.

6. Ribeiro P, Muthusamy R, Duran C. Right-sided endomyocardial fibrosis with recurrent pulmonary emboli leading to irreversible pulmonary hypertension. Br Heart J 1992;68:326–9.

7. da Costa F, Moraes C, Rodriques J, *et al*. Early surgical results in the treatment of endomyocardial fibrosis. A Brazilian cooperative study. Eur J Cardio-Thorac Surg 1989;3:408–13.

8. Schneider U, Jenni R, Turina J, *et al*. Long-term follow up of patients with endomyocardial fibrosis: effects of surgery. Heart 1998;79:362–7.

86

Postpartum cardiomyopathy

Susan E Wiegers MD

A 22-year-old woman was well until 8 weeks after the uncomplicated vaginal delivery of her third child. She came to the emergency room complaining of severe shortness of breath and orthopnea. In retrospect, she had experienced progressive exertional dyspnea since the birth of her child. On clinical examination there were rales in both lung fields. Cardiac auscultation revealed a normal S_1 and S_2 with a III/VI holosystolic murmur at the apex and a loud diastolic gallop. Pulmonary edema was present on chest X-ray. She was admitted to the coronary care unit where a Swan–Ganz monitor was placed.

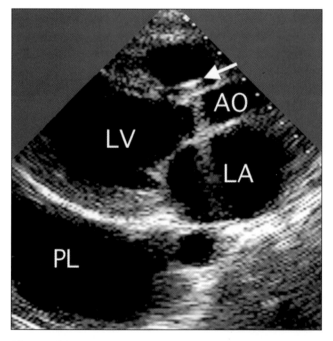

Figure 86.1
Parasternal long-axis view of the left ventricle (LV), which is markedly dilated, as is the left atrium (LA). A Swan–Ganz catheter (arrow) is seen as the echodense artifact in the right ventricle. A reverberation artifact from the catheter extends into the aortic root (AO) and the left atrium. A large pleural effusion (PL) is present posterior to the left ventricle. The effusion's relationship to the descending thoracic aorta distinguishes it from a pericardial effusion. In addition, the pericardium is visualized as an echodense border between the left ventricular posterior wall and the pleural effusion.

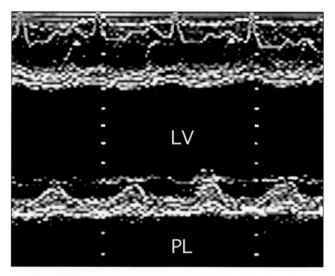

Figure 86.2
M-mode echocardiogram from the parasternal position. The pleural effusion (PL is the echolucent space posterior to the left ventricle (LV). The left ventricular cavity is severely dilated measuring 6.5 cm. The fractional area change is severely decreased consistent with profoundly decreased left ventricular systolic function.

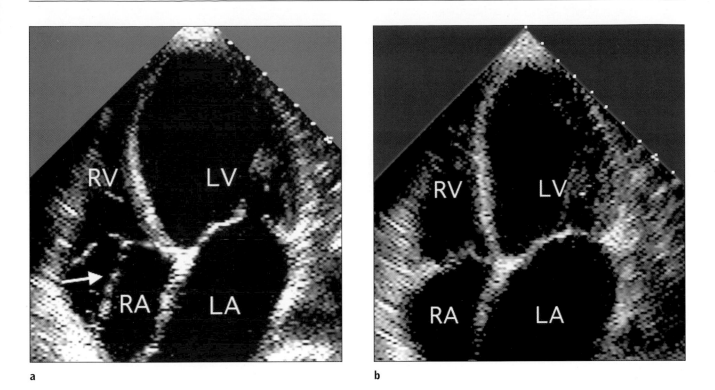

a   b

Figure 86.3
(a) Apical four-chamber view in diastole. The left ventricle is severely dilated and globular in shape. The major short-axis dimension approaches the long-axis dimension. The left atrium (LA) and the right atrium (RA) are dilated. The pulmonary artery catheter (arrow) is visualized in the right atrium.
(b) The same view in systole. The left ventricular ejection fraction is severely decreased. The left atrium demonstrates systolic expansion, which signifies severe mitral regurgitation. The right ventricle is not dilated, but comparison of the systolic and diastolic frames demonstrates decreased right ventricular systolic function.

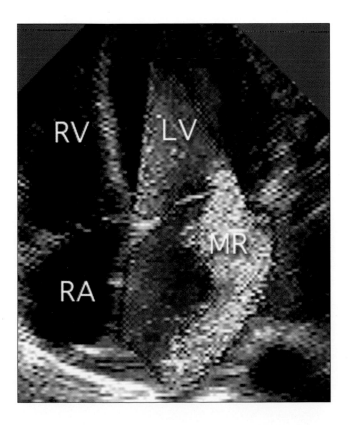

Figure 86.4
Apical four-chamber view in systole with color flow Doppler imaging of the high-velocity turbulent jet of mitral regurgitation in the left atrium. The mitral regurgitation jet is wide at the level of its origin at the mitral valve plane and extends into the pulmonary veins. By these criteria, the mitral regurgitation is severe.

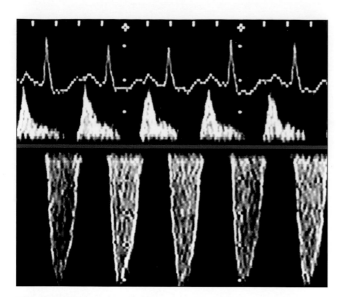

Figure 86.5
Spectral display of continuous-wave Doppler velocities across the mitral valve. The peak velocity of the diastolic inflow jet is approximately 1.7 m/s. The rapid deceleration slope of the mitral inflow rules out mitral stenosis as a cause of the elevated velocity. The mitral valve is demonstrated to be anatomically normal on the previous two-dimensional images. The severe mitral regurgitation results in markedly increased flow across the mitral valve in diastole which accounts for the increased velocity. The peak velocity of the mitral regurgitation is only 4 m/s which predicts a systolic gradient between the left ventricle and left atrium of 64 mmHg. Since the patient's systolic blood pressure was 108 mmHg, this is further evidence of increased left atrial pressure.

Discussion

Peripartum cardiomyopathy can occur in primigravida as well as during subsequent pregnancies. The presentation may occur prior to or coincident with delivery in up to one-half of the patients.[1] This patient demonstrates a severely dilated left ventricle which indicates that the left ventricular remodeling has been ongoing for some time. The left ventricular ejection fraction was estimated as 20% by real time two-dimensional imaging.

The echocardiogram demonstrates many features of severe mitral regurgitation. Left ventricular remodeling has resulted in severe dilatation of the mitral annulus.

The mitral valve leaflets are unable to coapt, resulting in severe mitral regurgitation.[2] This is best demonstrated in Figure 86.4, in which the mitral regurgitation jet appears to originate in the left ventricle, owing to the incomplete coaptation of the valve, resulting in tenting of the mitral valve leaflets. The sphericity of the left ventricle, a poor prognostic sign in dilated cardiomyopathy,[3] results in more severe mitral regurgitation.[4] Various methods of qualitative assessment have been proposed for color Doppler mapping. A color jet area of greater than 8 cm^2 in the left atrium has been shown to correlate with angiographically severe mitral regurgitation.[5] Similarly, the color jet area may be compared to the left atrial area. A color jet that encompasses 40% or more of the left atrium also signifies severe mitral regurgitation.[6] The diameter of the jet in the vena contracta is also correlated with the severity of the mitral regurgitation.[7] A number of other methods for quantifying the mitral regurgitation have been proposed, but are not in widespread clinical use.

References

1. O'Connell JB, Costanzo-Nordin MR, Subramanian R, *et al.* Peripartum cardiomyopathy: clinical, hemodynamic, histologic and prognostic characteristics. J Am Coll Cardiol 1986;8:52–6.

2. Kinney EL, Frangi MJ. Value of two-dimensional echocardiographic detection of incomplete mitral leaflet closure. Am Heart J 1985;109:87–90.

3. Douglas PS, Morrow R, Ioli A, *et al.* Left ventricular shape, afterload and survival in idiopathic dilated cardiomyopathy. J Am Coll Cardiol 1989;13:311–15.

4. Kono T, Sabbah HN, Stein PD, *et al.* Left ventricular shape as a determinant of functional mitral regurgitation in patients with severe heart failure secondary to either coronary artery disease or idiopathic dilated cardiomyopathy. Am J Cardiol 1991;68:355–9.

5. Spain MG, Smith MD, Grayburn PA, *et al.* Quantitative assessment of mitral regurgitation by Doppler color flow imaging: angiographic and hemodynamic correlations. J Am Coll Cardiol 1989;13:585–90.

6. Helmcke F, Nanda NC, Hsiung MC, *et al.* Color Doppler assessment of mitral regurgitation with orthogonal planes. Circulation 1987;75:175–83.

7. Hall SA, Brickner ME, Willett DL, *et al.* Assessment of mitral regurgitation severity by Doppler color flow mapping of the vena contracta. Circulation 1997;95:636–42.

87

Cardiac amyloidosis

Susan E Wiegers MD

A 55-year-old woman with mild hypertension noted the gradual onset of dyspnea on exertion over 3 months. A large transudative pleural effusion was drained. It recurred repeatedly over the next 2 months. Progressive pitting edema, which extended to thighs, developed. She complained of severe fatigue and incapacitating dyspnea. Two episodes of presyncope were associated with climbing stairs.

At the time of her echocardiographic study, the physical examination demonstrated decreased breath sounds halfway up the left posterior chest. The right side was clear. The jugular veins were distended to the angle of the jaw with the patient upright. The apical impulse was not palpable and the heart sounds were distant. No gallops were audible. Holosystolic regurgitant murmurs were heard at the apex and the right lower sternal border. There was marked pitting edema to the sacrum. The patient had several purpuric areas on her upper arms but did not recall trauma to the area.

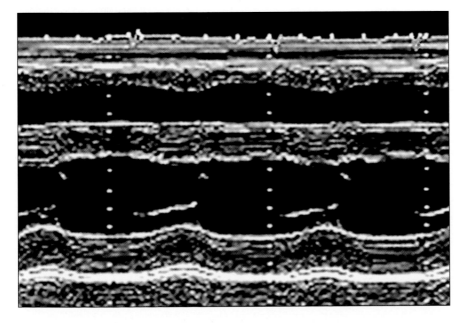

Figure 87.1
M-mode echocardiogram taken from the parasternal position. The small cavity size and marked hypertrophy are noted. The motion of both the septum and the posterior wall are severely decreased. Hypertrophy of the right ventricular free wall is also evident.

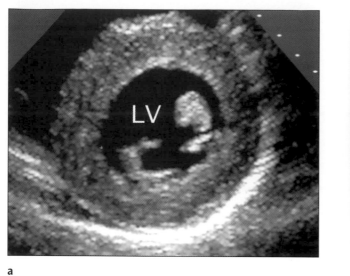

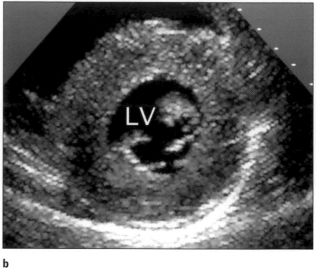

a   b

Figure 87.2

(a) Parasternal short-axis view in diastole. The left ventricular cavity is not dilated but the walls are markedly thickened. The thickening is concentric and the walls are almost 2 cm thick. Most characteristic of this disease process, the myocardium is noted to be highly granular or 'speckled'.

(b) Parasternal short-axis view in systole. The severely reduced ejection fraction is again evident with little systolic wall thickening and little change in cavity size.

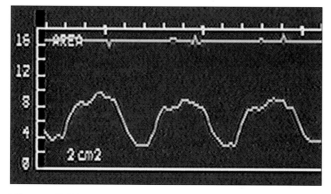

Figure 87.3

On-line analysis of the fractional area change from the parasternal short-axis. The fractional area change is severely diminished with a decrease from 9 cm² in diastole to 3 cm² at peak systole.

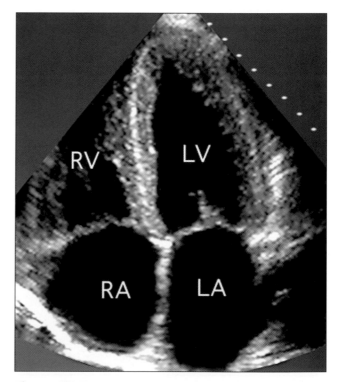

Figure 87.4

Apical four-chamber view in systole. Biventricular hypertrophy and biatrial enlargement are evident. The mitral valve is again seen to be diffusely thickened. The tricuspid valve is also abnormally thick. The interatrial septum is diffusely thickened (see subcostal view). The speckled pattern of the myocardium is again evident.

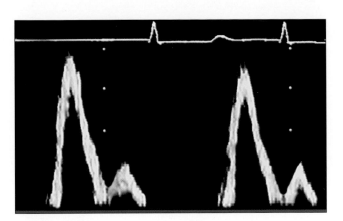

Figure 87.5
Spectral imaging of pulsed-wave Doppler flow velocities of the mitral inflow taken from the apical position. The A-wave is diminished and the E-wave demonstrates a steep deceleration slope characteristic of restrictive cardiomyopathy. A deceleration time of less than 150 ms is consistent with the diagnosis of restriction. On most systems, this analysis can be accomplished on-line.

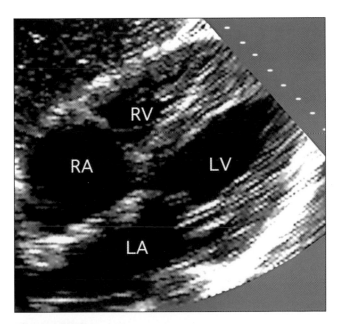

Figure 87.6
Subcostal four-chamber view. The interatrial septum is thickened. This thickening can be distinguished from the common pattern of lipomatous hypertrophy of the interatrial septum by the involvement of the foramen ovale. Lipomatous hypertrophy always spares the foramen ovale. The right ventricular hypertrophy is again appreciated.

Discussion

A number of features typical of cardiac amyloidosis are illustrated in this case. Amyloid fibrils composed of β-pleated sheets of immunoglobulin light chain infiltrate the myocardium, valvular structures and pericardium, causing thickening and loss of contractile function. Profound ventricular dysfunction without dilatation of the ventricular cavities is characteristic. The hypertrophy may be massive. The classic speckled pattern is believed to be secondary to the reflection of the ultrasound wave by individual amyloid fibrils. A similar speckled pattern may be seen in end-stage renal disease with hypertensive heart disease. Usually, however, ventricular function is not as profoundly affected as in amyloid heart disease. In addition, the myocardial infiltration in amyloidosis causes marked loss of voltage in the standard electrocardiogram, whereas the opposite is seen in hypertensive cardiomyopathy. In fact, normal or increased voltage on the electrocardiogram argues strongly against the diagnosis of cardiac amyloid. Ultrasound tissue characterization has been shown to be useful in the differentiation of amyloidosis from hypertensive heart disease and hypertrophic cardiomyopathy.[1,2]

Thickening of the valves, with resultant four-valvular regurgitation is common in amyloid. The restrictive pattern of the mitral valve inflow pattern is not specific for amyloidosis and can be seen in other infiltrative cardiomyopathies. However, the early loss of A-wave velocity is more commonly seen in amyloidosis and is thought to be due to contractile failure of the atrium.[3] This may occur earlier than ventricular failure, because of the relative thinness of the atrial wall. Dilatation of the atria is consistent with restrictive cardiomyopathy. Thickening of the pericardium and small pericardial effusions are not evident on this echocardiogram but are also common.[4] The thickening of the ventricular wall is progressive. An initial echocardiogram may show some of the features of amyloidosis without being diagnostic. The diastolic abnormalities are also progressive and correlate with wall thickening. A deceleration time of less than 150 ms is consistent with advanced amyloidosis and associated with a very poor short-term survival measured in months.[5]

A fat-pad biopsy confirmed the diagnosis of systemic amyloidosis in this patient. Cardiac biopsy was unnecessary, given the classic echocardiographic findings. Heart transplant was not offered, because of the recurrence of the disease in transplanted patients. Despite treatment with melphelan and prednisone, the patient died of sudden cardiac death 3 months after the echocardiogram.

References

1. Chandrasekaran K, Aylward PE, Fleagle SR, *et al.* Feasibility of identifying amyloid and hypertrophic cardiomyopathy with the use of computerized quantitative texture analysis of clinical echocardiographic data. J Am Coll Cardiol 1989;13:832–40.

2. Pinamonti B, Picano E, Ferdeghini EM, *et al.* Quantitative texture analysis in two-dimensional echocardiography: application to the diagnosis of myocardial amyloidosis. J Am Coll Cardiol 1989;14:666–71.

3. Plehn J, Southworth J, Cornwell GD. Brief report: atrial systolic failure in primary amyloidosis. N Engl J Med 1993;327:1570–3.

4. Falk R. Sensitivity and specificity of the echocardiographic features of cardiac amyloidosis. Am J Cardiol 1987;59:418.

5. Klein AL, Hatle LK, Taliercio CP, *et al.* Serial Doppler echocardiographic follow-up of left ventricular diastolic function in cardiac amyloidosis. J Am Coll Cardiol 1990;16:1135–41.

88

Non-obstructive hypertrophic cardiomyopathy

Elizabeth A Tarka MD

A 52 year-old man complained of severe exertional dyspnea and chest pain. He had noted a decrease in his exercise tolerance over the past several months and was unable to climb one flight of stairs. He denied palpitations and syncope. His cardiac examination demonstrated a regular rhythm, loud fourth heart sound and a sustained and laterally displaced point of maximal impulse (PMI). There was a prominent A wave in the jugular venous pulse, brisk carotid upstrokes, clear lung fields, benign abdomen and no edema of the lower extremities. A transthoracic echocardiogram was performed.

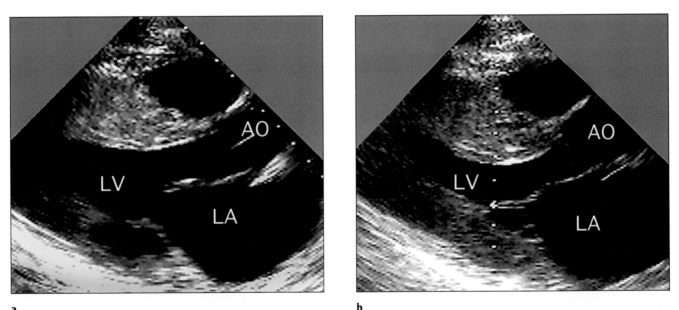

a   b

Figure 88.1
(a) Parasternal long-axis view in diastole. The left atrium (LA) is dilated. The mitral and aortic valves are normal, as is the aorta (AO). The left ventricular (LV) cavity is normal at 4.5 cm. There is marked asymmetric hypertrophy of the interventricular septum, which measures over 2 cm. The posterior wall is mildly hypertrophied. Asymmetric hypertrophy is defined by a septal/free wall thickness ratio of > 1.3–1.
(b) Parasternal long-axis view in systole. The left ventricular systolic function is hyperdynamic. The normal left ventricular systolic function distinguishes this condition from infiltrative diseases such as amyloidosis, in which the thickening of the ventricle may also be asymmetric. However, in restrictive disease the function is significantly decreased in all the cardiac walls involved by the infiltrative process. Note the normal location of the mitral valve leaflets. There is no evidence of systolic anterior motion of the mitral valve, and the left ventricular outflow tract is not obstructed.

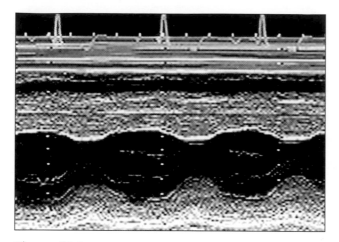

Figure 88.2
M-mode echocardiogram from the parasternal position taken just below the tips of the mitral valve leaflets. The asymmetric nature of the hypertrophy is apparent as is the normal left ventricular function. The M-mode should be used to measure the wall thickness. The septum measures 26 mm and the posterior wall 13 mm.

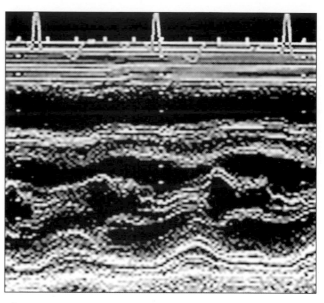

Figure 88.3
M-mode echocardiogram from the parasternal position at the level of the mitral valve leaflets. In systole, the mitral valve leaflets move anteriorly from their original coaptation point, owing to the motion of the posterior wall. However, the leaflets do not approximate the interventricular septum or move into the outflow tract which would be indicative of systolic anterior motion. This finding was confirmed by the two-dimensional images.

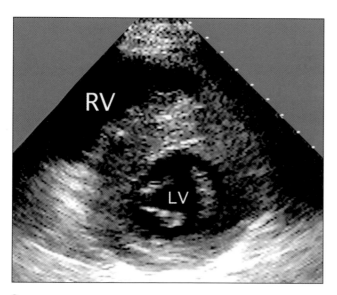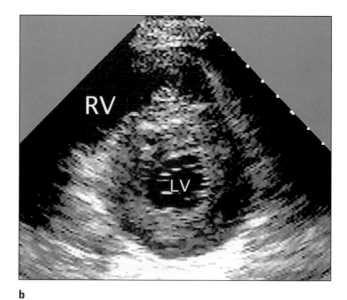

a   b

Figure 88.4
(a) Parasternal short-axis view at the level of the mitral valve chordae in diastole. Once again, the asymmetric pattern of hypertrophy is evident.
(b) Similar parasternal short-axis view in systole. The posterior wall thickens to a greater proportional extent than does the septum. This relative hypokinesis of the hypertrophied septum is characteristic of hypertrophic cardiomyopathy.

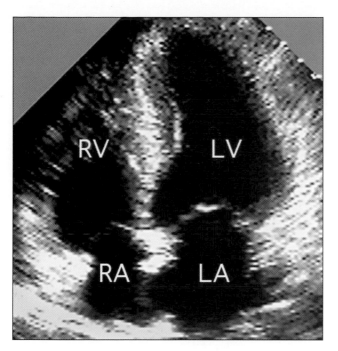

Figure 88.5

Apical four-chamber view in early diastole. The left atrium (LA) is again noted to be dilated but the right atrium (RA) is of normal size. The interatrial septum bows into the right atrium, indicating elevated left atrial pressures. Asymmetric hypertrophy of the entire muscular septum is visualized from the base to the apex. Pulsed-wave Doppler interrogation of the left ventricular outflow tract did not show evidence of an outflow tract gradient (not shown here).

Discussion

This patient has a non-obstructive form of hypertrophic cardiomyopathy. Hypertrophic cardiomyopathy is a primary myocardial abnormality characterized by hypertrophy of a non-dilated left ventricle.[1] The two primary echocardiographic features are asymmetric septal hypertrophy and systolic anterior motion of the mitral valve. In the classic description, the proximal interventricular septum is disproportionately greater in thickness than the posterior free wall in the ratio of at least 1.3 : 1. The two-dimensional echocardiographic appearance of this area is granular and speckled from myocardial fiber disarray and increased collagen content of the septum. The original diagnostic criteria for hypertrophic cardiomyopathy were described by M-mode and include asymmetric septal hypertrophy, systolic anterior motion of the mitral valve, septal hypomobility and premature closure of the aortic valve due to interruption of ventricular ejection by systolic anterior motion.

Obstructive and non-obstructive forms of hypertrophic cardiomyopathy exist. The obstructive form involves dynamic narrowing of the left ventricular outflow tract by abnormal systolic motion of the mitral valve.[2] This produces a resting left ventricular systolic pressure gradient which often worsens with provocative maneuvers. The gradient can be augmented by factors that decrease arterial pressure or ventricular volume such as the Valsalva maneuver. Conversely, squatting or the use of a handgrip increases ventricular volume or arterial pressure and may reduce or abolish the obstruction.

In non-obstructive forms of hypertrophic cardiomyopathy, such as is present in this patient, the left ventricular morphology differs. The left ventricular outflow tract is larger and the ventricular septum may not be disproportionately hypertrophied in comparison to the posterior wall. These patients do not have obstruction to left ventricular outflow under basal conditions, although intracavitary gradients may be recorded with continuous-wave Doppler. Profound hypovolemia or intense ionotropic stimulation with pharmacological agents may induce outflow tract obstruction in certain cases, although this is not the rule.

Most patients with non-obstructive hypertrophic cardiomyopathy are limited by diastolic dysfunction. While systolic function is normal or hyperdynamic, diastolic function is impaired. There is abnormal left ventricular relaxation, filling, and compliance. In approximately two-thirds of patients with hypertrophic cardiomyopathy, transmitral Doppler echocardiography reveals a decreased E wave and a prolonged deceleration time. These findings indicate a reduced peak velocity during rapid diastolic filling and abnormally slow left ventricular filling.[3] The E/A ratio is decreased or reversed in this group of patients. In contrast, a subset of patients with hypertrophic cardiomyopathy have a restrictive-type pattern. The E-wave deceleration time is shortened which reflects a more rapid equilibrium of ventricular and atrial pressures and represents the effects of increased myocardial stiffness.[4] The utility of echocardiography in the diagnosis and treatment of hypertrophic cardiomyopathy is well established.

This patient's dyspnea is secondary to an elevated left ventricular end-diastolic pressure and abnormal diastolic filling of the ventricle. A beta-blocker and low-dose diuretic were started and the patient reported some improvement in his symptoms.

References

1. Maron B, Epstein S. Hypertrophic cardiomyopathy: a discussion of nomenclature. Am J Cardiol 1979;43:1242–4.

2. Wigle E, Sasson Z, Henderson M, et al. Hypertrophic cardiomyopathy: the importance of the site and extent of hypertrophy. Prog Rev Cardiovasc Dis 1985;28:183.

3. Spirito P, Maron B. Relation between the extent of left ventricular hypertrophy and diastolic filling abnormalities in hypertrophic cardiomyopathy. J Am Coll Cardiol 1990;15:808–13.

4. Maron B, Spirito P, Green K, et al. Noninvasive assessment of left ventricular diastolic function by pulsed Doppler echocardiography in patients with hypertrophic cardiomyopathy. J Am Coll Cardiol 1987;10:733–42.

89

Left ventricular dysfunction after surgery in Marfan's syndrome

Martin St John Sutton MBBS

A 41-year-old woman complained of dull interscapular back pain of moderate intensity associated with shortness of breath and easy fatigue, symptoms that were exacerbated by lifting or straining. Her back pain had progressed over a 6-month period, during which time she had also noticed episodes of self-terminating palpitations for which she could not identify any triggers. A chest X-ray performed 3 years previously in an emergency room following a motor vehicle accident showed an enlarged heart, pectus excavatum, kyphoscoliosis and a fractured left seventh rib. She was advised to arrange an outpatient appointment visit, but was lost to follow-up.

She had a past medical history that included bilateral inguinal hernia repairs when aged 7, and spontaneous dislocation of her right patella and left shoulder joint. There was no family history of congenital or acquired heart disease and she had no risk factors for coronary artery disease.

On examination she was 6 foot tall and weighed 117 lbs, with marked mid-thoracic and thoracolumbar kyphoscoliosis, pectus excavatum, arachnodactyly and horizontal skin striae on her back, consistent with Marfan's syndrome. Her blood pressure was 110/65 mmHg, heart rate of 62 bpm in regular rhythm, with normal jugular venous pressure and normal peripheral pulses. Her apical impulse was laterally displaced and was left ventricular in type. There was a normal first heart sound and a normally splitting second heart sound with a soft immediate diastolic murmur at the left sternal border indicative of mild aortic regurgitation, multiple mid-systolic clicks and a holosystolic murmur at the apex radiating to the axilla, consistent with at least moderate mitral regurgitation associated with mitral valve prolapse.

An electrocardiogram revealed sinus rhythm, nonspecific interventricular conduction delay and left atrial enlargement. A chest X-ray showed a pectus, moderately severe kyphoscoliosis, a dilated aortic root and ascending aorta with cardiomegaly. A transesophageal echocardiogram was performed to evaluate the aorta.

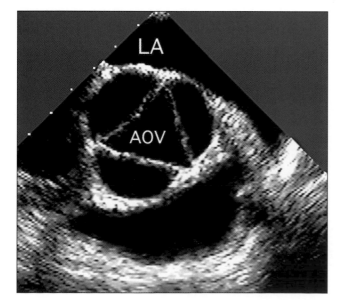

Figure 89.1
Short-axis view of the aortic valve (AOV) from the mid-esophageal position (imaging angle 35°). The aortic root is dilated. In this systolic view, the aortic cusps demonstrate a characteristic triangular orifice which is due to the dilatation of the root, preventing the tips of the leaflets from opening to the wall of the aorta.

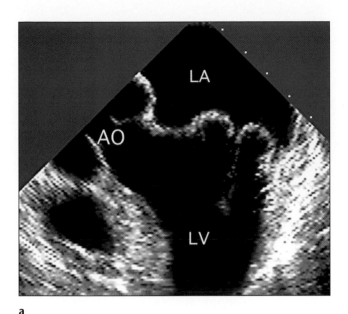

a

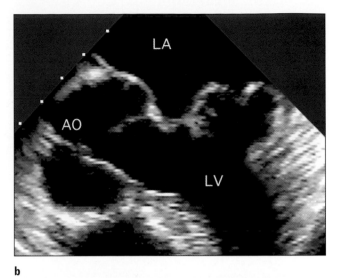

b

Figure 89.2

(a) Mid-esophageal echocardiogram in the transverse plane (imaging angle 0°). The left ventricular outflow tract is imaged in this modified four-chamber view. There is marked mitral valve prolapse of both anterior and posterior leaflets. The left atrium is enlarged. The left ventricular cavity is enlarged in this systolic frame, but the contractile function is vigorous.
(b) Close-up image of the mitral valve from the same imaging plane. The leaflets are myxomatous and redundant. Enlargement of the aortic root (AO) can be appreciated.
(c) Similar view with color Doppler flow imaging in systole. There is a moderate jet of mitral regurgitation (MR).

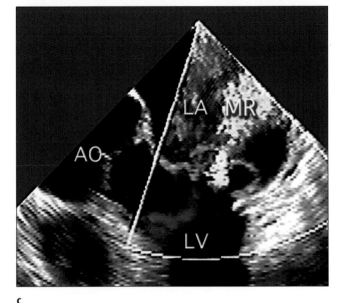

c

Magnetic resonance angiography demonstrated a 'tulip-shaped' ascending aortic aneurysm which had increased in size by 1.5 cm from the patient's chest X-ray 3 years previously. Her aortic arch and descending aorta were normal.

She underwent elective aortic valve homograft and aortic root replacement for an expanding aortic aneurysm and mitral valve replacement with a St Jude prosthesis. She developed complete atrioventricular dissociation which persisted for the first 5 days postoperatively and had a dual chamber pacemaker placed. She complained of shortness of breath on mild exertion postoperatively and repeat transthoracic two-dimensional echocardiography showed a dilated and poorly contracting left ventricle, which has improved only slightly with aggressive therapy with angiotensin converting enzyme (ACE) inhibitors and diuretics.

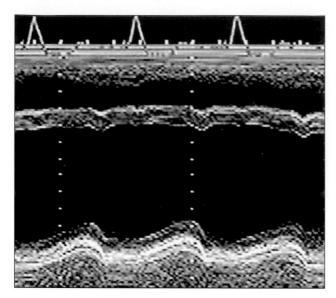
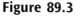

Figure 89.3
M-mode echocardiogram from the parasternal transthoracic window. The left ventricle is severely dilated and the fractional shortening is dramatically decreased.

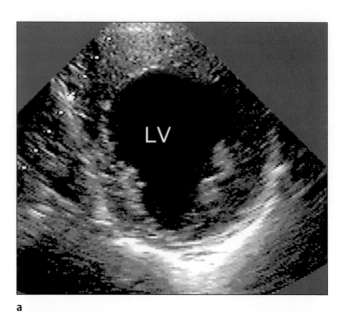

a

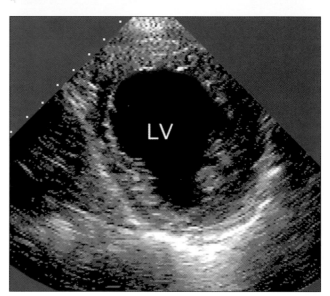

b

Figure 89.4
(a) Parasternal short-axis view of the left ventricle at the level of the papillary muscles in diastole. The walls are mildly hypertrophied. The ventricle is severely dilated.
(b) Similar systolic frame demonstrating the decreased left ventricular function. The left ventricular ejection fraction was estimated as 15–20%.

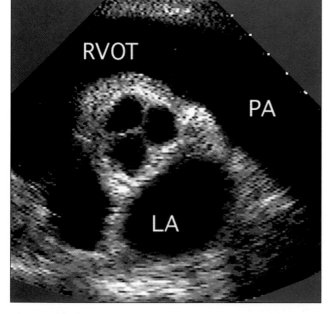
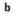

Figure 89.5
Parasternal short-axis view at the base of the heart in diastole. The aortic homograft is easily identified. The walls of the aortic root are thickened, owing to post-surgical change. The root itself is no longer dilated.

Discussion

The features of Marfan's syndrome are described in multiple reviews,[1] but the important prognostic information relates directly to the cardiac manifestations demonstrated in this patient. Aortic aneurysm formation is most frequently localized to the ascending aorta, but may occur throughout the aorta.[2] The material properties of the aortic wall are altered and form the substrate for dissection, which in the ascending and arch of the aorta is associated with poor prognosis from rupture into the thoracic cavity and retroperitoneum. Propagation of the dissection into the brachiocephalic vessels may cause stroke. The treatment of choice in patients with Marfan's syndrome and aortic aneurysm is beta-adrenergic receptor blockade and elective aortic valve and root replacement when the aortic diameter exceeds 5.5 cm or there is evidence of progressive enlargement. Emergency surgery is required for aortic dissection. Myxomatous prolapsing mitral valve leaflets with varying degrees of mitral regurgitation is common, as is present in this patient. Attempts at mitral repair are frequently unsuccessful and mitral valve replacement is required.

Symptoms are characteristically non-specific; examples are interscapular back pain and easy fatigue. The back pain experienced by our patient, who had not developed dissection, was probably due to expansion of the aortic root. The postoperative left ventricular dysfunction was due to preoperative left ventricular damage, which was masked by the normal ejection fraction that is often spuriously elevated because the left ventricle ejects partly into a low-pressure sink, namely the left atrium, and is inadequately hypertrophied to sustain normal ejection. In this patient left ventricular function remained moderately depressed at long-term follow-up, even on diuretic and ACE inhibitor therapy.

References

1. Simpson I, de Belder M, Treasure T, *et al.* Cardiovascular manifestations of Marfan's syndrome: improved evaluation by transoesophageal echocardiography. Br Heart J 1993;69:104–8.

2. Devereux R, Roman M. Aortic disease in Marfan's syndrome. N Engl J Med 1999;340:1358–9.

90

Left ventricular thrombus

Craig H Scott MD

A 63-year-old man with hypercholesterolemia and coronary artery disease presented at the emergency room with a transient ischemic attack. The patient had had a myocardial infarction 3 years previously. Coronary arteriography at that time revealed an occlusion of the mid-left anterior descending coronary artery.

Neurological examination in the emergency room was normal. An S_4 was audible on auscultation of the heart. There were no carotid bruits and the carotid upstroke was normal. His eye fields were unremarkable. An echocardiogram was ordered to evaluate the source of the embolus.

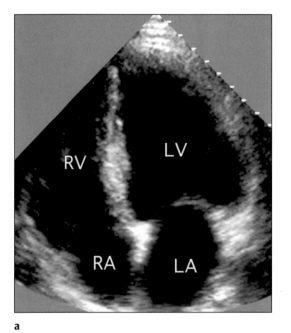

a

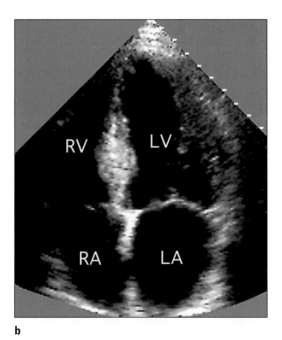

b

Figure 90.1
(a) Apical four-chamber view in diastole. The left ventricle (LV) is moderately dilated. Hypertrophy of the lateral wall is evident but the septum appears thinned. The apex is not completely visualized but there are echodensities at the apex that are suspicious for thrombus. However, trabeculations or artifact, rather than thrombus, might account for these findings. The left atrium (LA) is also mildly dilated. The right ventricle (RV) is not completely seen but appears enlarged as well.
(b) Apical four-chamber view in systole. Left ventricular systolic function is decreased. The septum from the mid-ventricular level to the apex does not thicken. The apex is also akinetic. The left atrium dilates in systole, which is consistent with significant mitral regurgitation (the color Doppler findings are not shown here but demonstrated moderate to severe mitral regurgitation). Note the dropout of the interatrial septum in the region of the fossa ovalis. This is the thinnest portion of the septum and may not be well seen when the ultrasound beam is parallel to the interatrial septum. A true atrial septal defect can be excluded by visualization of an intact septum in orthogonal views, such as the subcostal four-chamber view, and by the lack of color flow Doppler jets across the septum.

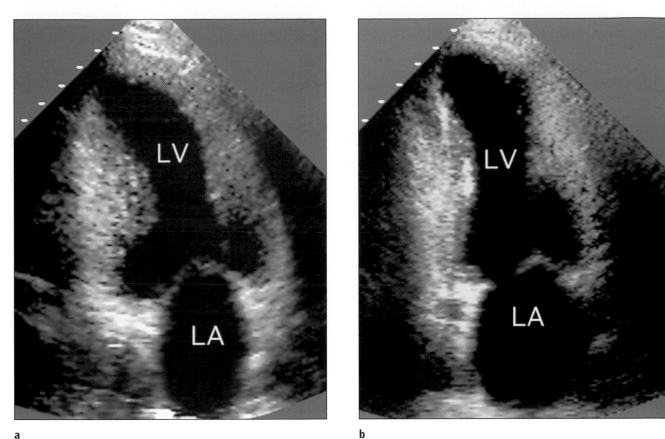

a

b

Figure 90.2

(a) Apical two-chamber view in diastole. Moderate left ventricular hypertrophy is evident. The papillary muscles are particularly prominent. The apex of the left ventricle is dilated, but once again endocardial details are not well seen. In diastole, the apparent bulging of the inferior wall at the base is artifactual and due to the prominent papillary muscles.

(b) Apical two-chamber view in systole. The apex is dyskinetic and actually expands in systole. The apical aneurysm is small but involves the lateral, posterior, and anterior walls of the apex. Both the inferior and anterior walls at the base are shown to contract normally.

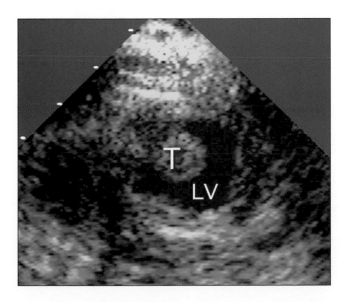

Figure 90.3

Short-axis view at the level of the apex. The transducer has been angled towards the left ventricular (LV) apex from the standard parasternal short-axis position. It may be necessary to move one or more intercostal spaces inferiorly to achieve this view. A smooth, round 1-cm mass (T) is attached to the endocardium. The apex is dilated and akinetic. None of the other standard echocardiographic views demonstrated the thrombus, emphasizing the importance of a complete study in every case. Trabeculation is not present and the echodensities apparent in the other views are confirmed to be thrombus. The mass appears to be of similar echodensity to the surrounding myocardium.

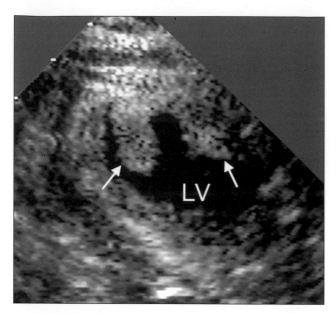

Figure 90.4
Off-axis parasternal view of the left ventricular (LV) apex.
A U-shaped mass attached to the endocardium of the apex
represents a thrombus. The two heads of the mass (arrows)
were highly mobile in real time. Only off-axis imaging
demonstrated the true size of the apical thrombus.

Discussion

Ventricular masses associated with hypokinetic segments
are most commonly thrombus. Included in the diagnosis
of an apical ventricular mass are heavy trabeculation or
false chordae tendinae (normal variants), endomyocardial
fibrosis, a rare, usually tropical disease of unknown etiology, intracardiac tumors (benign, malignant, primary or
metastatic), which are also rare and vary widely in presentation, and Chagas' disease, a parasitic infection endemic
in South America. Chagas' disease results in aneurysm
formation, often at the left ventricular apex, with associated thrombus. Patients with myocardial infarction,
especially in the left anterior descending coronary artery
territory, who are not on anticoagulation therapy, have a
40–60% incidence of mural thrombi.[1] Two-dimensional
echocardiography is the test of choice when mural thrombus is suspected. The most difficult task regarding assessment of apical thrombus is that artifact often obscures the

left ventricular apex. Phantom reverberations and side-
lobe artifacts make assessment of the apex difficult. The
use of higher-frequency transducers and multiple views of
the apex maximize the ability to diagnose thrombus.

An important distinction between thrombus and heavy
apical trabeculation is that thrombus is never contractile.
While it may move passively, it does not thicken. Trabeculations are linear while thrombus is a three-dimensional
structure that can be imaged in orthogonal views. Thrombus is more commonly associated with akinetic cardiac
segments, although local tumor infiltration can affect
contraction in the area surrounding the mass. As a thrombus ages, it may calcify, resulting in increased echodensity.
Transesophageal echocardiography is often not useful in
the assessment of the apex. The image is in the far field
of the esophageal transducer. Furthermore, the transesophageal transducer is more difficult to align with the
true long axis, given the limited mobility of the transducer
within the esophagus, and is thus likely to miss the apex.

Embolization is the major concern in patients with
ventricular thrombus. Echocardiographic criteria that
suggest an increased risk of embolization include
increased thrombus mobility, protrusion into the ventricular chamber, and the presence of a hyperkinetic segment
adjacent to the akinetic segment containing the thrombus.[2]

The incidence of systemic embolization with known
mural thrombus varies with the patient population.
Patients with ischemic cardiomyopathy are more likely to
develop mural thrombus but less likely to embolize than
patients with idiopathic cardiomyopathy.[3] The average
embolization rate is approximately 10% for all patients
with known ventricular thrombus.

References

1. Keeley E, Hillis L. Left ventricular mural thrombus after acute
   myocardial infarction. Clin Cardiol 1996;19:83.

2. Jugdutt B, Sivaram C, Wortman C, *et al.* Prospective two-dimensional echocardiographic evaluation of left ventricular thrombus and
   embolism after myocardial infarction. J Am Coll Cardiol
   1989;13:554.

3. Halperin J, Petersen P. Thrombosis in the cardiac chambers: ventricular dysfunction and atrial fibrillation. In: Fuster V, Verstraete M,
   eds. Thrombosis in Cardiovascular Disorders, WB Saunders:
   Philadelphia, 1992:215.

91

Left ventricular aneurysm and thrombus

Craig H Scott MD

A 54-year-old man with longstanding, poorly controlled hypertension, tobacco abuse and hypercholesterolemia developed substernal chest pain and shortness of breath which lasted for 8 hours before he sought medical attention. He was admitted to the hospital after thrombolysis was performed in the emergency room for electrocardio-gram changes consistent with an acute anterior myocardial infarction. The patient had an uneventful recovery. He continued to have difficulty controlling his blood pressure. Three years later, he had an episode of shortness of breath with some component of orthopnea and an echocardiogram was ordered to assess left ventricular function.

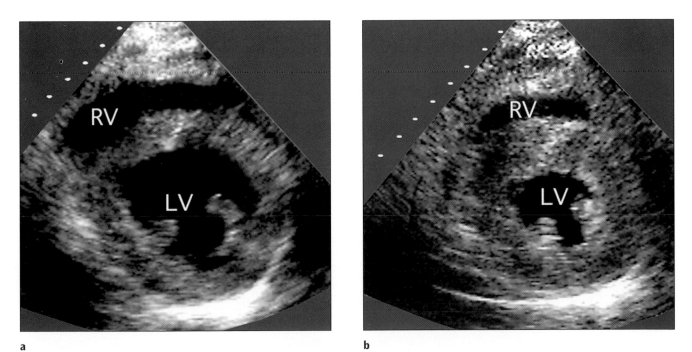

a   b

Figure 91.1
(a) Parasternal short-axis view of the left ventricle (LV) in diastole demonstrating moderate concentric left ventricular hypertrophy. The chamber sizes of the left ventricle and right ventricle (RV) appear to be normal.
(b) Similar short-axis view in systole. The left ventricular systolic function is normal and no wall motion abnormalities are seen at the mid-ventricular level. From this view alone, it would be estimated that the left ventricular ejection fraction was normal.

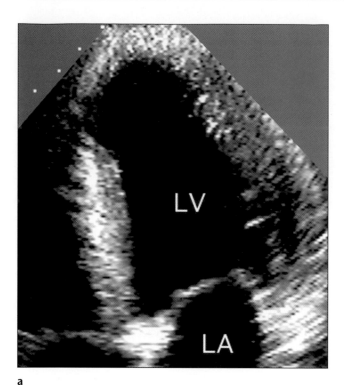

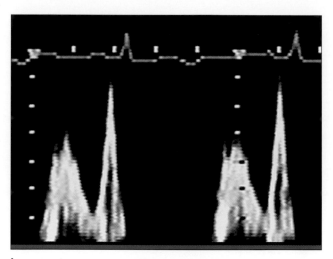

b

a

Figure 91.2

(a) Apical four-chamber view in late diastole. There is an abrupt change in the thickness of the distal septum with thinning and bulging of the apex. The distal lateral wall appears to be hypertrophied and is not involved in the aneurysm.

(b) Spectral Doppler display from the apical position at the tips of the mitral valve leaflets. The diastolic flow is abnormal with a reversal in the E-wave to A-wave amplitude ratio (E to A reversal). This finding is consistent with diastolic dysfunction and is not unexpected in a patient with this degree of hypertrophy.

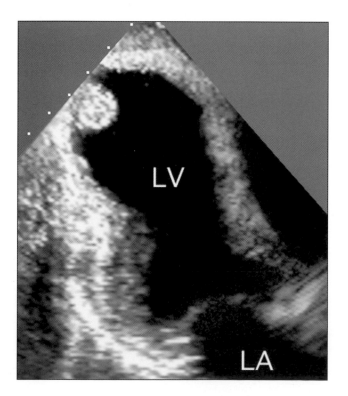

Figure 91.3

Apical long-axis view of the left ventricle in systole. It is evident that the function is normal at the mid-ventricular level. However, immediately distal to this there is abrupt thinning of the inferior wall and systolic bulging consistent with aneurysm formation. The involvement of the distal inferior wall, the distal septum, the distal anterior wall, and the apex is consistent with an infarction due to occlusion of a large 'wrap-around' left anterior descending artery in its middle or distal portion. There is a round, echo-bright mass that is approximately 1.3 cm in diameter within the aneurysm which is a calcified thrombus. It was a sessile mass that did not move during the cardiac cycle.

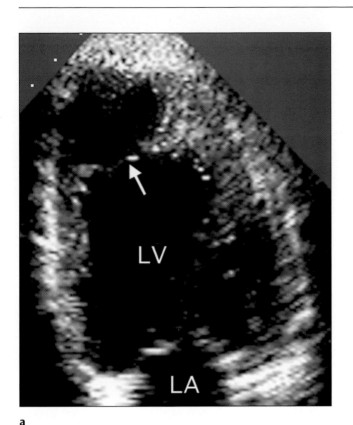

a

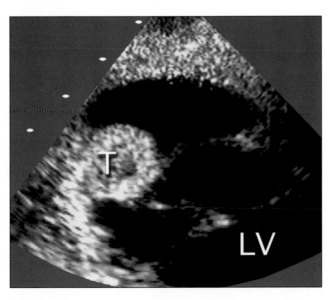

b

Figure 91.4
(a) Further imaging of the apex from the apical four-chamber plane revealing a false tendon (arrow) that extended from the septum to the lateral wall. The septal attachment is coincidentally at the junction between the normal myocardium and the infarction.
(b) Off-axis parasternal short-axis view at the level of the apex which demonstrates the apical thrombus (T). There are also several false chords or tendons that run across the apex. Their appearance is common for false chords and is not consistent with thrombus.

Discussion

Apical masses have a broad differential diagnosis. The finding of a thin filament in the four-chamber apical view may represent the leading edge of a cystic tumor or a mass with a necrotic center. Chordae tendinae typically connect the papillary muscles with the mitral valve leaflets. Occasionally, a chord will span the ventricle with no connection to either the papillary muscle or the mitral valve and is referred to as a false chord. In Figure 91.4a, a false chord is the most likely diagnosis. It may have a characteristic high-frequency motion during the cardiac cycle, mimicking a child's jump rope.

The patient also has a sessile, rounded mass seen in the apical two-chamber view. It probably represents a chronic thrombus because of its shape, location and echodensity. Poor apical images may be able to exclude a large thrombus, but may miss small masses. Body habitus and difficulty in imaging the near field may obscure the presence of apical thrombi. Given the relatively high rate of thrombus formation in anterior and apical akinetic or aneurysmal segments, anticoagulation should be considered in this situation, even if a thrombus is not visualized, since these segments act as a nidus for thrombus formation. Some patients have both an increased risk of anticoagulation and poor acoustic windows, so additional testing for left ventricular thrombus is warranted.

Presently, five imaging modalities have been considered for studying ventricular thrombus in cases where the transthoracic echocardiogram is inconclusive: contrast transthoracic echocardiography, transesophageal echocardiography, magnetic resonance imaging (MRI), ultrafast computerized tomography (CT), and labelled-platelet nuclear scans. Contrast injection using sonicated albumin can be used to highlight an apical thrombus. The signal that returns from the contrast agent is stronger than the tissue signal, so the thrombus appears as a dark protrusion into the left ventricular cavity, thereby outlining its extent. Transesophageal echocardiography is less sensitive for the diagnosis of apical thrombus than transthoracic echocardiography. The apex is in the far field of the esophageal transducer and the transgastric view cannot uniformly access the apex. It is also more difficult to assess whether the imaging plane includes the apex (the image may be subtly foreshortened) which may result in false negative readings. MRI can assess the amount of hemosiderin in the mass using tissue characterization. MRI with tissue tagging methods can assess contractility of the mass, also helping to delineate apical trabeculation from thrombus or tumor. A thrombus can also be characterized as acute or chronic by its appearance on T_1 weighted and gradient-recalled images.[1] Ultrafast CT with contrast has also been used to assess left ventricular thrombus. CT is valuable in patients with an equivocal or technically difficult chest wall echocardiogram.[2] Finally, indium-111 platelet imaging can detect a left ventricular thrombus. Multiple views in combination with late imaging at 48–72 hours after injection is essential to obtain reasonable results. The degree of platelet uptake is also dependent on the thrombus age. Fresh thrombi will take up the labelled platelets well, but established thrombi (older than 1 month) may be harder to recognize. Detection of a thrombus by platelet imaging predicts a higher embolization risk.[3]

References

1. Herfkens R, Marcus ML, Utz J, *et al.* Nuclear magnetic resonance assessment of valvular disease. In: Marcus M, et al., eds. Cardiac Imaging: a companion to Braunwald's Heart Disease, 3rd edn, WB Saunders: Philadelphia, 1988:903.

2. Love B, Struck L, Stanford W, *et al.* Comparison of two-dimensional echocardiography and ultrafast computer tomography for evaluating intracardiac thrombi in cerebral ischemia. Stroke 1990;21:1033–8.

3. Stratton J, Ritchie J. Indium-111 platelet imaging of the left ventricular thrombi: predictive value for systemic emboli. Circulation 1990;81:1182–9.

92

Chaga's disease

Martin St John Sutton MBBS

A 39-year-old male immigrant from Brazil complained of recurrent palpitations associated with shortness of breath and near syncope for which he could not identify any triggers. He had not experienced chest pain, had a normal exercise tolerance and had previously enjoyed good health. Other than being a current smoker he had no risk factors for heart disease and no family history of congenital or acquired heart disease.

On examination he was normotensive with a heart rate of 60 bpm in regular rhythm, a normal jugular venous pressure and normal central and peripheral arterial pulses. The cardiac apical impulse was normal, the first heart sound was split, the second sound was normal, and there were no cardiac murmurs. An electrocardiogram showed sinus rhythm, left axis deviation, and right bundle branch block with occasional premature ventricular contractions. A chest X-ray revealed mild cardiomegaly and clear lung fields. The echocardiogram revealed a dilated left ventricle with decreased systolic function and a discrete apical aneurysm with thrombus.

Four years later, he returned for a repeat examination, now with severe exercise intolerance and paroxysms of palpitations with exertion. He did not have chest pain or syncope. A repeat echocardiogram was performed.

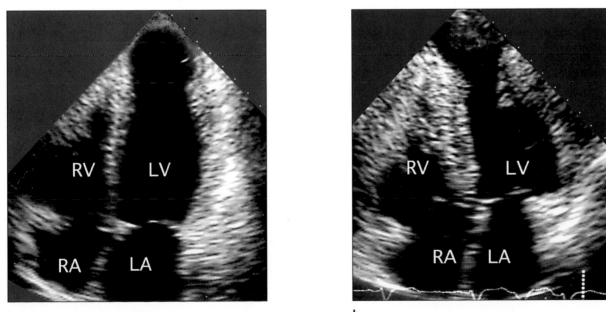

a   b

Figure 92.1
(a) Apical four-chamber view in late diastole. The left ventricle is dilated, as is the right ventricle. There is an aneurysm of the left ventricular apex with marked diastolic deformity.
(b) Similar view in systole. The right and left ventricular systolic function is mildly decreased, as evidenced by the decreased fractional area change compared to normal. The apical aneurysm expands in systole and a large thrombus is visualized within it. The mitral and tricuspid valves are normal and were competent.

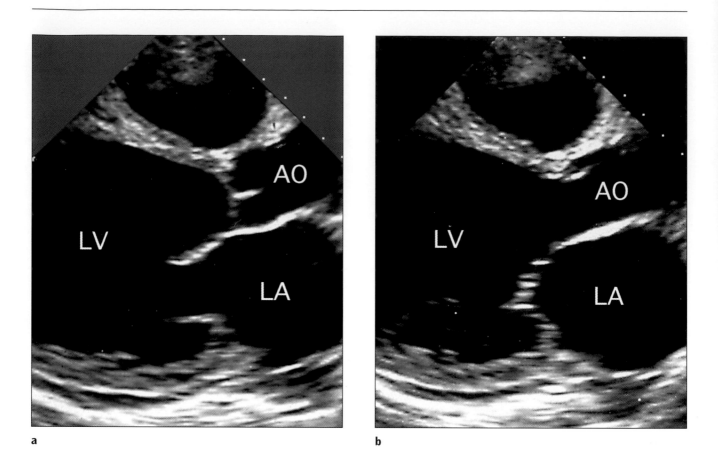

a   b

Figure 92.2
(a) Parasternal long-axis view of the ventricle in diastole from the second echocardiogram, four years after the previous images. The left ventricle is severely dilated and the left atrium is moderately so. There is a small posterior pericardial effusion.
(b) Parasternal long-axis view of the ventricle in systole. The left ventricular contractile function is severely diminished. The mitral valve demonstrates an incomplete closure pattern with the leaflets unable to coapt in their usual positions, owing to annular dilatation. Severe mitral regurgitation was present (not shown).

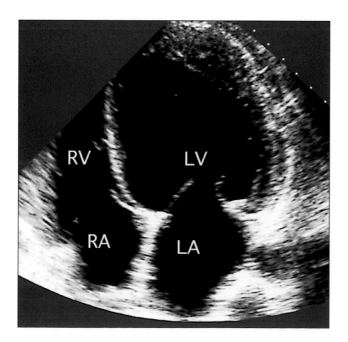

Figure 92.3
Apical four-chamber view in diastole. The left ventricle is enlarged with a globular cavity shape and no discernible segmental wall motion abnormalities, but a laminated mural thrombus adherent to the endocardium at the left ventricular apex. The thrombus appears to extend along the lateral wall towards the base of the heart. This picture is indistinguishable from that of dilated cardiomyopathy, although the extensive thrombus is unusual. Comparison with the echocardiogram of 4 years earlier demonstrates that the aneurysm has been replaced by massive left ventricular enlargement, which now appears to involve the entire ventricle.

Discussion

This patient presented with the classic symptoms of paroxysmal palpitations and exercise intolerance progressing to heart failure over a 4-year period. The electrocardiographic combination of left axis deviation and right bundle branch block without evidence of an intracardiac shunt and an apical left ventricular aneurysm on two-dimensional echocardiography in a previous inhabitant of Brazil should suggest Chagas' disease due to *Trypanosoma cruzi*. The diagnosis was confirmed in this patient by a complement fixation test.

Ventricular arrhythmias often feature prominently in Chagas' cardiomyopathy. The localized apical left ventricular aneurysm is gradually replaced by generalized severe left ventricular dilatation and deterioration in ventricular function, which may be complicated by formation of a mural thrombus with or without systemic embolization.[1,2] The time for the transition to the terminal phase of dilated cardiomyopathy varies, but once symptoms of dyspnea occur the deterioration in ventricular function is rapid.

References

1. Patel A, Lima C, Parro A, *et al*. Echocardiographic analysis of regional and global left ventricular shape in Chagas' cardiomyopathy. Am J Cardiol 1998;82:197–202.

2. Aquatella H, Schiller N. Echocardiographic recognition of Chagas' disease and endomyocardial fibrosis. J Am Soc Echocardiogr 1988;1:60–8.

93

Non-surgical septal ablation in hypertrophic obstructive cardiomyopathy

Susan E Wiegers MD

A 25-year-old man with a history of severe obstructive hypertrophic cardiomyopathy was markedly symptomatic despite maximal medical therapy. He had severe dyspnea on exertion and was unable to walk more than 100 yards. He had not responded to a dual chamber pacemaker. He

had been offered septal myectomy but refused surgery. Septal ablation in the catheterization laboratory was accomplished via injection of ethanol into the first septal perforator. Transthoracic echocardiography was performed during the procedure to monitor the results.

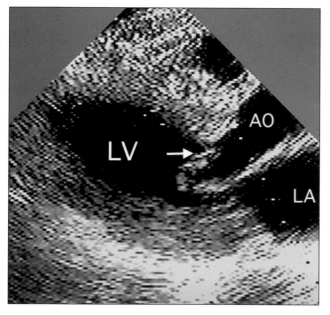

Figure 93.1
Parasternal long-axis view in systole. There is marked systolic anterior motion of the mitral valve (arrow) with contact of the septum by the anterior mitral valve leaflet. The septum is thicker than the posterior wall, which is also hypertrophied. The left atrium is mildly dilated.

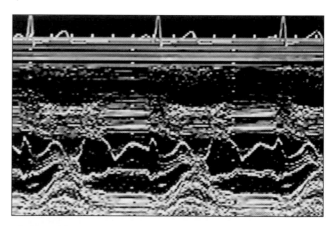

Figure 93.2
M-mode echocardiogram from the parasternal position at the level of the mitral valve leaflets. The systolic anterior motion of the anterior leaflet is evident. The disparity in the wall thickness of the posterior wall and the septum is demonstrated.

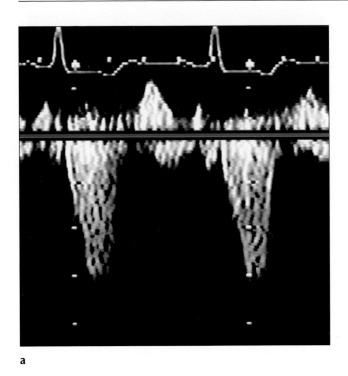

a

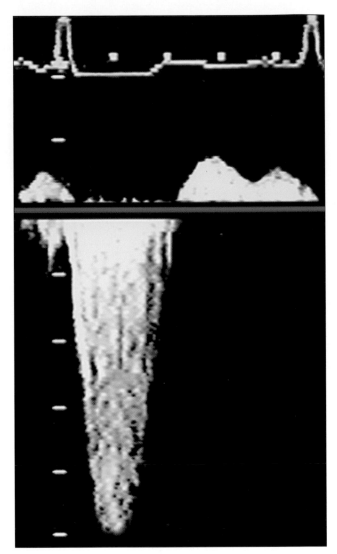

b

Figure 93.3

(a) Spectral display of continuous-wave Doppler across the left ventricular outflow tract in systole. The peak velocity at rest is 3 m/s which predicts a peak resting gradient of 36 mmHg. The spectral envelope demonstrates the late peaking pattern with an asymmetric 'dagger' shape characteristic of outflow tract obstruction.

(b) With the Valsalva maneuver, the peak velocity increased to 5 m/s and the gradient to 100 mmHg.

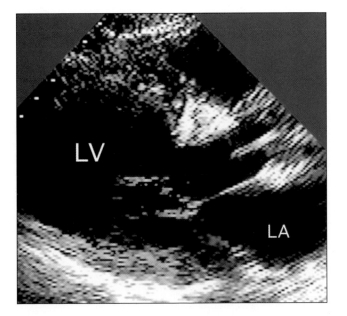

Figure 93.4

Parasternal long-axis view during injection of sonicated albumin into the septal perforator. The myocardium perfused by the vessel is opacified. This confirms that the septal perforator that has been cannulated supplies the target myocardium, the proximal septal knuckle that makes contact with the anterior mitral valve in systole.

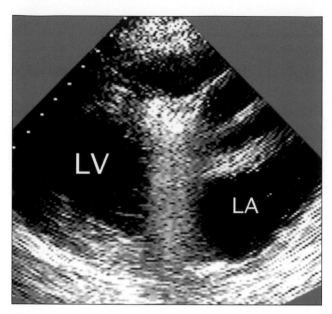

Figure 93.5
Similar parasternal long-axis view in systole after the alcohol injection. The ethanol creates a significant artifact which causes reverberation of the ultrasound beam and obscures posterior structures. This artifact was not permanent. The infarcted portion of the septum is clearly visible, with a marked difference in echodensity and a sharp demarcation from the normal tissue.

and then isolated with an occlusive balloon catheter. Ethanol is injected into the perforator after ascertaining that there is no back flow into the left anterior descending artery from the catheter in the artery of interest. Ethanol is a toxic substance that causes necrosis of the myocardium. The resulting scar decreases the mass of the proximal septum and remodels the septum toward a more normal configuration. This has proved to be of benefit to patients despite the production of a non-contracting scar in the proximal septum. Contrast echocardiography has proved very useful in delineating the portion of the septum subserved by the artery of interest.[1] There is an excellent correlation between the territory of the septum supplied by the perforating artery, the area of the enhancement by albumin injection, and the level of myocardial enzymes after the procedure.

This patient had a relatively low resting gradient before the procedure but a high provocable gradient. The best predictor of a significant provocable gradient is proximal septal bulging, as in this patient. Asymmetric septal hypertrophy alone is less often associated with a provocable gradient.[2]

The patient had an excellent response to the therapy with a decrease in the gradient to 10 mmHg at rest and no increase with maneuvers. The proximal septal bulge was eliminated on subsequent echocardiograms. He was able to increase his exertion significantly.

Discussion

Hypertrophic cardiomyopathy is a genetic disorder of the myocardium. Patients' symptoms may be due to diastolic abnormalities as well as outflow tract obstruction by the anterior mitral valve leaflet. Recently, non-surgical reduction therapy of the proximal interventricular septum has been undertaken in the invasive laboratory. The septal perforator supplying the proximal septum is identified

References

1. Nagueh S, Lakkis N, He Z, *et al.* Role of myocardial contrast echocardiography during nonsurgical septal reduction therapy for hypertrophic obstructive cardiomyopathy. J Am Coll Cardiol 1998;32:225–9.

2. Nakatani S, Marwick T, Lever H, *et al.* Resting echocardiographic features of latent left ventricular outflow obstruction in hypertrophic cardiomyopathy. Am J Cardiol 1996;78:662–7.

94

Restrictive cardiomyopathy

Martin St John Sutton MBBS
Susan E Wiegers MD

A 29-year-old woman was referred for consideration of tricuspid valve replacement for severe tricuspid regurgitation believed to be due to avulsion of the tricuspid valve leaflet by prior placement of a transvenous pacemaker. She complained of easy fatigue, progressive reduction in exercise capacity limited to walking one block or climbing five stairs, bilateral ankle edema and abdominal bloating. Her medical history included a viral illness at age 11 years with which she had noted dyspnea on minimal exertion and palpitations. One week later she developed sudden onset of pain and discoloration, first of her right hand and forearm and subsequently of her right leg, consistent with arterial embolism. Two-dimensional echocardiography showed a left atrial mass for which she underwent a sternotomy, but no mass was found in the left atrium. A thrombus was removed from her right subclavian and right common iliac arteries, both of which were occluded.

She improved symptomatically with diuretics, digitalis, propranolol and warfarin. At the age of 24 she had near syncope, intermittent bradycardias down to 20 bpm and tachycardias to 170 bpm; a permanent transvenous pacemaker was placed for sinoatrial dysfunction.

On examination she had acrocyanosis, oxygen saturation of 93% at rest, bilateral edema to her mid-calf, and marked elevation of her jugular venous pressure with a dominant 'v' wave consistent with tricuspid regurgitation. Her apical impulse was consistent with left ventricular predominance and there was an apical pansystolic murmur and a softer pansystolic murmur at the lower left sternal border that varied in intensity with respiration, indicating mitral and tricuspid regurgitation, respectively. An electrocardiogram showed electronic pacing throughout. A chest X-ray revealed biatrial enlargement and normal lung parenchyma without shunt vascularity.

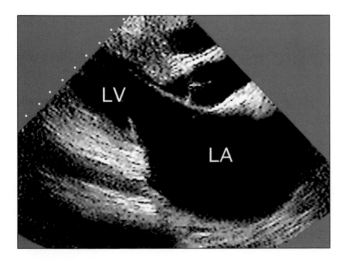

a

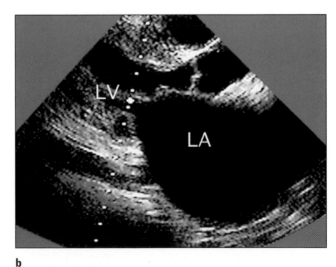

b

Figure 94.1
(a) Parasternal long-axis view in diastole. The left atrium is severely enlarged, the mitral valve is normal, but moderate mitral regurgitation was present (not shown here). The left ventricle is normal in size and mildly hypertrophied with abnormal septal motion in diastole. A posterior pericardial effusion is present and can be seen as a posterior echo-free space.
(b) Enlargement of the left atrium in systole, consistent with mitral regurgitation. The aortic valve has already closed in this late systolic frame.

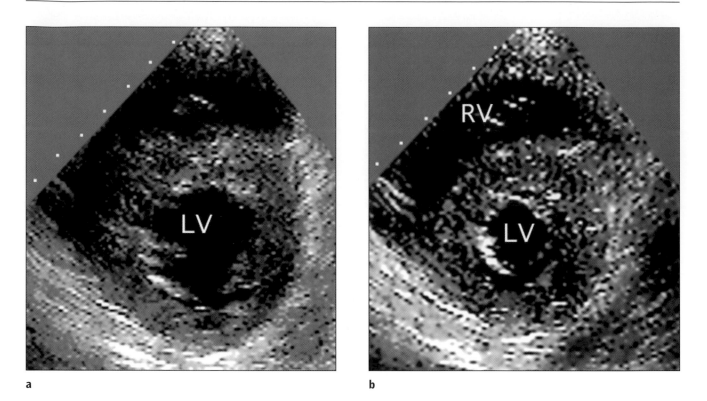

a
b

Figure 94.2
(a) Parasternal long-axis view in diastole. The ventricle is moderately hypertrophied and the right ventricular walls are not well seen but the cavity size is normal.
(b) Systolic function is preserved, as evidenced by the normal fractional area change.

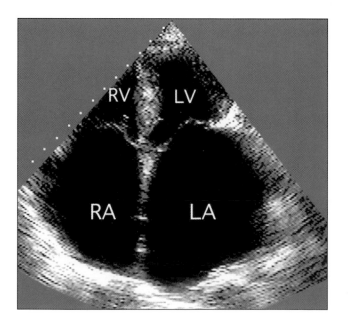

Figure 94.3
The apical four-chamber view shows normal-sized, hypertrophied right and left ventricles with preserved global systolic function. The right atrium is also massively dilated, and moderately severe tricuspid regurgitation was present.

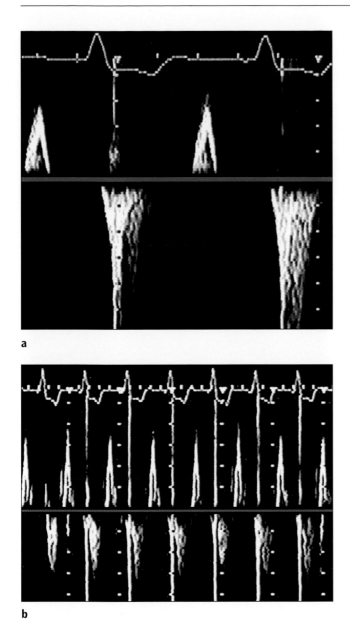

a

b

Figure 94.4
(a) Spectral display of pulsed-wave Doppler with the sample volume placed at the mitral valve leaflet tips. A short transmitral E-wave deceleration time consistent with restrictive physiology is present. The deceleration time is well under 100 ms. (Horizontal calibration marks represent 200 ms; vertical calibration marks represent 20 cm/s.) The systolic aliased flow away from the baseline is mitral regurgitation.
(b) Similar spectral display with the display time decreased so that respiratory variation may be assessed. The rapid deceleration is again noted, but there is little respirophasic variation in the inflow velocities.

Discussion

The important echocardiographic findings in this patient included massive biatrial dilatation, bilateral

atrioventricular valve regurgitation, two small moderately hypertrophied ventricles and, even during pacing, there was a very short transmitral E-wave deceleration time providing strong evidence for restrictive cardiomyopathy. Importantly, the pericardium was normal and did not appear thickened, although there is a small effusion. Constrictive pericarditis can produce similar massive biatrial enlargement and shortened deceleration times but would not produce the other echocardiographic characteristics of this case. In addition, there was no respirophasic variation in the tricuspid or mitral inflows, which would be expected with constriction.[1] Pulmonary artery systolic pressure estimated from the tricuspid regurgitant jet velocity was 35–40 mmHg which excluded pulmonary hypertension as the etiology of the right atrial dilatation. The patient underwent cardiac catheterization, which revealed markedly elevated right and left ventricular diastolic pressures with a dip and plateau configuration consistent with restrictive cardiomyopathy. Endomyocardial biopsy showed extensive non-specific interstitial myocardial fibrosis. A diagnosis of idiopathic restrictive cardiomyopathy was made, and she was treated with digitalis, diuretics, and angiotensin converting enzyme inhibitors, but continued to deteriorate symptomatically and is currently listed as status I for heart transplantation.

The diagnosis of idiopathic restrictive cardiomyopathy is made by demonstrating, by Doppler echocardiography, the resistance to filling that usually predominates on the left heart and consists of a continuous spectrum of abnormalities of E- and A-wave velocity profiles, indicating abnormal diastolic function.[2] Restrictive cardiomyopathy is relatively rare and has a varied course. The restrictive disease associated with amyloid heart disease generally produces decreased left ventricular function by the time the patient is severely symptomatic. A highly speckled pattern of the myocardium was also lacking in this case, and the diagnosis was ruled out by biopsy. This patient had quite a long course of disease since her childhood events, which were almost certainly associated. Idiopathic restrictive cardiomyopathy in children has been described and has a poor prognosis if the course is progressive.[3]

References

1. Hatle L, Appleton C, Popp R. Differentiation of constrictive pericarditis and restrictive cardiomyopathy by Doppler echocardiography. Circulation 1989;79:357–70.

2. Appleton CP, Hatle LK, Popp RL. Demonstration of restrictive ventricular physiology by Doppler echocardiography. J Am Coll Cardiol 1988;11:757–68.

3. Gewillig M, Mertens L, Moerman P, et al. Idiopathic restrictive cardiomyopathy in childhood. A diastolic disorder characterized by delayed relaxation. Eur Heart J 1996;17:1413–20.

95

Apical variant of hypertrophic cardiomyopathy

Martin St John Sutton MBBS
Susan E Wiegers MD

A 29-year-old man of Asian descent complained of pain and stiffness in the left side of his neck with restricted lateral rotation of his head and neck on account of pain for 10 days. He had been carrying his 3-year-old daughter on his back while back-packing the previous weekend. He sought medical attention because his symptoms had not resolved. He had no history of exercise intolerance, prior chest pain, palpitations or syncope. There was no history of congenital or acquired heart disease in his immediate or remote family. On physical examination a musical murmur was detected. An electrocardiogram was reported to show electrical criteria for left ventricular hypertrophy with biphasic 'T' waves in leads V1–V3, and a chest X-ray revealed mild cardiomegaly. He was referred for further investigation.

On examination, his blood pressure was 110/65 mmHg and heart rate 54 bpm with occasional ectopy. The jugular venous pulse was normal, and peripheral arterial pulses were brisk bilaterally. The apical impulse was sustained and unusually forceful, and a high-frequency ejection murmur was audible that did not appear to augment with the Valsalva maneuver. An electrocardiogram revealed sinus rhythm with occasional ventricular premature contractions, elevated ST segments and markedly abnormal T wave inversion in leads V1–V3 and left ventricular hypertrophy. A chest X-ray showed a top normal heart size and normal lung fields. A treadmill exercise test that he had brought with him showed ST segment depression in the anterior precordial leads which was not associated with symptoms. He had exercised for 15 min on a Bruce protocol, stopping on account of leg fatigue. A 48-hour ambulatory electrocardiogram revealed multiple episodes of asymptomatic non-sustained ventricular tachycardia.

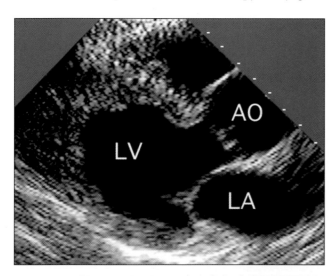
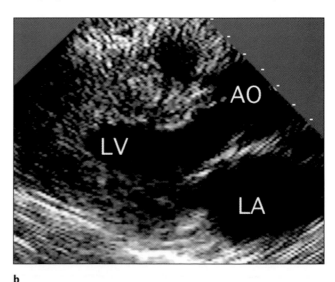

a

b

Figure 95.1
(a) Parasternal long-axis view in diastole. The left ventricular cavity is small. The mitral and aortic valves are normal. The interventricular septum is more hypertrophied than the posterior wall. The apical myocardium appears to be imaged but, in this standard transducer position, the appearance may be due to foreshortening of the ventricle.
(b) In systole, the apical hypertrophy is more apparent. There is no evidence of systolic anterior motion of the mitral valve or of left ventricular outflow tract obstruction. The left atrium is mildly enlarged.

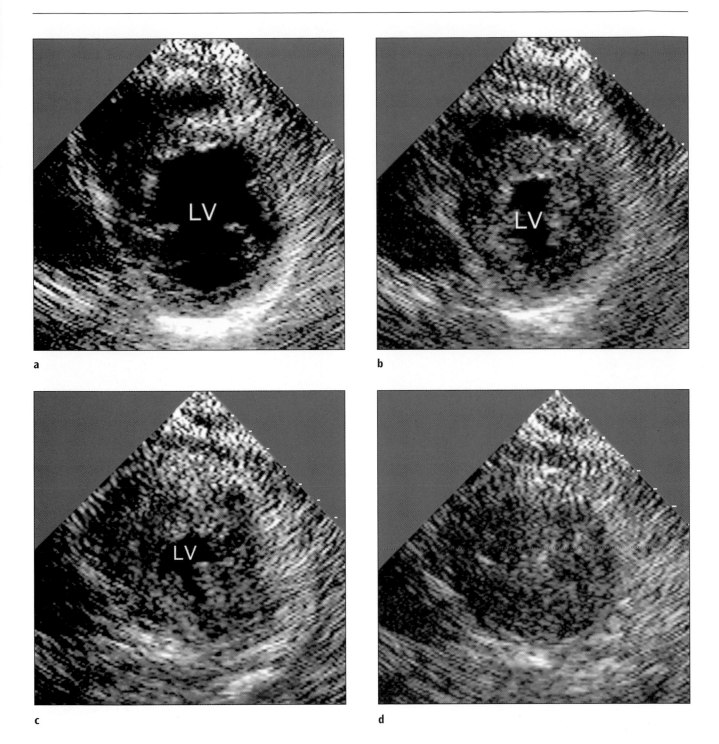

Figure 95.2

(a) Parasternal short-axis view at the level of the mitral valve leaflets in diastole. The ventricle is of normal size near the base of the heart.

(b) In systole, left ventricular function is supernormal with a small systolic cavity.

(c) The transducer had been angled towards the apex of the heart. There is near cavity obliteration in diastole and the papillary muscles appear to touch.

(d) Short-axis view at the same level in systole. The walls of the left ventricle are massively thickened. The cavity is completely obliterated in systole.

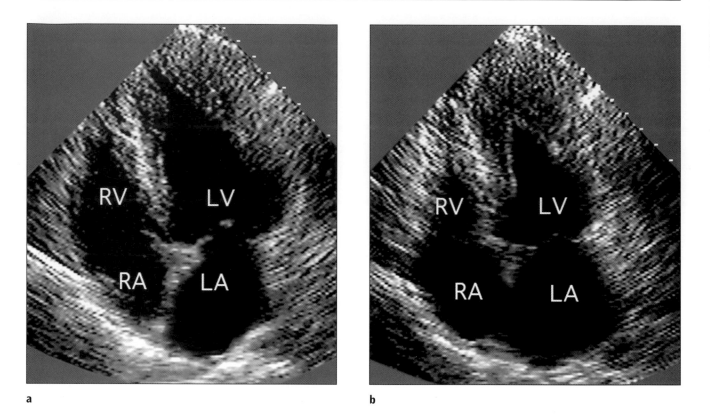

a

b

Figure 95.3
(a) Apical four-chamber view in diastole. There is severe apical hypertrophy. The left ventricular cavity has a spade shape. There is a marked disparity between the thickness of the walls at the mid-ventricular level and apex compared to the base.
(b) Similar view in systole. The cavity is obliterated at the apex, and left ventricular function is hyperdynamic. The right ventricular function is also supernormal.

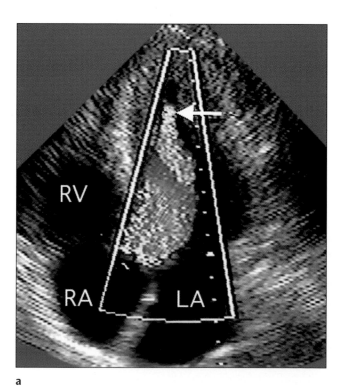

a

Figure 95.4
(a) Apical four-chamber view with color Doppler flow imaging in early systole. The left ventricular outflow jet is seen entering the left ventricular outflow tract where its velocity exceeds the Nyquist limit and the color jet aliases. There is no evidence of obstruction at this level, however, as the jet does not narrow or become turbulent. There is obliteration of the apical left ventricular cavity due to coaptation of the free wall and septum in early to mid-systole, and a turbulent color flow Doppler signal at the apex (arrow) which is due to obliteration of the cavity and mid-cavitary obstruction to flow.

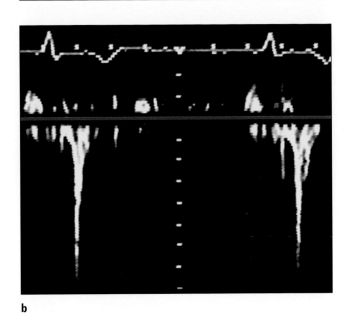

b

Figure 95.4
(b) Pulsed-wave Doppler spectral display (each calibration mark represents 20 cm/s). The sample volume has been placed in the high-velocity jet at the apex. There is a late-peaking high-velocity jet which is consistent with a small systolic gradient located close to the left ventricular apex.

Discussion

Hypertrophic cardiomyopathy primarily affecting the apex was first described in the Japanese in association with anterior and apical T-wave abnormalities on electrocardiography.[1] This pattern of hypertrophic cardiomyopathy is relatively uncommon in Europe.[2] Characteristically there is no systolic anterior motion of the mitral valve, because the papillary muscles are not usually involved in the hypertrophic process and therefore are not displaced into the left ventricular outflow tract. Because there is no left ventricular outflow tract obstruction, there is no mid-systolic closure of the aortic valve. The systolic gradient at the apex is late-peaking, and early diastolic apical flow towards the base may or may not be demonstrable. Occasionally in early diastole, when the free left ventricular wall initially separates from the septum at the onset of relaxation, there is a color flow Doppler signal close to the apex of the left ventricular cavity directed towards the base, indicating the release of blood trapped in the apex of the ventricle during systole. The optimal views to establish the diagnosis are the apical four-chamber and the apical long-axis planes combined with the Doppler signals at or within the apex.

Patients may be asymptomatic with this pattern but more often have exertional dyspnea secondary to diastolic dysfunction rather than to outflow obstruction. A variety of abnormalities of diastolic function have been reported in hypertrophic cardiomyopathy.[3,4]

This patient has remained asymptomatic. His siblings and child have been screened by echocardiography and no abnormalities were detected. Since the phenotypic manifestations of hypertrophic cardiomyopathy may not develop until adulthood, his child will require serial echocardiographic studies.[5]

References

1. Louie E, Maron B. Apical hypertrophic cardiomyopathy: clinical and two-dimensional echocardiographic assessment. Ann Intern Med 1987;106:663–70.

2. Klues H, Schiffers A, Maron B. Phenotypic spectrum and patterns of left ventricular hypertrophy in hypertrophic cardiomyopathy: morphologic observations and significance as assessed by two-dimensional echocardiography in 600 patients. J Am Coll Cardiol 1995;26:1699–708.

3. Severino S, Caso P, Galderisi M, et al. Use of pulsed Doppler tissue imaging to assess regional left ventricular diastolic dysfunction in hypertrophic cardiomyopathy. Am J Cardiol 1998;82:1394–8.

4. Spirito P, Maron B. Relation between the extent of left ventricular hypertrophy and diastolic filling abnormalities in hypertrophic cardiomyopathy. J Am Coll Cardiol 1990;15:808–13.

5. Fragola PV, Borzi M, Cannata D. The spectrum of echocardiographic and electrocardiographic abnormalities in nonaffected relatives of patients with hypertrophic cardiomyopathy: a transverse and longitudinal study. Cardiology 1993;83:289–97.

96

Complications of left ventricular assist device–right ventricular failure

Muredach P Reilly MB

A 55-year-old man with a 10-year history of dilated cardiomyopathy developed progressive cardiogenic shock despite maximal inotropic support while awaiting heart transplantation. He was taken to the operating room for urgent HeartMate TCI LVAD (left ventricular assist device) placement. The patient had preoperative coagulopathy due to hepatic dysfunction secondary to right heart failure. He received multiple perioperative blood transfusions. Intraoperative transesophageal echocardiography was performed during LVAD insertion.

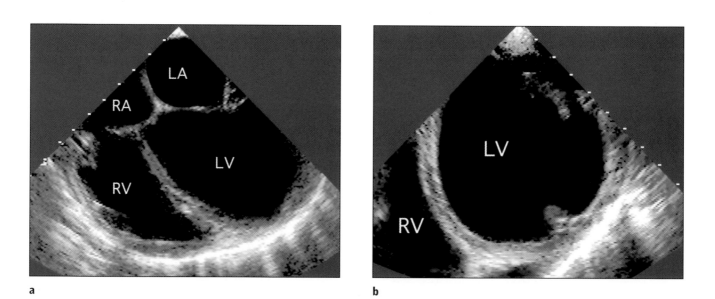

a   b

Figure 96.1
(a) Transesophageal echocardiogram in the transverse plane (imaging angle 0°). The four-chamber view demonstrates severe left ventricular (LV) dilatation and moderate right ventricular (RV) dilatation prior to LVAD placement. The left ventricular long axis is somewhat foreshortened in this view, but it is clear that the left ventricle is globular in shape. The valves are anatomically normal but the mitral valve demonstrates an incomplete closure pattern due to annular dilatation.
(b) Transgastric short-axis view in the transverse plane confirming severe left ventricular (LV) and right ventricular (RV) dilatation. The left ventricular dimension is greater than 7 cm and the ejection fraction was assessed as less than 10%.

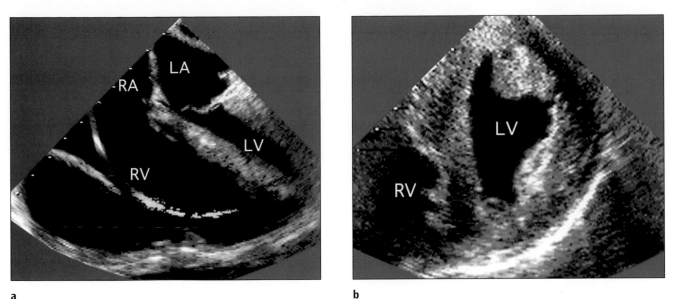

a
b

Figure 96.2

(a) Transesophageal echocardiogram in the transverse plane (imaging angle 0°), similar to Figure 96.1. Following LVAD placement the left ventricular cavity has been decompressed and is small and akinetic. There is now massive right venricular dilatation. The pulmonary artery catheter is present in the right atrium and ventricle.

(b) Transgastric short-axis view after LVAD placement confirming the marked reduction in left ventricular cavity size, now measuring less than 4 cm. The major portion of the right ventricular cavity is off the screen.

Despite LVAD placement the patient remained hypotensive, with high pulmonary artery pressures and low LVAD flow. Inhaled nitric oxide (NO) and intravenous prostaglandin E_1 and milrinone were administered for acute right ventricular failure with improvement in pulmonary pressures and LVAD flow. This was accompanied by a reduction in right ventricular size and improved right ventricular function as assessed by transesophageal echocardiography. Postoperatively, the patient was returned to the intensive care unit but developed elevation in pulmonary pressures, reduction in LVAD flows, and hypotension, despite an increased dose of inhaled NO. Emergency chest wall echocardiography was performed.

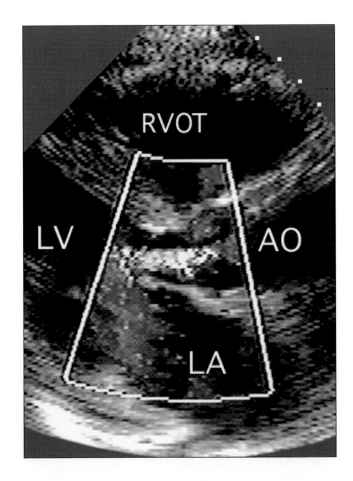

Figure 96.3

Parasternal long-axis view reveals the fact that the left ventricular cavity size is larger than it was immediately after the LVAD was placed. Furthermore, a moderate degree of previously undiagnosed aortic incompetence is present. This accounts for the inability of the LVAD to decompress the ventricle. The right ventricle remains dilated. Both ventricles appeared akinetic.

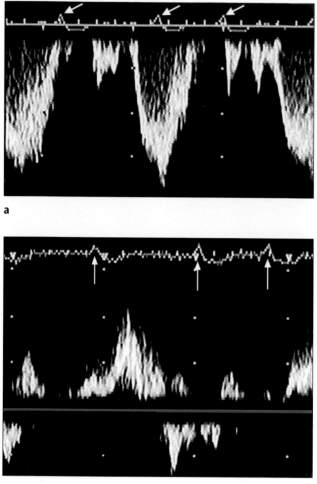

a

b

Figure 96.4
(a) Spectral display of pulsed-wave Doppler interrogation of the pulmonary valve from the parasternal position reveals flow that is asynchronous with cardiac electrical activity (arrows indicate QRS complex) but coincides with the respiratory rate, suggesting a totally failed, non-functioning right ventricle with passive filling.
(b) Spectral display of pulsed-wave Doppler across the tricuspid valve. Right ventricular filling does not occur during electrical diastole (arrows indicate QRS complex) but is related to the respiratory rate.

Discussion

Progressive heart failure with end-organ dysfunction despite maximal medical therapy is not uncommon (10–30%) in patients awaiting heart transplantation.[1] In this setting it is important to proceed to LVAD implantation prior to the development of multi-organ failure which is associated with a poor outcome despite LVAD support.[2]

Historically, acute right heart failure requiring RVAD placement occurred in 20–40% of LVAD recipients and was the leading cause of perioperative death in patients receiving LVAD support.[3,4] Transesophageal echocardiography during LVAD insertion is essential to assess the presence of this complication and to monitor cannula placement and function. The need for RVAD after LVAD placement has been reduced by the use of inhaled NO, a potent pulmonary vasodilator without significant systemic effects, which results in improved right heart function.[5,6] Perioperative hemorrhage and the need for blood transfusion, which may result in cytokine-mediated pulmonary hypertension, are major risk factors for the development of right-sided heart failure after LVAD placement.[7]

The presence of perioperative coagulopathy and bleeding, in addition to chronic pulmonary hypertension, placed this patient at increased risk of right heart failure after LVAD placement. The initial response to inhaled NO suggested that an RVAD would not be required. However, the subsequent intensive care unit course was notable for profound right ventricular dysfunction and new aortic regurgitation, which may have been unmasked by an LVAD-induced increased gradient across the valve due to a higher aortic diastolic pressure and a lower left ventricular diastolic pressure.[1] The acute reduction in end-organ perfusion resulted in rapid deterioration that did not respond to resuscitation attempts, including emergency RVAD placement.

References

1. Goldstein DJ, Oz MC, Rose EA. Implantable left ventricular assist devices. N Engl J Med 1998;339:1522–33.

2. Oz MC, Goldstein DJ, Pepino P, et al. Screening scale predicts patients successfully receiving long-term implantable left ventricular assist devices. Circulation 1995;92:II-169–73.

3. Frazier OH, Rose EA, Macmanus Q, et al. Multicenter clinical evaluation of the HeartMate 1000 IP left ventricular assist device. Ann Thorac Surg 1992;53:1080–90.

4. Oz MC, Argenziano M, Catanese KA, et al. Bridge experience with long-term implantable left ventricular assist devices. Are they an alternative to transplantation? Circulation 1997;95:1844–52.

5. Chen JM, Levin HR, Rose EA, et al. Experience with right ventricular assist devices for peri-operative right-sided circulatory failure. Ann Thorac Surg 1996;61:305–10.

6. Argenziano M, Choudhri AF, Moazami N, et al. Randomized, double-blind trial of inhaled nitric oxide in LVAD recipients with pulmonary hypertension. Ann Thorac Surg 1998;65:340–5.

7. Goldstein DJ, Seldomridge JA, Chen JM, et al. Use of aprotinin in LVAD recipients reduces blood loss, blood use, and perioperative mortality. Ann Thorac Surg 1995;59:1063–7.

97

Complications of left ventricular assist device–left ventricular thrombosis

Muredach P Reilly MB

A 56-year-old man with hypertension presented to an outside hospital with an anterior myocardial infarction and cardiogenic shock. He was taken directly to the cardiac catheterization laboratory where an intra-aortic balloon pump was placed, but angioplasty of his occluded left anterior descending artery was unsuccessful. He underwent emergency single-vessel bypass to the laft anterior descending artery but could not be weaned from bypass. An extracorporeal ABIOMED (ABIOMED Cardiovascular, Danvers, MA) left ventricular assist device

(LVAD) was placed via left atrial cannulation, and he was then successfully weaned from cardiopulmonary bypass and transferred to a heart transplantation center. There was extensive mediastinal bleeding in the postoperative period which required withholding of heparin and surgical re-exploration in the first 24 hours following implantation. Two days later the patient developed left hemiparesis and persistent reduction in LVAD flows associated with hypotension. Emergency transesophageal echocardiography was performed.

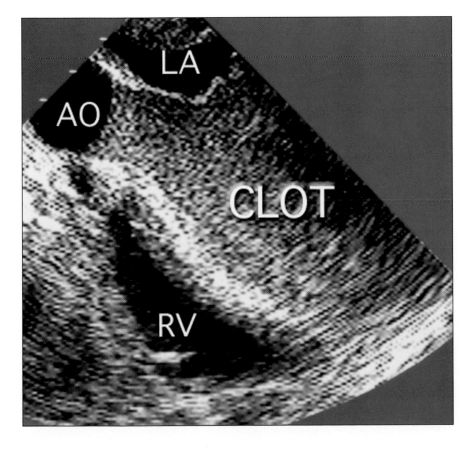

Figure 97.1
Transesophageal echocardiogram from the mid-esophagus in the transverse plane (imaging angle 0°). The modified four-chamber view demonstrates the left ventricle in long axis. The left ventricular outflow tract and a portion of the aortic root are demonstrated. The left ventricle is enlarged and completely obliterated by thrombus that extends into the left ventricular outflow tract. A separate thrombus is present in the left atrium (LA) which is decompressed, consistent with left atrial cannulation of the LVAD. The cannulation site is not imaged in this view. The right ventricle is normal in size and does not contain thrombus. A catheter is present within the right ventricle.

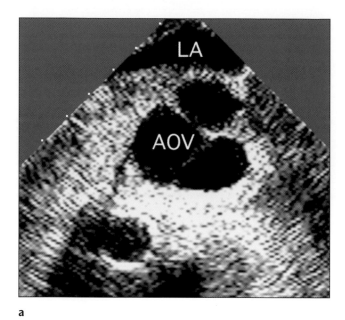

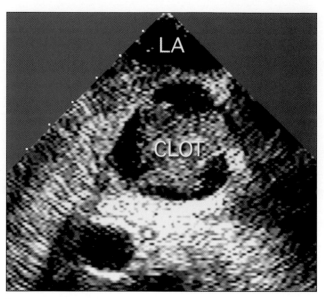

a   b

Figure 97.2
(a) Transesophageal image of the aortic valve from the mid-esophageal level (imaging angle 30°). In diastole, the aortic valve is closed and is trileaflet.
(b) Similar view in systole. The thrombus prolapses through the aortic valve which opens partially in systole.

The patient was returned to the operating room. The ABIOMED LVAD and a large amount of left atrial and left ventricular thrombus were carefully removed. An intracorporeal, Heartmate LVAD (Thermocardiosystems Inc., Woburn, MA) was placed via left ventricular apical cannulation.

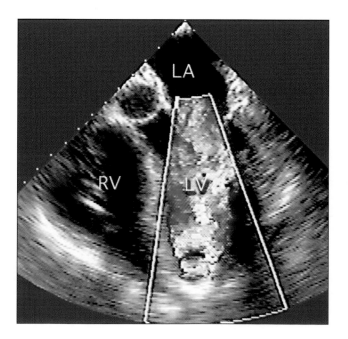

Figure 97.3
Intraoperative transesophageal echocardiogram with color Doppler flow imaging, from the mid-esophagus in the transverse plane (imaging angle 0°). The LVAD cannula has been placed at the left ventricular apex. The cannula itself is visualized only as a bright echodensity at the apex. However, the proximal flow convergence towards the cannulation site is visible at the apex.

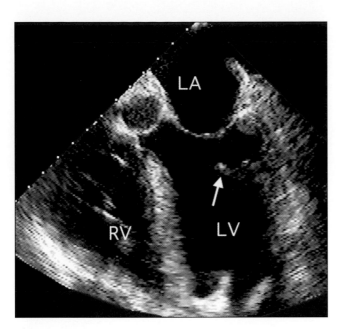

Figure 97.4
Similar view demonstrating residual thrombus (arrow) attached to the lateral wall of the left ventricle. The thrombus was mobile, but did not display the highly chaotic motion characteristic of pedunculated masses, because of the very abnormal flow pattern in the left ventricle.

Discussion

Increasing numbers of patients with end-stage heart failure are being supported with LVADs as a bridge to cardiac transplantation or recovery.[1] The success of the intracorporeal Heartmate TCI device has been partly due to the reduced incidence of thromboembolic events (approximately 4%) obviating the need for systemic anticoagulation in the long-term management of these patients.[2] Extracorporeal LVADs have been employed mainly as short-term support for postcardiotomy cardiogenic shock, and continue to be associated with significant heart-related thromboembolism (10–30%). Full systemic anticoagulation is therefore required.[3,4]

The extensive intracardiac thrombosis in this patient presumably obstructed LVAD inflow, resulting in decreased LVAD flows. Distal embolization of the thrombus resulted in stroke. Left ventricular blood stasis in the setting of recent extensive myocardial infarction and lack of anticoagulation in a patient with an extracorporeal LVAD may have precipitated thrombus formation. The diagnosis of left ventricular thrombosis by trans-esophageal echocardiography led to expeditious removal of thrombus and extracorporeal LVAD (under trans-esophageal echocardiography surveillance) and conversion to Heartmate TCI support, with subsequent successful transplantation.

We have recently examined the risk factors for LVAD-associated left ventricular thrombosis in consecutive patients ($n = 51$) receiving LVAD support at the Hospital of the University of Pennsylvania.[5] All cases ($n = 8$) of left ventricular thrombosis were seen in patients supported with short-term extracorporeal devices. Independent risk factors for left ventricular thrombosis included acute myocardial infarction prior to LVAD implantation, left atrial cannulation and post-implantation bleeding. Ischemic stroke was seen in seven of eight patients with left ventricular thrombosis. Despite this, most patients with LVAD-associated left ventricular thrombosis underwent successful transplantation following removal of thrombus and transition to Heartmate TCI devices. Left ventricular cannulation, when using short-term devices, combined with early transition to Heartmate TCI LVADs[6] may decrease the incidence of left ventricular thrombosis. Transesophageal echocardiography surveillance is essential in the management of these high-risk patients.

This patient's head computerized tomography scan demonstrated right parietal and left occipital cerebral infarcts. Postoperatively the patient's condition gradually improved and he underwent orthotopic heart transplantation 56 days later.

References

1. Goldstein DJ, Oz MC, Rose EA. Implantable left ventricular assist devices. N Engl J Med 1998;339:1522–33.

2. Slater JP, Rose EA, Levin HR, et al. Low thromboembolic risk without anticoagulation using advanced-design left ventricular assist devices. Ann Thorac Surg 1996;62:1321–8.

3. Korfer R, Elbanayosy A, Posival H, et al. Mechanical circulatory support. The Bad Oeynhausen experience. Ann Thorac Surg 1995;59;S56–63.

4. Guyton RA, Schonberger JP, Everts PA, et al. Post cardiotomy shock: clinical evaluation of the BVS-5000 biventricular support system. Ann Thorac Surg 1993;56:346–56.

5. Reilly MP, Wiegers SE, Cucchiara AJ, et al. Left ventricular assist-device associated ventricualr thrombosis: Risk factors and clinical outcomes. Am J Cardiol 2000 (in press).

6. DeRose JJ, Umana JP, Argenziano M, et al. Improved results for postcardiotomy cardiogenic shock with the use of implantable left ventricular devices. Ann Thorac Surg 1997;64:1757–63.

SECTION VIII

The Aortic Valve

98

Bicuspid aortic valve

Susan E Wiegers MD

Mild exercise intolerance brought this 35-year-old man to medical attention. He had known of a loud systolic murmur since childhood but had not been examined in 20 years. Physical examination revealed both a systolic ejection murmur and a holodiastolic murmur. The heart was enlarged and the peripheral circulation was hyperdynamic.

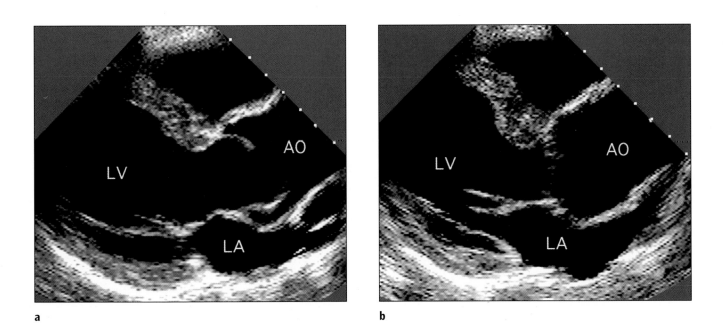

a   b

Figure 98.1
(a) Parasternal long-axis view in systole. Doming of the aortic valve leaflets within the dilated aortic root (AO) is demonstrated. The presence of doming and the unequal length of the leaflets are highly suggestive of a congenitally abnormal valve.
(b) In diastole, the eccentric coaptation point of the aortic valve is noted in the aortic root. This finding, on two-dimensional echocardiogram or on M-mode is again typical of a congenitally abnormal valve. Owing to severe aortic regurgitation (not seen in this figure), the aortic root is dilated and compresses the left atrium. This compression is not hemodynamically significant. The left ventricle (LV) is dilated. Comparison of the left ventricular diameter in diastole and systole indicates decreased fractional shortening.

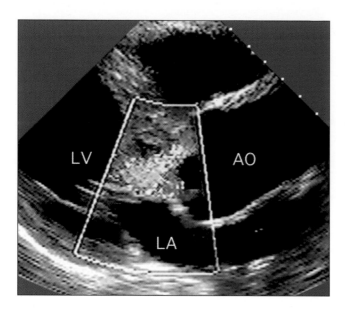

Figure 98.2
Parasternal long-axis view with color flow Doppler imaging in diastole. The turbulent, high-velocity jet of aortic regurgitation is seen as in the left ventricular outflow tract. The ratio of the height of the jet to the height of the outflow tract is approximately 40% consistent with moderately severe aortic regurgitation. This ratio must be measured at the level of the valve, since the regurgitation jet tends to splay out in the outflow tract and the diameter may increase further into the outflow tract.

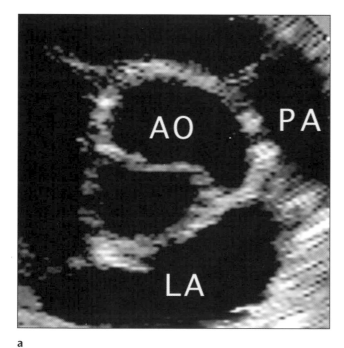

a

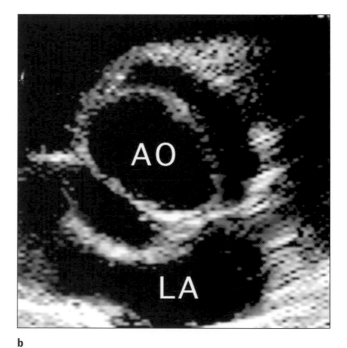

b

Figure 98.3
(a) Parasternal short-axis view in diastole. The aortic valve (AO) is bicuspid with a single, horizontal commissure. The coronary ostia are not well seen but both arise from the anterior sinus. Note that, in this valve, the normal sinus architecture is not seen. The usual arrangement of three sinuses of Valsalva is not present. Instead, the anterior sinus is abnormally large, and the posterior sinus is smaller.
(b) Parasternal short-axis view in systole. The typical ellipsoid shape of the orifice is identified. Incorrect angulation of the transducer may fail to image the three cusps of a normal aortic valve but the orifice is never made to appear ellipsoid with just two commissures. The configuration of this valvular orifice confirms the presence of a bicuspid aortic valve.

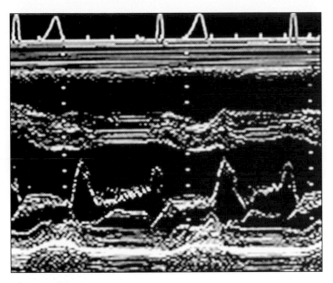

Figure 98.4
M-mode echocardiogram from the parasternal position. The mitral valve motion is well seen. High-frequency vibration of the mitral valve in diastole is diagnostic of significant aortic regurgitation. The mitral leaflets do not coapt until the QRS (seen at the top of the screen) has started. This indicates that early closure of the mitral valve is not present. When not caused by significant first-degree atrioventricular block, early closure of the mitral valve is a sign of acute decompensated aortic regurgitation.

Discussion

A bicuspid aortic valve is the most common congenital cardiac anomaly. The commissural arrangement is best described by the relation to the coronary ostia. In a valve with a horizontal commissure, both coronary ostia arise from the anterior sinus. With a vertical commissure, they arise from opposite sinuses. The horizontal arrangement is more common and more likely to calcify.[1] Accelerated stenosis of bicuspid valves is probably due to the normal ejection jets from the ventricle striking the abnormally arranged valve leaflets. All bicuspid valves are necessarily at least mildly regurgitant, but not necessarily stenotic.[2] Aortic regurgitation associated with a bicuspid aortic valve is more likely to be severe when discovered and to progress more rapidly than regurgitation in a congenitally normal valve.[3] The significant aortic regurgitation in this patient resulted in aortic root dilatation and thus in more severe aortic regurgitation.

In this case, significant aortic regurgitation had also resulted in left ventricular dilatation and decreased systolic function. The patient's symptoms were improved with diuresis and afterload reduction. However, because the decline in left ventricular function may be progressive and permanent, the patient underwent aortic valve replacement at this time.[4] This case illustrates the need for life-long surveillance once the diagnosis of bicuspid aortic valve is made. The need for antibiotic prophylaxis is ongoing. Serial echocardiographic exams will evaluate the presence of progressive aortic regurgitation or of premature calcification and stenosis. It should not be forgotten that there is a significant association between bicuspid aortic valve and coarctation of the aorta. Coarctation can be ruled out by imaging the proximal descending aorta from the suprasternal notch and sampling the velocities with pulsed-wave Doppler.

References

1. Beppu S, Suzuki S, Matsuda H, *et al*. Rapidity of progression of aortic stenosis in patients with congenital bicuspid aortic valves. Am J Cardiol 1993;71:322–7.

2. Pachulski R, Chan K. Progression of aortic valve dysfunction in 51 adult patients with congenital bicuspid aortic valve: assessment and follow up by Doppler echocardiography. Br Heart J 1993;69:237–40.

3. Padial LR, Oliver A, Vivaldi M, *et al*. Doppler echocardiographic assessment of progression of aortic regurgitation. Am J Cardiol 1997;80:306–14.

4. St John Sutton M, Plappert T, Hirshfeld J, *et al*. Assessment of left ventricular mechanics in patients with asymptomatic aortic regurgitation. Circulation 1984;69:259.

99

Moderate aortic regurgitation

Susan E Wiegers MD

A 55-year-old woman with hypertension had a history of a diastolic murmur. She was able to exercise vigorously and did not complain of any symptoms. An echocardiogram was performed to evaluate her left ventricular function and to follow the valvular lesion.

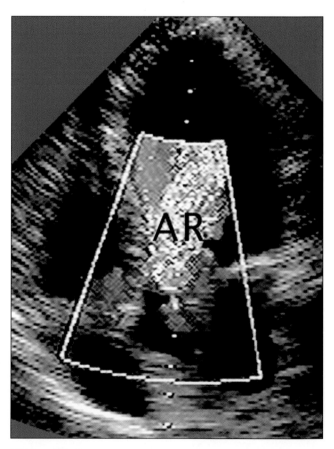

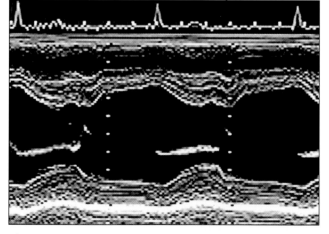

Figure 99.1
M-mode echocardiogram from the parasternal position. The left ventricle is dilated at 6 cm. The wall thickness is normal. The fractional shortening (LVID$_{diastole}$ −LVID$_{systole}$/LVID$_{diastole}$) is normal. The end-systolic dimension is 3.5 cm. A dense chord is visible in the center of the left ventricular cavity.

Figure 99.2
Apical five-chamber view with color flow Doppler display in diastole of the aortic regurgitation jet (AR). The high-velocity turbulent jet of aortic regurgitation arises from the level of the aortic valve and extends into the mid-left ventricular cavity. The spatial extent of the color disturbance is consistent with moderately severe aortic regurgitation. The left ventricular (LV) dilatation is noted in this view as well.

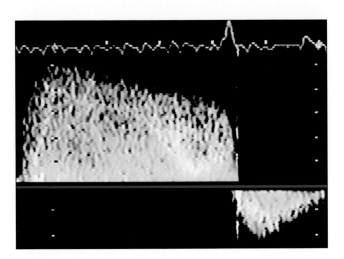

Figure 99.3
Spectral flow display of continuous-wave Doppler across the aortic valve. The aortic regurgitation is a positive jet above the baseline with a peak velocity of 5 m/s. The deceleration slope of the spectral envelope is 270 cm/s per second. A deceleration slope between 200 cm/s per second and 300 cm/s per second is predictive of moderate aortic regurgitation.

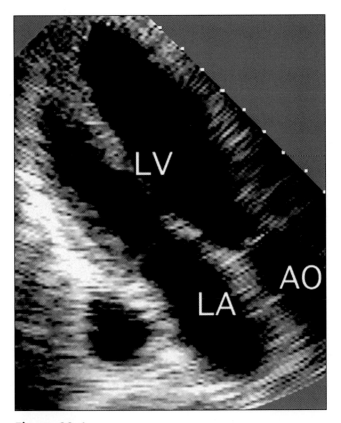

Figure 99.4
Apical long-axis view demonstrating an anomalous papillary muscle which is displaced apically. While of no clinical significance, apical papillary muscles have been mistaken for left ventricular tumors. The thick chordal attachment to the anterior mitral valve leaflet accounts for the dense interventricular echo on M-mode in Figure 99.1.

Discussion

Hypertension, with resultant aortic root dilatation, is one of the most common causes of aortic regurgitation. As the left ventricle adapts to the volume load, further enlargement of the chamber and the aortic root may occur. The parasternal long-axis is the best view in which to measure the size of the root. However, the apical five-chamber view (Figure 99.2) also demonstrates the mild root enlargement in this patient. The apical long-axis view does not usually demonstrate the aortic root well, because this structure is farther from the transducer than in the parasternal view.

The degree of aortic regurgitation continues to be qualitatively measured on echocardiography as well as aortography. The extent of the color Doppler jet into the left ventricular cavity has been correlated with angiographic grades of aortic regurgitation. Grade 1 (mild) regurgitant jets are present only in the left ventricular outflow tract immediately below the valve. Grade 2 extends to the tip of the mitral valve leaflets and Grade 3 (moderate) to the level of the papillary muscles tips. Grade 4 (severe) extends to the body of the papillary muscles or beyond. The jet in this case extends well into the ventricular cavity which is consistent with moderately severe aortic regurgitation. The deceleration slope is another method of estimating the severity of the aortic insufficiency.[1] The slope of the spectral envelope can be measured on-line with most ultrasound systems. A deceleration slope less than 200 cm/s per second is consistent with mild aortic regurgitation and a deceleration slope greater than 300 cm/s per second is considered to be severe aortic regurgitation. In this case, the deceleration slope of the spectral envelope of the aortic regurgitation is consistent with moderate aortic regurgitation. It is not uncommon for the qualitative measures of aortic regurgitation to disagree by a grade or more. The patient has a dilated ventricle which is best appreciated on the M-mode image in this study. The fractional shortening is preserved which indicates that the systolic function remains normal. However, the left ventricle is enlarged with a globular shape, commonly seen in hemodynamically significant aortic regurgitation.[2] In this patient, therefore, the aortic regurgitation appears to be moderately severe and is certainly the cause of the left ventricular remodeling.

Asymptomatic patients with severe aortic regurgitation should undergo aortic valve replacement if the left ventricular ejection fraction falls or the left ventricular end-systolic dimension reaches 50 mm or greater.[3] In this asymptomatic patient, neither is the case. However, it has recently been observed that these dimensions may not be appropriate when applied to women who have smaller left ventricular cavities and mass, based on their smaller body size.[4]

The anomalous papillary muscle in this study is an incidental finding but it is an important one to recognize. The nature of the apical mass can be determined by the attachment of the chords to the anterior mitral valve leaflet. The diagnosis is also confirmed by the echogenicity of the mass, which is identical to that of the surrounding myocardium, and the lack of any clear demarcation between the endocardium and the mass. However, it is the presence of the chordal attachments that is most helpful. This normal variant has not been associated with significant cardiac pathology or congenital abnormalities.

The patient was considered to have moderate to severe aortic regurgitation with no symptoms and no evidence of ventricular decompensation. Therefore, she was started on afterload reduction and will be followed with serial echocardiograms to evaluate ventricular size and function. She was educated about the symptoms of heart failure including orthopnea, exertional dyspnea and paroxysmal nocturnal dyspnea. She is being followed with the expectation that she will eventually require a valve replacement.

References

1. Labovitz A, Ferrara R, Kern M, *et al.* Quantitative evaluation of aortic insufficiency by continuous wave Doppler echocardiography. J Am Coll Cardiol 1986;8:1341–7.

2. Bonow R, Lakatos E, Maron B, *et al.* Serial long-term assessment of the natural history of asymptomatic patients with chronic aortic regurgitation and normal left ventricular systolic function. Circulation 1991;84:1625–35.

3. Tornos M, Olona M, Permanyer-Miralda G, *et al.* Clinical outcome of severe asymptomatic chronic aortic regurgitation: a long-term prospective follow-up study. Am Heart J 1995;130:333.

4. Klodas E, Enriquez-Sarano M, Tajik AJ, *et al.* Surgery for aortic regurgitation in women. Contrasting indications and outcomes compared with men. Circulation 1996;94:2472–8.

100

Aortic valve fibroelastoma

Monali Gupta MD

Susan E Wiegers MD

A 70-year-old woman, who was completely well, under-went stress echocardiography prior to starting an exercise program. A mass on the aortic valve was incidentally discovered. A transesophageal echocardiogram was performed to assess the mass. The patient had no history of fever, chills or systemic infection. She had no other medical problems and her physical examination was normal.

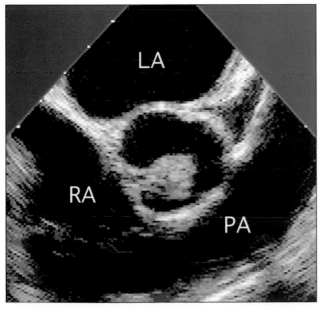

a

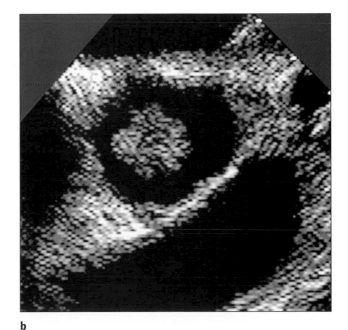

b

Figure 100.1

(a) Transesophageal echocardiogram from the mid-esophagus (imaging angle 40°). There is a large mass attached to the right coronary cusp of the aortic valve. This mass is lobulated and its edges were highly mobile. The commissure between the non-coronary and right coronary cusps is also thickened. The right ventricular outflow tract is imaged at the bottom of the screen. PA, pulmonary artery.

(b) Close-up image of the mass better demonstrates the lobulations with multiple small projections from the main portion of the mass. Both the lobes and the projections were highly mobile, a characteristic feature of this lesion.

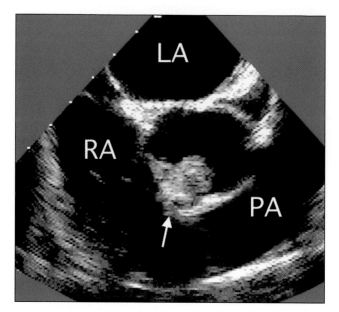

Figure 100.2

Transesophageal echocardiogram from the mid-esophagus in systole. A portion of the mass appears to engage the right coronary ostium (arrow). The attachment to the right coronary cusp is more evident in this view.

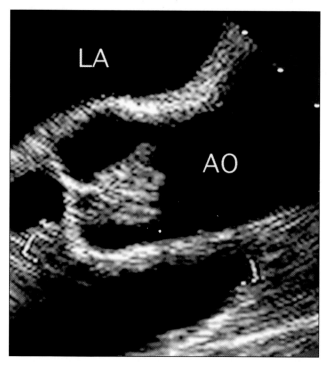

Figure 100.3

Transesophageal echocardiogram from the mid-esophagus in the longitudinal plane (imaging angle 135°). A thickened echodense stalk attaches the 1.5 cm by 1.2 cm mass to the right coronary cusp. In real time the edges of the mass were seen to be highly mobile, as was the entire mass. The leaflets themselves appear to be thickened but no significant aortic regurgitation was present.

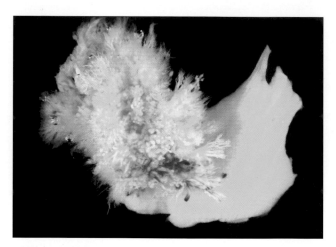

Figure 100.4

Gross histological view of the mass. The right aortic valve leaflet is shown with innumerable frond-like papillary projections. The entire mass measured 1.5 × 1.0 × 0.5 cm. A thin stalk (not demonstrated in this gross picture) attached it to the right coronary cusp.

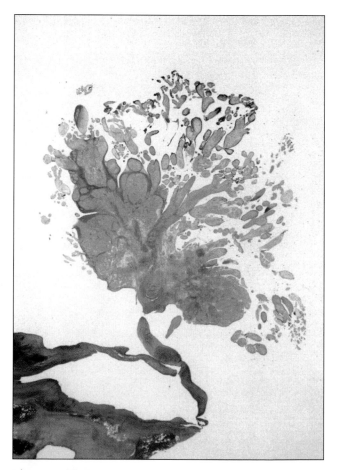

Figure 100.5

Low-power microscopic view (hematoxylin and eosin, ×1). Multiple homogeneous eosinophilic papillary projections contain loose connective tissue composed of collagen and elastic fibers, covered by a layer of endothelial cells.

Discussion

The echocardiographic and pathological findings are each diagnostic of fibroelastoma. These rare, benign lesions arise on the cardiac valves and consist of loose mucinous connective tissue with multiple fronds as seen on the gross pathology of this tumor. The nature of the tumor is not well understood but they are usually incidental findings rather than the cause of symptoms. The tumors generally arise in adulthood and may grow over many years.[1] Echocardiographically, fibroelastomas may resemble vegetations. However, the multiple projections which each exhibit chaotic motion are unusual for vegetations. It can be difficult to demonstrate the stalk attachment to the valve, since the stalk itself is thin and in constant motion, but the presence of a stalk is another argument against the mass being a vegetation. Most characteristically, fibroelastomas are generally present on the aortic side of the valve and are associated with surprisingly little valvular regurgitation even when quite large.[2] Both cerebral and systemic embolization have been reported[3,4] but most fibroelastomas are incidental findings on echocardiography or autopsy. Recurrence after excision has been reported and is due to incomplete removal of the lesion.

In this case, the size of the lesion and its proximity to the right coronary ostium led to the recommendation for surgical removal.[5] At surgery, a typical mass with multiple frond-like projections arose from the right coronary leaflet. The non-coronary and right coronary cusps were thickened and abnormal. Although the stalk attachment to the right coronary cusp was identified, there was concern that simple excision would not remove the entire lesion. Therefore, the patient underwent valve replacement.

References

1. Malik M, Sagar K, Wynsen J, et al. Evolution of a papillary fibroelastoma. J Am Soc Echocardiogr 1998;11:92–4.

2. Gopal A, Li Mandri G, King DL, et al. Aortic valve papillary fibroelastoma. A diagnosis by transthoracic echocardiography. Chest 1994;105:1885–7.

3. Etienne Y, Jobic Y, Houel JF, et al. Papillary fibroelastoma of the aortic valve with myocardial infarction: echocardiographic diagnosis and surgical excision. Am Heart J 1994;127:443–5.

4. Grote J, Mugge A, Schfers HJ, et al. Multiplane transoesophageal echocardiography detection of a papillary fibroelastoma of the aortic valve causing myocardial infarction. Eur Heart J 1995;16:426–9.

5. Howard R, Aleda G, Shapira O, et al. Papillary fibroelastoma: increasing recognition of a surgical disease. Ann Thorac Surg 1999;68:1881–5.

101

Radiation-induced valvular disease

Susan E Wiegers MD

An 87-year-old woman presented with a 1-year history of progressive dyspnea on exertion, and pedal edema. She had recently experienced two episodes of severe presyncope while scrubbing the floor. The patient had been generally well in recent years. Twenty years earlier she had received mantle radiation therapy for a lymphoma, which had not recurred.

On physical examination, she was comfortable at rest. Bibasilar pulmonary rales were auscultated. The neck veins were elevated with a rise in jugular venous pressure with inspiration. The PMI was not palpable. The heart sounds were quiet but a loud holosystolic murmur and a blowing diastolic murmur were present.

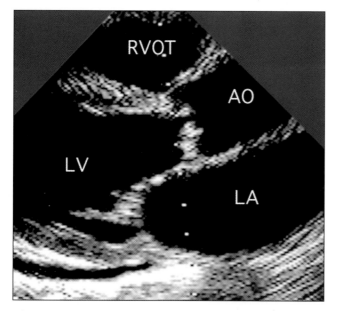

Figure 101.1
Parasternal long-axis view in early systole. The mitral valve is thickened, as are the subchordal structures. The aortic valve (AO) is also markedly thickened and opens poorly in systole consistent with significant aortic stenosis. A small pericardial effusion is present posterior to the left ventricle (LV). The two layers of the pericardium are markedly thickened. The pericardium is extremely echodense, suggesting calcification of the pericardium. LA, left atrium.

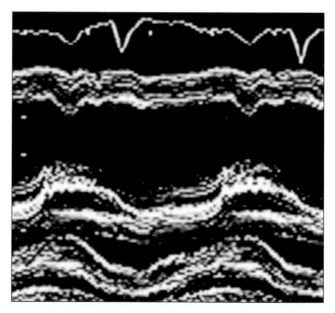

Figure 101.2
M-mode echocardiogram from the parasternal position at the level of the mitral valve. The mitral valve leaflets are severely thickened, with little separation between the two leaflets in diastole. There is paradoxical motion of the interventricular septum. The sharp posterior motion of the septum in early diastole is characteristic of constrictive pericarditis. The visceral pericardium is again noted to be markedly echodense. The posterior wall of the left ventricle, the visceral pericardium, and the parietal pericardium move together, indicating fusion of these structures.

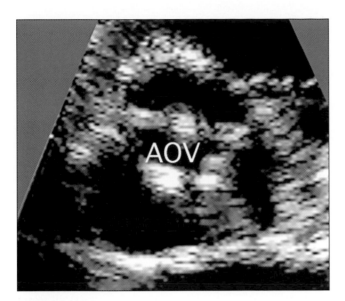

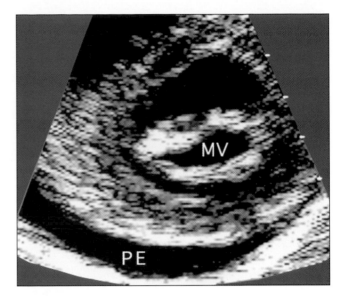

Figure 101.3

Parasternal short-axis view at the base of the heart. The close-up image of the aortic valve demonstrates the severe thickening of the aortic valve leaflets along the commissures and the abnormalities of the leaflets themselves. This systolic image demonstrates the markedly restricted motion of the aortic valve cusps which results in a severely stenotic aortic valve orifice (AOV).

Figure 101.4

Parasternal short-axis view of the mitral valve orifice (MV) which demonstrates the difference between this valvular abnormality and rheumatic disease. The leaflets are thickened and calcified. However, the commissures are not fused, as is particularly evident in the lateral commissure. The leaflet motion is restricted by the valvular thickening rather than the commissural fusion. The small posterior pericardial effusion (PE) is again evident between the two layers of the thickened pericardium.

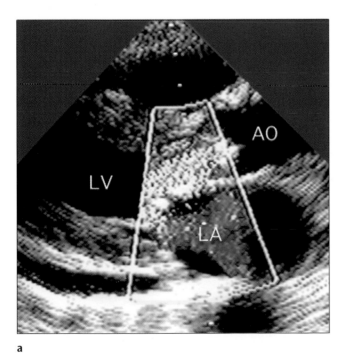

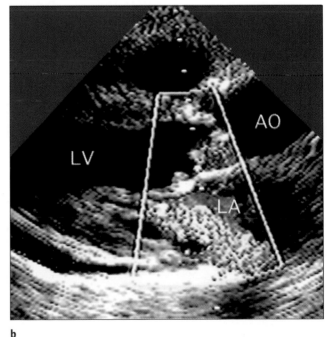

a   b

Figure 101.5

(a) Parasternal long-axis view with color flow Doppler imaging in diastole. A turbulent jet of aortic regurgitation fills the left ventricular outflow tract arising at the level of the aortic valve (AO). The aortic regurgitation is severe, as assessed by the width of the jet compared to the height of the outflow tract. The aortic valve leaflets were relatively fixed and did not coapt during diastole. (b) Similar view with color flow Doppler imaging in systole. There is a turbulent jet of mitral regurgitation arising from the mitral valve and extending into the left atrium (LA). The mitral valve and the sub-valvular apparatus are again seen to be thickened.

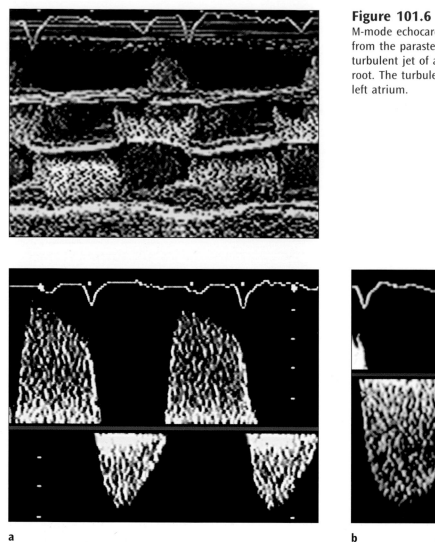

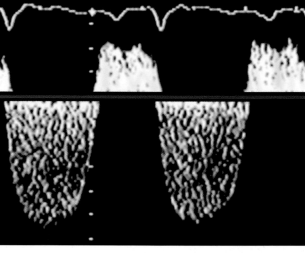

Figure 101.6
M-mode echocardiogram with color Doppler flow imaging from the parasternal position at the base of the heart. The turbulent jet of aortic regurgitation is seen within the aortic root. The turbulent jet of mitral regurgitation is seen in the left atrium.

a   b

Figure 101.7
(a) Spectral display of continuous-wave Doppler velocities from the apical position across the aortic valve. In diastole, the peak velocity of the aortic regurgitation is 4 m/s. The deceleration slope of the spectral envelope is steep (greater than 500 cm/s per second) which is consistent with severe aortic regurgitation. The peak systolic velocity across the valve is 2.8 m/s. Thus the peak aortic gradient is 31 mmHg.
(b) Spectral display of continuous-wave Doppler from the apical position across the mitral valve. In diastole, the peak velocity is slightly greater than 2 m/s and the deceleration slope is flat. This pattern is characteristic of significant mitral stenosis. The mitral regurgitation jet has a contour which is easy to distinguish from the aortic envelope. The spectral envelope of the mitral regurgitation is rounded and symmetric. The peak velocity is greater than 5 m/s which is typical for mitral regurgitation, reflecting the normal left ventricular–left atrial pressure gradient.

Discussion

Radiation therapy to the mediastinum commonly involves the cardiac structures. Acute radiation pericarditis has been reported. However, chronic changes are more common. All parts of the heart may be affected.[1] Constrictive and calcific pericarditis may occur. While pericardiectomy may relieve the constrictive physiology, this is high-risk surgery, owing to the difficulties in excising the thickened and adhesive pericardium from the epicardium while protecting the coronary vessels. The coronary arteries themselves are often involved in the fibrotic process. In one study, 15% of patients with mediastinal radiation developed thickened pericardium.[2] Coronary artery bypass surgery has been successfully performed in this situation, but it is technically challenging.

Significant myocardial fibrosis may develop over time in patients who have received over 3000 rad to the heart.[3] The right ventricle is more commonly affected than the left ventricle. Valvular fibrosis and calcification may also occur, but, in contrast, the aortic and mitral valves are more frequently affected than the right-sided valves. Restricted motion of the valves due to the fibrosis and calcification causes stenosis. Regurgitation may also develop in a fixed valve that is both stenotic and regurgitant. Up to 25% of patients may have valvular regurgitation on long-term follow-up. Women appear to be more susceptible to the radiation effects than men.[2] In one study, asymptomatic valvular disease was detected on average 11.5 years after mediastinal radiation, while symptomatic disease was detected by echocardiography an average of 16 years after the treatment. There was evidence in these patients of progression of the valvular lesions over time, with fibrosis and calcification of the valves.[4] Valve replacement can be very technically difficult in these patients. Radiation fibrosis results in massive adhesions, which hinder dissection of the cardiac structures. Seating of a prosthetic valve may also be difficult,

owing to severe annular calcification. Radiation changes in the cardiac tissues render suturing with usual techniques difficult or impossible. This patient would have required double valve replacement for definitive repair, but the surgery was judged to be too risky and she was treated medically.

References

1. Veeragandham R, Goldin M. Surgical management of radiation-induced heart disease. Ann Thorac Surg 1998;65:1014–19.

2. Lund M, Ihlen H, Voss B, et al. Increased risk of heart valve regurgitation after mediastinal radiation for Hodgkin's disease: an echocardiographic study. Heart 1996;75:591–5.

3. Veinot J, Edwards W. Pathology of radiation-induced heart disease: a surgical and autopsy study of 27 cases. Hum Pathol 1996;27:766–73.

4. Carlson R, Normann S, Alexander J. Radiation-associated valvular disease. Chest 1991;99:538–45.

102

Aortic valve ring abscess

Susan E Wiegers MD

A 40-year-old woman had become acutely ill with spiking fevers and malaise 2 to 3 days before admission. She had a long history of frequent and recent intravenous drug use.

The patient was tachypneic and diaphoretic. Her temperature was 102.5°F and she was tachycardic to 130 bpm. There were bilateral rales. The PMI was diffuse. A ventricular gallop and a soft, short diastolic murmur were audible. She was treated with vancomycin and gentamycin after the appropriate cultures were taken. Initially, the pulmonary congestion responded slightly to diuresis, but she developed increasing pulmonary edema the night of admission. Echocardiography confirmed the diagnosis of aortic valve endocarditis with severe, acute aortic regurgitation. Owing to hemodynamic instability, she was taken to the operating room the morning following admission.

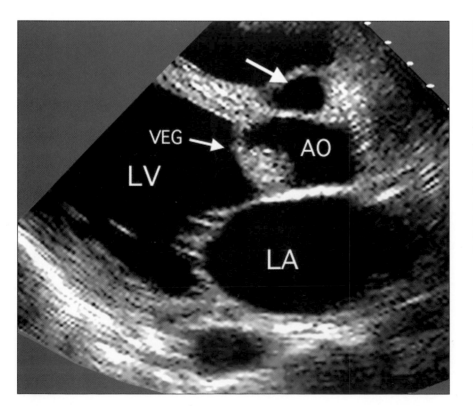

Figure 102.1
Parasternal long-axis view from a high parasternal window. The left ventricle (LV) is slightly dilated. The aortic valve is markedly abnormal. The anterior leaflet (right coronary cusp) prolapses into the left ventricular outflow tract. There is a large mass consistent with a vegetation (VEG) on the ventricular surface of the more posterior leaflet. This vegetation was attached to the left coronary cusp and measures approximately 12 mm by 20 mm. An echolucent structure anterior to the aortic root is highly suspicious for an abscess cavity (large arrow).

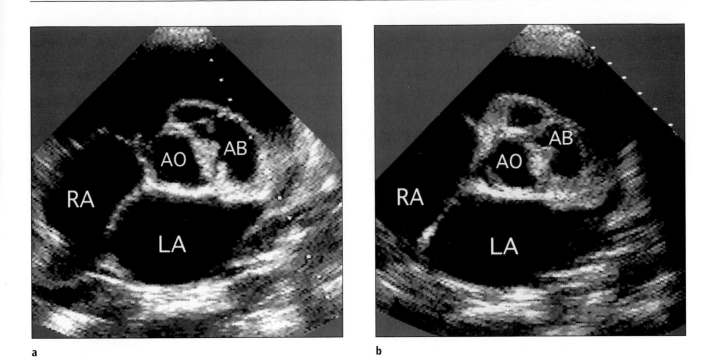

a   **b**

Figure 102.2
(a) Parasternal short-axis view at the base of the heart. This cross-section is taken superior to the plane of the aortic valve leaflets. The normal architecture of the aortic root (AO) is distorted by the large abscess cavity (AB) which surrounds it anteriorly. The normal shape of the three sinuses of Valsalva can be identified, although the large vegetation on the non-coronary cusp extends to this level (not marked). The abscess cavity is much larger than the root itself and could be mistakenly identified as an enlarged root. The abscess surrounds approximately 50% of the aortic annulus anteriorly. Large septa are seen within the cavity. The walls of the abscess are thickened, particularly the portion near the left atrial appendage.
(b) Superior angulation of the transducer demonstrates the extent of the abscess cavity which was not appreciated on the long-axis view. The abscess measures 6 cm by 2.3 cm and contains debris and several septa. There was no flow in the cavity itself demonstrated by color flow Doppler. LA, left atrium; RA, right atrium.

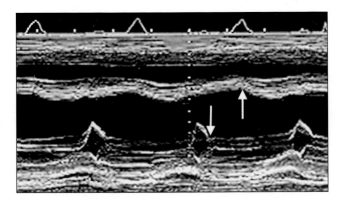

Figure 102.3
M-mode echocardiogram from the parasternal view at the level of the mitral valve. The left ventricle is dilated and, even at this level, it is apparent that the fractional shortening is reduced. Mitral valve motion is abnormal, with pronounced early closure of the valve. The first arrow demonstrates the time at which the mitral valve leaflets close. The second arrow represents the onset of mechanical systole, at which point the mitral valve normally closes. Note that mechanical systole, evidenced by posterior motion of the interventricular septum, begins a short time after electrical systole or the onset of the QRS complex at the top of the screen. Premature mitral valve closure is diagnostic, in the absence of marked first-degree atrioventricular block, of decompensated aortic insufficiency. The left ventricular diastolic pressure rises rapidly, owing to the regurgitant volume. The left atrial pressure is exceeded long before ventricular systole and the mitral valve closes prematurely.

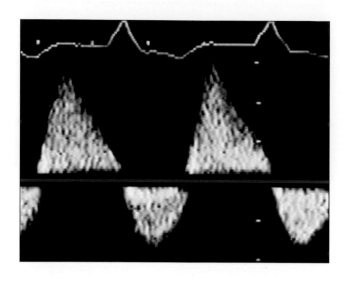

Figure 102.4
Continuous-wave Doppler spectral flow velocities across the aortic valve recorded from the apical position (each vertical mark represents 1 m/s). The diagnosis of severe aortic insufficiency is confirmed by the Doppler tracing. The peak velocity of the diastolic aortic insufficiency is only 3 m/s representing an initial diastolic gradient of only 36 mmHg across the aortic valve. The normal velocity of compensated aortic insufficiency is at least 4 m/s, owing to a usual initial diastolic gradient of more than 60 mmHg across the aortic valve. The extremely rapid deceleration slope of the aortic regurgitant jet is consistent with severe aortic insufficiency.

Discussion

Aortic annular abscess has been found to be a frequent complication of aortic valve endocarditis. While transthoracic echocardiography is fairly insensitive to the diagnosis, this abscess was so large that transesophageal echocardiography was not necessary to establish the diagnosis. Thickening of the aortic root to more than 3 mm on transthoracic studies should raise the question of valve ring abscess in the appropriate setting. However, even in cases in which the diagnosis is unequivocal, transesophageal echocardiography may demonstrate fistulous connections of the abscess cavity to the atria or the left ventricular outflow tract.[1] The new criteria for the diagnosis of endocarditis depends on the finding of characteristic vegetations on an echocardiogram as well as the previously accepted criteria of positive blood cultures and embolic lesions. Intraoperative transesophageal echocardiography is essential as well, to evaluate the postoperative results and the presence of remaining abscess cavity or fistulous connections. The diagnosis of aortic valve ring abscess carries an extremely poor prognosis, with some centers reporting a mortality of up to 45%.[2]

Acute severe aortic regurgitation is a poorly tolerated lesion. The peak velocity of the aortic regurgitation jet was 3 m/s. Thus the gradient between the aortic root and the left ventricle at the onset of diastole was only 36 mmHg. If the systemic diastolic pressure were 60 mmHg, this would represent an initial left ventricular diastolic pressure of 24 mmHg. The rapid deceleration slope of the aortic regurgitant envelope is evidence that the diastolic gradient falls to near zero by the end of diastole. In other words, the pressure difference between the aortic root and left ventricle equilibrates. The left ventricle does not have time to remodel in response to the overwhelming volume load, and depressed left ventricular function results. The finding of premature mitral valve closure heralds hemodynamic collapse.

This patient's blood cultures grew *Staphylococcus aureus* after 12 hours of incubation. Because of her deteriorating status, she was taken to the operating room. Extensive debridement of the aortic root was required and an aortic valve homograft was placed. The coronaries were reimplanted as buttons. The patient received intravenous antibiotic therapy for 6 weeks in a monitored setting because she was not a candidate for unsupervised use of central venous access. She was also enrolled in a drug rehabilitation program.

References

1. Afridi I, Apostolidou M, Saad R, *et al*. Pseudoaneurysms of the mitral–aortic intervalvular fibrosa: dynamic characterization using transesophageal echocardiographic and Doppler techniques. J Am Coll Cardiol 1995;25:137–45.

2. Leung D, Cranney G, Hopkins A, *et al*. Role of transoesophageal echocardiography in the diagnosis and management of aortic root abscess. Br Heart J 1994;72:175–81.

103

Calcific aortic stenosis

Susan E Wiegers MD

An 85-year-old woman had a heart murmur that had been diagnosed as calcific aortic stenosis 4 years earlier. At that time, the aortic valve area was estimated at 1.2 cm². She had been well and had undergone a total hip replacement at the age of 83 without complications. In the several months before her most recent hospitalization, she had noticed substernal chest pressure when walking through the grocery store. She saw her primary care physician who noted a blood pressure of 150/78 mmHg. She had a III/VI systolic ejection murmur, which was late peaking and radiated to the left carotid. S_2 was single. There were no diastolic murmurs or gallops. An electrocardiogram showed normal sinus rhythm, left ventricular hypertrophy with repolarization changes, inferior Q waves and left atrial abnormality. The inferior Q waves were new compared to the previous tracing from 4 years earlier. An echocardiogram was performed to assess her aortic valve.

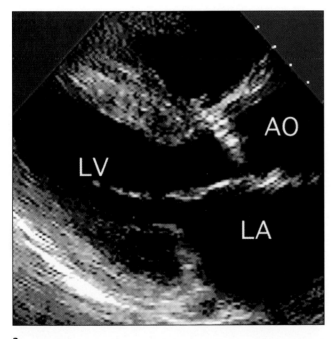

a

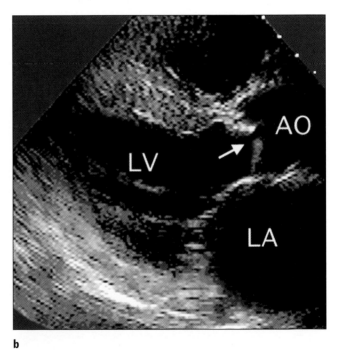

b

Figure 103.1
(a) Parasternal long-axis view in diastole. The left atrium is dilated. The left ventricular chamber is normal in diameter. There is moderate left ventricular hypertrophy which appears to involve the interventricular septum more than the posterior wall. The posterior mitral valve leaflet is thickened and the anterior leaflet is normal. The aortic valve is heavily calcified. The aortic root (AO) is normal in dimension but the ascending aorta is dilated.
(b) Parasternal long-axis view in systole. The aortic valve opens slightly and the very small orifice (arrow) is identified. The leaflets do not dome but have markedly restricted motion and are calcified and thickened. The left atrium is enlarged. The interventricular septum thickens normally, but the posterior wall at the base is severely hypokinetic. The distal posterior wall appears to have normal systolic function.

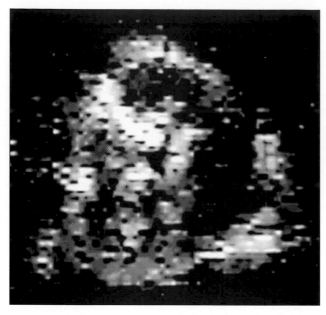
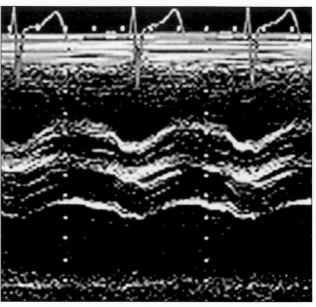

a   b

Figure 103.2

(a) Close-up view of the aortic valve from the parasternal short-axis view. The valve is trileaflet with normal sinuses of Valsalva. There is severe calcification of the cusps along the commissures and at the bases of the leaflets. This systolic frame shows the maximum opening of the aortic valve.

(b) M-mode echocardiogram from the parasternal position of the aortic valve and left atrium. The coaptation point of the aortic valve is in the middle of the aortic root. However, the systolic opening is severely restricted and appears as a small slit in the center of the aortic root.

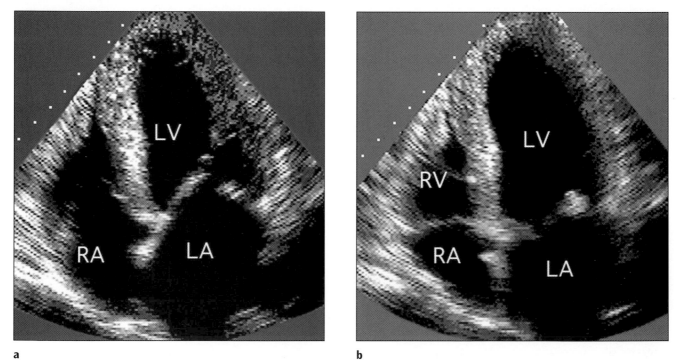

a   b

Figure 103.3

(a) Apical four-chamber view in diastole. The left atrium is dilated. The left and right ventricular cavities are normal but there is moderate left ventricular hypertrophy. There is no evidence of asymmetric septal hypertrophy in this view.

(b) Similar view later in diastole. The mitral valve is thickened and the mitral annular calcification is brought into view in this image. In real time, the overall left ventricular systolic function was moderately reduced, with an estimated ejection fraction of 40%.

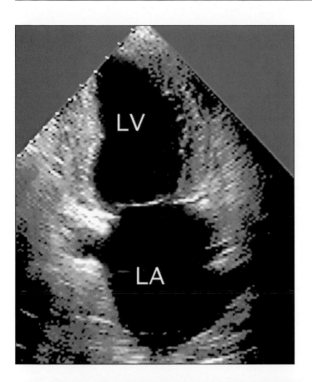

Figure 103.4
Apical two-chamber view in systole. The inferior wall is thinner than the anterior wall and the inferior wall did not contract at the base. The scalloping of the inferior wall is clearly visible in this image. The left atrium is dilated. The coronary sinus is cut obliquely and looks enlarged. It appears as an outpouching of the left atrium to the left of the image.

Figure 103.5
(a) Close-up image of the left ventricular outflow tract from the parasternal long-axis view. The outflow tract measures 2.1 cm in diameter.
(b) Spectral display of pulsed-wave Doppler from the apical view. The sample volume is in the left ventricular outflow tract. Digitization of the spectral display yielded a velocity–time integral of 19 cm.
(c) Continuous-wave Doppler across the aortic valve from the apical position. The peak velocity is 4.2 m/s. The velocity–time integral is 85 cm.
(d) Continuous-wave Doppler from the second right intercostal space. The signal was obtained using the non-imaging Doppler transducer. The systolic signal is positive as the ejection jet travels in the ascending aorta towards the transducer.

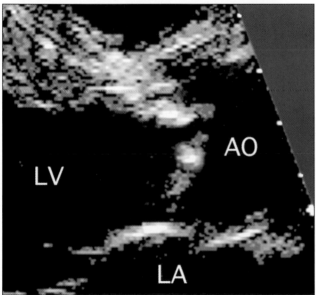

a

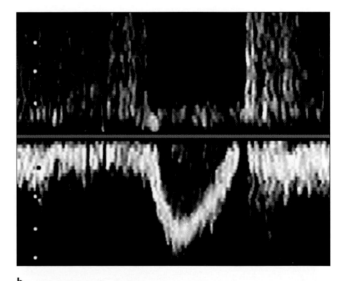

b

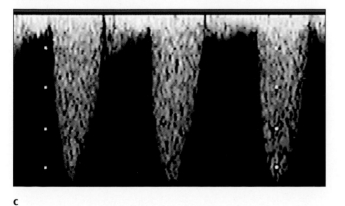

c

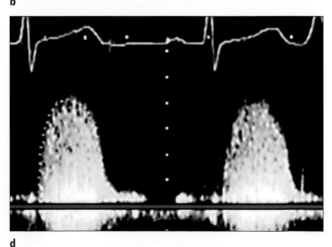

d

Discussion

The echocardiogram provided two reasons for this patient's anginal symptoms. Coronary artery disease is surely present, as there is an inferior wall motion abnormality. Additionally, severe aortic stenosis may cause exertional angina in the absence of epicardial artery disease. This patient had severe aortic stenosis with an aortic valve area of 0.7 cm². This is calculated using the continuity equation:

$$AVA = (D_{LVOT}/2)^2 \times \pi \times VTI_{LVOT}/VTI_{AO}$$

where AVA is the aortic valve area, D_{LVOT} is the diameter of the left ventricular outflow tract measured in the parasternal long-axis view, VTI_{LVOT} is the velocity–time interval of the pulsed-wave Doppler spectral envelope of the left ventricular outflow and VTI_{AO} is the velocity–time interval of the continuous-wave Doppler spectral envelope across the aortic valve. In this case the values obtained in Figure 103.5 can be substituted into the equation, giving:

$$AVA = (2.1/2)^2 \times 3.14 \times 18/85 = 0.7 \text{ cm}^2$$

The patient has critical aortic stenosis despite only moderately severe gradients. The continuity equation takes into account the decreased systolic function in the form of the left ventricular outflow tract velocity–time integral. The gradient across the aortic valve is dependent on flow as well as orifice area, a dependency that the continuity equation attempts to eliminate. The highest values of aortic and left ventricular outflow velocity–time integrals should be used. The Pedoff transducer has a smaller footprint than the imaging transducers. While adequate signals from the suprasternal notch can be difficult to obtain in many adults, the second right intercostal space often yields the highest velocities, as the jet may be highly eccentric.

Left ventricular hypertrophy gradually develops as the obstruction to outflow progresses with worsening degrees of aortic stenosis. There is individual variation in the degree and pattern of the hypertrophy.[1] Asymmetric hypertrophy in response to aortic stenosis can occur particularly in elderly patients with disproportionate septal hypertrophy. In this patient, the interventricular septum is significantly thicker than the posterior wall in the parasternal long-axis view. At first glance it appears that this may be due to an asymmetric pattern of hypertrophy in response to severe aortic stenosis. However, the systolic frame offers the true explanation for the difference in wall thickness. The posterior wall is thinned and hypokinetic, owing to a previous infarction. The other walls have hypertrophied in response to the pressure load.

The patient underwent cardiac catheterization with confirmation of the aortic valve area and demonstration of an occluded right coronary artery and important stenoses of the left anterior descending and circumflex arteries. Although the patient wished to avoid surgery, valvuloplasty was considered to be a poor alternative.[2] She underwent aortic valve replacement and four-vessel coronary bypass grafting. She was discharged on the 14th hospital day and after 3 months had returned to her previous level of functioning with relief of her anginal symptoms.

References

1. Carroll JD, Carroll EP, Feldman T, et al. Sex-associated differences in left ventricular function in aortic stenosis of the elderly. Circulation 1992;86:1099–107.
2. Lieberman EB, Bashore TM, Hermiller JB, et al. Balloon aortic valvuloplasty in adults: failure of procedure to improve long-term survival. J Am Coll Cardiol 1995;26:1522–8.

104

Aortic valve endocarditis and annular abscess

Susan E Wiegers MD

A 56-year-old man developed a urinary tract infection. Review of systems indicated that the patient had had pneumaturia on several occasions. His urine was foul smelling. Evaluation demonstrated a colonic–vesicular fistula with passage of small amounts of stool into the urinary bladder. This was eventually found to be due to a colon carcinoma that had eroded the bladder wall. The patient was treated with intravenous antibiotics but blood cultures remained positive for group D streptococcus. A transthoracic echocardiogram demonstrated aortic regurgitation but was technically limited. No vegetations were seen. When the patient remained febrile and moderately ill, a transesophageal echocardiogram was performed to evaluate the aortic valve with the concern that the patient had endocarditis.

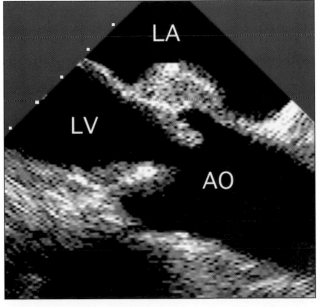

a

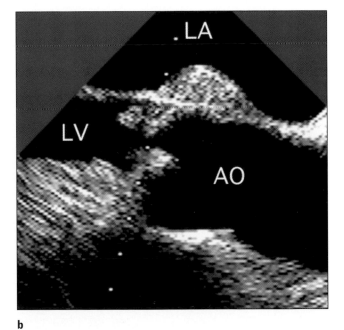

b

Figure 104.1
(a) Transesophageal echocardiogram in systole at the level of the mid-esophagus (imaging plane 130°). The ascending aorta (AO) is normal. The aortic valve leaflets are thickened, but no discrete mass is seen in this view. The left ventricular outflow tract (LV) also appears normal. There is an abnormal thickening of the posterior aortic root between the left sinus of Valsalva and the left atrium (LA).
(b) Similar transesophageal image in diastole. The aortic valve leaflets now appear more focally thickened. A mass is attached to the ventricular surface of the more posterior aortic valve leaflet (at the top of the screen) which is the non-coronary cusp. The vegetation prolapses into the left ventricular outflow tract in diastole. The marked thickening of the posterior root, suggestive of an abscess, is again seen.

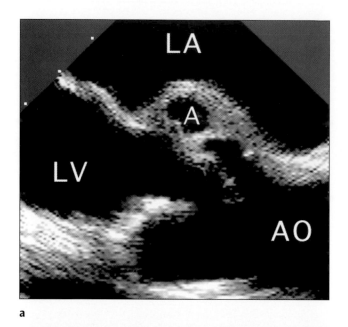

a

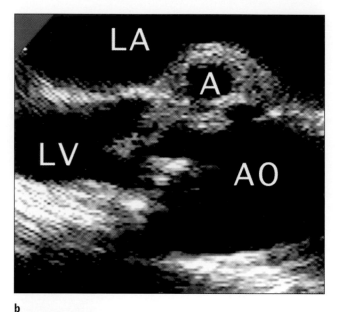

b

c

Figure 104.2

(a) Transesophageal echocardiogram from the level of the mid-esophagus in the same imaging plane (imaging angle approximately 130°) with the transducer rotated more towards the left of the patient than in Figure 104.1. An echolucent area (A) is evident within the thickened posterior root. This periannular cavity is highly suspicious for an abscess.

(b) Close-up image in diastole from the same orientation as (a). The more anterior aortic valve leaflet (seen towards the bottom of the screen) is the right coronary cusp. It is abnormal and markedly thickened at the tip, owing to an attached vegetation. The more posterior aortic valve leaflet, the left coronary cusp, is also thickened and prolapses with its attached vegetation into the left ventricular outflow tract. The thickening of the left coronary cusp extends to the base of the leaflet. Even in the absence of visualization of an abscess cavity, the presence of vegetation involving the base of the leaflet suggests involvement of the aortic valve ring.

(c) Similar diastolic frame as in (b) with color Doppler flow imaging. A turbulent jet of aortic regurgitation (AR) is present in the left ventricular outflow tract. In this view it appears that the regurgitation is not central but arises from the abscess cavity itself at the posterior commissure. The eccentric jet courses along the anterior mitral valve leaflet.

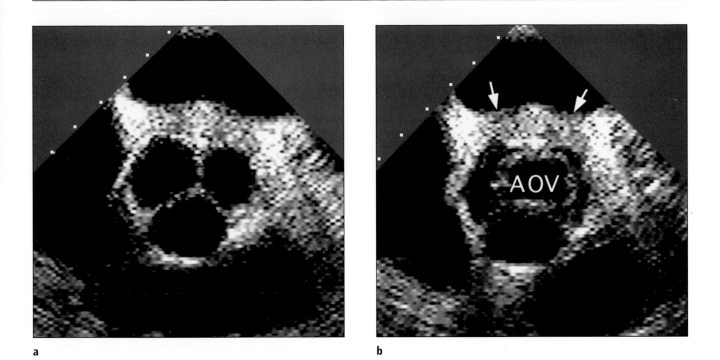

a   b

Figure 104.3

(a) Transesophageal echocardiogram from the level of the mid-esophagus of the aortic valve in diastole (imaging plane 33°). At this level the aortic valve leaflets themselves appear to be normal, although the thickening of the posterior root is again evident. (b) In systole and with advancement of the transducer slightly into the esophagus, the marked abnormality of the aortic valve is apparent. The edges of the leaflet are thickened, and severe thickening of the posterior annulus is again noted (arrows). The normal thickness of the aortic root is 3 mm or less. It is clear here that the posterior root measures over 1 cm.

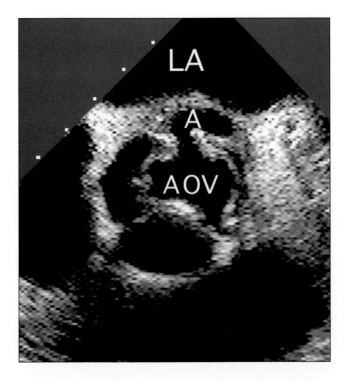

Figure 104.4

Transesophageal echocardiographic image from the level of the mid-esophagus of the aortic valve. The imaging plane is approximately 30°. This cross-section is taken just above the level of the aortic valve leaflets. The communication between the aortic root and the abscess cavity (A) is evident by the discontinuity leading from the aortic valve orifice (AOV) into the abscess cavity. The mechanism by which the aortic regurgitation appeared to arise from the abscess cavity as seen in Figure 104.2c is now evident. Note the shaggy abnormalities along the edges of the aortic valve leaflets which are vegetations.

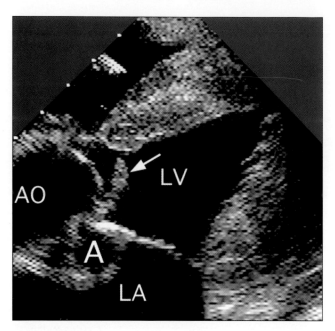

Figure 104.5
Transgastric image of the left ventricular outflow tract and aortic root (AO). The abscess cavity (A) between the left atrium (LA) and the aortic root is well seen. In addition, a large mass (arrow) prolapses into the left ventricle (LV) in diastole. This mass represents a vegetation attached to a prolapsing leaflet. The patient had longstanding hypertension prior to the development of his acute cardiac condition, and left ventricular hypertrophy is evident in this view.

Discussion

Transesophageal echocardiography is much more sensitive than transthoracic studies for the diagnosis of aortic annular abscess associated with endocarditis.[1] Thickening of the aortic root wall to more than 3 mm and involvement of the base of the aortic valve leaflet are signs that may be appreciated on transthoracic study and indicate the need for transesophageal echocardiography. In our laboratory, the final report of studies done to 'rule out endocarditis' indicate that endocarditis cannot be ruled out by transthoracic echocardiography and that transesophageal echocardiography should be done if clinically indicated.

Even on transesophageal echocardiography, vegetations and abscess cavities may be difficult to visualize. Initially, the aortic valve appeared to be normal on this patient's transesophageal study. The use of an omniplane probe and a careful and systematic examination are important to evaluate the possibility of endocarditis and

its complications. Perivalvular cavities seen on transesophageal studies may be abscess of the intervalvular fibrosa or may represent pseudoaneurysm. Echolucent cavities which demonstrate systolic expansion and diastolic collapse are more likely to represent pseudoaneurysms.[2] Pseudoaneurysms are more likely to be due to weakening of the wall of the aortic root by the infection with resultant dissection and rupture, rather than rupture of an already formed abscess cavity.[3] The pseudoaneurysms may rupture into the left ventricular outflow tract or into the left atrium. In either case, continuous flow will be visualized by color Doppler flow imaging. Abscess cavities are generally smaller than pseudoaneurysms and contain shaggy echodensities such as were seen in the areas of posterior root thickening in this patient. In general, they are not pulsatile. On occasion abscess cavities may be very large and obstruct a coronary artery.[4]

This patient probably had a primary abscess cavity that ruptured. Such an infection has a very low likelihood of responding to medical therapy and the disintegration of the intervalvular skeleton may continue despite antibiotics. In addition to these considerations, this patient had significant perivalvular aortic regurgitation. However, the colon carcinoma was presumed to be the source of his group D streptococcal bacteria. It was considered unwise to place a prosthetic heart valve in a patient with an ongoing risk of bacteremia. Luckily, the patient was hemodynamically stable. He underwent resection of the colon carcinoma and repair of the fistula, followed 3 weeks later by aortic valve replacement with a composite graft of the ascending aorta and reimplantation of the coronary arteries. He received a total of 6 weeks of intravenous antibiotics and is doing well 5 years later.

References

1. Daniel W, Mugge A, Martin R, et al. Improvement in the diagnosis of abscesses associated with endocarditis by transesophageal echocardiography. N Engl J Med 1991;324:795–800.

2. Afridi I, Apostolidou MA, Saad RM, et al. Pseudoaneurysms of the mitral–aortic intervalvular fibrosa: dynamic characterization using transesophageal echocardiographic and Doppler techniques. J Am Coll Cardiol 1995;25:137–45.

3. Tingleff J, Egeblad H, Gotzsche CO, et al. Perivalvular cavities in endocarditis: abscesses versus pseudoaneurysms? A transesophageal Doppler echocardiographic study in 118 patients with endocarditis. Am Heart J 1995;130:93–100.

4. Schlaifer JD, Martin TD, Hill JA, et al. Coronary artery obstruction caused by perivalvular abscess in aortic valve endocarditis. Am Heart J 1996;131:413–16.

105

Severe aortic regurgitation in a hypertensive patient

Susan E Wiegers MD

An 84-year-old man with a history of longstanding and poorly controlled hypertension went to see a new doctor for a complete physical examination. The patient had increasing difficulty caring for his wife who was ill, and he had recently developed pitting edema as well as dyspnea on exertion. Other medical problems included moderate renal insufficiency and chronic obstructive pulmonary disease. On physical examination his blood pressure was 170/60 mmHg with a pulse of 90 bpm. Rales were heard through the basilar half of the lung fields bilaterally. The cardiac impulse was laterally displaced. S_1 was normal and S_2 was normal. There was a III/VI holosystolic murmur heard at the apex and a II/VI systolic ejection murmur heard at the right upper sternal border. In addition, a loud blowing diastolic murmur was audible along the left lower sternal border. An echocardiogram was obtained to evaluate the patient's cardiac condition.

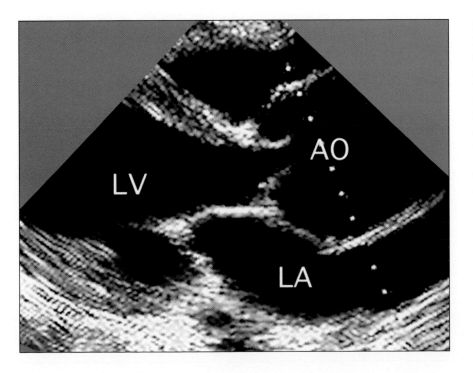

Figure 105.1
Parasternal long-axis view in systole demonstrating a severely dilated aortic root (AO), which measures over 6 cm. The upper limit of normal measurement for the aortic root is 3.7 cm in an adult. The aortic root appears to compress the left atrium (LA); however, this compression was not hemodynamically significant. The aortic valve leaflets are anatomically normal and are partially opened at the beginning of systole in this frame. The left ventricle (LV) is enlarged.

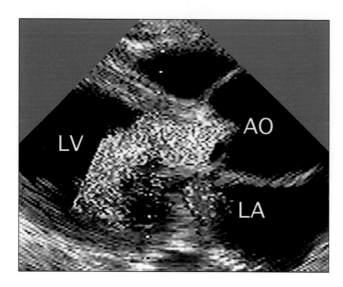

Figure 105.2
Parasternal long-axis view in diastole with color Doppler flow imaging. A jet of aortic regurgitation (AR) is visualized in the left ventricular outflow tract arising from the level of the aortic valve leaflets. This high-velocity turbulent jet extends past the mitral valve leaflets to the mid-ventricular cavity. The jet fills the left ventricular outflow tract immediately below the aortic valve, indicating the severe nature of the regurgitation.

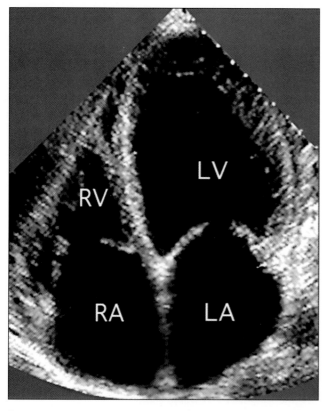

a

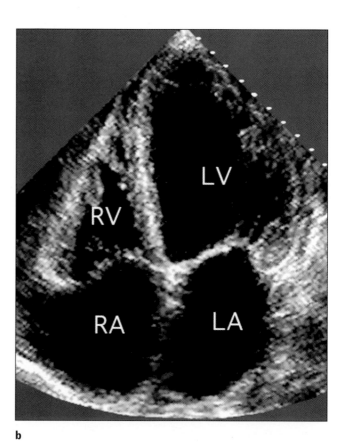

b

Figure 105.3
(a) Apical four-chamber view in diastole. The left ventricle (LV) is moderately dilated and hypertrophied. The right ventricle (RV) is also mildly dilated. Biatrial enlargement is also evident. The left ventricular dilatation has resulted in a globular shape, which is characteristic of ventricular remodeling due to severe aortic regurgitation. The major short axis of the left ventricle approaches the length of the long axis.
(b) Similar apical four-chamber view in systole. Global hypokinesis is demonstrated. There is dyskinesis of the lateral wall at the base in systole which was due to an old myocardial infarction. The systolic bulging was also evident in the short-axis (not shown here). The left ventricular ejection fraction was severely decreased and estimated to be 20%. The right ventricle is mildly dilated but the systolic function is normal. The mitral valve leaflets are normal.

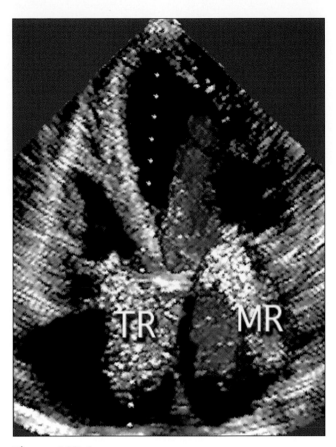

Figure 105.4
Apical four-chamber view in systole with color Doppler flow imaging. A turbulent jet of mitral regurgitation (MR) is seen in the left atrium. Tricuspid regurgitation (TR) is also present in the right atrium. The chronic, severe aortic regurgitation has resulted in left ventricular remodeling. The cavity enlargement associated with the eccentric hypertrophy of the left ventricle caused mitral annular dilatation leading to moderate mitral regurgitation. The color sample area is large in this view for illustration purposes. However, employment of a wide color Doppler scan area in clinical practice would result in an unacceptably low temporal resolution.

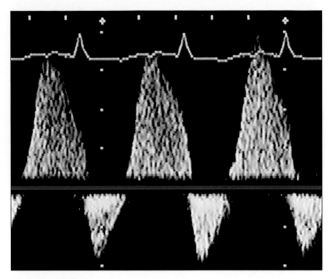

Figure 105.5
Spectral display of continuous wave Doppler velocities across the aortic valve taken from the apical position. The aortic regurgitation is severe, as evidenced by its rapid deceleration slope. Peak velocity of the aortic insufficiency is approximately 3.3 m/s, which suggests left ventricular systolic failure. The initial diastolic gradient is less than 44 mmHg between the aortic root and the left ventricle which would occur with an elevated left ventricular diastolic pressure.

Discussion

The patient has echocardiographic evidence of decompensated valvular heart disease. The aortic, mitral and tricuspid valves appear to be anatomically normal. Therefore, the aortic regurgitation is due to aortic root dilatation, which is the result of chronic and poorly controlled hypertension. Hypertension is the most common cause of aortic root dilatation in the elderly population. The aortic root is normally larger in men than in women and is correlated somewhat with height and weight. However, mean and diastolic blood pressures have been shown to be related to aortic root dilatation.[1] The aortic valve leaflets are unable to coapt normally in the dilated root, resulting in regurgitation. As the aortic regurgitation progresses, left ventricular remodeling will result in left ventricular enlargement and further aortic annular dilatation. Eventually the annulus may dilate enough to allow prolapse of one of the aortic valve leaflets, resulting in even more severe aortic insufficiency.

In this case the dilatation of the left ventricle has also resulted in mitral annular dilatation and moderate mitral regurgitation. The tricuspid regurgitation, on the other hand, is more likely to be due to progressive pulmonary hypertension from the left ventricular failure. Although one would expect the patient to improve somewhat with diuresis and afterload reduction, it is unlikely that either of these therapies would lead to a significant decrease in his mitral or aortic regurgitation. This patient clearly had longstanding aortic regurgitation which was asymptomatic despite a decline in his left ventricular systolic function until severe left ventricular systolic failure occurred. The decreased contractile function may be permanent in spite of valve replacement and relief of the left ventricular volume overload.[2]

This patient also had evidence of coronary artery disease as indicated by the lateral wall motion abnormality. Not unexpectedly, the patient did poorly despite maximal medical therapy including aggressive diuresis, digoxin, and afterload reduction with an angiotensin converting enzyme inhibitor. He was not a candidate for double valve replacement because of his poor left ventricular function, high pulmonary artery pressure, and concomitant medical problems. He died of congestive heart failure within a year of this echocardiographic study.

References

1. Vasan RS, Larson MG, Levy D. Determinants of echocardiographic aortic root size. The Framingham Heart Study. Circulation 1995;91:734–40.

2. Bonow R, Lakatos E, Maron B, *et al*. Serial long-term assessment of the natural history of asymptomatic patients with chronic aortic regurgitation and normal left ventricular systolic function. Circulation 1991;84:1625–35.

106

Aorta to left atrial fistula

Bonnie Milas MD

A 48-year-old man presented with nausea and vomiting, fever, chills, a temperature of 102.1°F, and a white blood cell count of 14 500. He had undergone an aortic valve replacement 2 years previously, for treatment of aortic stenosis due to a congenitally bicuspid aortic valve. He was a poor candidate for anticoagulation, and a bioprosthesis had been placed. Within 24 hours of admission, blood cultures were positive for *Staphylococcus aureus*.

The patient denied recent invasive or dental procedures. His physical examination was normal. Antibiotic therapy was initiated for treatment of suspected prosthetic valve endocarditis. A transthoracic echocardiogram was non-diagnostic for endocarditis. Owing to the presence of a prosthetic valve and positive blood cultures, a transesophageal echocardiogram was obtained.

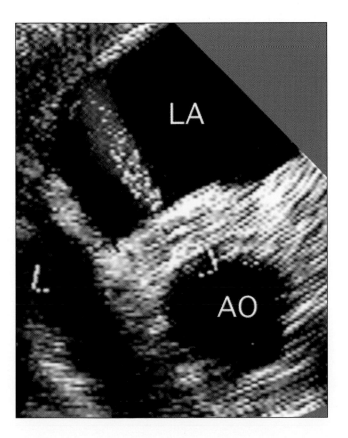

Figure 106.1
Transesophageal basal short-axis view, color Doppler image. The ascending aorta (AO) appears to be normal, although the posterior annulus is thickened, which may represent results of the previous surgery. The left atrium is slightly enlarged. There is an abnormal color jet in the left atrium which was continuous and appeared at a distance from the mitral valve. The location and the timing rule out a small jet of mitral regurgitation.

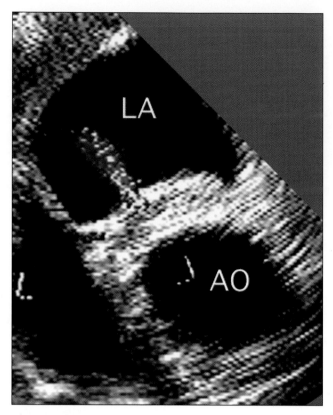

Figure 106.2
Transesophageal basal short-axis view, color Doppler image. The probe has been advanced into the esophagus. The proximal ascending aorta (AO) is visualized; however, the image does not demonstrate the structure of the prosthetic valve. The posterior aortic annulus is severely thickened, beyond what would usually be expected from 'surgical change'. The left atrium is noted posteriorly, with abnormal color flow from the aortic annulus into the left atrium. This is consistent with a fistulous left atrial connection. A thorough survey of the aortic root and left atrium is needed to discern the lead point of the fistula. This is important from a surgical standpoint to direct a surgical repair. This fistula may originate from the ascending aorta or the aortic annulus, which would be managed differently from a surgeon's perspective.

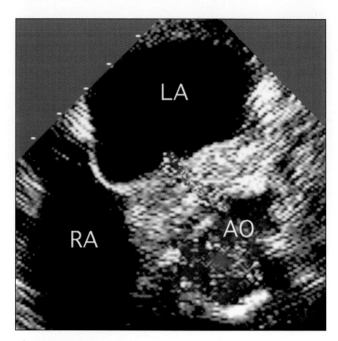

Figure 106.3
Transesophageal basal short-axis view, color Doppler image. The orientation and the views are similar to those in Figure 106.2, but the probe has been advanced slightly. Again the distinctive features of the prosthetic aortic valve are not discernible (nor is the detection of a vegetation possible). There is a direct communication between the aortic root (AO) and the left atrium consistent with an aortic–left atrial fistula. The severe thickening of the posterior sewing ring is highly suggestive of abscess formation, despite the fact that no vegetations are visualized.

Discussion

Infective endocarditis is caused by a microbial infection of the endothelial lining of the heart. Most patients who develop this have a pre-existing cardiac condition that affects the valves. Cardiac lesions pose differing degrees of risk for the development of infective endocarditis. Prosthetic heart valves, previous infective endocarditis, cyanotic congenital heart disease, patent ductus arteriosus, aortic regurgitation and/or stenosis, mitral regurgitation, mitral stenosis with regurgitation, ventricular septal defect, and coarctation of the aorta confer a relatively high risk. Gram-positive cocci predominate as the causative organisms. Streptococci or staphylococci cause more than 80% of infective endocarditis on native valves. Of the streptococci, alpha hemolytic (viridans) streptococci from the mouth cause most cases of sub-acute bacterial endocarditis. The etiological organism in the presence of a prosthetic heart valve varies, depending on the time from the surgical implantation of the valve. Early prosthetic valve endocarditis is caused predominantly by staphylococcus, while late-occurring prosthetic valve endocarditis is caused equally by staphylococci and streptococci.

Echocardiography is essential in the diagnosis of infective endocarditis. The detection of a vegetation, abscess, new partial dehiscence of a prosthetic valve, or new valvular regurgitation are considered major criteria for the diagnosis for infective endocarditis. The predominant goal of echocardiography is to identify the presence, size, location, and mobility of a vegetation. The affected valve(s) must be assessed for functional abnormalities (regurgitation or obstruction/stenosis). In addition, the valve(s) must be evaluated for underlying, coincident anatomic abnormalities that may have predisposed to the development of infective endocarditis. The effect of the valvular lesion on chamber size should be assessed. An evaluation for complications of endocarditis (abscess, fistula, aneurysm, perforation, pericardial effusion, prosthetic valve dehiscence) is also performed. In the setting of prosthetic valve endocarditis a complete echocardiographic examination must be performed to assess for: vegetation, prosthetic valve leaflet motion to detect stenosis, regurgitation or a 'frozen' leaflet, fistula or abscess formation, annulus disruption or an unseated prosthetic valve, perivalvular leak, concomitant involvement of the mitral valve through contiguous spread or pulmonary/tricuspid valve via hematogenous seeding, and response of the cardiac chambers to the resultant pressure or volume overload.[1,2]

Findings that can mimic infective endocarditis include papillary fibroma, myxomatous mitral valve disease (especially with a flail leaflet or ruptured chordae), healed (old) vegetation, systemic lupus cardiac involvement with Libman–Sacks endocarditis, prosthetic valve thrombosis, and artifact from calcium deposits or prosthesis. On the aortic valve, Lambl's excrescence or prominent nodules of Arantius may be mistaken for vegetations. When feasible, a comparison of findings should be made with previous initial postoperative echocardiograms.

The use of transthoracic versus transesophageal echocardiography for the diagnosis of infective endocarditis is controversial. Transesophageal echocardiography offers superior sensitivity and specificity compared to transthoracic echocardiography, but is more invasive. A conservative approach is to use transesophageal echocardiography only in the presence of a prosthetic valve when a transthoracic examination was technically limited or indicated an intermediate probability of endocarditis.[3] Transesophageal echocardiography is not recommended to make the diagnosis of endocarditis in patients with a low probability of the disease.[4]

This patient did not have a vegetation that could be identified. However, the presence of an abscess was strongly suggested by the fistulous connection. Concomitant involvement of the mitral valve with perforation of a leaflet or the annulus can produce a similar and deceptive color flow jet and had to be excluded. Review of the post-bypass images from the intraoperative transesophageal echocardiogram performed during his original valve surgery demonstrated a normal annulus and no fistula tract or abnormal flow. On this basis, the diagnosis of prosthetic valve endocarditis with aortic root abscess was made and the patient was returned to the operating room for placement of an aortic valve homograft.[5]

References

1. Ananthasubramaniam K, Karthikeyan V. Aortic ring abscess and aortoatrial fistula complicating fulminant prosthetic valve endocarditis due to *Proteus mirabilis*. [Review] J Ultrasound Med 2000;19:63–6.

2. Kelion AD, Chambers JB, Deverall PB. Aorto-left atrial fistula in prosthetic aortic endocarditis. J Heart Valve Dis 1993;2:481–4.

3. Khandheria BK. Transesophageal echocardiography in the evaluation of prosthetic valves. [Review] Am J Cardiac Imag 1995;9:106–14.

4. Shapiro SM, Young E, De Guzman S, *et al*. Transesophageal echocardiography in diagnosis of infective endocarditis. Chest 1994;105:377–82.

5. Brecker SJ, Jin XY, Yacoub MH. Anatomical definition of aortic root abscesses by transesophageal echocardiography: planning a surgical strategy using homograft valves. Clin Cardiol 1995;18:353–9.

107

Congenitally dysplastic aortic valve

Susan E Wiegers MD

A 15-year-old boy came to his cardiologist for a regular evaluation. The patient had been born with severe congenital aortic stenosis which had been diagnosed at 3 months. He underwent percutaneous aortic balloon valvuloplasty at the age of 4 and again at the age of 10 for symptoms of dyspnea on exertion. His mother now believes his exercise tolerance to have decreased. The patient has a sedentary lifestyle, but is doing well in school and appears to be comfortable with his peers. Physical examination demonstrated a harsh, late-peaking systolic ejection murmur heard across the precordium. S_2 was single. There was a holodiastolic blowing murmur audible at the lower left sternal border.

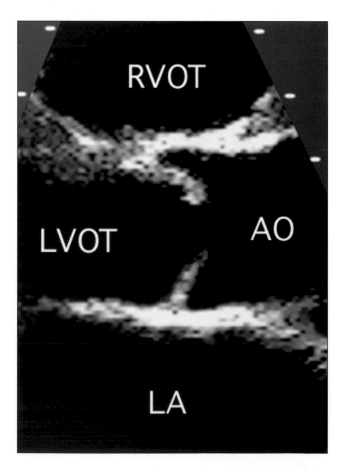

Figure 107.1
The parasternal long-axis view of the aortic valve demonstrates a thickened valve which domes in systole. The apparent maximum systolic opening of the valve is demonstrated. The left atrium (LA) is dilated. LVOT, left ventricular outflow tract; RVOT, right ventricular outflow tract; AO, ascending aorta.

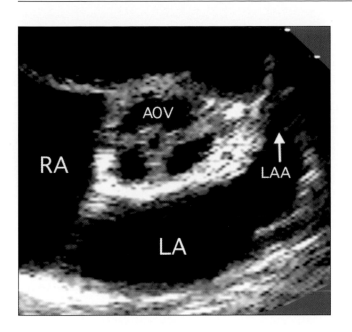

Figure 107.2
Parasternal short-axis systolic view of the congenitally abnormal aortic valve. The systolic orifice is very small in the center of a dysplastic valve. The true orifice is considerably smaller than that appreciated in the long-axis view. When the valve leaflets are pliable, the movement of the leaflets may artifactually create the appearance of normal or only mildly restricted leaflets when viewed from the long axis. The actual orifice may be extremely restricted, owing to fusion of the leaflet tips. This image of the true systolic orifice was obtained by scanning across the left ventricular outflow tract and aortic root in short-axis until the smallest orifice was visualized. Owing to the elevated left atrial pressure, the left atrial appendage (LAA) is dilated and well seen. The echodensity within the appendage (arrow) represents a normal pectinate muscle rather than a thrombus. RA, right atrium.

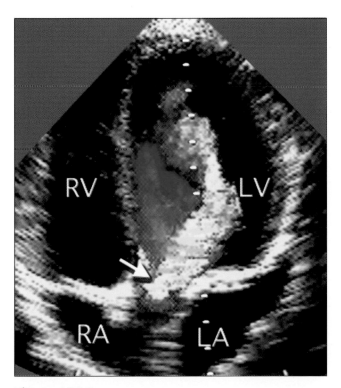

Figure 107.3
Color flow Doppler image of the apical five-chamber view in diastole. A large jet of aortic regurgitation is seen arising from the aortic valve and extending into the left ventricle (LV). The proximal flow convergence of the aortic regurgitation is seen in the aorta. The narrowest diameter (arrow) of the color flow represents the level of the aortic valve. The triangular left atrial appendage is again appreciated at the level of the atrioventricular groove. RA, right atrium; RV, right ventricle.

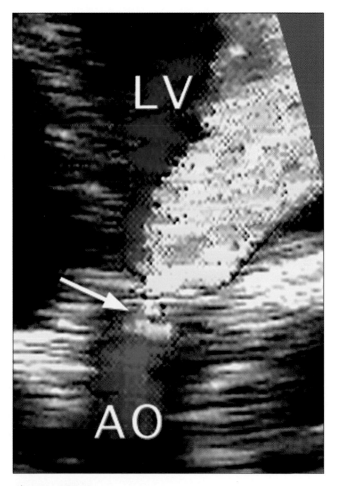

Figure 107.4
Close-up image of the proximal flow convergence on the aortic (AO) side or the aortic valve from the apical five-chamber view. The diameter of the regurgitant orifice is seen clearly in this image.

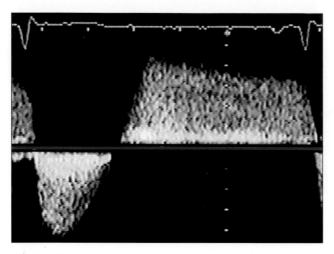

Figure 107.5
Continuous-wave spectral Doppler across the aortic valve from the apical position. The peak systolic velocity is approximately 4 m/s which predicts a peak transvalvular gradient of 64 mmHg. The peak velocity of the diastolic aortic regurgitation, seen above the baseline is also 4 m/s, which is normal for compensated aortic regurgitation. The deceleration slope of the aortic regurgitation envelope is approximately 325 m/s per second, which is consistent with moderate aortic regurgitation.

Discussion

The degree of aortic stenosis associated with congenitally abnormal valves may often be underestimated. In these cases, the stenosis is caused not by calcified and immobile leaflets but rather by a membrane formed by the dysplastic leaflets across the aortic root. The actual orifice is a perforation in the center of the membrane. If the aortic root is visualized in short axis below the true orifice of the valve, the valve motion may appear to be enough to exclude severe aortic stenosis. Additionally, the ejection jets from the valve may be extremely eccentric. These difficulties emphasize again the need for a complete imaging and Doppler study. The short-axis image should be obtained by sweeping through the entire valve plane to obtain the true valvular orifice. Finally, Doppler interrogation of the valve must be obtained not only from the apical five-chamber view, but also from the right parasternal and the supraclavicular view. In some difficult cases, turbulent color Doppler flow in the ascending aorta may be the initial clue that the valve is stenotic.

Percutaneous valvuloplasty is often successful for the relief of congenital aortic stenosis. It is rarely performed in cases of acquired calcific aortic stenosis because of poor long-term results due to high rates of rapid restenosis. In one study of elderly patients with calcific aortic stenosis, the 3-year event-free survival was 6% and was similar to the survival of untreated end-stage aortic stenosis.[1] In contrast, percutaneous valvuloplasty may be very successful in the treatment of congenital aortic stenosis, and the procedure may be repeated if restenosis occurs. Comparison with surgical valvotomy yields similar rates and degrees of aortic regurgitation as assessed by echocardiography.[2]

This patient was considered to have had a progression of his symptoms with echocardiographic evidence of severe aortic stenosis. In addition, the ventricle was dilated and the regurgitation was also hemodynamically significant. The two prior valvuloplasties and this degree of valvular regurgitation ruled out a repeat attempt. The patient was thought to be near his adult height and he underwent the Ross procedure with placement of his pulmonary valve autograft in the aortic position and a homograft in the pulmonary position.

References

1. Lieberman EB, Bashore TM, Hermiller JB, et al. Balloon aortic valvuloplasty in adults: failure of procedure to improve long-term survival. J Am Coll Cardiol 1995;26:1522–8.

2. Justo RN, McCrindle BW, Benson LN, et al. Aortic valve regurgitation after surgical versus percutaneous balloon valvotomy for congenital aortic valve stenosis. Am J Cardiol 1996;77:1332–8.

108

Aortic valve prolapse

Susan E Wiegers MD

A 50-year old man with a long history of untreated hypertension had developed insomnia several months before seeking medical therapy. On close questioning, his sleeplessness was found to be due to multiple episodes of breathlessness and sweating which woke him from sleep and required him to sit up for 10 minutes each time it occurred. He rarely climbed stairs and had given up bowling, which had been his only exercise, owing to chronic back pain. On the day he came to the emergency room, he had been unable to catch his breath despite sitting with his feet over the edge of the bed. He was unable to talk in full sentences and finally sought medical assistance. Physical examination revealed a laterally displaced PMI and water hammer pulses throughout. There was a 3/6 systolic ejection murmur and a loud diastolic murmur heard across the precordium. An echocardiogram was done to evaluate the degree of aortic insufficiency which was thought to be severe on clinical grounds.

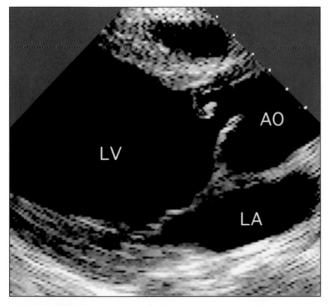

Figure 108.1
Parasternal long-axis view in diastole. The right coronary cusp of the aortic valve prolapses into the left ventricular outflow tract. The non-coronary cusp, seen posterior to the right cusp, is in the normal position but is unable to coapt normally with the prolapsing cusp. The aortic root (AO) is dilated and measures over 4 cm at the level of the sinuses of Valsalva. The left ventricle (LV) is markedly dilated.

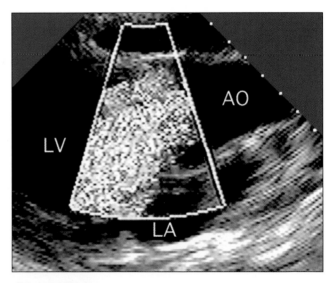

Figure 108.2
Similar parasternal long-axis view with color flow Doppler. The turbulent jet of aortic regurgitation originates from the level of the aortic valve and fills the left ventricular outflow tract. The ratio of the jet height to the left ventricular outflow height is greater than 60%, which is consistent with severe aortic regurgitation. The anterior leaflet of the mitral valve appears to be in the closed position in this diastolic frame. The jet is clearly directed against the leaflet, which may result in the early closure of the mitral valve.

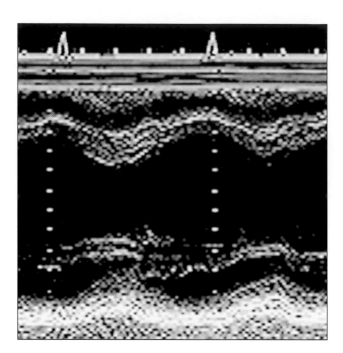

Figure 108.3
M-mode echocardiogram from the parasternal position at the level of the mitral valve leaflets. The M-mode is particularly helpful in measuring the timing of cardiac events. The early closure of the mitral valve is readily apparent in this echocardiogram. The mitral leaflets coapt well before the onset of the QRS and mechanical systole. Early closure of the mitral valve, in absence of first degree atrioventricular block, is a sign of decompensated, severe aortic regurgitation. The left ventricle is dilated to over 7.5 cm in diastole.

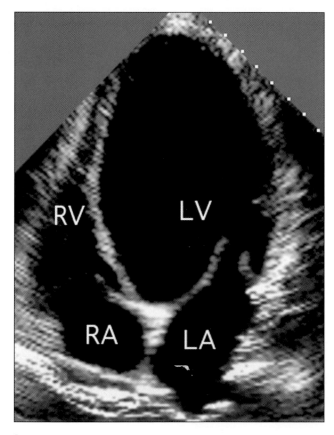

a

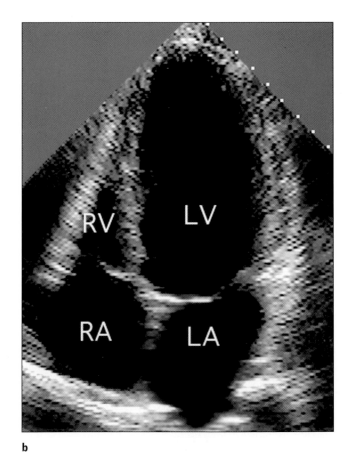

b

Figure 108.4
Apical four-chamber view in diastole (a) and systole (b): The left ventricle is severely dilated while the right heart chambers are normal. The diastolic minor axis approaches the long axis of the left ventricle which is characteristic of the globular left ventricular remodeling in severe chronic aortic regurgitation. Comparison between systolic and diastolic left ventricular areas indicates abnormal left ventricular function.

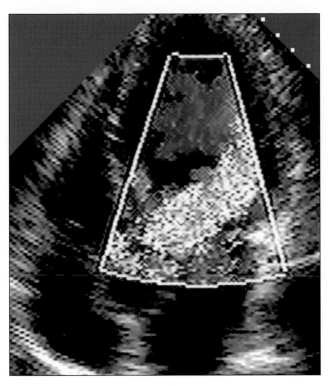

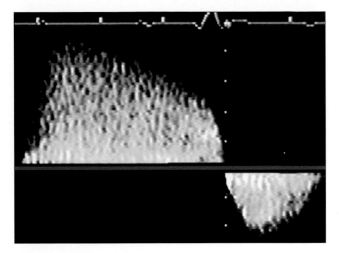

Figure 108.6
Continuous-wave Doppler spectral flow pattern: the Pedoff continuous-wave Doppler transducer is placed at the apex. The spectral pattern of the aortic regurgitation is above the baseline in diastole, indicating flow towards the transducer. The deceleration slope of the aortic regurgitation envelope is rapid, consistent with significant aortic regurgitation. The systolic velocity is increased, owing to the increased flow across the aortic valve as a result of the aortic regurgitation, rather than to valvular obstruction.

Figure 108.5
Apical five-chamber view with color flow Doppler imaging. The turbulent high-velocity jet of aortic regurgitation is seen arising from the aortic valve. The jet is wide and extends past the level of the papillary muscles, again indicating severe aortic regurgitation.

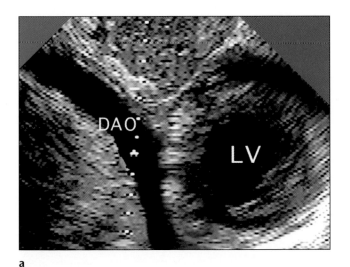

a

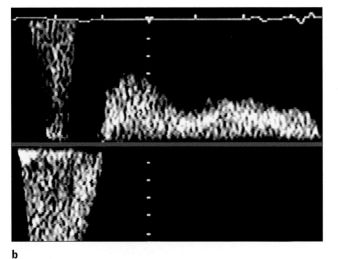

b

Figure 108.7
(a) Flow in the aorta may be sampled at multiple levels. In the subcostal view, the pulsed-wave Doppler sample volume may be placed in the abdominal aorta. In this position, normal systolic flow will be a laminar signal directed towards the transducer and displayed above the baseline. There should be no evidence of diastolic flow in the abdominal aorta, however, significant aortic regurgitation may cause reversed diastolic flow which will be below the baseline in the spectral display (not shown here).
(b) Spectral display of pulsed-wave Doppler flow in the descending thoracic aorta. The diastolic signal represents reversal of flow towards the transducer which is in the suprasternal notch. The area under the curve of the diastolic signal correlates with the severity of the aortic regurgitation.

Discussion

The patient has evidence of chronic aortic regurgitation which has now decompensated hemodynamically. The multiple episodes of paroxysmal nocturnal dyspnea were the cause of his complaint of insomnia. Patients on occasion may complain of nightmares or restlessness rather than dyspnea. The chronicity of the aortic regurgitation is evidenced by the eccentric left ventricular hypertrophy resulting in severe ventricular dilatation and a globular shape to the heart. Aortic root dilatation is most commonly caused by hypertension. The dilatation interrupts the normal coaptation of the valve cusps. As the ventricle remodels in response to the volume load, the aortic annulus dilates further, which results in further aortic regurgitation. Prolapse of a cusp of the valve has been identified in echocardiographic studies as a further cause of aortic regurgitation.[1] In this case, disruption of the support of the right coronary cusp occurred because of annular dilatation, allowing the cusp to prolapse in diastole. Other common causes of aortic valve prolapse include aortic dissection extending to the valve annulus and endocarditis. Neither were present in this patient. He had probably recently developed more severe aortic regurgitation due to development of prolapse which resulted in the acute presentation. Prolapse of a leaflet is best visualized in the parasternal long-axis view. The apical five-chamber view is not reliable for detecting prolapse, since the leaflets may appear to be in the left ventricular outflow tract even in a normal valve. Transesophageal imaging in the transverse plane may also be valuable in documenting the presence of prolapse.

Grading of aortic regurgitation remains qualitative both by echocardiography and angiography. A number of criteria should be examined and correlated, to establish the severity of the aortic regurgitation. The length and extent of the color Doppler jet may appear to give an exact picture of the aortic regurgitation. However, the size of the color jet is also dependent on gain settings, pulse repetition frequency, transmission frequency, and left ventricular compliance.[2] The ratio of the width of the color Doppler jet in the left ventricular outflow tract to the width of the outflow tract itself is more reliable in grading the degree of regurgitation.[3] This must be measured in the parasternal long-axis view. Since the jet of aortic regurgitation splays out as it travels down the outflow tract, the width of the jet should be taken immediately below the valve. A ratio of less than 25% indicates mild regurgitation, and greater than 40% represents severe regurgitation. In this patient, the ratio is greater than 60%, which is consistent with very severe regurgitation. Reversal of flow in the descending thoracic aorta, imaged from the suprasternal notch, can be demonstrated with pulsed-wave Doppler in patients with severe aortic regurgitation.[4] This patient has very severe aortic regurgitation, as demonstrated by the reversal of flow in the abdominal aorta in diastole.

By echocardiography, this patient has evidence of systolic dysfunction that was probably present for some months. The severe congestive heart failure on presentation may have been due to end-stage decompensation or to a further increase in volume load due to the development of aortic cusp prolapse. The presence of premature closure of the mitral valve is an ominous sign. Although the premature closure was suspected on the two-dimensional images, it should be confirmed by M-mode, which has a much higher temporal resolution. While it is possible that the jet of aortic regurgitation physically impinges on the anterior leaflet of the mitral valve, forcing it closed, the markedly elevated left ventricular diastolic pressure is probably responsible for the phenomenon.

The patient was treated aggressively with diuresis but did not tolerate afterload reduction because of a marginal blood pressure. He received a mechanical aortic valve replacement and was left with a residual left ventricular ejection fraction of 40%. His symptoms were markedly improved.

References

1. Kai H, Koyanagi S, Takeshita A. Aortic valve prolapse with aortic regurgitation assessed by Doppler color-flow echocardiography. Am Heart J 1992;124:1297–304.

2. Smith M, Kwan O, Spain M, et al. Temporal variability of color Doppler jet areas in patients with mitral and aortic regurgitation. Am Heart J 1992;123:953–60.

3. Dolan M, Castello R, St. Vrain J, et al. Quantitation of aortic regurgitation by Doppler echocardiography: a practical approach. Am Heart J 1995;129:1014–20.

4. Tribouilloy C, Shen W, Slama M, et al. Assessment of severity of aortic regurgitation by M-mode colour Doppler flow imaging. Eur Heart J 1991;12:352–6.

109

Endocarditis of an aortic valve bioprosthesis

Susan E Wiegers MD

An 80-year-old man complained of malaise, fever, and chills for 4 days before being admitted to the hospital with right arm paralysis. He had undergone an aortic valve replacement 5 years earlier for critical aortic stenosis, which was due to senile calcification. On clinical examination the patient was alert and comfortable but febrile. There was a systolic ejection murmur that had been present since the valve replacement. A new diastolic murmur was also present, but no ventricular gallop was heard. The rest of the examination was unremarkable. Within 24 hours, three sets of blood cultures were reported to be positive for Gram-positive cocci in clusters. A transthoracic echocardiogram revealed aortic insufficiency but the bioprosthetic valve was poorly seen. A transesophageal study was performed to rule out complications of bacterial endocarditis.

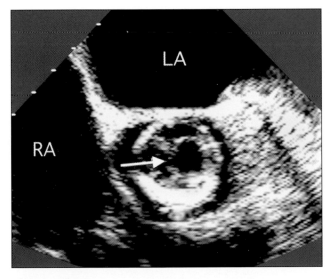

Figure 109.1
Transesophageal image of the bioprosthetic aortic valve in the transverse plane (imaging angle 0°). The left atrium (LA) is at the top of the image and is mildly dilated. The sewing ring of the aortic valve is seen as an echodense structure in the aortic root. The leaflets of the bioprosthesis are markedly thickened. Disruption of the leaflets is evident (arrow). An abnormal echolucent area surrounds the sewing ring except the most posterior portion of the annulus, which is adjacent to the left atrium. This echolucent area represents a large root abscess. Echodensities within the abscess cavity, such as are present anteriorly (towards the bottom of the screen), are highly suggestive of the diagnosis. RA, right atrium.

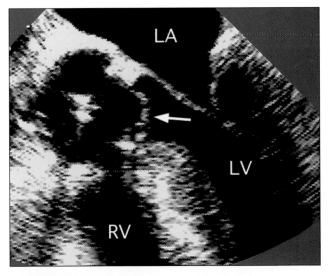

Figure 109.2
Transesophageal image of a modified four-chamber view from the mid-esophagus. One of the leaflets of the aortic bioprosthesis (arrow) prolapses into the left ventricular outflow tract. A linear structure associated with a bioprosthesis is most likely to be a flail leaflet but a vegetation is also a possibility. LA, left atrium; LV, left ventricle; RV, right ventricle.

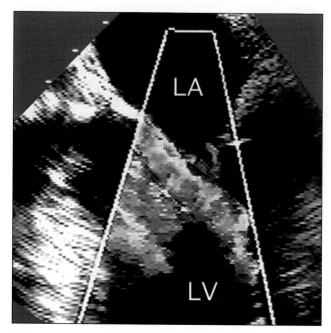

Figure 109.3

Similar transesophageal image as in Figure 109.2 with color Doppler flow imaging demonstrating significant aortic regurgitation in diastole. Note the jet of aortic regurgitation tracks along the anterior mitral leaflet, extending to the level of the anterolateral papillary muscle. The color Doppler jet obscures the image of the prolapsing leaflet. This degree of regurgitation with a bioprosthesis should always raise the question of endocarditis.

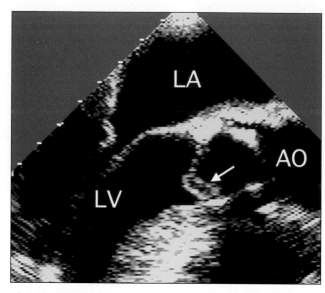

Figure 109.4

Transesophageal image in the longitudinal plane (imaging angle 130°). The more posterior stent of the bioprosthesis is the echodense structure which projects into the aortic root (AO). The prolapsing leaflet of the bioprosthesis with attached vegetation (arrow) is seen in the left ventricular outflow tract. While the posterior aortic annulus is unremarkable in this view, the abnormal anterior annular echo-free space representing the abscess cavity is easily appreciated. Note the normal mitral valve leaflets.

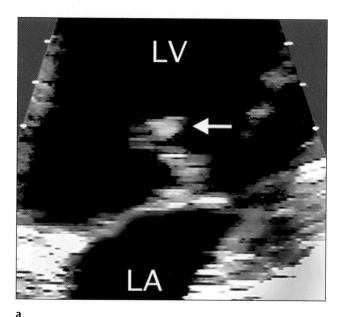

a

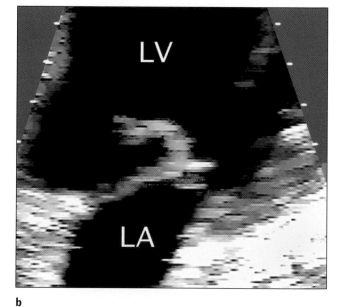

b

Figure 109.5

(a) Close-up image from the transthoracic study in the apical four-chamber view demonstrates a vegetation (arrow) on the chords to the anterior mitral valve leaflet. This was a metastatic infection due to the jet of aortic regurgitation from the infected bioprosthesis striking this area.

(b) The vegetation is approximately 1 cm in length and was highly mobile. The anterior leaflet of the mitral valve itself is normal and there is only trivial mitral regurgitation.

Discussion

Transesophageal echocardiography is far more sensitive than transthoracic studies for the evaluation of prosthetic valves.[1] Any significant abnormality of a prosthetic valve should raise the question of endocarditis. Many cases are initially missed because of an inappropriately low level of suspicion. Acoustic shadowing obscures the anatomic findings in transthoracic studies. In this case, the transthoracic study did provide evidence of aortic regurgitation and the unusual vegetation on the mitral valve chords, but the aortic valve vegetation, prolapse of the aortic bioprosthesis leaflet, and the associated abscess were only visualized on transesophageal echocardiography. Criteria for the diagnosis of endocarditis have recently been modified to include the presence of vegetation on echocardiographic examination.[2] Since the vegetations associated with aortic valve endocarditis tend to be located on the ventricular surface of the valve, it is mandatory to visualize the outflow tract in patients suspected of having endocarditis. On transesophageal studies, this view is best achieved in the modified four-chamber view from the transverse plane (Figure 109.2) or from the longitudinal plane (imaging angle approximately 120°) as in Figure 109.4.

Transesophageal echocardiography is also more sensitive than transthoracic studies in demonstrating complications of endocarditis. Abscess formation is best assessed from this approach.[3] The metastatic involvement of the mitral valve chordal apparatus was also easily identified on transesophageal study.[4] Owing to the superiority of transesophageal echocardiography in the diagnosis of prosthetic endocarditis, this study is strongly recommended for evaluation of infected prosthetic valves.

Despite the patient's age and clinical status, it was clear that the abscess would not be effectively treated with antibiotics alone. The cerebral embolism did not recur and the patient underwent repeat aortic valve replacement with a bioprosthesis one week after being admitted to the hospital. He did well post-operatively and was left with a small neurological deficit.

References

1. Daniel W, Mugge A, Grote J, et al. Comparison of transthoracic and transesophageal echocardiography for detection of abnormalities of prosthetic and bioprosthetic valves in the mitral and aortic positions. Am J Cardiol 1993;15:210–15.

2. Lamas C, Eykyn S. Suggested modifications to the Duke criteria for the clinical diagnosis of native valve and prosthetic valve endocarditis: analysis of 118 pathologically proven cases. Clin Infect Diss 1997;25:713–19.

3. Daniel W, Mugge A, Martin R, et al. Improvement in the diagnosis of abscesses associated with endocarditis by transesophageal echocardiography. N Engl J Med 1991;324:795–800.

4. Karalis D, Chandrasedaran K, Wahl J, et al. Transesophageal echocardiographic recognition of mitral valve abnormalities associated with aortic valve endocarditis. Am Heart J 1990;119:1209–11.

110

Sub-aortic stenosis

Susan E Wiegers MD

A 42-year-old man with a history of a loud systolic murmur for many years presented with symptoms of congestive heart failure. He had not sought medical follow-up in the past. No workup had been undertaken for a 3/6 systolic ejection murmur which had been noted since at least adolescence. He currently was complaining of worsening orthopnea and significant dyspnea with mild exertion.

Physical examination was remarkable for a laterally displaced cardiac impulse and 4/6 systolic ejection murmur, which radiated to the carotids. S_2 was normally and physiologically split. An echocardiogram was undertaken to assess the sources of the murmur. His parasternal images were very poor and are not reproduced.

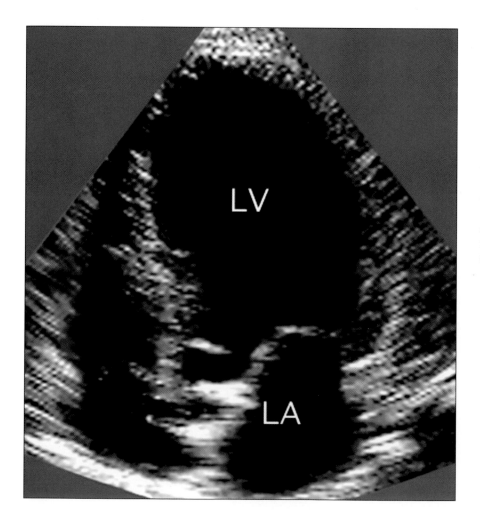

Figure 110.1
Apical five-chamber view demonstrating a calcified ridge which is attached to the interventricular septum and extends into the left ventricular outflow tract (arrow). The aortic valve is not well seen in the apical five-chamber view but appears calcified. The left ventricle (LV) is moderately dilated and the right ventricular size is normal. In real time, left ventricular systolic dysfunction was evident. The right ventricle was normal. Mild left atrial (LA) dilatation cannot be appreciated in this view, which is not a standard view for assessment of atrial size.

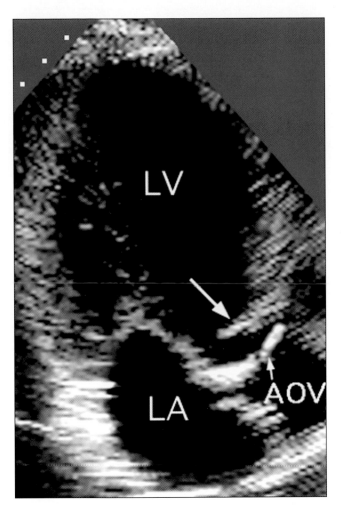

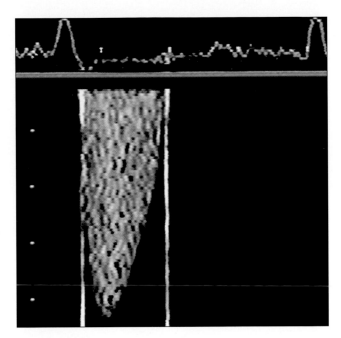

Figure 110.3

Spectral display of continuous-wave Doppler across the aortic valve from the apical position. In systole, there is a high-velocity jet with a peak velocity of approximately 4.2 m/s representing a peak systolic gradient of 71 mmHg across the left ventricular outflow tract and aortic valve. These two obstructions are in series and it is not possible to separate their relative contribution to the total gradient. The two high-velocity signals at the beginning and end of ejection represent motion of the aortic valve.

Figure 110.2

Apical long-axis view. Once again, the calcified ridge extending into the left ventricular outflow tract from the interventricular septum is noted (arrow). The ridge arises from the septum and extends towards the anterior mitral valve leaflet but does not appear to attach, in this view, to the leaflet. This aortic valve (AOV) is heavily calcified and does not open normally in the systolic view. The left ventricle (LV) is dilated. There was mild global hypokinesis of all walls and moderate hypokinesis of the anterior septum.

Figure 110.4

Continuous-wave Doppler spectral display across the aortic valve from the suprasternal notch. In this case the systolic flow across the aortic valve is towards the transducer and is thus displayed as a positive signal. Once again the peak velocity is approximately 4 m/s. Because the jet across the sub-valvular obstruction may be quite eccentric, it is necessary to sample the aortic valve Doppler signal from multiple vantage points including the apical position, the right parasternal position, and the suprasternal notch.

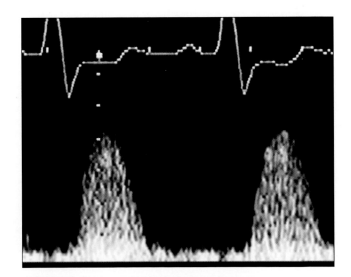

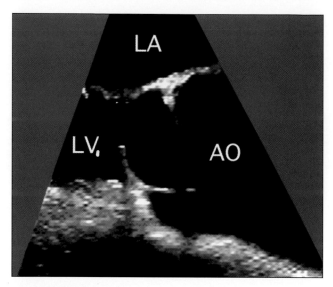

Figure 110.5
Transesophageal echocardiogram from the mid-esophageal level in the longitudinal plane (imaging angle 130°). The subvalvular membrane (arrow) is seen in the left ventricular outflow tract immediately below the right coronary cusp of the aortic valve (AO). This membrane arises from the interventricular septum of the left ventricle (LV) but does not extend all the way across the left ventricular outflow tract to the anterior mitral valve leaflet in this view. There is some restriction of motion of the aortic valve in this early systolic image. However, in real time, adequate motion of the aortic valve excluded significant aortic stenosis. The gradient demonstrated by transthoracic echocardiography was entirely due to obstruction of the outflow tract by the sub-valvular membrane.

Discussion

Discrete sub-aortic membranes cause variable degrees of obstruction to left ventricular outflow, depending on the anatomy of the membrane. The membrane may encircle the entire left ventricular outflow tract, being connected to the interventricular septum, the anterior wall of the ventricle, and the anterior mitral valve leaflet. Alternatively, a crescent-shaped membrane may be attached primarily to the interventricular septum. The high-velocity ejection jet will be eccentrically directed and over time damages the aortic valve resulting in aortic regurgitation. Aortic regurgitation was present in this patient, although not pictured, but was mild and is not likely to have contributed to the left ventricular dilatation and dysfunction. While sub-aortic stenosis usually presents in infancy

or early childhood, it may occasionally be first diagnosed in adulthood. In this case, calcification of the aortic membrane may have led to progressive obstruction of the outflow tract.

A sub-aortic membrane is usually best visualized in the parasternal long-axis view, although not in this particular patient, who had a very poor parasternal window. The apical five-chamber and apical long-axis views are also helpful in assessing fixed obstruction of the left ventricular outflow tract. The aortic membrane may be closely associated with the aortic valve leaflets themselves, leading to further valvular dysfunction. Transesophageal echocardiography provides better visualization of the attachments to the aortic valve and can be used to direct surgical therapy.[1–3] Surgical resection of the membrane often requires concomitant aortic valve replacement to correct the defect. Regrowth of the membrane has been reported in a minority of patients in some cases many years after the original surgery.[4] While continuous-wave Doppler can measure the outflow tract pressure gradient, the continuity equation cannot be used, because of the inability to measure an appropriate left ventricular outflow tract diameter. As noted, contributions of sub-valvular and valvular obstruction cannot be separated by continuous-wave Doppler.

In this case, close attachment of the membrane to the aortic annulus and the right coronary cusp of the aortic valve made simple resection difficult. Aortic regurgitation was also present, although not pictured in these images. A St Jude's aortic valve was placed after debridement of the interventricular septum and resection of the severely calcified and severely obstructing membrane. The patient had adequate left ventricular function to be weaned from bypass and has symptomatically improved since surgery.

References

1. Essop M, Skudicky D, Sareli P. Diagnostic value of transesophageal versus transthoracic echocardiography in discrete subaortic stenosis. Am J Cardiol 1992;70:962–3.

2. Decoodt P, Kacenelenbogen R, Viart P, et al. Evaluation of membranous subaortic stenosis using biplane transesophageal echocardiography. Report of two cases. Acta Cardiol 1991;46:479–84.

3. Gnanapragasam J, Houston A, Doig W, et al. Transoesophageal echocardiographic assessment of fixed subaortic obstruction in children. Br Heart J 1991;66:281–4.

4. Maron BJ, Graham KJ, Poliac LC, et al. Recurrence of a discrete subaortic membrane 27 years after operative resection. Am J Cardiol 1995;76:104–5.

111

Aortic valve endocarditis

Susan E Wiegers MD

A 36-year-old man who abused intravenous drugs came to the hospital complaining of myalgias, low-grade fever and a headache. He had not received medical attention since early childhood and did not know of any medical history. He injected both heroin and cocaine several times a day. He had no other complaints and denied chest pain or shortness of breath.

Physical examination was remarkable for a temperature of 100°F, a pulse of 110 bpm and a blood pressure of 149/95 mmHg. The lungs were clear. There was a loud systolic ejection murmur at the right upper sternal border and a blowing diastolic murmur at the left lower sternal border. A single conjunctival hemorrhage was present, as

well as multiple track marks consistent with chronic intravenous drug use, but there were no stigmata of endocarditis. A transthoracic echocardiogram was performed to evaluate the patient's murmur. The images were technically limited, but there was a suspicion of a bicuspid valve, and moderate aortic regurgitation was present. No vegetations were identified. The blood cultures grew *Staphylococcus epidermidis* in only one out of six bottles. The patient continued to have low-grade fevers on combination antibiotics. A transesophageal echocardiogram was done to determine whether the patient had endocarditis. The patient had agreed to the study but had difficulty co-operating with the examination.

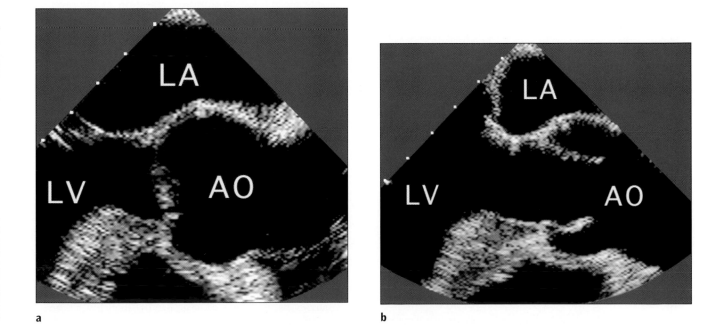

a   b

Figure 111.1
(a) Transesophageal echocardiogram from the longitudinal plane (imaging angle 137°). The aortic valve appears essentially normal, perhaps being slightly thickened. The other structures are also normal.
(b) In systole, the anterior leaflet domes slightly. The leaflets themselves appear normal and the annulus is also of normal thickness.

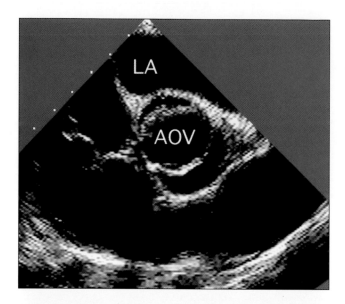

Figure 111.2
Short-axis view of the aortic valve from an imaging angle of approximately 50°. The aortic valve is bicuspid, demonstrating the typical ellipsoid orifice associated with this anomaly. The edges of the leaflets are mildly thickened. The tricuspid valve is normal. The pulmonary artery is imaged anteriorly at the bottom of the screen, although the pulmonary valve is not well seen.

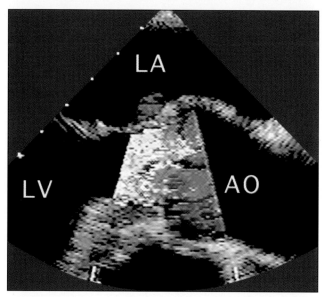

a

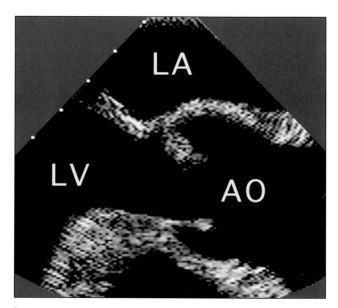

b

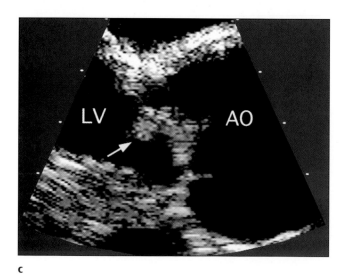

c

Figure 111.3
(a) Transesophageal echocardiogram from the longitudinal plane (imaging angle 110°) with color flow Doppler imaging in diastole. The probe has been rotated to the patient's left to obtain this image. There is a broad jet of aortic regurgitation that fills the posterior left ventricular outflow tract. The ratio of the jet height to the left ventricular outflow tract diameter is almost 50%, which is consistent with severe aortic regurgitation.
(b) Same view without color Doppler imaging. The posterior leaflet in this view is abnormal and thickened.
(c) Close-up view of the aortic valve in diastole. There is a mass (arrow) attached to the ventricular surface of the aortic valve which prolapses into the left ventricular outflow tract in diastole. Chaotic motion of the mass was evident in real time.

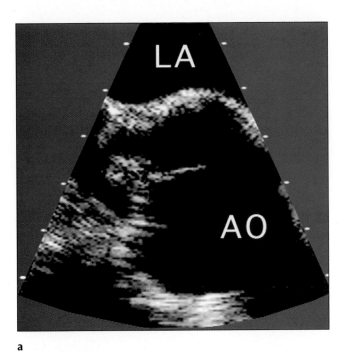

a

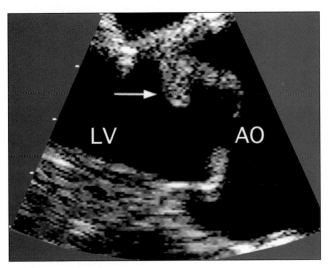

b

Figure 111.4

(a) In another diastolic frame, the posterior aortic valve leaflet is perforated. Comparison with Figure 111.3a reveals that much of the aortic regurgitation may be through the leaflet perforation.

(b) In systole, the mass (arrow) attached to the posterior leaflet of the aortic valve reaches the annulus. This raises the concern of annular involvement by the infectious process. The systolic doming of the leaflets is more clearly demonstrated in this view.

Discussion

This patient was eventually proved unequivocally to have bacterial endocarditis. However, the transthoracic study showed only a bicuspid valve and aortic regurgitation. Since most bicuspid valves are regurgitant, it was not obvious that the patient had endocarditis.[1] It was possible that this patient, who had never had primary medical care, had longstanding aortic regurgitation due to the bicuspid valve, and that the positive blood culture was the result of contamination in one bottle. The transesophageal echocardiogram was undertaken to further define the valvular abnormality. The patient was not co-operative and the initial images did not show a significant abnormality of the bicuspid valve. It was only with extensive imaging that the vegetation was detected. Although in the still frames the vegetation is easily seen, the real-time study was far more difficult. A cursory study would have missed the vegetation and led to a serious diagnostic error.

Many studies have demonstrated the utility of transesophageal echocardiography in the diagnosis of endocarditis.[2] The criteria for the diagnosis have been revised to include echocardiographic features.[3] This case illustrates the need for careful evaluation of the valve from multiple planes, to ensure that a focal abnormality is not overlooked. A strategy of particular merit is to locate the view in which the valvular regurgitation appears the most severe with color flow Doppler and then examine the valve in that plane without color Doppler imaging. This may allow for detection of small vegetations that are not easily imaged in the standard planes. The patient was treated with 4 weeks of antibiotics with improvement in symptoms and negative blood cultures. The aortic regurgitation continued to appear to be severe on echocardiography and the left ventricle was mildly dilated. The patient has not yet had aortic valve replacement.

References

1. Pachulski R, Chan K. Progression of aortic valve dysfunction in 51 adult patients with congenital bicuspid aortic valve: assessment and follow up by Doppler echocardiography. Br Heart J 1993;69:237–40.

2. Yvorchuk K, Chan K. Application of transthoracic and transesophageal echocardiography in the diagnosis and management of infective endocarditis. J Am Soc Echocardiogr 1994;7:294–308.

3. Durack D, Lukes A, Bright D. New criteria for diagnosis of infective endocarditis: utilization of specific echocardiographic findings. Duke Endocarditis Service. Am J Med 1994;96:200–9.

112

Unicuspid aortic valve

Susan E Wiegers MD

A 25-year-old woman with a history of severe congenital aortic stenosis had chronic presyncope with mild exertion. The patient had undergone balloon valvuloplasty of her aortic valve at the age of 10. Her symptoms initially improved but then recurred, and at the age of 15 she had a conduit placed between her left ventricular apex and her descending thoracic aorta. On physical examination she had a hyperdynamic left ventricular impulse. There was a very loud systolic ejection murmur at the left upper sternal border with a single S_2. In the posterior thorax a harsh bruit was heard at the level of the mid-thoracic spine on the left. An echocardiogram was performed to evaluate left ventricular function.

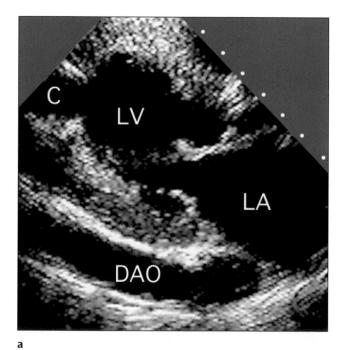

a

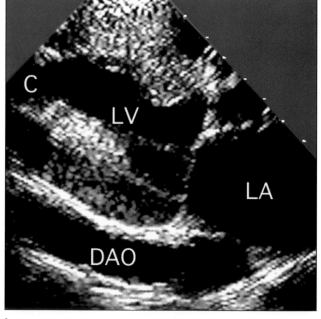

b

Figure 112.1
(a) Parasternal long-axis view of the left ventricle in diastole. The left atrium (LA) is dilated. There is moderate left ventricular (LV) hypertrophy. The left ventricular outflow tract is narrowed, but the aortic annulus is more severely narrowed. The aortic valve is echodense and the normal structures are not visible. At the apex of the left ventricle an out-pouching, which represents the surgical conduit (C), is visualized. The descending thoracic aorta (DAO) is seen in long-axis posterior to the heart in this slightly off-axis view.
(b) The same view in systole. The aortic valve demonstrated no motion with systole. This lack of motion of the aortic valve throughout the cardiac cycle is consistent with critical aortic stenosis. The left ventricular systolic function is seen to be normal. The opening to the conduit remains patent in systole and measures approximately 1 cm at its ventricular anastamosis.

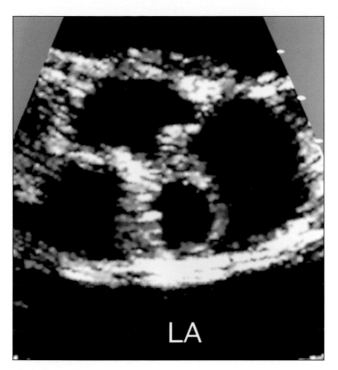

Figure 112.2
Parasternal short-axis view of the aortic valve. Once again, the aortic sinus dimension is well below normal. While the sinuses of Valsalva have a normal arrangement, the unicuspid nature of the valve is noted by a single commissure which is visualized at the posterior annulus. The raphes between the incompletely formed coronary cusps are well seen. The valvular orifice is present between the non-coronary and left coronary cusps, which are not fused. The aortic valve area by planimetry was less than 0.5 cm^2. In this case the aortic stenosis was caused by anatomical malformation of the valve rather than by calcification.

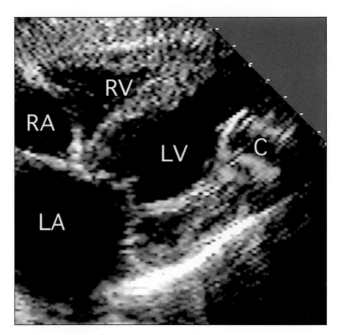

Figure 112.3
Subcostal four-chamber view of the left ventricular conduit (C) anastamosis. The distal anastamosis of the conduit to the descending thoracic aorta is not visualized. This view could not be obtained on transthoracic echocardiography despite attempts with off-axis imaging.

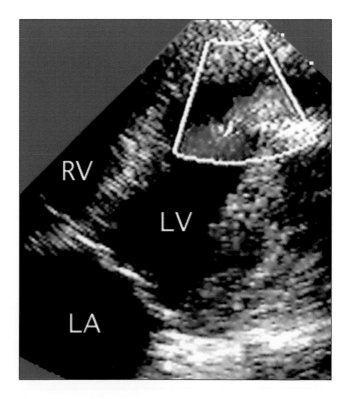

Figure 112.4
Off-axis apical four-chamber view with color Doppler flow imaging demonstrating non-aliased flow into the left ventricular apical conduit in systole. The connection between the left ventricle and the surgical conduit is clearly visualized. It is non-stenotic as evidenced by its wide patency and the low-velocity non-turbulent flow into it from the ventricle. However, the attachment to the mid-descending thoracic aorta could not be visualized.

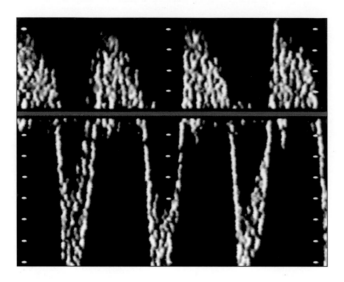

Figure 112.5
Spectral display of pulsed-wave Doppler taken from the off-axis subcostal four-chamber view of flow into the apical conduit (see Fig. 112.3). In systole the laminar flow below the baseline demonstrates non-turbulent flow from the left ventricular apex into the conduit. In diastole, the low-velocity flow above the baseline demonstrates reflux of blood from the conduit into the left ventricle. The conduit contains a bioprosthetic valve which prevents retrograde flow in diastole from the aorta to the conduit. There is a small amount of low-velocity retrograde flow from the conduit into the left ventricular in diastole.

Discussion

The patient is suffering from inadequate perfusion to the cerebral vessels, especially with exercise, owing to the placement of the shunt into the descending thoracic aorta. There is little antegrade flow across the stenotic aortic valve and dysplastic outflow tract. Echocardiographic evaluation failed to show evidence of conduit obstruction or significant regurgitation from the aorta to the left ventricular apex in diastole. The patient had received the conduit some years previously, before the evolution of surgical procedures which successfully addressed the dysplastic outflow tract and valve. If she had had evidence of left ventricular failure, cardiac transplantation would have been the only possible surgical option. However, given the reasonable ventricular volumes and good systolic function, a modified Ross–Konno procedure was undertaken with aortoventriculoplasty to enlarge the aortic annulus.[1] A pulmonary homograft was successfully placed and the conduit was taken down. The patient had excellent relief of her symptoms. This procedure also made it possible for the patient to consider a pregnancy, which had been her goal.

Reference

1. Reddy VM, Rajasinghe HA, Teitel DF, *et al.* Aortoventriculoplasty with the pulmonary autograft: the 'Ross–Konno' procedure. J Thorac Cardiovasc Surg 1996;111:158–65; discussion 165–7.

SECTION IX

The Aorta

113

Coronary artery embolism

Susan E Wiegers MD

An echocardiogram was performed on a 62-year-old woman 2 days after an inferior myocardial infarction in order to assess her right ventricular function. She had received thrombolytic therapy, but had remained relatively hypotensive despite volume infusion. She was presumed to have right ventricular involvement, and an echocardiogram was ordered. An unexpected abnormality was noted in the ascending aorta on the transthoracic study. A transesophageal echocardiogram was immediately performed to evaluate the abnormality in the aorta.

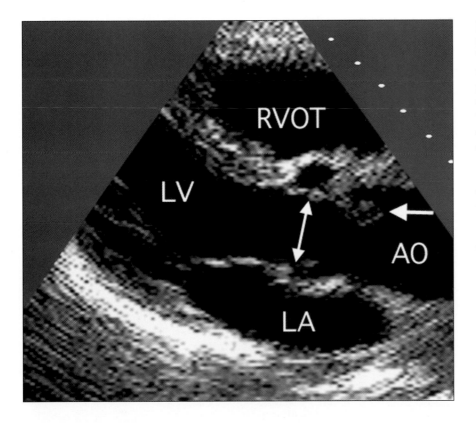

Figure 113.1
Parasternal long-axis view in systole. The ascending aorta is well seen from the standard transducer position in this patient. The aortic valve leaflets are demonstrated in systole at the level of the sinuses of Valsalva (double-headed arrow). There is a mass (arrow) in the ascending aorta (AO) which appears to be attached to the wall of the aorta near the sinotubular junction. In this systolic image, it is not clear whether or not the mass is associated with the right coronary cusp. In real time the mass was highly mobile, reaching to the posterior wall of the aorta. The differential diagnosis includes an incompletely imaged dissection flap, and a mass associated with the valve such as a vegetation or tumor.

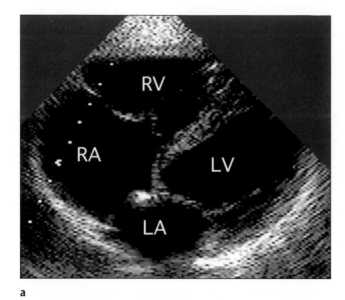

a

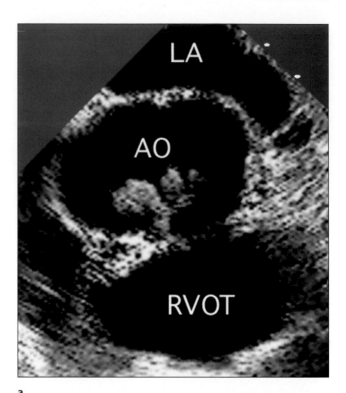

a

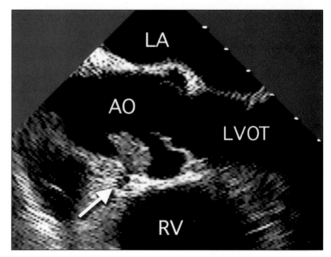

b

Figure 113.2

(a) Subcostal four-chamber image in diastole. The right ventricle (RV) and the right atrium (RA) are dilated. No significant abnormalities are seen in the left ventricle (LV) or atrium (LA).

(b) Similar view in systole. Marked right ventricular dysfunction is noted. The right ventricular apex contracts slightly but the free wall is immobile. The regional wall motion abnormality with significant systolic dysfunction is diagnostic of right ventricular dysfunction. The left ventricle contracts normally and the area of the left ventricle has significantly decreased. Both the septum and the lateral wall of the left ventricle appear to thicken normally.

b

Figure 113.3

(a) Transesophageal image from the high esophagus in the transverse plane, at the level of the ascending aorta (AO). A bilobed mass is freely mobile in the aortic lumen and appears to be attached to the anterior wall of the aortic root. The walls of the aorta are normal at this level and there is no evidence of a dissection flap.

(b) Transesophageal image from the high esophagus in the transverse plane in a modified five-chamber view. The left ventricular outflow tract (LVOT) and aortic valve leaflets are well seen. The 1.5 cm by 1 cm mobile mass is not attached to the aortic valve leaflets and appears to arise from the aortic wall in close proximity to the right coronary ostium (arrow). While a tumor might have such an appearance, the site of attachment is distinctly unusual.

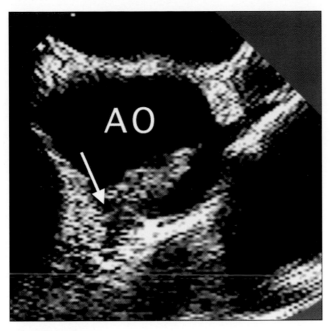

Figure 113.3
(c) Magnified transesophageal image from the high esophagus (imaging angle 35°) at the level of the aortic root. The mass protrudes into the right coronary artery ostium (arrow) and can be followed for approximately 1 cm distally into the artery.

Discussion

The unusual mass in the aortic root demonstrated on the transthoracic study was thought possibly to be a dissection flap, and a transesophageal echocardiogram was immediately undertaken to assess the diagnosis. Dissection flaps may occasionally have unusual appearances, particularly if there is overlying atheroma on the intimal flap. Dissection can also involve the coronary arteries. If the right coronary artery is dissected, the patient may survive long enough to sustain an inferior myocardial infarction. Dissection of the left coronary artery is, of course, more routinely fatal. However, the transesophageal images clearly ruled out the diagnosis of dissection while demonstrating the highly unusual finding of a mass lodged in the right coronary ostium. The complete obstruction of the right coronary artery was responsible for the inferior and right ventricular infarctions.

The nature of the mass was not clear from the images. The mass had the 'fluffy' appearance of a vegetation, but the aortic valve appeared entirely normal and there was no aortic regurgitation. Thus, embolization of a vegetation would be extremely unlikely. The edges of the mass were highly mobile and had a frond-like appearance,

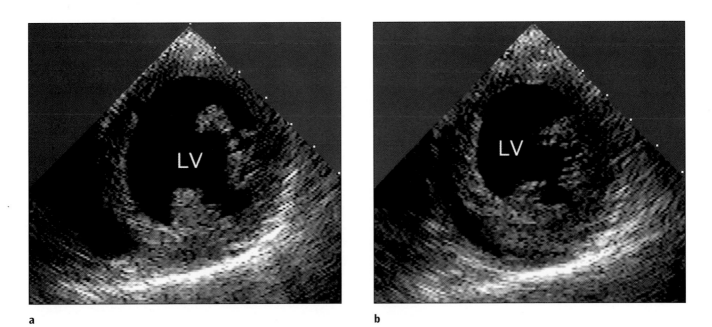

a   b

Figure 113.4
(a) Transgastric diastolic echocardiogram in the transverse plane (imaging angle 0°). The inferior and posterior walls are slightly thinner than the other walls.
(b) Similar view in systole. The posterior and inferior walls are clearly hypokinetic compared to the other walls, and do not thicken to any significant extent.

which is reminiscent of a fibroelastoma. These benign tumors have not been reported on the aortic walls and this mass appeared to be firmly lodged in the right coronary ostium. Any tumor or process involving the wall of the right coronary itself would not have been expected to become so large without producing any previous ischemic symptoms. While fibroelastomas have been reported to cause myocardial infarctions, the attachment to the aortic valve is always apparent.[1] Coronary artery embolism from an intracardiac thrombus is a potential mechanism for the patient's presentation. Transesophageal echocardiography is a sensitive tool for the detection of a cardiac source of embolism.[2] However, in this case, there was no left ventricular or atrial thrombus and the interatrial septum was intact. Aortic atheroma may also be a source of embolus, although distal embolism is far more common than retrograde embolism. In one study performed during coronary artery bypass grafting surgery, a mean of 535 emboli was detected within the aortic arch in 20 patients undergoing the procedure.[3] This patient had minimal atherosclerotic plaquing of the descending thoracic aorta and no other evidence of systemic emboli, nor had she undergone manipulation of the aorta.

Surgery to remove the mass was performed because of concern that it could embolize into the left coronary ostium. Pathology confirmed that the mass was a thromboembolism which had lodged in the right coronary ostium, causing an infarction with severe right ventricular involvement. The origin and etiology of the clot could not be determined. The patient has subsequently been maintained on oral anticoagulation.

References

1. Pasteuning WH, Zijnen P, van der Aa MA, *et al.* Papillary fibroelastoma of the aortic valve in a patient with an acute myocardial infarction. J Am Soc Echocardiogr 1996;9:897–900.

2. Lethen H, Flachskampf F, Schneider R, *et al.* Frequency of deep vein thrombosis in patients with patent foramen ovale and ischemic stroke or transient ischemic attack. Am J Cardiol 1997;80:1066–9.

3. Yao FS, Barbut D, Hager DN, *et al.* Detection of aortic emboli by transesophageal echocardiography during coronary artery bypass surgery. J Cardiothorac Vasc Anesth 1996;10:314–17.

114

Sinus of Valsalva aneurysm

Martin St John Sutton MBBS
Susan E Wiegers MD
Kuo-Yang Wang MD

A 34-year-old Oriental woman sought medical attention following an episode of upper substernal chest pain which was initially accompanied by a tearing sensation and shortness of breath 5 weeks previously. The discomfort had recurred intermittently with exertion, and she had noticed palpitations consisting of skipped and extra beats. She did not have sustained tachycardia, syncope or light-headedness. She had no risk factors for cardiovascular disease and no history of congenital heart disease even in her remote family.

On examination she had a heart rate of 94 bpm, blood pressure of 110/55 mmHg. There was no elevation of her jugular venous pressure, no edema and normal periph-eral pulses. The apical impulse was normal. On auscul-tation a systolic click varied in intensity and a soft systolic murmur was heard best mid-way between the left sternal border and the apex. The clinical diagnosis of mitral valve prolapse was made with mild mitral regur-gitation. An electrocardiogram showed sinus rhythm, normal intervals and non-specific inferior T wave flattening. Transthoracic two-dimensional echocardiog-raphy was technically limited, but a mobile right atrial mass was visualized which appeared to be arising from the tricuspid valve. A transesophageal echocardiogram performed as an outpatient procedure revealed the definitive diagnosis.

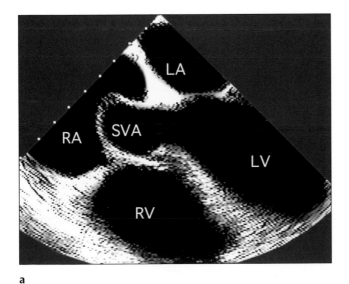
a

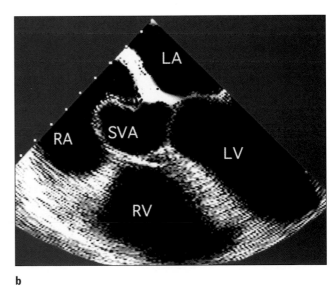
b

Figure 114.1
(a) Transesophageal image from the modified four-chamber view in the transverse plane (imaging angle 0°). The cardiac chambers are of normal size. A thin-walled chamber (SVA) that protrudes into the right atrium occupies the usual location of the aortic root. (b) Angulation of the probe demonstrates the same blind-ended sac taking origin from the crest of the interventricular septum and projecting into the right atrium. The sac appears to be contiguous with the interatrial septum superiorly. One of the cusps of the aortic valves is seen in the aortic root and identifies the chamber as arising from the aortic root rather than the outflow tract. The mitral valve was normal and there was no mitral prolapse.

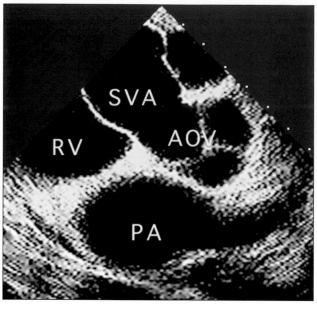
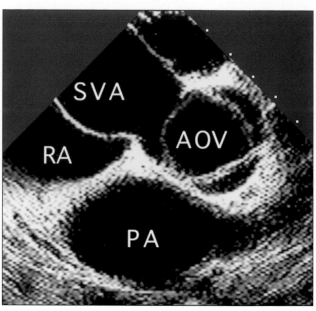

a   b

Figure 114.2
(a) In the short-axis view of the aorta (imaging angle 35°), the aortic valve is trileaflet with normal commissural anatomy demonstrable in diastole. The region of the non-coronary cusp is deficient and the sinus is contiguous with a thinned-walled, fluid-filled blind sac projecting into the right atrium.
(b) In systole, unrestricted leaflet opening is demonstrated. It is clear from this image that the sac originates from the aortic root rather than the left ventricular outflow tract.

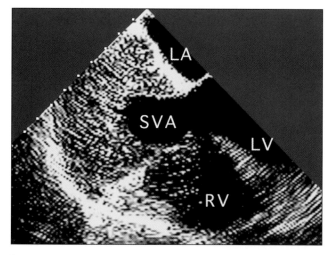
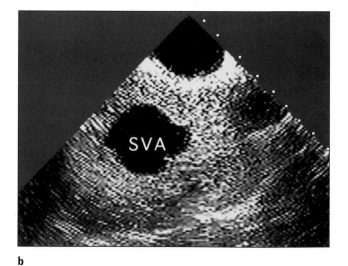

a   b

Figure 114.3
(a) Contrast injection into a peripheral vein opacifies the right atrium and right ventricle defining the contour of the blind-ended sac which projects into the right atrium immediately proximal to the tricuspid valve. The sac neither fills with contrast nor produces disturbance of the distribution of the right atrial contrast, making a left to right shunt unlikely.
(b) In the transverse plane the superior vena cava is to the right of the image and the interatrial septum is at the top of the image. The sinus of Valsalva aneurysm (SVA) is demonstrated in short-axis as it projects into the right atrium. The injected contrast circumscribes the sac.

Discussion

The patient was originally thought to have a right atrial mass and the transesophageal echocardiogram was undertaken to assess the nature of the mass. Sinus of Valsalva aneurysms can be highly mobile and may mimic tricuspid valve vegetations.[1] However, transesophageal echocardiography diagnosed a large unruptured sinus of Valsalva aneurysm taking origin from the non-coronary aortic sinus. In this location, sinus of Valsalva aneurysms most commonly rupture into the right atrium and less commonly into the right ventricle. Our patient had a further episode of upper sternal chest pain the day prior to elective surgical repair and intraoperatively was noted to show rupture into the right atrium.

Sinus of Valsalva aneurysms are usually diagnosed following acute rupture into the right heart chambers and the symptoms relate to the size of the shunt and the associated hemodynamic compromise. Sinus of Valsalva aneurysms usually occur after puberty and rupture usually occurs in the second or third decade, and is more frequent in Oriental patients. There is a defect in the media of the aortic wall at the site of the aneurysm which causes it to be classified as a congenital lesion. Mutations of connective tissue formation such as Ehlers–Danlos syndrome are associated with sinus of Valsalva aneurysms.[2,3] They may rupture spontaneously or secondarily to endocarditis. Treatment is surgical and accurate diagnosis is imperative,

as they may progress with death resulting within a year from rupture.[4] Color flow Doppler readily identifies the site and magnitude of the left to right shunt. Transesophageal echocardiography is especially helpful in delineating the anatomy of the aneurysm and its connections to other chambers.[5]

References

1. Atay A, Alpert M, Bertuso J, et al. Right sinus of Valsalva aneurysm presenting as an echocardiographic right atrial mass. Am Heart J 1986;112:169–72.

2. Cupo LN, Pyeritz RE, Olson JL, et al. Ehlers–Danlos syndrome with abnormal collagen fibrils, sinus of Valsalva aneurysms, myocardial infarction, panacinar emphysema and cerebral hctcrotopias. Am J Med 1981;71:1051–8.

3. Takahashi T, Koide T, Yamaguchi H, et al. Ehlers–Danlos syndrome with aortic regurgitation, dilation of the sinuses of Valsalva, and abnormal dermal collagen fibrils. Am Heart J 1992;123:1709–12.

4. Burakovsky V, Podsolkov V, Sabirow B, et al. Ruptured congenital aneurysm of the sinus of Valsalva. Clinical manifestations, diagnosis and results of surgical corrections. J Thorac Cardiovasc Surg 1988;95:836–41.

5. McKenney P, Shemin R, Wiegers S. Role of transesophageal echocardiography in sinus of Valsalva aneurysm. Am Heart J 1992;123:228–9.

115

Stab wound to the chest

Susan E Wiegers MD

A 19-year-old man was brought to the emergency department by the police after being involved in an altercation. The man had been found lying on the ground with blood on his shirt. He had bruises to his head and a laceration on his right hand. The police had no available witnesses. The patient stated that he had been stabbed. However, he was highly combative and intoxicated and could not describe the size of the weapon or the length of the blade.

Physical examination revealed an entrance wound on the chest, in the left third intercostal space. There was dried blood but no active oozing. The depth could not be determined. The patient's blood pressure was 100/60 mmHg and his pulse was 120 bpm. The oxygen saturation was 98% in room air. The patient required physical restraint. A toxicological screen was positive for cocaine. The alcohol level was 306. A chest X-ray did not show widening of the mediastinum. One examiner believed that there was a loud systolic murmur but others could not confirm this finding. A transthoracic echocardiogram was attempted but was of limited quality and was also limited by the patient's delirium. The patient was admitted to an intensive care unit bed and observed. He became more co-operative but could recall none of the events of the previous evening. He remained tachycardic and the blood pressure fell slightly. The presence of a loud continuous murmur was confirmed. A transesophageal echocardiogram was performed.

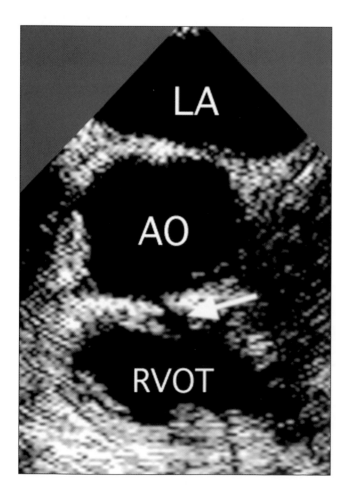

Figure 115.1
Transesophageal image from the mid-esophagus in the transverse plane (imaging angle 0°) modified four-chamber view. The left atrium (LA) is at the top of the screen. The aortic root (AO) is visualized directly anterior to the left atrium (below the left atrium in the transesophageal image). The aortic valve leaflets are out of plane in this image. There is a discontinuity of the wall (arrow) between the aortic root and the right ventricular outflow tract (RVOT). A flap is seen in the right ventricular outflow tract that represents tissue prolapsing from the laceration.

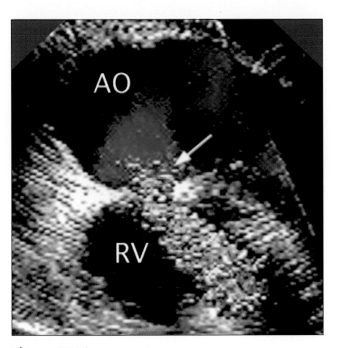

Figure 115.2
Similar transesophageal view with color Doppler flow imaging in systole. This is a close-up image of the area of discontinuity. A high-velocity, turbulent jet (arrow) passes from the aortic root into the distal right ventricular outflow tract. The proximal flow convergence of the jet can be seen in the aortic root.

Discussion

Patients who have sustained a cardiac injury from penetrating chest trauma may on occasion escape initial hemodynamic collapse. A patient who stabilizes after the administration of intravenous fluid presents a diagnostic dilemma. Often, transthoracic studies are done to evaluate the heart.[1] The absence of a pericardial effusion is a favorable sign, although it does not definitively rule out cardiac injury. Patients with normal transthoracic echocardiogram after penetrating chest injury may be admitted to a monitored unit.[2] Significant cardiac trauma may be delayed in presentation and the diagnosis may not be made in the emergency room. In one study, 23% of patients with penetrating chest wounds had severe cardiac injury that was not diagnosed initially.[3] The most common lesions are ventricular septal defects, but atrial septal defects, and aortic and tricuspid valve trauma can also occur. In addition, a patient with a ventricular laceration and tamponade should undergo immediate repair of the life-threatening lesion. Occasionally, additional lesions are discovered postoperatively and may require a second thoracotomy.

This patient was hemodynamically stable in the emergency room, with no definite evidence of injury to the heart or great vessels. The tachycardia was thought to be secondary to his drug intoxication. While it was hoped that the knife blade had not penetrated to the level of essential mediastinal structures, he was admitted to the hospital and carefully observed. In fact, the knife had penetrated the anterior surface of the right ventricular outflow tract and the aortic root. Both the aortic and the pulmonary valves had escaped injury which would have been recognized by significant regurgitation. The laceration to the anterior surface of the pulmonary artery had sealed, preventing significant mediastinal bleeding. However, the gradient between the aortic root and the pulmonary root throughout the cardiac cycle led to a continuous left to right shunt, which may have increased the size of the defect and the degree of shunting over time. Aortic to right-sided fistulas have been described after penetrating trauma. They lead to progressive heart failure and cardiac decompensation if unrepaired. This patient underwent thoracotomy and closure of the defect on the third hospital day with excellent results.

References

1. Bolton JW, Bynoe RP, Lazar HL, *et al.* Two-dimensional echocardiography in the evaluation of penetrating intrapericardial injuries. Ann Thorac Surg 1993;56:506–9.

2. Freshman SP, Wisner DH, Weber CJ. 2-D echocardiography: emergent use in the evaluation of penetrating precordial trauma [see comments]. J Trauma 1991;31:902–5; discussion 905–6.

3. Cha EK, Mittal V, Allaben RD. Delayed sequelae of penetrating cardiac injury. Arch Surg 1993;128:836–9; discussion 839–41.

116

Aortic disease–descending and abdominal aortic aneurysm

Frank E Silvestry MD

A 67-year-old African-American woman presented with upper back and left shoulder pain of several months' duration. She described the pain as a dull intermittent ache, which did not limit her activities, and was not associated with exertion. Her medical history was remarkable for longstanding poorly controlled hypertension, and moderate tobacco abuse. Her physical examination revealed blood pressure of 155/98 mmHg in both arms, and a soft S$_4$ gallop on cardiac auscultation. On abdominal examination, there was a 6-cm pulsatile non-tender mass. Chest radiography revealed a widened mediastinum, and a top normal cardiac silhouette. A screening transthoracic echocardiogram was obtained.

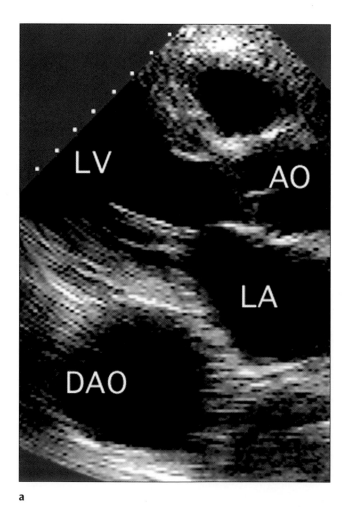

a

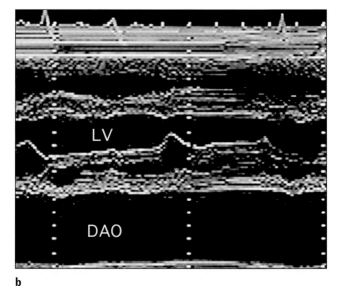

b

Figure 116.1
(a) Two-dimensional echocardiogram in the parasternal long-axis view demonstrating the left ventricle (LV), left atrium (LA), and ascending aorta (AO). The descending thoracic aorta (DAO) is seen in short-axis posteriorly to the left ventricle and left atrium. It is significantly enlarged, measuring approximately 6 cm in diameter. The aortic root and ascending aorta are normal in size.
(b) M-mode echocardiogram at the level of the mitral valve, demonstrating a descending thoracic aortic aneurysm of 6 cm in diameter, posterior to the left ventricle. Note that the large echo-free space might be mistaken for a pericardial effusion on M-mode.

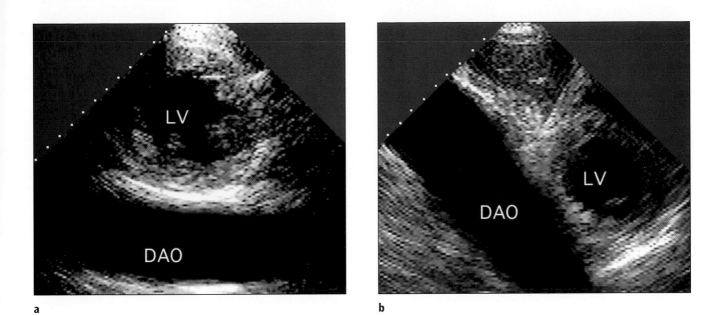

a   b

Figure 116.2

(a) Parasternal short-axis view of the left ventricle (LV) at the level of the papillary muscles. The descending thoracic aorta (DAO) is seen in long-axis posterior to the left ventricle, and is significantly enlarged. The walls of the aorta are smooth and no definite dissection flap is seen within the aorta.

(b) Off-axis view of the aorta from the subcostal short-axis position. The descending thoracic and proximal abdominal aorta are markedly dilated throughout its course. The dimension of the aorta is consistent with aneurysmal dilatation. The aneurysm does not appear to be discrete and involves the entire descending aorta that is visualized. The walls of the aorta now appear somewhat shaggy, consistent with moderate atherosclerosis.

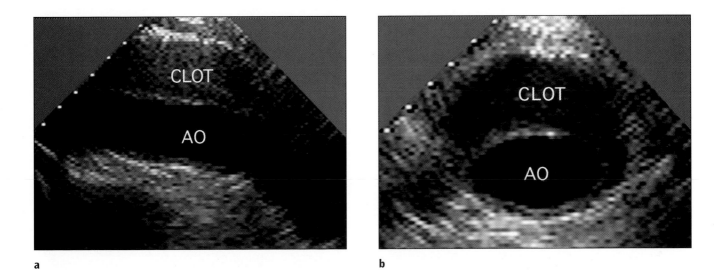

a   b

Figure 116.3

(a) Sub-xiphoid view of the mid-abdominal aorta (AO) shown in long-axis. The level of the aorta is more distal than that imaged in Figure 116.2. The lumen of the abdominal aorta is largely filled with thrombus (CLOT), which is at least 3 cm thick anteriorly.

(b) Sub-xiphoid view of the abdominal aorta (AO) shown in short-axis. Note the aneurysmal dilatation, with prominent thrombus (CLOT) seen anteriorly, which significantly encroaches on the luminal diameter.

Discussion

This patient presents with both a descending thoracic aneurysm and an abdominal aortic aneurysm. The echocardiographic appearance of aneurysmal aortic dilatation and atherosclerosis produces a characteristic echocardiographic appearance. Enlargement of the descending thoracic aorta and abdominal aorta can usually be visualized by transthoracic echocardiography; however, disease in the ascending aorta and transverse aorta often requires transesophageal echocardiography for a complete evaluation. Biplanar or omniplanar transesophageal echocardiography offers the ability to image almost the entire aorta in multiple planes. A short portion of the distal ascending aorta and proximal transverse arch is usually not visible; this is a 'blind' area, due to the carina passing between the aorta and the esophagus. The superior sensitivity and specificity of transesophageal echocardiography for aortic disease including aneurysm, dissection, atherosclerosis, mobile plaque, and traumatic aortic disruption make it the test of choice in many clinical situations.[1] Transthoracic echocardiography has evolved as an initial screening test, however, and attempts to visualize the entire thoracic aorta should be included in every clinical study. Transesophageal echocardiography can then be performed in selected patients with either abnormal transthoracic echocardiograms, or a high clinical index of suspicion for significant aortic disease.

Within aortic aneurysms, stagnant blood flow may result in spontaneous echo contrast (or 'smoke'), as well as frank thrombus formation, as seen in this patient.[2] Both of these entities may be seen on transthoracic echocardiography, although transesophageal echocardiography again offers superior sensitivity and greater definition in the thoracic aorta. Intraluminal thrombus must be differentiated from aortic dissection, where thrombus may be present in the false lumen. Features such as a mobile intimal flap and flow into and out of the space that contains the thrombus through a defect in the dissection flap favor dissection over intraluminal thrombus within an aortic aneurysm.

Marfan's syndrome may result in characteristic aortic pathology, including symmetrical enlargement of the aortic root and sinuses of Valsalva, aortic aneurysms, and aortic dissection.[3] Enlargement of the aortic root and annulus, as well as abnormal aortic leaflet tissue, may result in significant aortic regurgitation. Again transesophageal echocardiography offers superior sensitivity and specificity in detecting and defining aortic root pathology as well as aortic aneurysms and aortic dissection in Marfan's syndrome.

References

1. Simpson IA, de Belder MA, Treasure T, et al. Cardiovascular manifestations of Marfan's syndrome: improved evaluation by transesophageal echocardiography. Br Heart J 1993;69:104–8.

2. Castello R, Pearson AC, Fagan L, Labovitz AJ. Spontaneous echocardiographic contrast in the descending aorta. Am Heart J 1990;120:915–9.

3. Fox R, Ren JF, Panidis IP, et al. Annuloaortic ectasia: a clinical and echocardiographic study. Am J Cardiol 1984;54:177–81.

117

Pseudoaneurysm of the aorta after aortic valve reoperation

Susan E Wiegers MD

A 44-year-old man with Marfan's syndrome had under-gone an aortic valve replacement with a Starr Edward's valve in his early twenties for severe aortic regurgitation. He had subsequently developed an ascending aortic aneurysm which required an aortic root replacement with a surgical conduit 10 years later. At the age of 44 he was noted to have a markedly aneurysmal aorta distal to the conduit site. In addition, there were high velocities across his Star Edward's valve which was now 20 years old. He underwent replacement of a bileaflet mechanical valve

with a composite graft to the high ascending aorta. He did well in the immediate postoperative period. He was discharged on anticoagulation for the prosthetic valve. Four weeks after surgery, while at home, he had the sudden onset of severe chest pain, and shortness of breath, followed by loss of consciousness. He was taken to another hospital and transferred directly to the operating room at our hospital. A transesophageal echocardiogram was performed in the operating room to evaluate the cause of his cardiogenic shock.

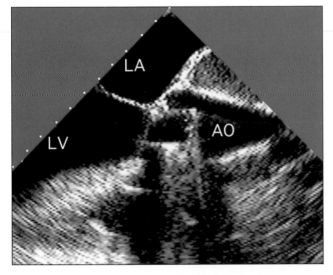 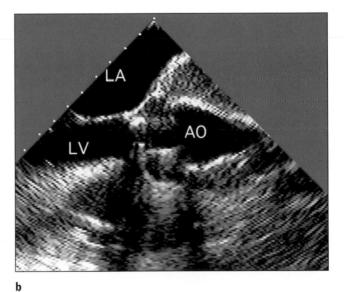

a   b

Figure 117.1
(a) Transesophageal echocardiogram from the mid-esophageal position (imaging angle 130°). The left atrium (LA) and left ventricle (LV) are incompletely visualized. The bileaflet mechanical valve is seen in systole in the open position. The composite graft appears to be normal posteriorly but a large hematoma is visible posterior to the posterior wall of the conduit. The distal portion the conduit is seen to be narrowed and there is echodense material anterior to the conduit (at the bottom of the screen), which appears to represent hematoma as well.
(b) Similar transesophageal echocardiogram (imaging angle 130°) with rotation of the transducer towards the right side of the patient. The highly refractile leaflets of the mechanical valve are out of plane, allowing imaging of the anterior structures. Again, compression is noted of the distal portion of the aortic conduit. There is an echolucent area anterior to the conduit and homogeneous material, consistent with thrombus. Note that anterior structures are imaged at the bottom of the screen and posterior structures at the top in the transesophageal image. This echolucent area with surrounding hematoma is consistent with pseudoaneurysm of the aorta.

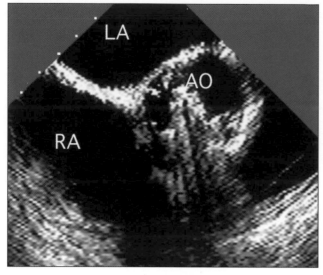

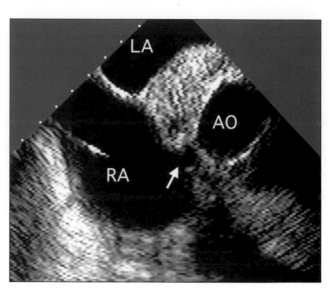

a

b

Figure 117.2

(a) Transesophageal echocardiogram in the transverse plane (imaging angle 0°). The probe has been withdrawn slightly and is at the level of the aortic valve leaflet. The root and conduit appear essentially normal at this level, although the anterior portion of the conduit, that is the portion adjacent to the right atrium, appears to have a break in it. Because the mechanical valve leaflets are interposed between the ultrasound beam in this structure it is not clear whether this is shadowing from the leaflets or a true defect. Reverberation lines and lines of shadowing are visible arising from the aortic valve leaflets and extending towards the bottom of the image along the path of the ultrasound beam.

(b) Similar transesophageal image in the transverse plane (imaging angle 0°). The probe has been withdrawn slightly to image the aortic conduit. The hematoma within the pseudoaneurysm is visible posteriorly. While the wall of the surgical conduit appears to be intact at this level, there is a defect in the wall of the pseudoaneurysm (arrow), which appears to communicate with the right atrium. In addition, a catheter is present in the right atrium.

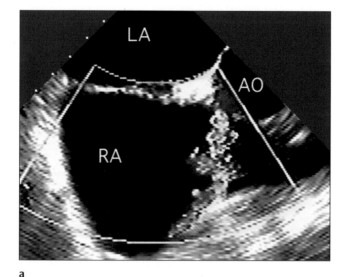

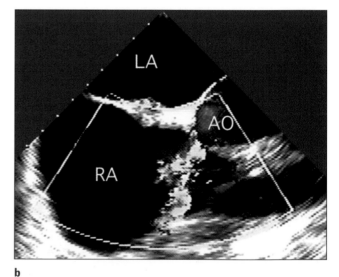

a

b

Figure 117.3

(a) and (b) Transesophageal echocardiogram from the mid-esophageal position in the transverse plane. The probe has been advanced slightly compared to Figure 117.2b. There is a high-velocity jet in the right atrium which was continuous throughout the cardiac cycle. At this level it did not appear to be arising from within the aortic conduit itself. Note that the wall of the aortic conduit (AO) is outlined by the jet and there is no proximal acceleration on the aortic side of the jet. This jet arose from the pseudoaneurysm which had a very small leak into the right atrium. The other clue that this jet does not arise directly from the aorta is the velocity.

Although the jet is turbulent and aliases, it is neither severely turbulent nor of very high velocity, as indicated by the absence of a mosaic pattern. This again suggests that the pressure of the originating chamber is not that of the systolic aorta.

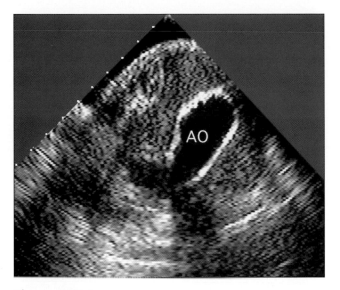

Figure 117.4
Transesophageal echocardiogram from the high esophageal
position in the transverse plane (imaging angle 0°). The aortic
conduit (AO) is surrounded by a massive pseudoaneurysm
containing hematoma which appears to be compressing the
aorta.

Discussion

Pseudoaneurysm of the aorta is a rare complication after
aortic valve replacement, repair of aortic dissections and
surgical replacement of the ascending aorta. It has also
been reported to occur at the site of aortic cannulation for
coronary artery bypass graft surgery. Pseudoaneurysms of
the aorta may reach massive proportions and can be a
chronic condition. However, the propensity for sudden
rupture mandates immediate repair when the diagnosis is
made. In the setting of chronic pseudoaneurysms, surgical mortality has been reported to be acceptable.[1]

Cystic medial necrosis of the aorta predisposes to development of aortic pseudoaneurysm after aortic surgery.[2]
Infection of the conduit or valve prosthesis may also
predispose to the development of a pseudoaneurysm.
Multiple surgical procedures on the aorta also appear to
be a risk factor. No doubt, the repeated surgeries lead to
fibrosis and scar tissue which are able to contain an aortic
rupture. If this were not the case, aortic rupture would
lead to immediate exsanguination into the mediastinum.
As demonstrated in this patient, the hematoma was
contained within the native aortic tissue that had been
wrapped around the surgical conduit. The patient's shock
state was due not only to acute blood loss but also to acute
aortic compression, which resulted in supravalvular aortic
stenosis.

Echocardiography is an important tool for the diagnosis of the condition. Transesophageal imaging is particularly helpful. In the less acute setting, magnetic resonance
imaging may be used to assess the aorta and the site of
rupture. A spiral computerized tomography scan with
contrast and aortography are also useful modalities.[3] This
patient's hemodynamic condition precluded any evaluation outside the operating room. It is most important to
diagnose the site of rupture, in order to accomplish a
successful repair. Periannular dehiscence appears to be the
most common site of leakage but some patients have
more than one site of rupture. The site of rupture may be
distinguished by a high-velocity systolic jet into the
pseudoaneurysm.[4] Subsequent rupture of the pseudoaneurysm has been reported into another mediastinal
structure, including the bronchus, esophagus, and the
right atrium. The resulting bleeding is less severe than that
associated with a direct fistula from the aorta to the
bronchus or esophagus. However, the bleeding may be
brisk enough to produce complications on its own.

The site of the rupture in this patient's case could not
be definitively seen by transesophageal echocardiography,
owing to interference from the prosthetic mechanical
valve. It was suspected that the rupture must be close to
the right coronary artery anastamosis, owing to the
finding of an echolucent collection in this area with more
solid hematoma in other parts of the pseudoaneurysm. At
surgery, a dehiscence was found at the site of the right
coronary artery anastamosis to the surgical conduit. The
site was repaired and a vein graft placed to the right
coronary artery. The fistula to the right atrium was not
specifically addressed, but the flow was not visible on
immediate post-pump echocardiogram. The patient's
course was complicated by inferior myocardial infarction
with right ventricular infarction and acute renal failure,
which did not require dialysis. The patient has not been
reanticoagulated despite a fall in his ejection fraction. Two
years after the event he has returned to limited physical
activity.

References

1. Sato O, Tada Y, Miyata T, *et al*. False aneurysms after aortic opera-
    tions. J Cardiovasc Surg 1992;33:604–8.

2. Albat B, Leclercque P, MessnerPellenc P, *et al*. False aneurysm of the
    ascending aorta following aortic valve replacement. J Heart Valve Dis
    1994;3:216–19.

3. Lasorda D, Power T, Dianzumba S, *et al*. Diagnosis of aortic
    pseudoaneurysm by echocardiography. Clin Cardiol 1992;15:773–6.

4. Barbetseas J, Crawford E, Safi H, *et al*. Doppler echocardiographic
    evaluation of pseudoaneurysms complicating composite grafts of the
    ascending aorta. Circulation 1992;85:212–22.

118

Marfan's syndrome and acute aortic dissection

Martin G Keane MD

21-year-old man with a history of lenticular dislocation and 'double-joints' presented with 3 hours of mid-scapular back pain. He had been in his usual state of health until attempting to move heavy equipment in his office. On physical examination, he was in severe distress. His blood pressure was 144/50 mmHg. The lungs were clear and he had a decrescendo diastolic murmur, heard best at the left sternal border.

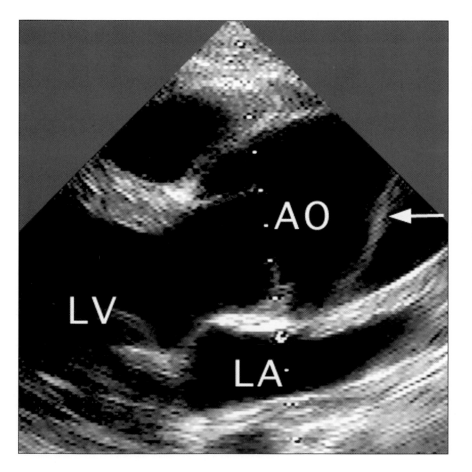

Figure 118.1
Parasternal long-axis view of the ascending aorta. The proximal aorta (AO) is moderately dilated, a common finding in patients with Marfan's syndrome. The aortic leaflets are open in systole but do not reach the walls of the aortic root, owing to the severe dilatation. The left atrium appears to be compressed by the ascending aorta, although this is not a hemodynamically significant finding. A dissection flap (arrow) originates just distal to the non-coronary sinus of Valsalva, and extends upwards into the ascending aorta.

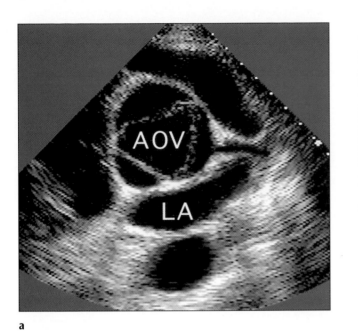

a

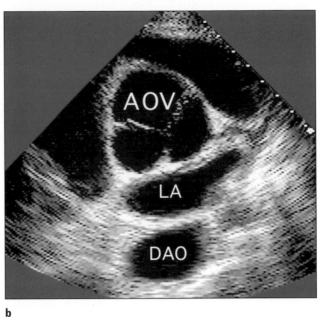

b

Figure 118.2

(a) Parasternal short-axis view at the level of the aortic valve leaflets. The aortic root dilatation and left atrial (LA) compression are again evident. The trileaflet aortic valve demonstrates normal systolic opening, but the leaflets are thin and redundant. This image is taken below the level of the dissection flap, as can be appreciated from the previous image. The left main ostium is normally patent arising from the left coronary sinus. The descending thoracic aorta, visible posterior to the left atrium at this level, is of normal caliber. (b) Similar view in systole. There is uniform enlargement of all sinus segments, a common feature of patients with Marfan's syndrome. Leaflet coaptation is not perfectly symmetrical, consistent with leaflet redundancy and possibly prolapse. DAO – descending thoracic aorta.

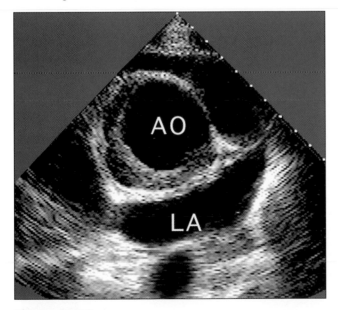

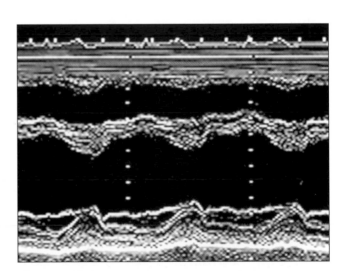

Figure 118.3

Parasternal short-axis view of the ascending aorta (AO) above the level of the sinuses of Valsalva. The false lumen of the dissection is clearly visualized, forming a hemi-arc in the lower left-hand portion of the aorta. There is increased echodensity within this lumen, consistent with early thrombus or dense spontaneous echo contrast. The aneurysmal dilatation of the aorta was present prior to the acute dissection.

Figure 118.4

M-mode echocardiogram from the parasternal position of the left ventricle. There is moderate dilatation of the left ventricular cavity (6 cm). During early diastole, a second inward motion of the interventricular septum is noted. This is known as a diastolic dip, and is consistent with severe aortic insufficiency.

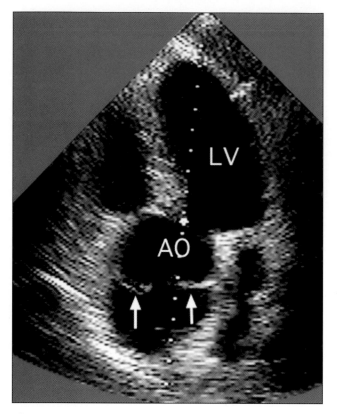

Figure 118.5
Apical five-chamber view. The aortic root dilatation is
prominent. The transverse structure (arrows) in the proximal
ascending aorta is well above the usual plane of the aortic
valve leaflets. This is the proximal extent of the dissection
flap. Although it is incompletely seen, this appearance of the
aorta in the five-chamber view should raise the question of
aortic dissection, particularly in association with aortic
regurgitation. The dilated aorta obstructs the view of the right
atrium and compresses the left atrium.

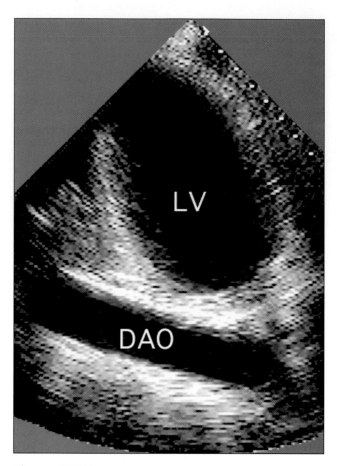

Figure 118.7
Off-axis apical view with the transducer directed posteriorly
and slightly inferiorly from the standard two-chamber view.
The descending aorta (DAO) appears to be normal and there
is no clear dissection flap.

Figure 118.6
Spectral display of continuous-wave Doppler across the aortic
valve from the apical position. Diastolic flow towards the
transducer in this position is consistent with aortic
insufficiency. The magnitude of the velocity deceleration slope
is a measure of the severity of insufficiency, which is
moderate in this case.

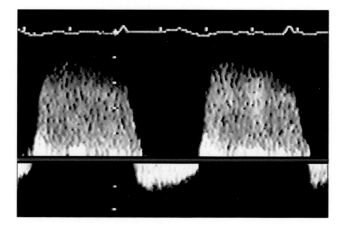

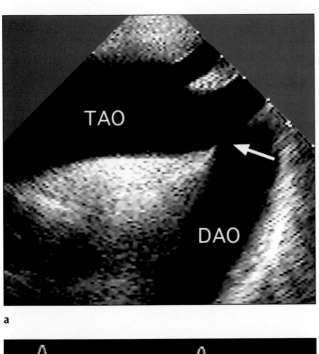

a

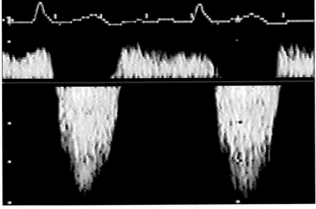

b

Figure 118.8

(a) Suprasternal notch view of the transverse aortic arch (TAO) and the descending thoracic aorta (DAO). The arch is dilated but the dissection flap, which was seen in the parasternal images of the ascending aorta, is not visualized. The caliber of the descending aorta is more normal. There is apparent narrowing of the aorta at the level of the ligamentum arteriosum (arrow) which probably represents the transition between the dilated and the normal aorta. There is no obstruction to flow at this level. It is possible that there is a dissection flap at this level which is being incompletely visualized.

(b) Spectral display of continuous-wave Doppler across the narrowing in the descending aorta. The velocity of systolic flow is elevated at 3 m/s. Diastolic reversal of flow is also seen. In this case, the reversed flow is most likely to be due to the significant aortic regurgitation. However, this finding should be confirmed with pulsed-wave Doppler well away from the left subclavian take-off. Diastolic run-off into the great vessels may give the appearance of diastolic flow reversal in the absence of important aortic regurgitation.

Discussion

Marfan's syndrome, an autosomal dominant disorder of connective tissue, is characterized by a fairly classic constellation of clinical findings, including abnormalities of the eye, skeleton, heart, and aorta.[1] Specific cardiovascular manifestations of the syndrome include myxomatous degeneration of the mitral valve and chordal apparatus, mitral valve prolapse, dilatation of the aortic root, and myxomatous degeneration of the aortic valve leaflets.[2] These anomalies tend to be progressive over time and can lead to serious cardiovascular complications in the fourth or fifth decade of life. Aortic dissection is a common cause of death in these patients.[3]

Echocardiographic examination of the proximal aorta in patients with Marfan's syndrome most commonly demonstrates symmetric dilatation of the valve annulus and sinuses of Valsalva. The ascending aorta is often dilated as well. The degree of dilatation can range from mild to massive; it may be present at birth but can also develop and progress in adulthood.[4] Compression of surrounding structures can be seen in multiple echocardiographic views. Most characteristically, the left atrium appears to be compressed in its anteroposterior dimension in either the parasternal long-axis or short-axis views. The aortic valve itself is also abnormal in these patients. The aortic leaflets are often elongated and mildly thickened in a myxomatous pattern. This gives them a classically redundant appearance on two-dimensional imaging. The abnormalities of aortic leaflet structure, combined with enlargement of the aortic root, lead to poor coaptation of the leaflets which ultimately results in varying degrees of aortic insufficiency. Frank leaflet prolapse may also be present and can be detected best in the parasternal long-axis views. In such cases, the jet of aortic insufficiency may be eccentric, and more difficult to quantitate.

When complicated by acute proximal dissection, transthoracic echocardiograms may show the presence of a free intimal dissection flap within the lumen of the aorta. This extra echodensity moves freely within the aortic lumen, and is clearly separated from the singular echoes from the aortic wall. The flap motion may be appreciated on two-dimensional or on M-mode imaging. Occasionally, the intimal flap extends to the level of the aortic annulus, undermining the annular supports of the aortic valve itself. With dehiscence of the aortic valve commissures a severe degree of aortic insufficiency is usually present.

Assessment of the extent of distal dissection of the aorta is occasionally possible on transthoracic studies. Right-sided intercostal views may image the mid-ascending aorta. Turning the patient to the right lateral decubitus position may be helpful in obtaining these images. The suprasternal notch images allow visualization of the distal ascending aorta, the transverse arch, the head vessels, and the proximal descending thoracic aorta. The distal extent of the intimal flap may be identified. Subcostal views and off-axis apical views can often be used to visualize the distal descending thoracic aorta. Despite these abilities, transthoracic imaging has limited sensitivity and specificity for the presence of aortic dissection. In general, the diagnosis of and clear localization of dissection relies on confirmation by more sensitive techniques such as magnetic resonance imaging or transesophageal echocardiography.[5]

References

1. De Paepe A, Devereux R, Hennekam R, et al. Revised diagnostic criteria for the Marfan's syndrome. Am J Med Genet 1996;62:417–26.

2. Marsalese D, Moodie D, Vacante M, et al. Marfan's syndrome: natural history and long-term follow-up of cardiovascular involvement. J Am Coll Cardiol 1989;14:422.

3. Devereux R, Roman M. Aortic disease in Marfan's syndrome. N Engl J Med 1999;340:1358–9.

4. Kornbluth M, Schnittger I, Eyngorina I, et al. Clinical outcome in the Marfan's syndrome with ascending aortic dilatation followed annually by echocardiography. Am J Cardiol 1999;84:753–5.

5. Laissy J, Blanc F, Soyer P, et al. Thoracic aortic dissection: diagnosis with transesophageal echocardiography vs MR imaging. Radiology 1995;194:331.

119

Kawasaki's disease

Martin St John Sutton MBBS
Susan E Wiegers MD

A 29-year-old man complained of a band-like episode of chest discomfort which occurred intermittently associated with moderate exertion, relieved by rest, and associated with nausea. His risk factors for coronary heart disease included current tobacco use and a family history of myocardial infarction and stroke in his father in his late fifties. There was no history of congenital heart disease in his extended family. An electrocardiogram showed normal sinus rhythm, and a treadmill exercise test using a Bruce protocol was normal at high workload. A chest X-ray demonstrated a normal cardiac silhouette and normal lung fields.

On examination, he was normotensive and in regular rhythm with a resting heart rate of 58 bpm. The jugular venous pressure and peripheral arterial pulses were equal bilaterally and on auscultation there was a normal first heart sound and a normally split second heart sound. A soft ejection systolic murmur was audible at the base. Review of his electrocardiogram and chest X-ray were both within normal limits.

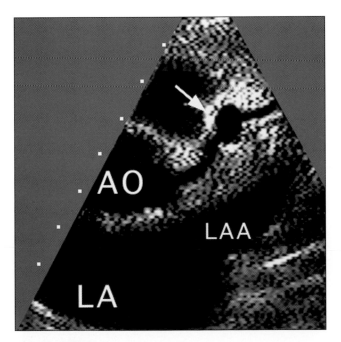

Figure 119.1
In the left parasternal short-axis view of the aorta, rotated to visualize the origin of the left coronary artery, a large aneurysm (arrow) approximately 7–8 mm in diameter, involves the origin of the left anterior descending branch. AO – aortic root; LAA – left atrial appendage.

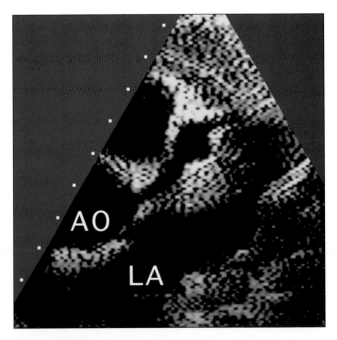

Figure 119.2
Using the zoom feature, the coronary aneurysm can be seen in continuity with the lumen of the proximal left coronary artery lumen, and this was confirmed with color flow Doppler. The rest of the echocardiogram was normal and there were no wall motion abnormalities.

Discussion

This patient had never had the diagnosis of Kawasaki's disease prior to the demonstration of coronary artery aneurysm. The syndrome includes fever, bilateral conjunctivitis and extensive cervical adenopathy. Erythema of the tongue and lips with cracking of the lips may also be prominent. Early echocardiography can demonstrate the presence of coronary artery ectasias or aneurysm. However, wall motion abnormalities in the early period are probably due to myocarditis rather than to epicardial coronary disease.[1] Myocardial infarctions and sudden death have been reported in association with coronary artery aneurysms.[2] Presumptive diagnosis of Kawasaki's disease is made with demonstration of coronary artery aneurysms in the adult. Giant coronary artery aneurysms may predispose to thrombus formation and resultant ischemia.[3] Both regression and enlargement of the aneurysms have been reported. Transesophageal echocardiography may be helpful in defining the proximal coronary artery anatomy. The patient underwent coronary arteriography, which demonstrated multiple coronary artery aneurysms involving the right and left coronary arteries consistent with Kawasaki's disease. A workup for other causes of arteritis was negative. The patient was treated with warfarin and low-dose aspirin.

References

1. Vogel M, Smallhorn JF, Freedom RM, Serial analysis of regional left ventricular wall motion by two-dimensional echocardiography in patients with coronary artery enlargement after Kawasaki disease. J Am Coll Cardiol 1992;20:915–19.

2. Suzuki A, Tizard EJ, Gooch V, *et al.* Kawasaki disease: echocardiographic features in 91 cases presenting in the United Kingdom. Arch Dis Child 1990;65:1142–6.

3. Habon T, Toth K, Keltai M, *et al.* An adult case of Kawasaki disease with multiplex coronary aneurysms and myocardial infarction: the role of transesophageal echocardiography. Clin Cardiol 1998;21:529–32.

120

Ruptured sinus of Valsalva aneurysm

Susan E Wiegers MD

Λ 27-year-old woman with no past medical history developed shortness of breath and orthopnea which progressed over 2 weeks. Her physician noted a new continuous murmur that was loudest at the left lower sternal border.

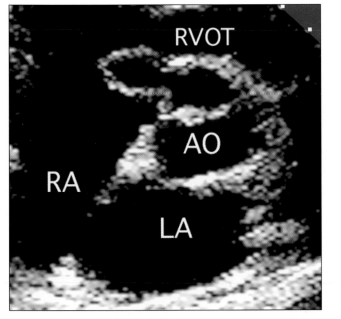

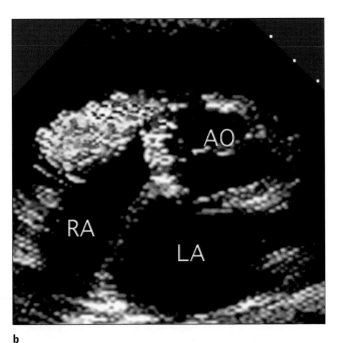

a   b

Figure 120.1
(a) Transthoracic echocardiogram of the parasternal short-axis of the base of the heart in diastole. The aortic valve (AO) is tricuspid, although the left coronary cusp is not imaged. The off-axis projection allows imaging of the right sinus of Valsalva which is enlarged (arrow) and projects into the right atrium (RA) at the level of the tricuspid valve. The aneurysm was highly mobile and was initially mistaken for a vegetation attached to the tricuspid valve. RVOT, right ventricular outflow tract; LA, left atrium.
(b) Similar view with color Doppler flow imaging of the left to right shunt. The flow originates in the aortic root and is seen in the right atrium as a turbulent jet. The peak systolic velocity of 5 m/s distinguished it from possible tricuspid regurgitation. The peak pulmonary systolic pressure would have to be suprasystemic to result in a tricuspid regurgitation jet with such a velocity.

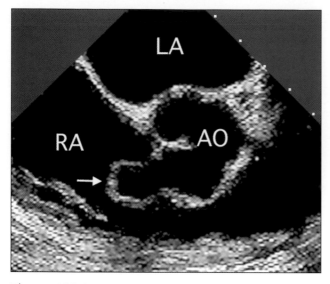

Figure 120.2
Transesophageal echocardiogram from the level of the mid-esophagus (imaging angle 30°). The right sinus of Valsalva aneurysm (arrow) projects into the right atrium. Its origin from the aortic root is clearly defined in this image. The walls of the aneurysm are thin and mobile. The structure resembles a windsock.

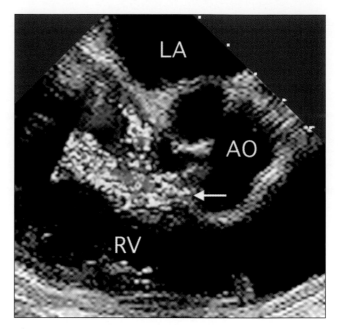

Figure 120.3
Transesophageal echocardiogram with color flow Doppler mapping. The orientation is approximately the same as in Figure 120.2. Several jets of shunt flow from the aortic root to the right atrium are present as turbulent, high-velocity jets. The largest jet is marked by an arrow. Multiple perforations may be present in the aneurysm, resulting in several jets of shunt flow.

Discussion

Sinus of Valsalva aneurysm is a congenital lesion. The walls of the aneurysm are generally thinner than the normal aortic root. Shunt flow is uncommon at birth. However, the sinus of Valsalva aneurysm enlarges with time and may eventually rupture. The rupture is usually sudden and may be accompanied by sharp chest pain. Rupture may occur spontaneously or be precipitated by endocarditis or blunt chest trauma. Right sinus aneurysms usually rupture into the right atrium, while left sinus aneurysms rupture into the left ventricle or the left atrium. Non-coronary sinus aneurysms most commonly result in shunt flow into the left atrium.

A new continuous murmur is usually audible. High output failure may result from the large shunt flow. The site of the rupture determines the degree of hemodynamic instability associated with the shunt, but all sites may eventually result in high output failure. Rupture into the left atrium is the least well tolerated acutely, although very small perforations in the aneurysm can occasionally be asymptomatic. On transthoracic examination, the shunt may be mistaken for severe atrioventricular valve regurgitation. However, the diastolic component of the shunt flow should be evident.[1] The velocity of the jet in the case of rupture into the right atrium is another clue that tricuspid regurgitation is not present. Finally, the turbulent jet will be eccentric and will not appear to arise from the valvular plane. However, transesophageal echocardiogra-

phy may be necessary to delineate the diagnosis and the level of the shunt.[2] Echocardiography obviates the need for angiography in young patients with ruptured sinus of Valsalva aneurysms.[3]

The Q_P/Q_S ratio may be easily calculated from the transthoracic study. The flow across the pulmonary circuit (Q_P) is equal to the $VTI_{PA} \times CSA_{PA}$, where the VTI_{PA} is the velocity–time integral obtained from the main pulmonary artery and the CSA is the cross-sectional area of the pulmonary artery at the same level. This is calculated by measuring the diameter (D) of the pulmonary artery and using the formula $CSA = \pi D/2$. Similarly, the VTI_{LVOT} of the left ventricular outflow tract is measured in the apical five-chamber view and the diameter of the left ventricular outflow tract is measured from the parasternal long-axis view. The shunt flow calculation simplifies to:

$$Q_P/Q_S = VTI_{PA}(D_{PA})^2/VTI_{LVOT}(D_{LVOT})^2$$

In this patient, the left to right shunt flow was significant and signs of right heart failure quickly ensued. Multiple blood cultures were negative. She underwent primary closure with excision of the aneurysm and closure of the defect with a pericardial patch. Her symptoms completely resolved and she has done well.

References

1. Chiang C, Lin F, Fang B, *et al.* Doppler and two-dimensional echocaridographic features of sinus of Valsalva aneurysms. Am Heart J 1988;116:1283–8.

2. McKenney P, Shemin R, Wiegers S. Role of transesophageal echocardiography in sinus of Valsalva aneurysm. Am Heart J 1992;123:228–9.

3. Sahasakul Y, Panchavinnin P, Chaithiraphan S, *et al.* Echocardiographic diagnosis of a ruptured aneurysm of the sinus of Valsalva: operation without catheterisation in seven patients. Br Heart J 1990;64:195–8.

121

Mycotic aneurysm of the ascending aorta

Susan E Wiegers MD

A 71-year-old patient underwent five-vessel bypass surgery for severe coronary artery disease. He was diabetic and had mild renal insufficiency. Several weeks after discharge he developed increasing chest pain and was diagnosed with a superficial sternal wound infection. After several months of persistent fevers, he had a computerized tomography scan which demonstrated a significant retrosternal fluid collection. He was admitted to the hospital, where wound cultures grew methicillin-resistant *Staphylococcus aureus*

(MRSA). The patient had an elevated white count and a fever as high as 102°F. On the third hospital day, he acutely developed severe substernal chest pain associated with hypotension and a decrease in the hematocrit. The electrocardiogram demonstrated ST elevation in the inferior and lateral leads. A chest X-ray showed a new widening of the mediastinum and he was transferred via helicopter to a tertiary care hospital. A transesophageal echocardiogram was done to assess the aorta.

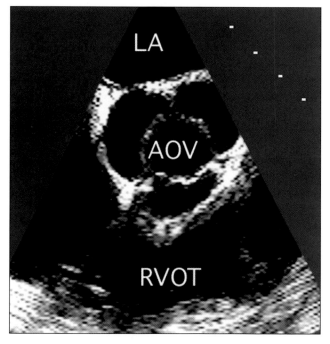
a

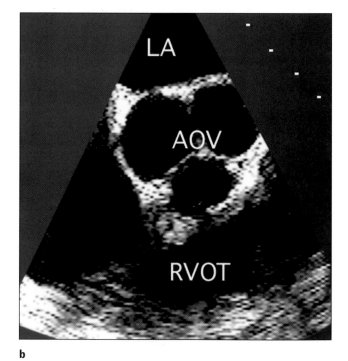
b

Figure 121.1
(a) Transesophageal echocardiogram from the mid-esophageal view (imaging angle 40°). The aortic valve is shown in systole in short axis. The valve leaflets are mildly thickened. The commissures between the right and non-coronary cusps are mildly calcified. The aortic root is normal. The other heart structures including the left atrium (LA) and the right ventricular outflow tract (RVOT) are normal.
(b) In diastole, the leaflets of the aortic valve coapt normally. The anterior root (towards the bottom of the screen) is mildly thickened, but no other significant abnormalities are seen.

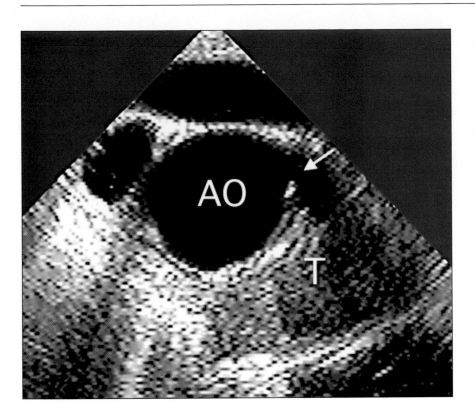

Figure 121.2
Transesophageal echocardiogram from the transverse plane (imaging angle 0°). Compared to the previous image, the probe has been withdrawn to a higher esophageal position. The ascending aorta (AO) is imaged in short-axis and the superior vena cava is seen in short-axis parallel to the aorta. The right pulmonary artery is imaged posteriorly (at the top of the screen) as it passes behind the aorta. There is a break (arrow) in the posterolateral wall of the ascending aorta which is large. A sizable thrombus (T) is present anterior to the aorta.

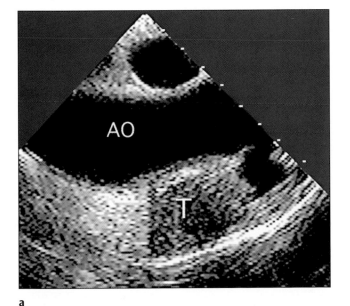

a

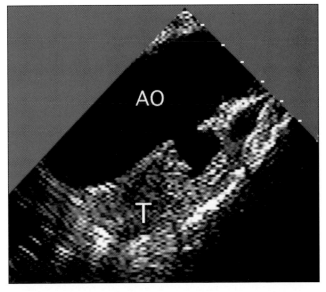

b

Figure 121.3
(a) Transesophageal echocardiogram from the longitudinal plane (imaging angle 130°). The transducer has been rotated towards the right to image the right pulmonary artery in short axis behind the ascending aorta. The neck of the pseudoaneurysm is visible in the anterior wall of the aorta. The break in the aortic wall occurred at the aortic cannulation site from the previous bypass surgery. The defect in the aorta was seripiginous and occurred at several levels of the ascending aorta. The thrombus is due to contained hemorrhage from the ruptured aorta. The echolucent area in the thrombus adjacent to the tear in the aortic wall represents uncoagulated blood from ongoing hemorrhage.
(b) Similar view with the transducer withdrawn further. The defect in the aortic wall is large and involves a significant proportion of the circumference of the aorta. The intima of the aorta at other levels appears to be normal. The defect is an abrupt transection in the aortic wall at that level. The normal aorta at other levels makes dissection or intramural hematoma unlikely.

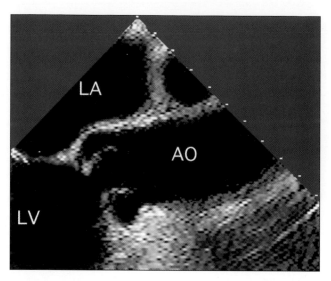

Figure 121.4
Postoperative image of the aorta. The friable aortic wall was resected and replaced by an aortic homograft. The anterior fluid collection was drained and was found to consist of purulent material and fresh thrombus. There was no residual bleeding.

Discussion

Aortic pseudoaneurysm is most frequently a complication of traumatic injury to the aorta in deceleration injuries. Surgical technique may be responsible for damage to the aortic wall and be the resultant nidus for an aortic tear or infection.[1] Cross-clamping of the aorta during coronary artery bypass surgery has been implicated as a predisposing factor in the development of aortic dissection, since the intima may be damaged at this site. Cannulation of the aorta involves a full thickness violation of the wall and can be the site of pseudoaneurysm formation. In this setting, there is a contained rupture of the aorta which is tamponaded by the surrounding periaortic tissue. Immunosuppressed patients who have undergone heart transplantation may be more susceptible to the development of infection of the aortic wall at the site of intimal disruption due to surgical technique.[2,3]

Echocardiography is an essential technique for the diagnosis of aortic pseudoaneurysm.[4] The disruption of the aortic wall allows hemorrhage into the surrounding mediastinum. The degree of bleeding depends on the size of the hole in the aorta, the patient's coagulation status, and the tension exerted by the periaortic tissue. Our patient had a severe sternal wound infection resulting in mediastinitis. The resultant scarring probably prevented exsanguination when the aortic tear developed. It is possible that the disruption of the aorta was due to the external infection, but it is more likely that the cannulation site was the nidus for hematogenous infection of the aortic wall. This patient did well after placement of the homograft and sternal wound closure with muscle flaps.

References

1. Sato O, Tada Y, Miyata T, *et al.* False aneurysm after aortic operation. J Cardiovasc Surg 1992;33:604–8.

2. Palac R, Strausbargh L, Antonovic R, *et al.* An unusual complication of cardiac transplantation – infected aortic pseudoaneurysm. Ann Thorac Surg 1991;51:479–81.

3. Taylor D, Rehr R, Thompson J, *et al.* Aortic pseudoaneurysm occurring after cardiac transplantation. Am Heart J 1990;120:1222–5.

4. Lasorda D, Power T, Dianzumba S, *et al.* Diagnosis of aortic pseudoaneurysm by echocardiography. Clin Cardiol 1992;15:773–6.

122

Aortic dissection

Frederick F Samaha MD

A 58-year-old woman with a history of hypertension and peripheral vascular disease presented with a 3-hour history of excruciating chest pain which radiated to her back. Her blood pressure was 170/80 mmHg, and pulse rate 90 bpm. She appeared uncomfortable. Her cardiac examination was normal and pulses were symmetric. A chest X-ray revealed clear lungs and a mildly widened mediastinum. ST elevation consistent with acute infarction was present in the inferior leads on electrocardiography. Dissection was suspected due to the character of the patient's pain.

Emergency transesophageal echocardiography was performed.

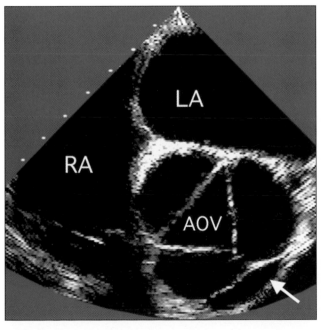

a

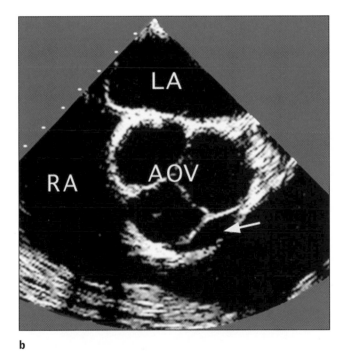

b

Figure 122.1
(a) Transesophageal echocardiogram from the upper esophageal position, at approximately 30° from the true horizontal plane. The aortic root is seen in short-axis view. The aortic valve (AOV) is open in systole. The root itself is enlarged and the leaflets are unable to open fully to the aortic wall. An intimal flap is present in the root and has dehisced the commissure between the right and left coronary cusps. The false lumen (arrow), while small, appears to involve the region of the origin of the right coronary artery (at the bottom of the screen). The ostium is not visualized at this level. The origin of the left main coronary artery is clearly seen, and originates from the true lumen.
(b) Similar view in diastole. The aortic valve leaflets coapt but a portion of the left and right coronary cusps are no longer attached to the aortic root wall. This resulted in severe eccentric aortic regurgitation which is not pictured here.

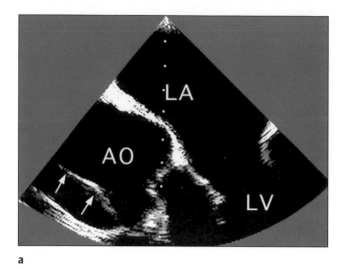
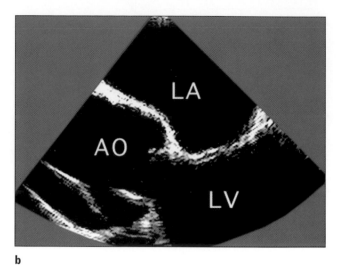

a   b

Figure 122.2
(a) Transesophageal echocardiogram from the mid-esophageal position from a modified close-up view of the left ventricular outflow tract. The enlarged aortic root is imaged in this view, although this is not usually the case. The probe has been retroflexed to achieve this view. The intimal flap (arrows) extends longitudinally along the length of the aortic root and ascending aorta. The proximal extent of the flap terminates in the right sinus of Valsalva. The distal extent of the dissection flap is not seen at this level. There is prolapse of the right coronary cusp in this diastolic view. The non-coronary cusp, adjacent to the anterior mitral valve leaflet, does not prolapse.
(b) Similar view in systole. The true lumen has expanded, owing to the systolic ejection of blood, causing mild compression of the false lumen, which can be appreciated in this image.

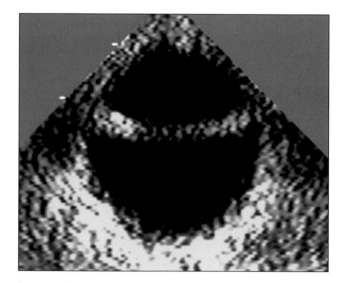
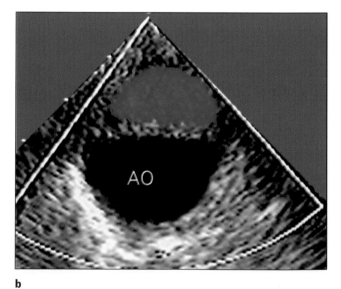

a   b

Figure 122.3
(a) Transesophageal echocardiogram from the mid-esophageal position in the transverse plane. The probe has been turned posteriorly to image the descending thoracic aorta. The aorta itself is not dilated but an intimal flap is clearly visible at this level.
(b) Similar view with color flow Doppler imaging. The true lumen is identified in this systolic frame by the flow present within the lumen. The false lumen is larger and does not appear to contain thrombus but does not have significant systolic flow at this level.

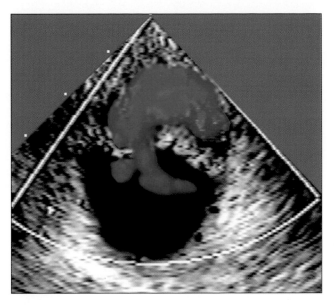

Figure 122.4
The probe has been further withdrawn with color Doppler flow imaging. At the level of the proximal descending thoracic aorta, there is a break in the intimal flap allowing flow between the true and false lumen. Again the true lumen is seen at the top of the screen. Several such entry sites may be present and it is not always possible to identify the original culprit site at which the dissection process began.

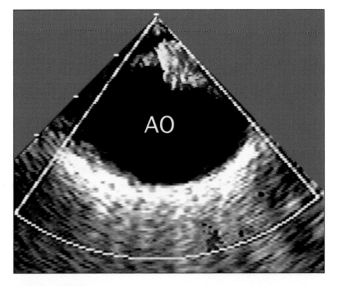

Figure 122.5
The transesophageal probe has been further withdrawn to image the aortic arch. There is another entry site between the true and false lumen. The dissection spiraled up the aorta so that the true lumen is now seen at the bottom of the screen with systolic flow from the true to the false lumen.

Discussion

There is considerable variability in presenting symptoms in patients with acute aortic dissection. In one study, based on a retrospective chart review, only 54 of 83 patients with aortic dissection were correctly suspected clinically by the examining physician.[1] In another study, the most common presenting symptom was found to be chest pain (41%) or chest pain together with back pain (31%).[2]

Patients who are clinically suspected of having an aortic dissection need urgent diagnostic evaluation. The information needed includes the presence and extent of the dissection, the location of the entry site, the formation of thrombus in the false lumen, whether or not there is a pericardial effusion or aortic regurgitation, and whether or not there is involvement of the coronary arteries. Transesophageal echocardiography is an accurate primary diagnostic tool, in experienced hands, for patients with a clinical presentation suggestive of aortic dissection. Its logistical advantages include the ability to perform the procedure at the bedside anywhere in the hospital, and the small number of hospital personnel required. The diagnostic advantages include rapidity of diagnosis, simultaneous assessment of cardiac wall motion and aortic valve involvement, identification of pericardial effusions, identification of uncommon aortic to right atrium or right ventricular fistulas, and its semi-invasive nature. The entire thoracic aorta can usually be well visualized, with the exception of the proximal portion of the aortic arch. Potential disadvantages include a higher false-positive rate and difficulty in identifying the relationship of the dissection to major aortic branches compared to magnetic resonance imaging.

The definitive diagnosis of aortic dissection by transesophageal echocardiography is based on the identification of an intimal flap, which divides the true aortic lumen from the false lumen. If there is complete thrombosis of the false lumen, a central displacement of intimal calcifications is considered to be diagnostic.[3] As demonstrated in the above images, the pulsatile nature of the true lumen can be helpful in distinguishing the true lumen from the false lumen. This particular patient had a relatively small false lumen in the ascending aorta. In patients with a large false lumen, one may see complete collapse of the true lumen during diastole.

Color flow Doppler is also helpful in the diagnosis of an aortic dissection. Since the flow characteristics are different in the true and false lumen, one will see the difference in flow velocity and direction reflected in the color flow Doppler. Alternatively, one may see no flow or only spontaneous echo contrast in the false lumen. The site of entry is identified by the disruption of the dissected membrane or by a communication between the true and false lumens on color flow Doppler echocardiography.

Dissections that involve the ascending aorta are classified as type A, regardless of the site of the primary intimal tear. All other dissections are classified as type B.

There have been two major studies evaluating the diagnostic accuracy of the various modalities for aortic dissection. In one large multi-center study, sensitivity and specificity for the diagnosis of aortic dissection by transesophageal echocardiography of 99% and 98% were reported.[4] In the only large, randomized and blinded study, the sensitivity of transesophageal echocardiography for type A dissections was found to be 97.7% versus 98.3% for magnetic resonance imaging (MRI), and specificity of 76.9% versus 97.8% for MRI.[3] In this study, transesophageal echocardiography was accurate in identifying an entry site, but less useful in demonstrating thrombus formation in the ascending aorta and arch. The relatively lower specificity of transesophageal echocardiography in this study was notable, and the authors recommended consideration of MRI in patients deemed stable enough to undergo this procedure. However, specificity may be better with the current use of multi-plane probes compared to the single-plane probe used in that study. It has recently been proposed that definitive diagnosis of an aortic dissection by transesophageal echocardiography requires the demonstration of an intimal flap plus Doppler color flow evidence for a dissection, and that transesophageal echocardiographic demonstration of an intimal flap only, with no other supportive evidence for dissection, requires another imaging modality to confirm the diagnosis.[5]

This patient had involvement of the right coronary artery ostium by the dissection. This is a relatively rare complication, which has been noted to occur in 1.5 to 7.5% of cases.[3,6] Selective coronary angiography may be risky in type A dissections, and should be avoided in most cases, since surgical intervention is almost always indicated. The decision regarding bypass or reimplantation of the coronary artery(s) can be made at the time of surgical inspection of the coronary ostia.

This patient had no phenotypic or historical markers for a connective tissue disorder. She underwent emergency surgery for tube-graft replacement of the ascending aorta, with resuspension and preservation of the native aortic valve. The right coronary artery was noted intraoperatively to originate from the false lumen, and reimplantation of the right coronary ostium into the graft was performed. The surgery was successful, and the patient was ultimately discharged to home in good condition.

References

1. Rosman HS, Patel S, Borzak S, et al. Quality of history taking in patients with aortic dissection. Chest 1998;114:793–5.

2. Armstrong WF, Bach DS, Carey LM, et al. Clinical and echocardiographic findings in patients with suspected acute aortic dissection. Am Heart J 1998;136:1051–60.

3. Nienaber CA, von Kodolitsch Y, Nicolas V, et al. The diagnosis of thoracic aortic dissection by noninvasive imaging procedures. N Engl J Med 1993;328:1–9.

4. Erbel R, Engberding R, and Daniel W, et al. Echocardiography in diagnosis of aortic dissection. Lancet 1989;1:457.

5. Cigarroa JE, Isselbacher EM, DeSanctis RW, Eagle KA. Diagnostic imaging in the evaluation of suspected aortic dissection: old standards and new directions. N Engl J Med 1993;328:35.

6. DeSanctis RW, Doroghazi RM, Austen WG, Buckley MJ. Aortic dissection. N Engl J Med 1987;317:1060–7.

123

Postoperative tamponade after aortic valve replacement

Susan E Wiegers MD

A transesophageal echocardiogram was requested as an emergency in the surgical intensive care unit to evaluate hypotension in a 48-year-old man who had undergone aortic valve replacement with aortic composite graft placement for a stenotic tricuspid aortic valve and ascending aortic aneurysm. The patient had done well in the first few postoperative hours but then developed progressive hypotension. There was no significant output from the chest tube. The patient's blood pressure was 60 mmHg systolic despite the infusion of large volumes of blood products and triple pressor agents intravenously. The heart rate was 150 bpm. He had not yet regained consciousness. Physical examination was otherwise remarkable for an intubated white male with normal respiratory sounds and good oxygenation. A transesophageal echocardiogram was immediately performed to evaluate the cause of the patient's hypotension.

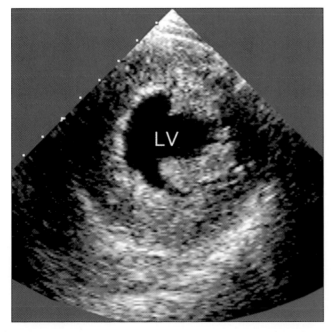

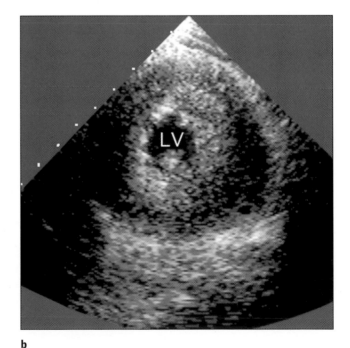

a   b

Figure 123.1
(a) Transgastric cross-sectional view of the left ventricle in the transverse plane (imaging angle 0°). Moderate left ventricular hypertrophy is present, consistent with the patient's history of aortic stenosis. The left ventricular cavity is small and underfilled.
(b) Similar transgastric view in systole. There is near systolic cavity obliteration which demonstrates that cardiac systolic failure is not the cause of this patient's hypotension. The small ventricular cavity area coupled with the finding of systolic cavity obliteration are strongly suggestive of hypovolemia.

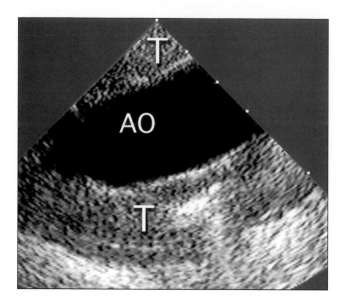

Figure 123.2
Withdrawal of the transesophageal probe to the high esophageal level in the longitudinal plane (imaging angle 130°). The conduit has surgically replaced the ascending aorta (AO). There is a large mass consistent with mediastinal thrombus (T) which surrounds the aortic conduit. Pulsation within the mass in real time suggested ongoing bleeding.

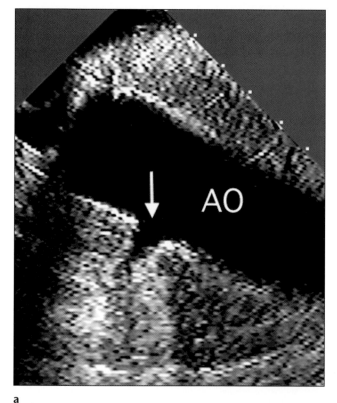

a

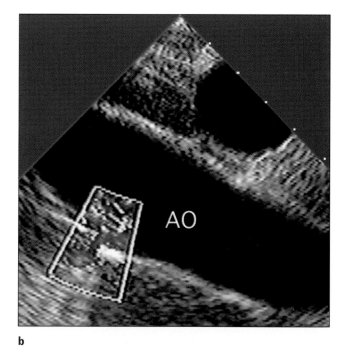

b

Figure 123.3
(a) Rotation of the probe towards the patient's right imaged a break in the conduit wall (arrow). This discontinuity is at the level of the right coronary artery anastamosis to the conduit. However, the opening is larger than that seen with coronary anastamosis and is distorted by the surrounding thrombus.
(b) Color flow Doppler imaging in a similar view demonstrates turbulent flow into this area which should not be evident if the flow was solely into the right coronary artery anastamosis. Note that the probe has been further rotated from the previous figure. The right pulmonary artery at the top of the image is surrounded by the thrombus, attesting to the massive nature of the process.

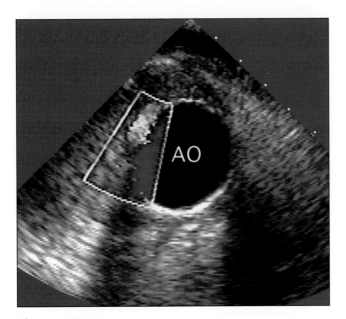

Figure 123.4
Transesophageal echocardiogram from the high esophageal level in the transverse plane (image angle 0°) taken near the level of the right coronary artery anastamosis. The right coronary artery ostium is out of plane, but a high-velocity jet is seen along the wall of the ascending aorta. The anastamosis site was leaking, resulting in brisk bleeding under high pressure into the mediastinum.

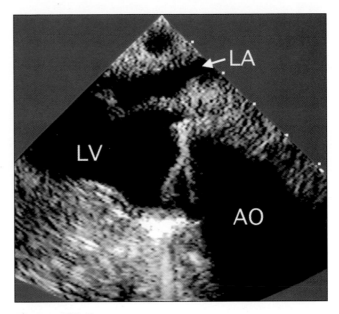

Figure 123.5
Transesophageal echocardiogram from the mid-esophagus in the transverse plane (imaging angle 90°). The path of the aorta is distorted by the mediastinal hematoma, which is not well visualized. Note that the left atrial chamber (LA) is severely compromised by the thrombus, which extends into the posterior mediastinum and is compressing the left atrium from behind.

Discussion

The patient had an unusual anastamotic leak at the site of the right coronary anastamosis to the aortic conduit. The initial images of the transesophageal study identified an underfilled left ventricle and echocardiographic evidence of hypovolemia.[1] The cause of the hypovolemia was two-fold, as revealed by further imaging. A massive mediastinal hematoma which had accumulated over several hours contained a significant portion of the patient's blood volume. However, fluid resuscitation had not been successful because the hematoma had produced localized tamponade of the left atrium. Localized tamponade is far more common after cardiac surgery than in medical conditions and may be impossible to diagnose on transthoracic study.[2]

In this patient, the large hematoma was high in the mediastinum and was not evident on initial transthoracic images, which suggested only hyperdynamic left ventricular function. Transesophageal echocardiography is a critical tool in the evaluation of the aorta in acutely ill patients with suspected aortic disease, including dissection, ruptured aneurysms and trauma. While the magnetic resonance imaging may have a slight edge in defining aortic abnormalities in selected patients, it cannot be performed in the critically ill patient with any degree of safety, and transesophageal echocardiography remains the preferred imaging modality.

The hematoma was pulsating in a manner that suggested active hemorrhage. Careful imaging of the entire surface area of the ascending aorta allowed visualization of the bleeding site. This was accomplished by slow withdrawal of the probe to image all levels of the ascending aorta and with omniplane examination at all levels. The identification of the bleeding site was not immediately obvious (as opposed to the case of aortic dissection, where the diagnosis is often instantly apparent). Once the rent in the ascending aortic conduit was visualized, color flow Doppler imaging allowed confirmation that the bleeding was systolic and passed outside of both the conduit and the coronary anastamosis into the surrounding hematoma.

As an emergency, the patient was returned to the operating room, where the mediastinal hematoma was evacuated and a hole in the aortic conduit was repaired. The patient sustained a small perioperative inferior myocardial infarction but was discharged in stable condition.

References

1. Cheung AT, Savino JS, Weiss SJ, *et al.* Echocardiographic and hemodynamic indexes of left ventricular preload in patients with normal and abnormal ventricular function. Anesthesiology 1994;81:376–87.

2. Chandraratna PA. Echocardiography and Doppler ultrasound in the evaluation of pericardial disease. Circulation 1991;84:I303–10.

124

Aortic atheroma

Eileen MacDonald MD
Susan E Wiegers MD

A 67-year-old man presented to the emergency department with paresis of the left upper and lower extremities. He had a history of poorly controlled hypertension and elevated cholesterol. He lived a vigorous life and was fully independent. Upon presentation to the emergency department, he denied chest pain, palpitations, headache or shortness of breath. His blood pressure was 132/78 mmHg and the heart rate was 80 bpm. Room air oxygen saturation was 98%. His neurological examination was significant for a right-sided facial droop and flaccid paralysis of the left upper and lower extremities with increased reflexes. His speech was slurred. There were no carotid bruits and the cardiac examination was normal. There was a soft abdominal bruit over the aorta in the epigastrium, but no pulsatile mass or tenderness. A head computerized tomogram revealed an area of infarct in the distribution of the right middle cerebral artery thought to be secondary to an embolus. Carotid Doppler ultrasound revealed minimal stenoses bilaterally. A transthoracic echocardiogram was performed to look for an embolic source and none was found.

On the third hospital day, the patient's right great toe became painful and blue, worrisome for systemic embolization. A transesophageal echocardiogram was performed to further look for an embolic source.

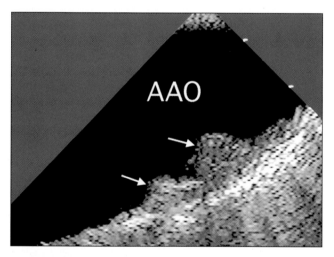

Figure 124.1
Transesophageal echocardiogram from a high esophageal position in the transverse plane (imaging angle 135°). The probe has been withdrawn and rotated to the left of the patient to image the ascending aorta, which is of normal caliber. The anterior wall of the aorta contains two masses (arrows) which protrude into the lumen. The larger projects approximately 8 mm into the lumen of the aorta. The proximal wall of the aorta (to the left of the image) appears of normal thickness and consistency. The wall distal to the protruding atheroma is diffusely thickened.

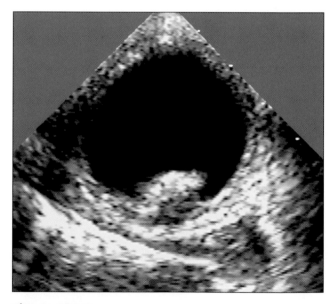

Figure 124.2
Transesophageal echocardiogram from a high esophageal position in the transverse plane (imaging angle 0°). The ascending aorta is seen in short-axis. The atheroma is large and projects into the aorta. The posterior wall of the ascending aorta appears to be normal.

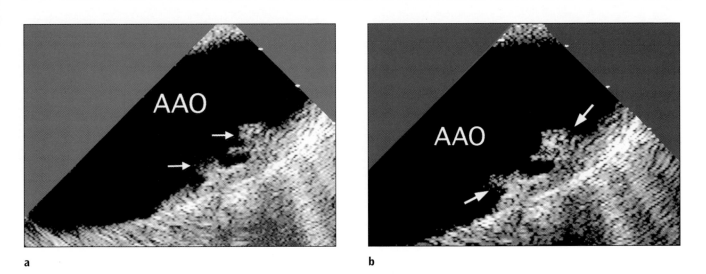

a   b

Figure 124.3
(a) Transesophageal echocardiogram from a high esophageal position in the transverse plane (imaging angle 135°). The probe has been rotated slightly in this image, which is taken later in systole. Both atheromas are visualized (arrows). The smaller of the two no longer appears smooth and has an indistinct luminal margin. The larger atheroma consists of at least two portions which project from the base of the atheroma. The marked thickening of the aortic wall is again demonstrated and atherosclerotic thickening of the proximal aorta has been brought into view.
(b) Similar image from a later portion of the cardiac cycle. The atheromas are complex structures with shaggy edges and were highly mobile (arrows). These atheromas are classified as grade V (see below).

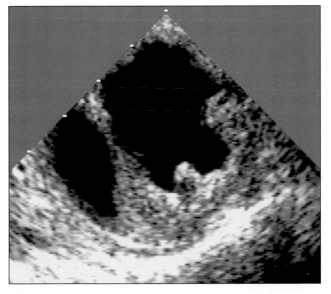

Figure 124.4
Transesophageal echocardiogram from the mid-esophagus in the transverse plane (imaging angle 0°). The probe has been rotated posteriorly to visualize the junction between the distal transverse aorta and the proximal descending thoracic aorta. The oval shape of the lumen is a clue to the level of the image. This image demonstrates severe atherosclerosis with a mildly dilated aorta and atheromas which involve the entire wall and protrude more than 1 cm into the lumen of the vessel. The apparent bridging mass is due to off axis imaging of the wall of the distal transverse aorta.

Discussion

Aortic atheromas are considered to be a sign of generalized atherosclerotic disease. They are now commonly identified with the increased use of transesophageal echocardiography, which also provides imaging of the left atrium and its appendage along with the thoracic aorta. Aortic atheromas have a significant potential for embolization and have been implicated as the cause of embolic stroke and transient ischemic attack as well as systemic embolization. These events may occur spontaneously or in association with manipulation of the aorta during catheterization or cross-clamping during cardiac surgery.[1,2] The presence of aortic atheroma in the absence of evidence of an intracardiac thrombus, patent foramen ovale, or carotid pathology, should raise concern regarding the pathophysiological role of aortic atheroma in embolic stroke. However, in the presence of these co-morbidities, the role of the atheroma may not be entirely clear. The French Study Group evaluated atherosclerosis of the aortic arch as a risk factor for recurrent ischemic stroke. Patients with plaques greater than 4 mm in depth had a recurrence rate of 11.9 per 100 patient-years despite treatment.[3] This study also demonstrated an increasing risk of vascular events with increasing severity of aortic atheroma. The presence of aortic atheroma on transesophageal echocardiography is also a powerful predictor of coronary artery disease, although this relationship is less strong in the elderly.[4]

Aortic atheromas are rarely well demonstrated on transthoracic studies. Therefore, the most common grading system should be applied only to transesophageal studies. Grade I atherosclerosis represents a normal aortic wall or minimal intimal thickening; grade II represents intimal thickening less than 4 mm; grade III represents distinct atheromas that protrude < 5 mm into the aortic lumen; grade IV represents atheromas that protrude > 5 mm into the lumen; and grade V represents any mobile atheroma. This grading system is highly reproducible between observers.[5] There is some difficulty imaging the true dimensions of the wall of the distal aortic arch where the curvature of the aorta may produce the appearance of intimal thickening. In addition, gain artifacts may produce apparent severe thickening of the descending thoracic aorta in the absence of true disease.

While it is well established that aortic atheromas are implicated in strokes, it is not clear whether therapeutic interventions are helpful. Additionally, little is known about the natural history of the different grades of atherosclerosis. A recent study sought to determine the influence of plaque morphology and warfarin anticoagulation on the risk of recurrent emboli in patients with mobile aortic atheroma. This study concluded that patients presenting with systemic emboli and a mobile aortic atheroma have a high incidence of recurrent vascular events. Warfarin therapy appeared to be effective in significantly decreasing the incidence of these events independently of the size of the mobile component of the atheroma.[6] Another study recently reported a better outcome among patients treated with anticoagulation as compared to antiplatelet agents.[7] However, neither study was randomized and both contained small numbers of patients.

This patient was started on anticoagulation with warfarin and did not have any further evidence of emboli at one year of follow-up, but remained functionally incapacitated by his stroke. This patient's course reflects the significance of aortic atheroma and the need for further data to better treat and hopefully prevent complications of this condition.

References

1. Shmuely H, Zoldan J, Sagie A, et al. Acute stroke after coronary angiography associated with protruding mobile thoracic aortic atheromas. Neurology 1997;49:1689–91.

2. Royse C, Royse A, Blake D, et al. Assessment of thoracic aortic atheroma by echocardiography: a new classification and estimation of risk of dislodging atheroma during three surgical techniques. Ann Thorac Cardiovasc Surg 1998;4:72–7.

3. The French Study of Aortic Plaques in Stroke Group. Atherosclerotic disease of the aortic arch as a risk factor for recurrent ischemic strokes. N Engl J Med 1996;334:1216–21.

4. Khoury A, Schwartz R, Gottlieb S, et al. Relation of coronary artery disease to atherosclerotic disease in the aorta, carotid and femoral arteries evaluated by ultrasound. Am J Cardiol 1997;80:1429–33.

5. Hartman G, Peterson J, Konstadt S, et al. High reproducibility in the interpretation of intraoperative transesophageal echocardiographic evaluation of aortic atheromatous disease. Anesth Analg 1996;82:539–43.

6. Dressler F, Craig W, Castello R, et al. Mobile aortic atheroma and systemic emboli: efficacy of anticoagulation and influence of plaque morphology on recurrent stroke. J Am Coll Cardiol 1998;21:134–8.

7. Ferrari E, Vidal R, Chevallier T, et al. Atherosclerosis of the thoracic aorta and aortic debris as a marker of poor prognosis: Benefit of oral anticoagulants. J Am Coll Cardiol 1999;33:1317–22.

125

Acquired supravalvular aortic stenosis

Susan E Wiegers MD

A 32-year-old woman complained of exertional chest pressure to her family physician. Her parents had both died in their forties of myocardial infarction. She had a brother who had sustained his first myocardial infarction at the age of 27. She was found to have a total cholesterol level of 700 mg/dl. Her brother's cholesterol level was 1000 mg/dl. As part of her evaluation, an echocardiogram was done to assess left ventricular function and to evaluate the etiology of a systolic murmur.

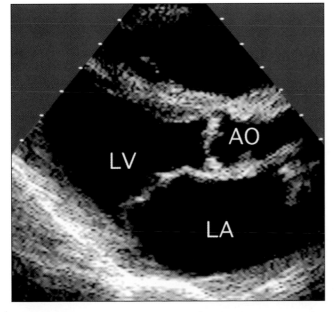

Figure 125.1
Parasternal long-axis view. The left ventricle (LV) and left atrium (LA) are of normal size. The aortic valve is thickened and echodense. The walls of the aortic root (AO) are markedly thickened, owing to deposition of atherosclerotic plaque. The lumen of the proximal ascending aorta is significantly narrowed. Supravalvular stenosis is present in a long segment of the proximal ascending aorta. The gradient associated with a long moderate stenosis may be similar to that associated with a more severe discrete lesion.

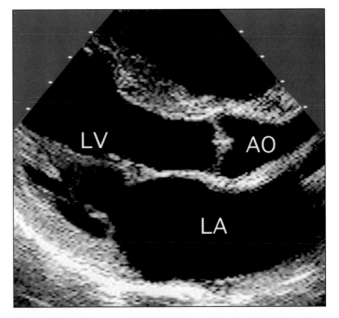

Figure 125.2
Parasternal long-axis view from a more superior intercostal space. The ascending aorta is well seen. An 'hourglass' narrowing of the aorta above the sinotubular junction results in moderately severe supravalvular stenosis.

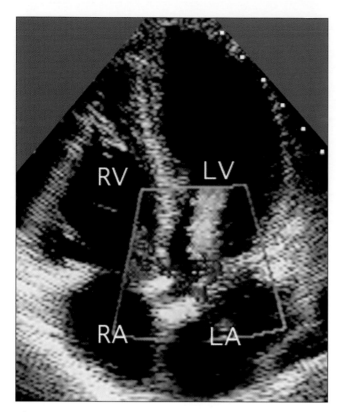

Figure 125.3
Apical five-chamber view with color Doppler imaging in diastole. Moderate aortic regurgitation is present as the result of the valvular thickening. The turbulent jet of aortic regurgitation extends from the left ventricular outflow tract to the level of the papillary muscle tips. In this case, the valvular thickening had not resulted in significant aortic valvular stenosis.

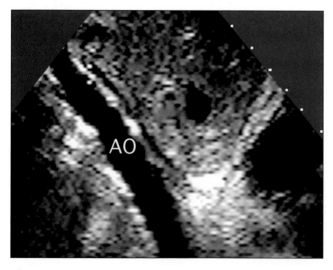

Figure 125.4
Subcostal view of the abdominal aorta. The liver (not labelled) lies anteriorly to the abdominal aorta (AO). The walls of the aorta are thickened and calcified, demonstrating the same accelerated atherosclerotic process that is present in the ascending aorta.

Discussion

The patient had familial homozygous hypercholesterolemia, as did her sibling. Supravalvular aortic stenosis may occur with atherosclerotic plaquing of the aortic wall and the aortic root, leading to narrowing of the ascending aorta.[1,2] The atherosclerotic depositions may obstruct or extend into the coronary ostia, leading to high-grade ostial stenoses. Sudden death is a significant risk for this population. Unlike congenital supravalvular stenosis, the acquired supravalvular stenosis is rarely of hemodynamic significance, although it may occasionally be severe enough to require surgical intervention. The degree of stenosis is signified by the peak and mean gradient as measured by continuous-wave Doppler from the apical position similar to the gradients reported with valvular stenosis. More rarely, valvular aortic stenosis may develop.[3] The gradients may be followed by Doppler echocardiography to assess the degree of stenosis and predict the need for intervention.[4,5] Thickening of the aortic valve leaflets often leads to mild or moderate aortic regurgitation, as in this case.

The more common cause of supravalvular aortic stenosis is William's syndrome, a congenital lesion in which supravalvular stenosis is associated with typical facies, mental retardation, and hypercalcemia.[6]

This patient had a 95% ostial stenosis of her right coronary artery and obtained complete relief of symptoms with a single-vessel coronary artery bypass graft.

References

1. Brook GJ, Keidar S, Boulos M, *et al.* Familial homozygous hypercholesterolemia: clinical and cardiovascular features in 18 patients. Clin Cardiol 1989;12:333–8.

2. Beppu S, Minura Y, Sakakibara H, *et al.* Supravalvular aortic stenosis and coronary ostial stenosis in familial hypercholesterolemia: two-dimensional echocardiographic assessment. Circulation 1983; 67:878–84.

3. Rallidis L, Nihoyannopoulos P, Thompson GR. Aortic stenosis in homozygous familial hypercholesterolaemia. Heart 1996;76:84–5.

4. Braunstein P, Sade R, Crawford F, *et al.* Repair of supravalvular aortic stenosis: cardiovascular morphometric and hemodynamic results. Ann Thorac Surg 1990;50:700–7.

5. French J. Aortic and pulmonary artery stenosis: improvement without intervention? J Am Coll Cardiol 1990;15:1631–2.

6. Wren C, Oslizlok P, Bull C. Natural history of supravalvular aortic stenosis and pulmonary artery stenosis. J Am Coll Cardiol 1990;15:1625–30.

126

Dilated ascending aorta and descending aortic plaque

Frederick F Samaha MD

An 80-year-old woman had an outpatient echocardiogram because of the detection of a diastolic murmur by her new physician. She was asymptomatic.

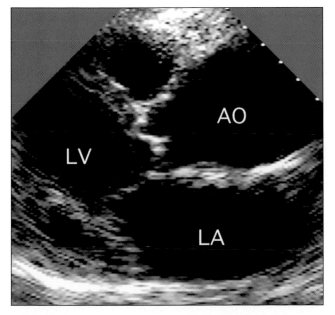

Figure 126.1
Transthoracic two-dimensional echocardiogram of the parasternal long-axis view. The transducer has been moved up an interspace to image the proximal ascending aorta (AO), which is aneurysmal. The aortic valve leaflets demonstrate mild thickening and calcific changes. The left ventricle (LV) is mildly enlarged at 5.7 cm and the left atrium (LA) is normal.

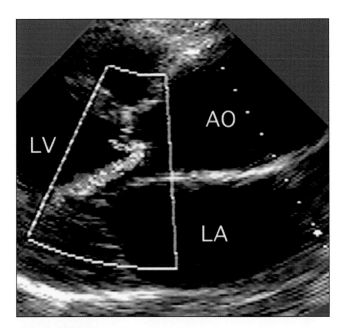

Figure 126.2
Color flow Doppler imaging in the same view. A turbulent, high-velocity jet of aortic insufficiency extends centrally, from the aortic valve, along the length of the anterior leaflet of the mitral valve towards the posterior wall of the left ventricle. A smaller second jet is seen to originate close to the first, but passes out of the plane, and its extent is not visualized in this view. The widths of the color jets at their proximal origins are small, and the diameters of the two jets comprises less than 25% of the left ventricular outflow tract diameter. These findings are consistent with mild aortic insufficiency of grade I.

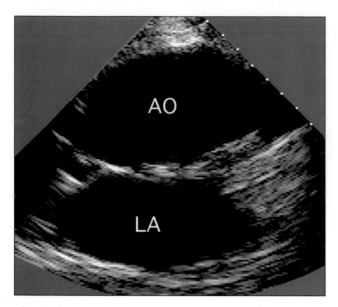

Figure 126.3
Transthoracic two-dimensional echocardiogram of the parasternal long-axis view. The transducer has been moved further in a cranial direction to visualize the ascending aorta (AO). The maximum diameter is enlarged, at 5.5 cm. There is a plaque along the posterior wall of the aorta.

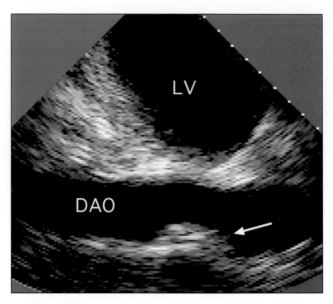

Figure 126.4
Transthoracic two-dimensional echocardiogram of the descending thoracic aorta (DAO). The off-axis view from a low parasternal window allows visualization of the descending aorta posterior to the left ventricle. A large sessile atheromatous plaque or thrombus (arrow) is present along the wall of the aorta. The more proximal aorta (on the right of the picture) is dilated and the wall is irregular.

Discussion

It is not always possible to image the ascending and descending aorta in such detail from the transthoracic approach. However, these views can be obtained in many patients by off-axis imaging. Two-dimensional echocardiographic measurements of ascending aortic size have an excellent correlation with those obtained by cineangiographic measurements in normal patients and those with ascending aortic aneurysms. The aortic root and proximal ascending aorta may be assessed from the standard parasternal long-axis transducer position. By moving the transducer superiorly one or two intercostal spaces, more of the ascending aorta may be visualized. The ascending aorta may be better evaluated from a high right intercostal space along the right sternal edge with the patient in the right lateral decubitus position, although it is not always possible to obtain adequate images from the right parasternal region, since the right lung may intervene between the heart and chest wall at this site. However, when there is aneurysmal dilatation of the ascending aorta, it may encroach upon the right lung, and cross the midline to the right side of the chest. In such patients, right parasternal scanning has been shown to correlate better with angiographic root diameters than left parasternal scanning.[1]

Both invasive and non-invasive evaluation of the severity of aortic regurgitation remain largely qualitative. The ratio of the width of the regurgitant jet to the left ventricular outflow diameter has been found to have a > 90% correlation with angiographic assessments. In one study, four grades of aortic regurgitation by color flow Doppler imaging using this ratio were described: grade I corresponded to a ratio of less than 0.25; grade II of 0.25–0.46; grade III of 0.47–0.64; and grade IV of 0.65 or greater.[2] The severity of aortic insufficiency can also be estimated by deriving the deceleration slope (or pressure half-time) from the continuous-wave Doppler signal.[3] The continuous-wave Doppler signal is obtained from the apical window, with regurgitant flow velocity directed towards the transducer and displayed above the baseline. The continuous-wave Doppler signal of the aortic regurgitation may also be obtained from the second right intercostal space, in which case it will be displayed below the baseline. A deceleration rate that exceeds 3 m/s per second (300 cm/s per second) or a pressure half-time of less than 300 ms are consistent with severe aortic regurgitation. Other parameters to consider in assessing the severity of aortic insufficiency include thoracic or abdominal aortic flow reversal, late diastolic or presystolic mitral regurgitation, and premature closure of the mitral valve.

When examining atheromatous plaques, the size, complexity, and morphology of the lesions should be assessed. In a study by Karalis, a descriptive definition of plaque morphology was presented.[4] Simple atherosclerotic plaques are those first, with focal increased echodensity and thickening of the intima extending < 5 mm from the aortic wall into the aortic lumen; and second, without overlying shaggy echogenic material or disruption or irregularity of the intimal surface. Complex lesions are characterized by disruption or marked irregularities of the intimal surface, with focal increased echodensity and thickening of the adjoining intimal; and overlying irregular echogenic material extending > 5 mm from the wall of the aorta into the aortic lumen. In this same study, aortic plaques were subdivided into those that were layered, broad-based and immobile, or pedunculated and highly mobile. Embolic events were more common in those with protruding, highly mobile lesions than in those with layered, immobile plaques.

In this case, the decision was made to continue medical management for the patient's hypertension, mild aortic insufficiency, and moderately dilated ascending aorta. Serial echocardiograms were performed to evaluate the size of the aorta. Coumadin was started, as the plaque in the descending aorta was felt to present a high risk for embolization.

References

1. DiCruz I, Jain D, Hirsh L, et al. Echocardiographic diagnosis of dilatation of the ascending aorta using right parasternal scanning. Radiology 1978;129:465–9.

2. Perry G, Helmcke F, Nanda N, et al. Evaluation of aortic insufficiency by Doppler color flow mapping. J Am Coll Cardiol 1987;9:952–9.

3. Grayburn P, Handshoe R, Smith M, et al. Quantitative assessment of the hemodynamic consequences of aortic regurgitation by means of continuous wave Doppler recordings. J Am Coll Cardiol 1987;10:135.

4. Karalis D. Recognition and embolic potential of intraaortic atherosclerotic debris. J Am Coll Cardiol 1991;17:73.

127

Coarctation of the aorta

Martin St John Sutton MBBS
Susan E Wiegers MD

A healthy male infant was noted to have a murmur at 6 weeks of age. This was initially thought to be a ventricular septal defect and was managed conservatively, awaiting spontaneous closure. He underwent cardiac catheterization at the age of 7. Aortography demonstrated an enlarged ascending aorta and aortic arch with an incomplete tubular post-ductal coarctation, a small descending thoracic aorta and mild aortic regurgitation. He underwent surgical reconstruction of the coarcted segment with a Dacron interposition graft, and was followed up for treatment of mild persistent hypertension. Aged 28 he presented with a grand mal seizure, but also complained of progressively easy fatigue, exercise intolerance due to leg cramps and intermittent headaches of one year's duration. He had no chest pain or palpitations.

On examination, right and left arm blood pressures were equal, at 150/100 mmHg; the blood pressure in his legs was 95/60 mmHg. There was delay between the radial and femoral pulses, and pulses in the legs and feet were diminished compared to pulses in the arms but were equal bilaterally. He had an apical impulse suggesting left ventricular hypertrophy and enlargement. There was an ejection click, an ejection systolic murmur and an immediate diastolic murmur consistent with aortic regurgitation. In addition there was a harsh murmur audible over the left upper chest and between the scapulae but no continuous murmurs to suggest the presence of collaterals. Electrocardiography revealed sinus rhythm and left ventricular hypertrophy with repolarization changes. A chest X-ray showed an enlarged ascending aorta and mild cardiomegaly. A head computerized tomography scan showed a large sacular cerebral aneurysm arising from the anterior communicating artery.

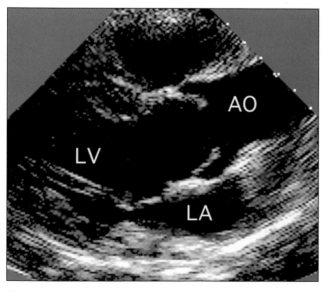

Figure 127.1
Parasternal long-axis view in systole. The aortic valve domes in systole, consistent with a bicuspid valve. The aortic root is enlarged, although the ascending aorta is of normal caliber. There is left ventricular hypertrophy.

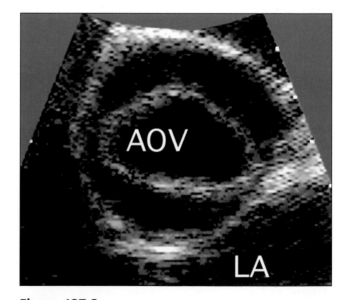

Figure 127.2
Parasternal short-axis close-up image of the aortic valve. It is bicuspid, with a single complete commissure with two equal-sized cusps. The ellipsoid shape of the orifice is characteristic of bicuspid valves.

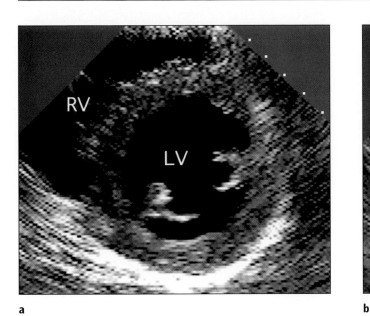
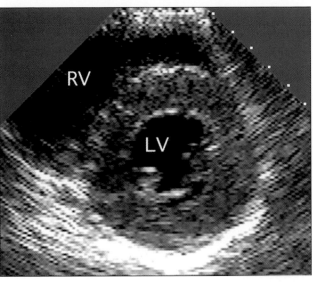

a

b

Figure 127.3
(a) Parasternal short-axis view at the level of the papillary muscles in diastole. The ventricle is mildly dilated and hypertrophied.
(b) Similar systolic view demonstrating preserved systolic function.

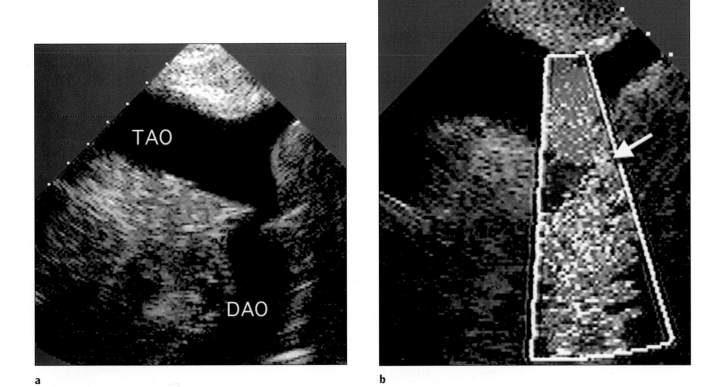

a

b

Figure 127.4
(a) Suprasternal notch view with the transducer directed leftward to image the descending thoracic aorta (DAO). The ascending and transverse aorta (TAO) are enlarged. The post-ductal coarctation is evident as bilateral ridges intruding into the lumen of the aorta. The origin of the left subclavian artery is not visualized in this image.
(b) Similar view with color flow Doppler. The flow is laminar until it reaches the site of the restenosis, at which point it becomes turbulent. The width of the color jet (arrow) reflects the significant restenosis in this area.

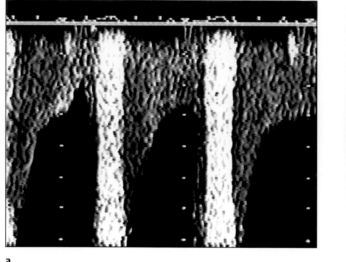

a

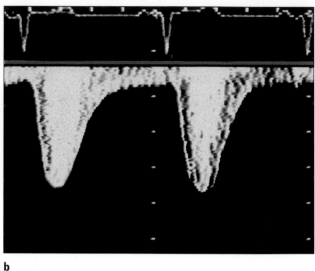

b

Figure 127.5

(a) Spectral display of pulsed-wave Doppler with the sample volume placed just distal to the coarctation. The transducer is in the suprasternal notch. There is aliased systolic flow (each calibration mark represents 20 cm/s). Continuous diastolic flow away from the transducer indicates that there is a diastolic gradient at the coarctation site. Normally, there is no detectable flow in mid- to late diastole in the thoracic aorta.

(b) Spectral display of continuous-wave Doppler across the obstruction (each calibration mark represents 1 m/s). The peak velocity is 3.7 m/s which predicts a systolic gradient of 55 mmHg. Note the classic feature of coarctation, a continuous gradient peaking in systole.

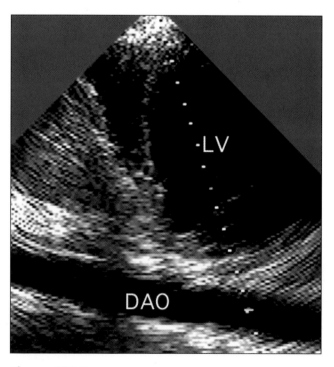

Figure 127.6

Off-axis image of the descending thoracic aorta distal to the site of the coarctation. This view is obtained by directing the transducer medially and inferiorly from the apical two-chamber view. The aorta at this level is diminutive.

Discussion

Bicuspid aortic valves are commonly associated with coarctation. They may be stenotic but are more frequently regurgitant. The ascending aorta and aortic arch are moderately dilated and the hypertensive upper body circulation and collaterals results in large brachiocephalic branch arteries. The diameter of the descending aorta correlates well with that measured on magnetic resonance imaging and angiography.[1] The Doppler velocity signal across the coarctation is characteristic in continuing throughout systole and diastole. The peak velocity across the coarctation correlates well with the degree of narrowing. In general, a peak velocity of less than 2 m/s is not associated with significant stenosis.[2] Development of a gradient during exercise may also reveal significant stenosis that is not detected at rest.[3] In our laboratory, the suprasternal notch view is recorded in every patient with Doppler sampling of the descending thoracic aorta.

Coarctation is associated with cerebral aneurysms arising from the circle of Willis and more rarely with multiple left-sided stenotic lesions including supra-mitral valve ring, sub-aortic stenosis, and supra-valvular aortic stenosis consisting of Shone's syndrome. The patient underwent repair of his coarctation and subsequent successful clipping of his anterior communicating cerebral aneurysm.

References

1. Stern HC, Locher D, Wallnofer K, *et al*. Noninvasive assessment of coarctation of the aorta: comparative measurements by two-dimensional echocardiography, magnetic resonance, and angiography. Pediatr Cardiol 1991;12:1–5.

2. Muhler EG, Neuerburg JM, Ruben A, *et al*. Evaluation of aortic coarctation after surgical repair: role of magnetic resonance imaging and Doppler ultrasound. Br Heart J 1993;70:285–90.

3. Cyran SE, Grzeszczak M, Kaufman K, *et al*. Aortic 'recoarctation' at rest versus at exercise in children as evaluated by stress Doppler echocardiography after a 'good' operative result. Am J Cardiol 1993;71:963–70.

128

Chronic aortic dissection

Martin G Keane MD

An 83-year-old woman with a history of hypertension complained of fevers, malaise, and weight loss. She vaguely recalled a prolonged episode of substernal chest pain radiating to the back 6 months previously, which she attributed to 'rheumatism'. Physical examination revealed a blood pressure of 150/90 mmHg in the right arm, and 134/72 mmHg in the left. There were no other significant positive findings. Chest radiograph demonstrated clear lung fields, a prominent aortic knob and blunting of the left costophrenic angle.

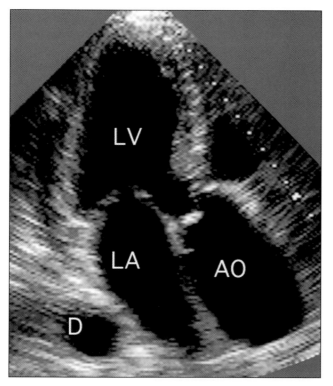

Figure 128.1
Apical long-axis view. There is moderate dilatation of the aortic root and ascending aorta (AO). The ascending aorta is similar in dimension to the left ventricle. The descending thoracic aorta (D) is also seen in cross-section, but is of normal size. There is no clear evidence of a dissection flap in this image, although the aortic root and ascending aorta are in the far-field. The left ventricle (LV) is of normal size and the left atrium (LA) is mildly dilated.

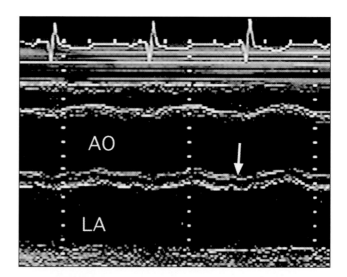

Figure 128.2
M-mode echocardiogram from the parasternal position at the level of the aortic root (AO) and left atrium (LA). The aortic root is moderately dilated, as was detected in two-dimensional images. With the greater resolution of directed M-mode, a second echogenic structure (arrow) is now detected within the ascending aorta. This represents a dissection flap, with a small false lumen present at the posterior wall of the aorta.

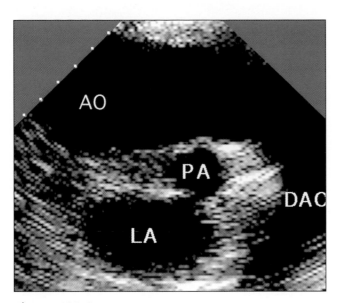

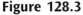

Figure 128.3
Suprasternal notch view of the aorta and pulmonary artery (PA). The aneurysmal dilatation of the ascending aorta (AO) is better appreciated in this view, with a diameter of more than 5 cm. The arch and proximal descending aorta (DAO) are less impressively enlarged. Once again, no dissection flap is seen in this view.

Discussion

Proximal aortic dissection is typically a catastrophic illness, with a dramatic symptomatic presentation associated with hemodynamic collapse, myocardial infarction or stroke. Early mortality is as high as 75% within the first 48 hours, and urgent surgical repair is generally the treatment of choice. Overall morbidity and mortality decrease to a low level in those who survive the acute phase. A dissection that has been present for 2 weeks or more is therefore classified as 'chronic'. As much as 33% of all dissections may actually be chronic at the time of initial diagnosis.[1] In some series, 50% of patients with proximal dissection did not undergo surgical repair until the chronic phase.[2] Furthermore, patients with acute dissection may not undergo operative management, either because of the presence of significant co-morbidity or because of patient refusal.[3]

The majority of patients (68%) with chronic dissection are unrecognized acutely, owing to either a failure to seek medical attention, or misdiagnosis.[3] More subtle forms of dissection, such as a localized dissection or intramural hematoma, may not be detected upon acute presentation because of the atypical presentation.[4,5] The residual descending aortic dissection flap after surgical repair of the ascending aorta and arch is sometimes classified as a 'chronic' dissection.[6] In cases of unrecognized dissection, the diagnosis is usually made fortuitously on echocardio-

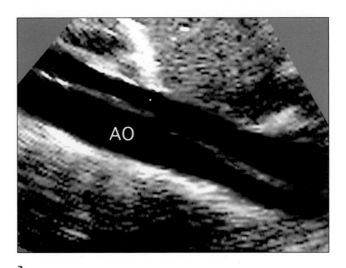

a

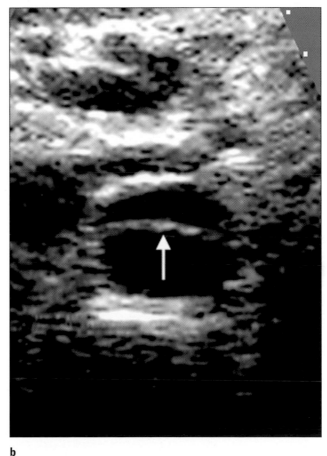

b

Figure 128.4
(a) Subcostal view of the aorta. The distal segments of the descending thoracic aorta are more clearly visualized in long axis. A dissection flap extending downward throughout this section of the aorta is clearly visualized in this case. The intimal flap is thin and exhibited motion independent of the other walls.
(b) Subcostal view of the aorta in short-axis. The dissection flap is noted within the lumen (arrow).

graphy or magnetic resonance imaging performed for other indications in an asymptomatic patient. Some patients may present chronically with symptoms of systemic disease attributable to the dissection, including fever, night sweats, pleural effusions, anemia of chronic disease, or elevated erythrocyte sedimentation rate.[7,8]

Transthoracic echocardiograms of patients with chronic proximal dissections most typically demonstrate aneurysmal dilatation of the ascending aorta. The presence of an intimal dissection 'flap' is detected on two-dimensional images as an extra echodensity within the aortic lumen, distinct from the echoes of the aortic wall. Proximal dissection can be seen within the sinuses or proximal ascending aorta in the parasternal long-axis view. M-mode echocardiography may detect dissection that is not apparent on two-dimensional images. Like acute dissection, proximal chronic dissections may undermine the annular structure of the aortic valve, resulting in varying degrees of aortic insufficiency. Assessment of the distal extent of dissection of the aorta is possible, using suprasternal notch, subcostal, off-axis apical, and right parasternal views to visualize the entire thoracic aorta from the root to the distal descending thoracic aorta.

Transthoracic imaging has limited sensitivity (58–85%) and specificity (63–96%) for the detection of acute aortic dissection.[9] Chronic dissections are often more organized and harder to detect, with progressive hematoma formation and partial or complete obliteration of the false lumen. In general, the diagnosis of and clear localization of such chronic dissections relies on confirmation by more sensitive techniques such as magnetic resonance imaging or transesophageal echocardiography. More subtle forms of dissection, including localized intimal tears or intramural hematomas, may require a combination of advanced imaging techniques.[10]

References

1. Spittell PC, Spittell JA Jr, Joyce JW, et al. Clinical features and differential diagnosis of aortic dissection: experience with 236 cases (1980 through 1990). Mayo Clin Proc 1993;68:642–51.

2. Safi HJ, Miller CC, Reardon MJ, et al. Operation for acute and chronic aortic dissection: recent outcome with regard to neurologic deficit and early death. Ann Thorac Surg 1998;66:402–11.

3. Scholl FG, Coady MA, Davies R, et al. Interval or permanent nonoperative management of acute type A dissection. Arch Surg 1999;134:402–5.

4. O'Gara PT, DeSanctis RW. Acute aortic dissection and its variants: towards a common diagnostic and therapeutic approach. Circulation 1995;92:1376–8.

5. Nienaber CA, von Kodolitsch Y, Petersen B, et al. Intramural hemorrhage of the thoracic aorta: diagnostic and therapeutic implications. Circulation 1995;92:1465–72.

6. Masani ND, Banning AP, Jones RA, et al. Follow-up of chronic thoracic aortic dissection: comparison of transesophageal echocardiography and magnetic resonance imaging. Am Heart J 1996:131:1156–63.

7. Schattner A, Klepfish A, Caspi A. Chronic aortic dissection presenting as a prolonged febrile disease and arterial embolization. Chest 1996;110:1111–14.

8. Geppert AG, Mahvi A, Hainaut P, Lambert M. Chronic aortic dissection masquerading as systemic disease. Acta Clin Belg 1998;53:19–21.

9. Cigarroa JE, Isselbacher EM, DeSanctis RW, Eagle KA. Medical progress: diagnostic imaging in the evaluation of suspected aortic dissection – old standards and new directions. N Engl J Med 1993;328:35–43.

10. Svensson LG, Labib SB, Eisenhauer AC, Butterly JR. Intimal tear without hematoma: an important variant of aortic dissection that can elude current imaging techniques. Circulation 1999;99:1331–6.

129

Traumatic aortic rupture

Bonnie Milas MD

A 29-year-old man presented with multiple long-bone fractures and soft-tissue injuries secondary to a motor vehicle accident. There was no anterior chest wall trauma noted. His blood pressure was 140/60 mmHg, heart rate 120 bpm, and his electrocardiogram demonstrated sinus tachycardia. His chest radiograph was remarkable for a normal cardiac silhouette, normal mediastinum, and multiple left-sided rib fractures. While in the operating room for repair of long-bone fractures the patient became acutely hypotensive and developed sinus tachycardia at a rate of 145 bpm. An emergency transesophageal echocardiogram was requested.

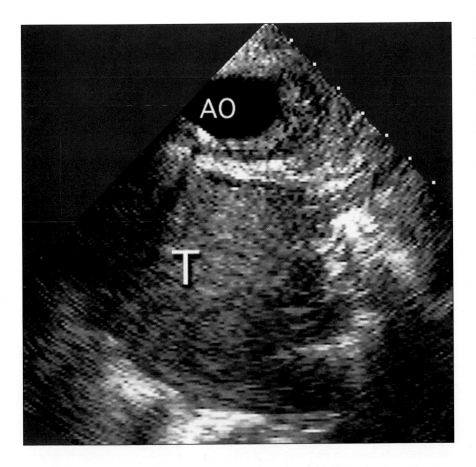

Figure 129.1
Transesophageal view of the aorta at the level of the distal aortic arch at the origin of the left subclavian artery (aortic isthmus). The level can be identified by the non-circular appearance of the aorta. Identification of the left subclavian artery would confirm the anatomic level of the aorta. The diameter of the aorta is noted to be normal, and not aneurysmal. Within the lateral wall of the aorta (to the right of the screen) is a well-circumscribed echodensity, consistent with an intramural hematoma. There is no intimal flap. Anterior to the aorta is a large heterogeneous collection suggestive of a clot. The non-uniform clotting of blood causes the heterogeneous nature of this collection. The above findings, in conjunction with the history of a deceleration injury, are consistent with aortic transection with aortic intramural hematoma and contained mediastinal clot.

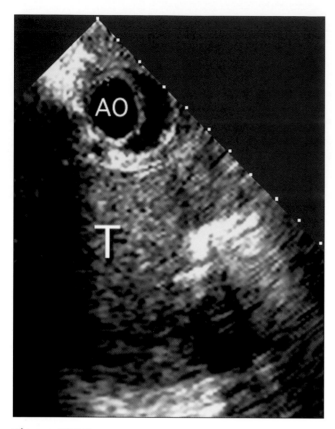

Figure 129.2
Transesophageal view of the descending thoracic aorta. The aortic wall is nearly circumscribed by an echolucent space. This is consistent with a periaortic hematoma. Its echolucent quality probably represents non-clotted blood. Color flow Doppler can be used to detect blood flow within this structure. The large anterior collection of heterogeneous material is again noted (clotted blood). This clinical situation requires immediate surgical intervention.

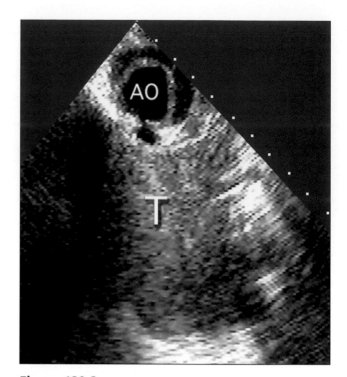

Figure 129.3
Transesophageal view of the descending thoracic aorta. The transducer has been advanced another 1 cm. The view is similar to that in Figure 129.2 but there is a tear in the anterior wall of the aorta characterized as a discontinuity in the wall of the vessel. The outpouching anterior to the hole is unclotted blood at the site of active bleeding. The large mediastinal thrombus is again seen.

Discussion

There are several different syndromes associated with traumatic injury to the aorta. Blunt chest trauma can cause rupture of a sinus of Valsalva, usually into the left or right atrium. Aortic disruption with formation of a fistula between the aorta and the inferior vena cava has also occurred. Motor vehicle accidents are a particular type of blunt trauma referred to as deceleration injuries. The base of the heart is tethered by the great vessels while the ventricles are relatively unrestrained within the pericardium. The aorta is fixed to the posterior chest wall by the intercostal branches while anteriorly the ligamentum arteriosum secures it to the pulmonary artery. Deceleration injury at the level of the aortic root is routinely fatal, owing to the aortic rupture and the abrupt onset of cardiac tamponade. The most common site of injury is the aortic isthmus. This type of aortic disruption or transsection is usually fatal; however, the patient may survive until hospitalization by containment of the bleeding within the parietal pleura and adjacent structures or by the development of an aortic pseudoaneurysm. A high index of suspicion for concurrent cardiac or great vessel injury should be maintained in the setting of severe blunt trauma or deceleration injury. Penetrating injuries to the chest and mediastinum can result in fistula formation, cardiac chamber perforation, pseudoaneurysm formation, pericardial effusion, or cardiac tamponade.

A comprehensive echocardiogram should be performed in the setting of a suspected traumatic aortic injury.[1] Transesophageal imaging is far more sensitive than transthoracic studies and is the study of choice.[2,3] Occasionally, severe facial trauma will preclude passage of the probe. Often the most difficult aspect of the examination is the determination of the type and extent of the aortic injury. Two-dimensional images are used to determine the confines of the aortic lumen, and anatomic landmarks are used to locate the site of aortic injury. A complete trans-section of the aorta may produce a 'double-barrel' or a discontinuous aortic lumen. Focal calcifications and the presence of atherosclerosis can be used to distinguish the wall of the aorta from a false lumen of an aortic dissection, a hematoma, or a collection of blood.[4] Two-dimensional imaging may demonstrate spontaneous echo contrast (smoke) representing stagnant blood flow adjacent to the aortic lumen. The size of the aorta and the presence of pre-existing aortic disease should be assessed. The lack of a thin, mobile intimal flap associated with aortic dissection should be documented. Color flow Doppler imaging can be used to establish blood flow from the aorta to contiguous structures (hematoma or pleural effusion) and may identify the lead point of an aortic free wall rupture.[5] A complete examination would also include an evaluation for pericardial effusion/tamponade, cardiac contusion (global and regional ventricular function), and the integrity of the aortic valve. The adequacy of volume resuscitation can also be assessed at that time.

References

1. Chirillo F, Totis O, Cavarzerani A, et al. Usefulness of transthoracic and transesophageal echocardiography in recognition and management of cardiovascular injuries after blunt chest trauma. Heart 1995;75:301–6.

2. Mollod M, Felner JM. Transesophageal echocardiography in the evaluation of cardiothoracic trauma. Am Heart J 1996;132:841–9.

3. Saletta S, Lederman E, Fein S, et al. Transesophageal echocardiography for the initial evaluation of the widened mediastinum in trauma patients. J Trauma-Injury Crit Care 1995;39:137–41; discussion 141–2.

4. Berenfeld A, Barraud P, Lusson JR, et al. Traumatic aortic ruptures diagnosed by transesophageal echocardiography. J Am Soc Echocardiogr 1996;9:657–62.

5. Vignon P, Gueret P, Vedrinne JM, et al. Role of transesophageal echocardiography in the diagnosis and management of traumatic aortic disruption. Circulation 1995;92:2959–68.

SECTION X

Congenital Disease

130

Perimembranous ventricular septal defect

Susan E Wiegers MD

A 50-year old man was referred to the echocardiography laboratory for evaluation of a loud murmur noted by his new primary care giver. The patient recalled several visits to a hospital clinic as a child, but did not know the nature of his condition. Further history was not available and he was unaware of the existence of a murmur. On physical examination, he had a palpable systolic thrill and a 4/6 harsh holosystolic murmur, which was heard everywhere across the precordium including the right sternal edge. The patient's other medical problems included untreated hypertension, tobacco use and untreated diabetes.

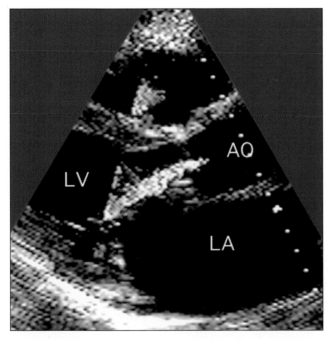

Figure 130.1
Parasternal long-axis view with color Doppler flow imaging. The left atrium (LA) is moderately enlarged and the left ventricular cavity (LV) is mildly dilated. The ascending aorta (AO) appears to be normal. There is a turbulent high-velocity jet of aortic insufficiency arising from the aortic valve and extending into the left ventricular outflow tract. Comparison of the width of the jet at its origin to the diameter of the left ventricular outflow tract demonstrates a ratio of less than 25%. This is an indication that the aortic regurgitation is mild.

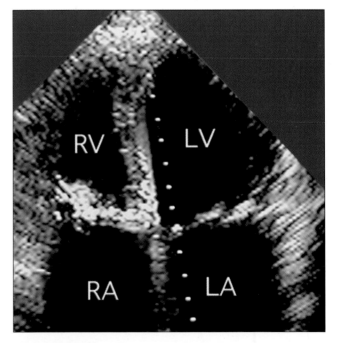

Figure 130.2
Apical four-chamber view in systole demonstrates biatrial enlargement. The left ventricular systolic function is moderately globally reduced. Right ventricular (RV) function appears to be normal. A high-velocity, narrow, turbulent jet crosses the interventricular septum at the level of the tricuspid annulus.

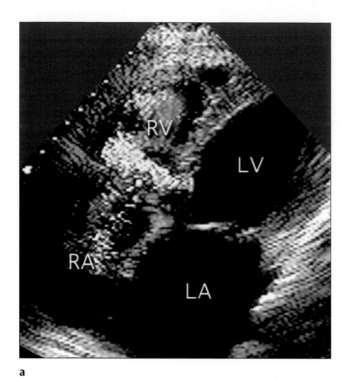

a

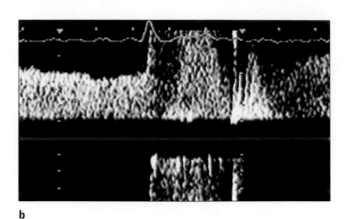

b

Figure 130.3

(a) Off-axis apical four-chamber view of the systolic jet. The high-velocity jet crosses the perimembranous septum from the left ventricle to the right ventricle. The jet size is small, consistent with a restrictive ventricular septal defect. Tricuspid regurgitation is visualized in the right atrium (RA).

(b) Spectral display of pulsed-wave Doppler from a similar transducer position. The sample volume has been placed on the right ventricular side of the ventricular septal defect jet. There is systolic aliased flow which represents the high-velocity left to right flow across the defect. In addition, low-velocity continuous diastolic flow is present, indicating persistent left to right flow across the ventricular septal defect in diastole.

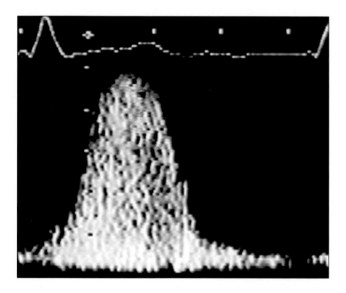

Figure 130.4

Spectral continuous-wave Doppler taken from the parasternal position. The ventricular septal defect jet characteristically reaches peak velocity in mid-systole. The peak velocity of 4.9 m/s indicates a systolic gradient between the left and right ventricles of 96 mmHg. The patient's systolic blood pressure was 140 mmHg. Therefore, the peak right ventricular systolic pressure is estimated to be 44 mmHg.

Discussion

The patient had a perimembranous ventricular septal defect that had been present since birth. He had received little in the way of medical care over the years and the shunt flow was insignificant. The incidental finding had several important clinical implications. The aortic insufficiency in this patient might have been caused by the high-

velocity ventricular septal defect jet passing in close proximity to the right coronary cusp of the aortic valve. Over the years, prolapse of the right cusp may have resulted in aortic insufficiency. In most cases of ventricular septal defect associated with aortic regurgitation, prolapse of the right coronary cusp of the aortic valve can be identified.[1,2] It has recently been demonstrated by serial echocardiographic studies that mild aortic regurgitation is not necessarily an indication for surgical closure in patients with insignificant shunt flow through the ventricular septal defect. Only significant aortic regurgitation with evidence of progressive left ventricular dilatation is an indication for closure.[3] This patient is also at increased risk for endocarditis and requires antibiotic prophylaxis for dental procedures and the like. The high-velocity jet of the ventricular septal defect impacts on the right ventricular free wall. Vegetations are most likely to form in this situation on the right ventricular wall and can be identified by transthoracic imaging.

The confounding condition of untreated hypertension may also have been the cause of this degree of aortic regurgitation. The left ventricular dysfunction was due to hypertensive heart disease, diabetes and coronary artery disease. Mild pulmonary hypertension was the result of left ventricular dysfunction rather than a response to the trivial left to right shunt flow. Several weeks after this echocardiogram was performed the patient sustained a large anteroseptal myocardial infarction again unrelated to the congenital condition.

References

1. Ogino H, Miki S, Ueda Y, *et al.* Surgical management of aortic regurgitation associated with ventricular septal defect. J Heart Valve Dis 1997;6:174–8.

2. Craig B, Smallhorn J, Burrows P, *et al.* Cross-sectional echocardiography in the evaluation of aortic valve prolapse associated with ventricular septal defect. Am Heart J 1986;112:800–7.

3. Butter A, Duncan W, Weatherdon D, *et al.* Aortic cusp prolapse in ventricular septal defect and its association with aortic regurgitation – appropriate timing of surgical repair and outcomes. Can J Cardiol 1998;14:833–40.

131

Eisenmenger ventricular septal defect

Martin St John Sutton MBBS
Susan E Wiegers MD

A 44-year-old man with trisomy 21 mosaic living in the community with his mother had cyanotic congenital heart disease and carried the diagnosis of tetralogy of Fallot. He has never undergone cardiac catheterization or shunt procedure but had a poor quality two-dimensional echocardiogram in the distant past. He was referred for advice regarding the utility of venesection and to determine 'if anything else needed to be done'.

He was well able to give an account of his symptoms, which included shortness of breath on walking more than 50 feet on the flat at a moderate pace or climbing half a flight of stairs. Both of these activities resulted in fatigue and light-headedness. He had never experienced chest pain, palpitations or syncope. He was able to help his mother with minor household chores.

On examination, he was centrally cyanosed with an oxygen saturation of 83% on room air at rest falling to 72% with mild exertion. He had digital clubbing, an elevated jugular venous pressure with a predominant 'v' wave, regular rate and rhythm and a blood pressure of 126/72 mmHg. There was a prominent left parasternal lift consistent with right ventricular hypertrophy, a loud pulmonary component of the second heart sound and an immediate diastolic murmur consistent with pulmonary regurgitation. A pansystolic murmur of tricuspid regurgitation was audible as well. There was no murmur of pulmonary stenosis. His chest X-ray showed cardiomegaly, large proximal pulmonary arteries and increased vascular markings. The electrocardiogram revealed sinus rhythm, right axis deviation and severe right ventricular hypertrophy with repolarization abnormalities consistent with chronic right heart strain. An echocardiogram was performed to establish the diagnosis.

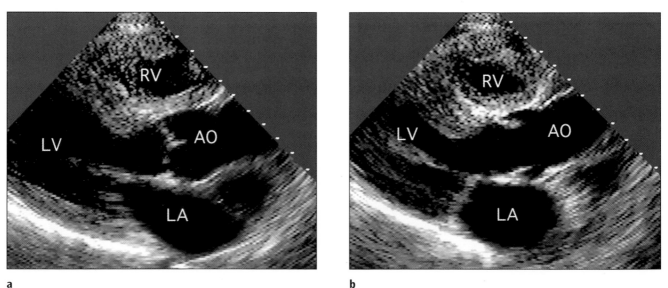

a   b

Figure 131.1
(a) Parasternal long-axis view in diastole. The left ventricle, mitral valve and aortic valve are normal. The right ventricle is severely hypertrophied. The attachment of the aortic root to the interventricular septum is normal, and there is no evidence of an overriding aorta.
(b) In systole, normal left ventricular systolic function is identified. The right ventricular outflow tract is nearly obliterated during systole.

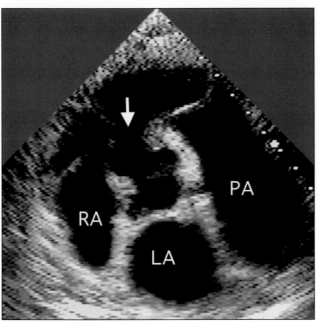

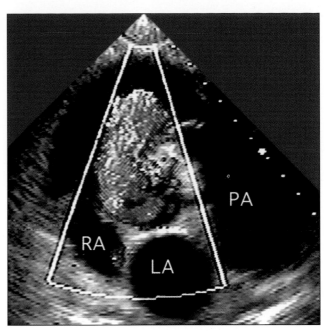

a   b

Figure 131.2

(a) Parasternal short-axis view of the aorta shows a large perimembranous ventricular septal defect (arrow), which measures over 2 cm in diameter. There is no infundibular stenosis and the pulmonary valve is normal. In contrast to the situation in tetralogy of Fallot, the main pulmonary artery is markedly dilated.

(b) Similar view in systole with color flow Doppler imaging. There is a low-velocity red jet that passes from the left ventricular outflow tract into the right ventricle. The low velocity indicates a loss of the normal pressure gradient between the ventricles due to severe elevation of right ventricular systolic pressures.

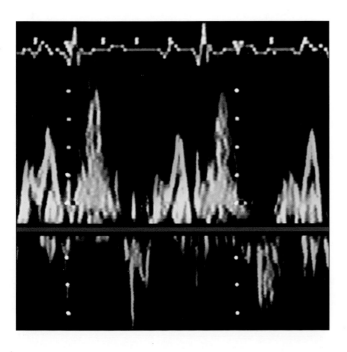

Figure 131.3

Spectral display of pulsed-wave Doppler with the sample volume in the ventricular septal defect. The transducer is in the parasternal position. There is low-velocity bidirectional flow which is predominantly left to right across the defect (each calibration mark represents 20 cm/s).

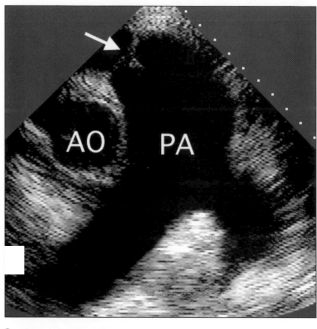

a

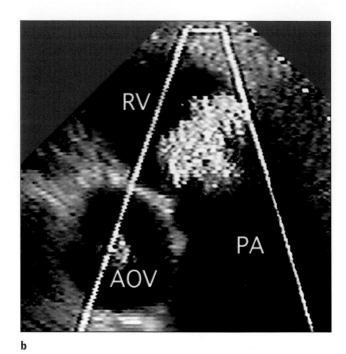

b

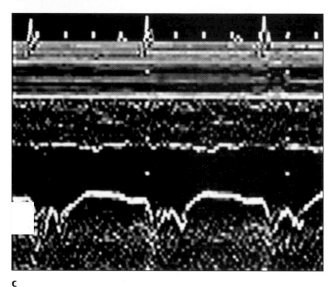

c

Figure 131.4

(a) Parasternal short-axis view at the base of the heart. The transducer has been angled superiorly and to the patient's left compared to Figure 131.2a. The main pulmonary artery and both branches are severely enlarged. The pulmonary valve (arrow) is normal. The valve opened normally in systole.

(b) Close-up image of the pulmonary valve with color flow Doppler imaging in diastole. A high-velocity jet of pulmonary regurgitation arises at the level of the valve and extends into the right ventricular outflow tract. The jet is wide at its inception consistent with severe pulmonary regurgitation. The peak velocity of this jet by continuous-wave Doppler was 4.8 m/s (not shown) representing a pulmonary artery to right ventricular diastolic pressure gradient of 92 mmHg.

(c) M-mode echocardiogram from the parasternal position. One of the pulmonary valve leaflets is demonstrated. The valve opens fully in early systole but demonstrates mid-systolic notching, a sign of pulmonary hypertension.

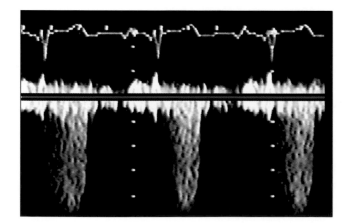

Figure 131.5

Spectral display of continuous-wave Doppler across the tricuspid valve. The peak velocity is approximately 4.9 m/s (each calibration mark represents 1 m/s). This indicates a gradient between the right atrium and right ventricle of nearly 100 mmHg in systole.

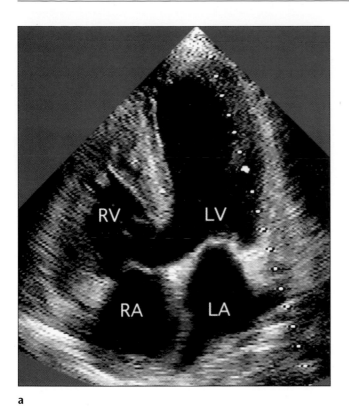

a

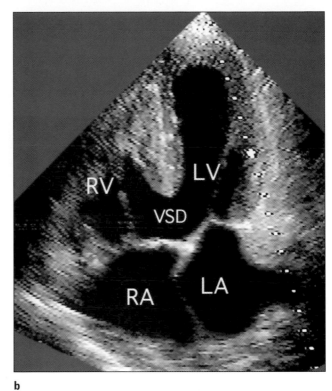

b

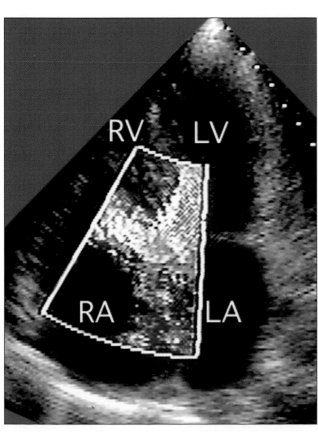

c

Figure 131.6

(a) Apical four-chamber view in diastole demonstrates normal left ventricular size and marked right ventricular hypertrophy (RVH). The ventricular septal defect is easily demonstrated. Note that the interatrial septum is intact.

(b) In systole, biventricular function is normal. The ventricular septal defect is large and non-restrictive.

(c) Similar systolic view with color flow Doppler imaging showing flow through the ventricular septal defect.

Discussion

The results of the echocardiogram were discordant with the referral diagnosis. The diagnosis of tetralogy of Fallot which the patient had carried for more than 20 years was incorrect. There was no right ventricular outflow tract obstruction due to posterior deviation of the outlet septum which is the fundamental structural abnormality in tetralogy of Fallot. This patient had a large non-restrictive ventricular septal defect. In childhood, a large left to right shunt would have been present with very high pulmonary pressures, because there was no infundibular or valvular stenosis to protect the pulmonary circulation. The patient developed systemic level pulmonary hypertension or Eisenmenger ventricular septal defect. The pulmonary artery progressively enlarged. Severe pulmonary hypertension and the altered geometry of the pulmonary root caused pulmonary regurgitation.

In patients with ventricular septal defects, the right ventricular systolic pressure can be estimated by recording cuff systolic blood pressure and subtracting the systolic gradient across the defect calculated from the modified Bernoulli equation, provided that the aortic valve is not stenotic. The magnitude of the right ventricular systolic pressure can be confirmed by assessing the right atrial to right ventricular gradient from the peak velocity of the tricuspid regurgitant jet. The absence of aliasing across the ventricular septal defect indicates that there is no gradient and therefore small and equivalent right to left and left to right shunt flow which is typical of Eisenmenger's reaction in association with ventricular septal defect.[1] Progression of pulmonary hypertension can occur in some patients who have undergone closure of non-restrictive ventricular septal defects at a young age.

The patient was not a candidate for a single lung transplantation with closure of the ventricular septal defect. He continued to experience exertional symptoms. He was found dead in bed several years after these images were taken.

Reference

1. Stojnic B, Pavlovic P, Ponomarev D, *et al.* Bidirectional shunt flow across a ventricular septal defect: pulsed Doppler echocardiographic analysis. Pediatr Cardiol 1995;16:6–11.

132

Holt–Oram heart–hand syndrome

Martin St John Sutton MBBS

A 33-year-old man had been noted to have a harsh pansystolic murmur soon after birth heard best midway between the cardiac apex and the lower left sternal border. He underwent cardiac catheterization at the age of 7 years which demonstrated an apical muscular ventricular septal defect with a 1.3 : 1.0 left to right shunt and normal pulmonary artery systolic pressure. He was treated medically with antibiotic prophylaxis for dental therapy. Aged 30 he had an insurance medical examination and was referred to the adult congenital heart disease clinic for re-evaluation. He had no symptoms of dyspnea, palpitations, syncope or chest pain but did complain of intermittent fatigue for which he could identify no triggers. He worked out in a gym for one or two days per week without difficulty. He had no family history of congenital heart disease.

On examination, the most striking feature was the abnormal upper body habitus which included short clavicles, short humeri, radioulnar synostoses and digitization of the thumbs bilaterally. Cardiovascular examination revealed an oxygen saturation in room air of 96% at rest, normal jugular venous pulse, a normal apical impulse, and a moderately loud apical pansystolic murmur. The second heart sound was widely split without augmentation of pulmonary closure. An electrocardiogram showed sinus rhythm, first-degree atrioventricular block and right bundle branch block with normal QRS axis.

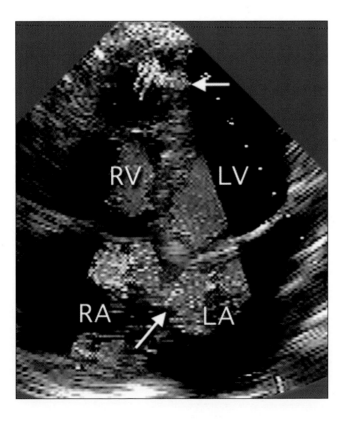

Figure 132.1
Apical four-chamber view with color flow Doppler in systole. The left ventricle is normal-sized with normal function. The mitral and aortic valves are also normal. The right ventricle is dilated and hypertrophied. There is a muscular ventricular septal defect at the apex (arrow) with systolic flow from the left to the right ventricle. In addition, there is an enlarged right atrium with a secundum atrial septal defect over 1 cm in diameter (lower arrow). Left to right flow is present at this level as well.

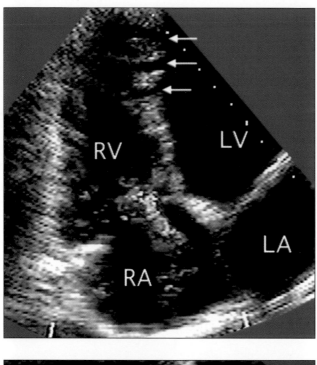

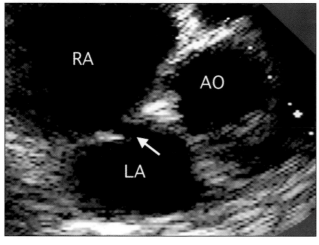

a

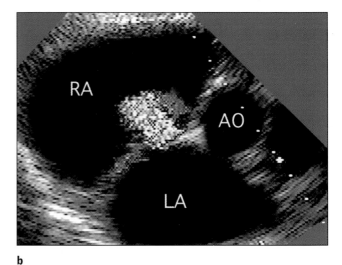

b

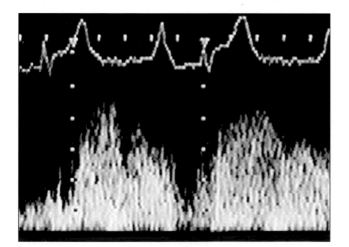

c

Figure 132.2
Off-axis apical image demonstrating multiple fenestrations of the interventricular septum (arrows).

Figure 132.3
(a) The patient has been placed in the right lateral decubitus position and the transducer is in short-axis orientation in the second right intercostal space. From this view, the interatrial septum is more perpendicular to the ultrasound beam than in the standard left parasternal short-axis view. A defect is visualized in the secundum atrial septum (arrow).
(b) Color flow Doppler demonstrates flow across the atrial septum from left to right.
(c) Spectral display of pulsed-wave Doppler from the right parasternal view. The sample volume has been placed in the right atrium adjacent to the atrial septal defect. Continuous left to right flow with a systolic peak is demonstrated.

Discussion

The patient had congenital heart–hand or Holt–Oram syndrome which is an autosomal dominantly inherited condition with varying penetrance consisting of secundum atrial septal defects and anomalies of the upper limb girdle.[1,2] In its most extreme form it may include phocomelia, but the syndrome is more commonly expressed as described in this patient. The most frequently associated cardiac lesion in heart–hand syndrome is a muscular ventricular septal defect, as in our patient. The gene locus has recently been identified. Our patient had no other member of his family pedigree affected, and his condition probably reflects a sporadic mutation. He is routinely followed medically with antibiotic prophylaxis for dental therapy, and with serial echocardiograms to assess pulmonary artery pressure.

References

1. Basson CT, Solomon SD, Weissman B, *et al.* Genetic heterogeneity of heart–hand syndromes. Circulation 1995;91:1326–9.

2. Basson CT, Cowley GS, Solomon SD, *et al.* The clinical and genetic spectrum of the Holt–Oram syndrome (heart–hand syndrome) [see comments] [published erratum appears in N Engl J Med 1994; 330:1627]. N Engl J Med 1994;330:885–91.

133

Complete atrioventricular canal

Martin St John Sutton MBBS
Susan E Wiegers MD

A 22-year-old man with cyanotic congenital heart disease and severe pulmonary hypertension was referred for heart and lung transplantation evaluation. He was noted to have a murmur at birth but was lost to follow-up until the age of 11 years when he developed pneumonia. He was admitted to hospital, where severe cyanosis was noted and he was finally diagnosed with congenital heart disease and underwent non-invasive testing and cardiac catheterization. A diagnosis of atrial and ventricular septal defects with severe pulmonary hypertension was made, and the mother was informed that he was inoperable on account of irreversible pulmonary vascular disease. Since that time he had developed insidiously progressive dyspnea and polycythemia with two episodes of hemoptysis. He had intermittent venesections when he complained of leg cramps and/or his hematocrit exceeded 65% with some symptomatic relief of his hyperviscosity syndrome. He could walk 50 meters before having to stop because of fatigue, dyspnea and light-headedness. He complained of intermittent central chest discomfort occurring with exercise, and transitory palpitations.

On examination he had severe central cyanosis with an oxygen saturation in room air of 79%, digital clubbing, elevation of his jugular venous pressure but no extremity edema, blood pressure of 90/60 mmHg, and a heart rate of 78 bpm. He had a pectus carinatum, a prominent right ventricular heave, and on auscultation there was an immediate diastolic murmur at the upper sternal border of pulmonary regurgitation and a loud pulmonary second heart sound consistent with pulmonary hypertension. An electrocardiogram demonstrated sinus rhythm with first-degree atrioventricular block, left axis deviation, right bundle branch block, and right ventricular hypertrophy with strain.

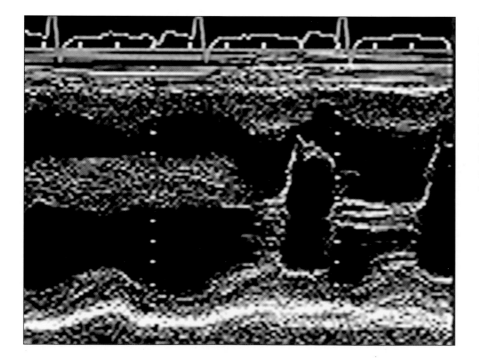

Figure 133.1
M-mode echocardiogram from the parasternal position. The beam is swept from the ventricular to the valvular level. On the left of the image, at the ventricular level, there is marked right ventricular free wall and septal hypertrophy. As the beam is angled cephalad, there is an interruption in the interventricular septum and the common atrioventricular valve fills both ventricles.

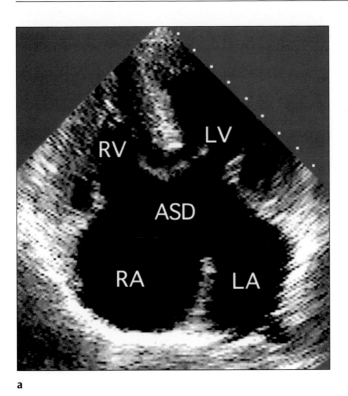

a

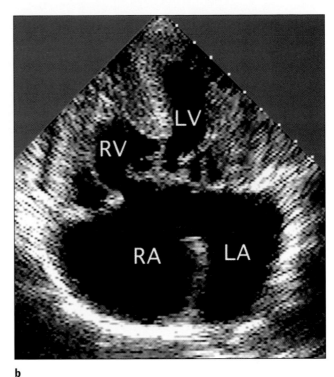

b

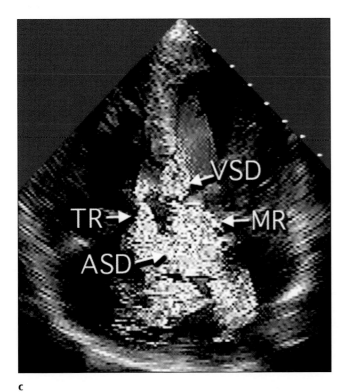

c

Figure 133.2

(a) Apical four-chamber view in diastole. A large primum atrial septal defect is well seen. The common atrioventricular valve has chordal attachments to both ventricles and to the crest of the interventricular septum. The septal leaflets of the mitral and tricuspid valves are contiguous, which is diagnostic of a common atrioventricular valve. A ventricular septal defect is present.

(b) In systole, the chordal attachments are clearly demonstrated. There are chordal structures present in the ventricular septal defect but these did not close the defect. It is clear in this view that the tricuspid valve leaflets do not coapt normally. Biatrial enlargement is present. The left ventricular systolic function is normal but the right ventricular systolic function is decreased.

(c) Similar systolic view with color flow Doppler imaging. There is severe tricuspid regurgitation (TR), mitral regurgitation (MR), and flow through the atrial septal defect (ASD) and ventricular septal defect (VSD).

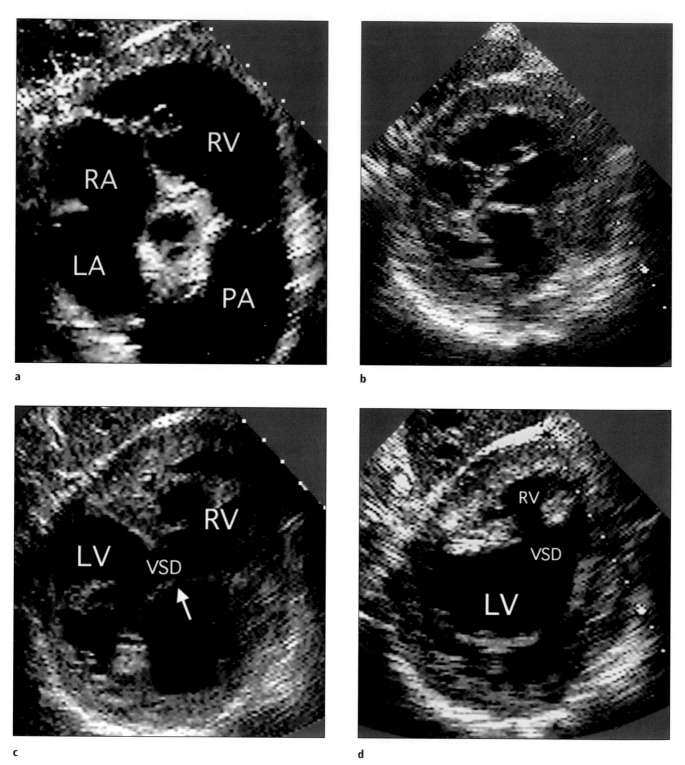

a

b

c

d

Figure 133.3

(a) Subcostal short-axis view at the base of the heart. The pulmonary artery (PA) is dilated. The defect in the interatrial septum between the left and right atria is clearly visible. The tricuspid valve leaflets are redundant but not severely abnormal in this view.

(b) Subcostal short-axis view. The transducer has been angled towards the apex of the heart to obtain this view at the level of the five leaflet common atrioventricular valve. Significant right ventricular hypertrophy is present.

(c) With further apical angulation, the ventricular septal defect is imaged. There is a complex papillary muscle arrangement with anomalous chordal attachments (arrow).

(d) Subcostal short-axis view at the mid-ventricular level. The true size of the ventricular septal defect (VSD) is better demonstrated and the diameter is over 2 cm. Once again, the multiple abnormal papillary muscles are seen.

Discussion

This patient had a complete atrioventricular canal defect with absence of the true atrioventricular septum, a large ventricular septal defect and a large primum atrial septal defect. Over the years, advanced pulmonary hypertension developed, causing irreversible pulmonary vascular disease. This is a common complication of unrestricted shunt flow in pulmonary vasculature exposed to systemic level pressures due to the non-restrictive ventricular septal defect. Echocardiography is essential in the diagnosis of the syndrome and associated abnormalities.[1] Contrast injection can be helpful to document the presence of the two defects, one in the atrial and one in the ventricular septum. Visualization of the cleft mitral valve is additionally helpful in establishing the diagnosis of atrioventricular septal defects. On occasion, repair of the canal defect results in left ventricular outflow tract stenosis and systolic anterior motion of the mitral valve.[2] This complication is suggested by development of left ventricular hypertrophy and a loud precordial murmur which progresses until the inflow tract is hemodynamically compromised.

References

1. Cabrera A, Pastor E, Galdeano JM, *et al.* Cross-sectional echocardiography in the diagnosis of atrioventricular septal defect. Int J Cardiol 1990;28:19–23.

2. Ebels T, Meijboom EJ, Anderson RH, *et al.* Anatomic and functional 'obstruction' of the outflow tract in atrioventricular septal defects with separate valve orifices ('ostium primum atrial septal defect'): an echocardiographic study. Am J Cardiol 1984;54:843–7.

134

Ventricular septal defect with retained pulmonary artery band

Martin St John Sutton MBBS
Susan E Wiegers MD

A 27-year-old woman with lipodystrophy presented for treatment 16 weeks pregnant complaining of fatigue. She had had a spontaneous abortion 8 months previously due to failed placentation. She complained of palpitations and tiredness that she was able to distinguish from dyspnea which she ascribed to the stage of her gestation. Previous history revealed that a cardiac murmur was detected in the first few weeks after her birth. She was subsequently admitted to hospital with failure to thrive and congestive heart failure. Cardiac catheterization demonstrated a large non-restrictive ventricular septal defect, for which she underwent pulmonary artery banding to obviate development of pulmonary vascular disease. At the age of 7 years she had closure of the ventricular septal defect but attempts to de-band the pulmonary artery were unsuccessful. Prior to her current pregnancy she had had a normal exercise tolerance and had participated in a vigor-

ous exercise program at a gymnasium for one hour 4 days a week, which she accomplished without difficulties.

On examination she was neither cyanosed nor clubbed, with an oxygen saturation of 96% in room air at rest. Blood pressure was 100/55 mmHg, heart rate was 92 bpm with normal peripheral arterial pulses but prominent 'a' and 'v' waves in the jugular venous pulse. There was a left parasternal lift indicating right ventricular hypertrophy and a harsh ejection systolic murmur audible throughout the entire precordium but loudest in the pulmonary area without any detectable diastolic murmur. There was an additional pansystolic murmur at the lower sternal border which varied with respiration. An electrocardiogram showed sinus rhythm, right bundle branch block, right axis deviation and right ventricular hypertrophy. A chest X-ray revealed mild cardiomegaly and an enlarged main pulmonary artery.

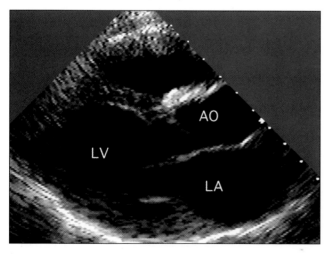

a

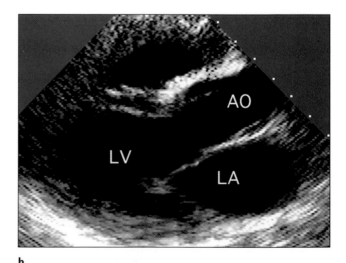

b

Figure 134.1
(a) Left parasternal long-axis view in diastole. The left ventricle is normal in size and the mitral and aortic valves are normal. Right ventricular hypertrophy is present. The anterior wall of the aortic root and the proximal interventricular septum are brightly reflective. This is due to the marked difference in acoustic impedance between the material used to patch the ventricular septal defect and the surrounding tissue.
(b) The diastolic image further demonstrates the patch material in the proximal septum and abnormal interventricular septal motion.

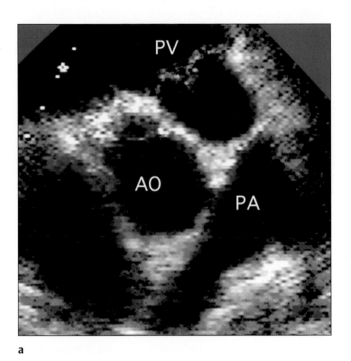

a

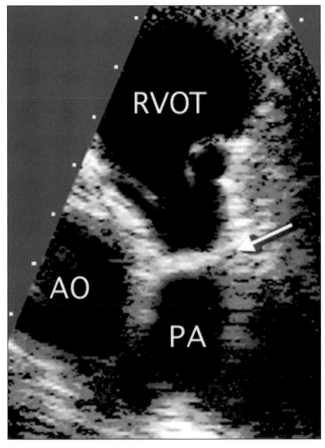

b

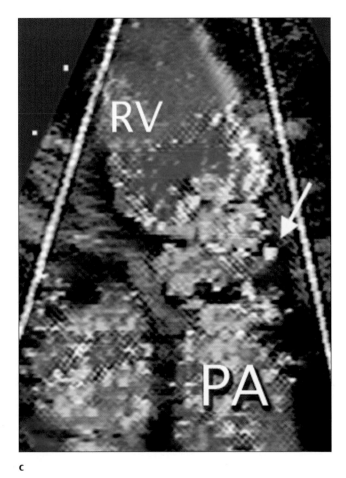

c

Figure 134.2

(a) The parasternal short-axis at the base of the heart demonstrates the pulmonary artery (PA) in long axis. The very echodense band around the main pulmonary artery is approximately 2 cm from the pulmonary valve. The pulmonary valve is normal. The surgical patch used to close the membranous ventricular septal defect is also visible between the left ventricular outflow tract and the right ventricle.

(b) A similar view of the pulmonary artery in systole shows that the pulmonary valve opens normally but the surgical band is immobile.

(c) Same as the previous view with color Doppler flow imaging. The flow in the proximal pulmonary artery is normal. However, proximal flow convergence prior to the band is observed. The diameter of the pulmonary artery (PA) at the level of the band is demonstrated by the narrow turbulent jet at this level. The jet is less than 5 mm in diameter.

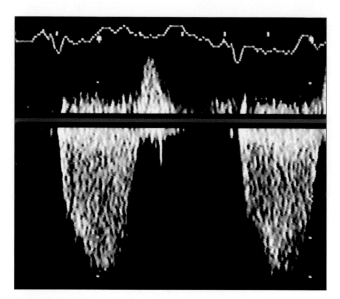

Figure 134.3
Continuous-wave Doppler across the pulmonary band with a peak velocity of 4 m/s (each calibration mark represents 1 m/s). There was a 60–70 mmHg systolic gradient across the pulmonary artery band and mild pulmonary regurgitation.

Discussion

This patient received the conventional therapy that was current 20 years ago for a large ventricular septal defect presenting with heart failure. The rationale for pulmonary artery banding was to reduce pulmonary arterial blood flow and minimize the risk of pulmonary vascular disease; when the child was larger, direct or patch closure of the ventricular septal defect would be performed and the band removed from the pulmonary artery. Complications of pulmonary artery banding include inadequate protection of the pulmonary circulation, residual stenosis once the band is removed, and pseudoaneurysm formation.[1] In this female patient who was pregnant, it was of pivotal importance to determine pulmonary artery pressure beyond the band. The increased intravascular volume that occurs in pregnancy exacerbates pulmonary hypertension. Severe pulmonary hypertension from pulmonary vascular disease is poorly tolerated by both the mother and the fetus and is an indication for termination of pregnancy. The echocardiogram demonstrated that the high right ventricular pressure was due to suprapulmonary stenosis and not from pulmonary hypertension. The long-axis views of the main pulmonary artery were essential in locating the level of right heart obstruction, and the apical and subcostal four-chamber views were important to exclude the presence of an intracardiac shunt at ventricular level and localize the ventricular septal defect patch repair.

The other remaining clinical issue in this patient was whether the right ventricle operating at a developed systolic pressure of 80 mmHg could tolerate a full-term pregnancy and labor, or whether it would be irreversibly damaged with the onset of congestive heart failure before term and compromise fetal viability. Successful delivery at term has been reported in patients with severe pulmonary stenosis.[2] Residual shunt flow across the surgically closed ventricular septal defect was easily ruled out by transthoracic echocardiography. The patient was advised to rest and not participate in her former exercise program. She successfully delivered a healthy infant at term and is currently without any symptoms of heart failure.

References

1. Foale RA, King ME, Gordon D, *et al.* Pseudoaneurysm of the pulmonary artery after the banding procedure: two-dimensional echocardiographic description. J Am Coll Cardiol 1984;3:371–4.

2. Ransom DM, Leicht CH. Continuous spinal analgesia with sufentanil for labor and delivery in a parturient with severe pulmonary stenosis. Anesth Analg 1995;80:418–21.

135

Brock procedure for tetralogy of Fallot

Martin St John Sutton MBBS
Susan E Wiegers MD

A 29-year-old African American male complained of chest pain and dyspnea on moderate exertion which was progressive over an 18-month period. Eight weeks previously he had an admission for *Pseudomonas* pneumonia presenting with fevers, pleuritic pain and hemoptysis which responded slowly to intravenous antibiotics. His history was that at 21 months of age he had had a series of squatting attacks during which he appeared grayish with impaired mentation; he was found to have a harsh systolic murmur for which he underwent cardiac catheterization. This revealed tetralogy of Fallot with absent left pulmonary artery. A Brock procedure was performed which consisted of a partial resection of the right ventricular outflow tract and infundibulum; the ventricular septal defect was not closed. He improved symptomatically but was advised to avoid competitive sporting activities at school. He was recatheterized at the age of 16 years. The right and left ventricular pressures were equal at the systemic level. A large non-restrictive ventricular septal defect was present along with a short muscularized infundibulum and a dysplastic, stenotic pulmonary valve. The pulmonary artery systolic pressure was in the low twenties. There was a normal sized main pulmonary artery but the left pulmonary artery was absent. He was advised to have further corrective surgery but declined, because of the quoted high perioperative mortality.

On examination he was not cyanosed or clubbed, his blood pressure was 90/65 mmHg, his heart rate was 78 bpm and regular. There was no dependent edema but the jugular venous pressure was elevated with a 'v' wave visible. There was a left parasternal lift consistent with right ventricular hypertrophy, and on auscultation there was a loud systolic murmur at the upper sternal border and a single second heart sound. An electrocardiogram showed sinus rhythm, first-degree heart block, right bundle branch block, right axis deviation and right ventricular hypertrophy. A chest X-ray showed cardiomegaly, elevation of the cardiac apex and interstitial opacities in both middle and lower lung fields suggestive of resolving bronchopneumonia.

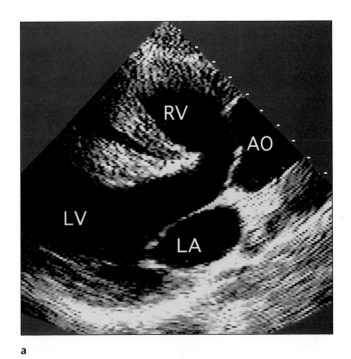

Figure 135.1
(a) Parasternal long-axis view in diastole. The aorta is enlarged and over-riding, creating a large malalignment ventricular septal defect. The left ventricle is of normal size but the right ventricle is enlarged and severely hypertrophied. The mitral and aortic valves were anatomically normal and competent.

a

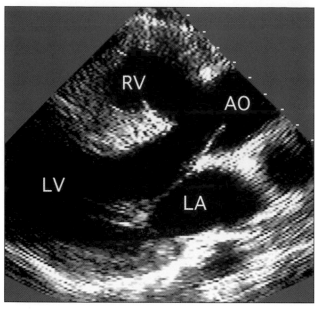

b

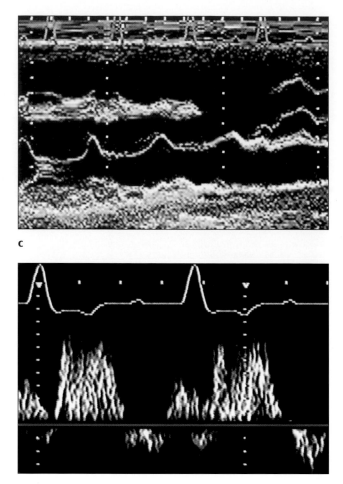

c

d

Figure 135.1

(b) In systole, there is abnormal septal motion.

(c) M-mode echocardiogram from the parasternal position. On the left of the image, the ultrasound beam is at the level of the mitral valve leaflets and is swept cephalad. The right ventricle is hypertrophied and dilated. There is an abrupt discontinuity in the interventricular septum and then imaging of the over-riding aorta.

(d) Pulsed-wave Doppler across the ventricular septal defect. There is low-velocity bidirectional flow.

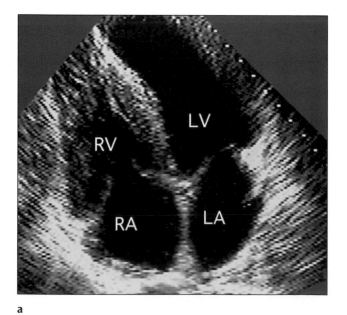

a

Figure 135.2

(a) Diastolic apical four-chamber view showing a normal-sized left ventricle and a severely hypertrophied right ventricle. The ventricular septal defect is out of plane in this image.

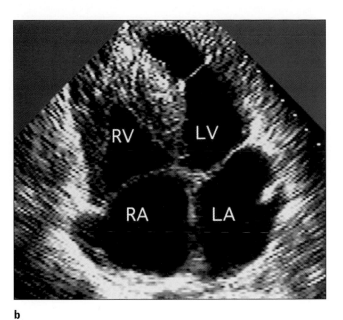

b

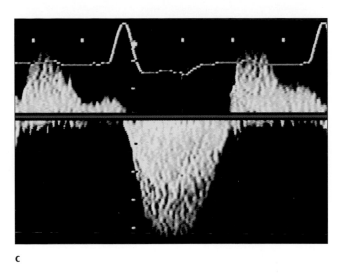

c

Figure 135.2

(b) In systole, decreased right ventricular contractile function is evident. There is a false chord in the left ventricle.

(c) Continuous-wave Doppler spectral display of tricuspid regurgitation. The peak velocity is 4.2 m/s (each calibration mark represents 1 m/s) which predicts a gradient of 71 mmHg between the right ventricle and atrium in systole.

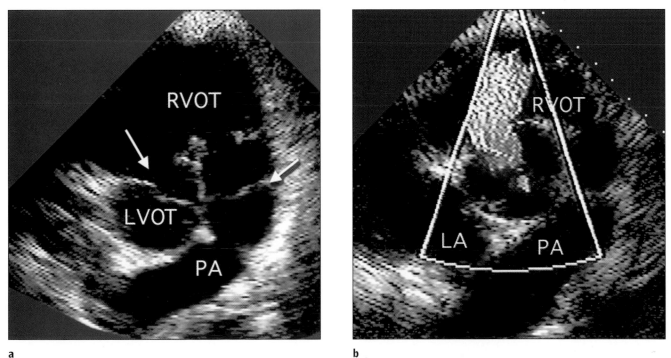

a

b

Figure 135.3

(a) Parasternal short-axis view at the base of the heart. The large ventricular septal defect (larger arrow) is demonstrated between the left ventricular outflow tract (LVOT) and the right ventricle. The right ventricular outflow tract (RVOT) is dilated. The pulmonary valve (smaller arrow) is thickened and abnormal. There is tissue at the level of the infundibulum projecting into the right ventricular outflow tract.

(b) Similar view with color flow Doppler imaging in systole. There is free flow across the ventricular septal defect between the left ventricular outflow tract and the right ventricle. The flow is turbulent but of low velocity.

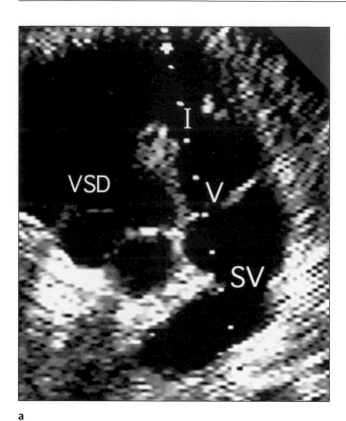

a

Figure 135.4

(a) Close-up image of the pulmonary valve from the parasternal view. The infundibular stenosis (I) is clearly demonstrated and is due to muscle bundles projecting into the right ventricular outflow tract, causing significant narrowing. The pulmonary valve (V) is dysplastic and did not open normally. The main pulmonary artery narrows, producing a supravalvular stenosis (SV) at the level of what should be the bifurcation. However, only the right main pulmonary artery is demonstrated. The left pulmonary artery was congenitally absent. The ventricular septal defect (VSD) is clearly seen.

(b) Similar systolic view with color Doppler flow imaging. There is turbulence at the level of the infundibulum, indicating obstruction to flow at that level.

(c) In this image, the narrowing of the high-velocity jet can be seen at the level of the supravalvular stenosis (larger arrow). The ventricular septal defect is again demonstrated (smaller arrow).

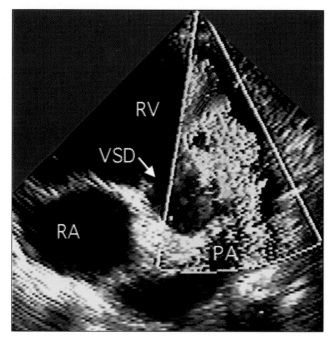

b

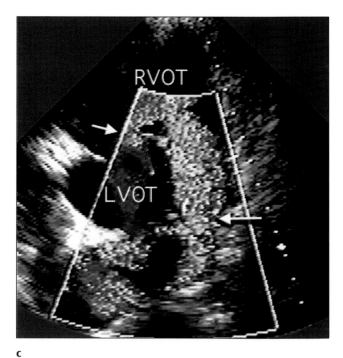

c

Discussion

Tetralogy of Fallot is a complex of abnormalities that derive from the fundamental anomaly of malalignment of the outlet septum. It is this anomaly that results in narrowing and underdevelopment of the right ventricular outflow tract due to the aortic over-ride and the non-restrictive ventricular septal defect.[1] Coronary artery anomalies are common in tetralogy and should be assessed echocardiographically.[2] This patient had fortuitously residual infundibular and serial stenosis which, in the presence of a large ventricular septal defect, had protected the lungs from pulmonary vascular disease. The right ventricular hypertrophy also contributed to the stenosis which can be progressive in these patients.[3] The result was similar to surgical banding of the pulmonary artery for large ventricular septal defects which was the procedure in use during this patient's childhood. The gradient between the right ventricle and right atrium was 71 mmHg during systole. Assuming a right atrial pressure of 15 mmHg, the right ventricular systolic pressure would be 85 mmHg. The patient's systemic blood pressure was 90 mmHg by blood pressure cuff. Thus, the right ventricle and left ventricle had equalized pressures, owing to the non-restrictive ventricular septal defect.

The echocardiographic features of tetralogy of Fallot were all demonstrated in this patient, who was finally persuaded to undergo total surgical correction.

References

1. Gatzoulis M, Soukias N, Ho S, et al. Echocardiographic and morphological correlations in tetralogy of Fallot. Eur Heart J 1999;20:221–31.

2. Berry JM, Jr, Einzig S, Krabill KA, et al. Evaluation of coronary artery anatomy in patients with tetralogy of Fallot by two-dimensional echocardiography. Circulation 1988;78:149–56.

3. Geva T, Ayres N, Pac F, et al. Quantitative morphometric analysis of progressive infundibular obstruction in tetralogy of Fallot. A prospective longitudinal echocardiographic study. Circulation 1995;92:886–92.

136

Subaortic stenosis after repair of an atrioventricular canal defect

Martin St John Sutton MBBS

Susan E Wiegers MD

A 33-year-old female nurse with insulin-dependent diabetes complained of two near-syncopal episodes lasting for seconds only but followed by profuse diaphoresis, which she initially ascribed to hypoglycemic episodes. Her history was relevant for type I diabetes mellitus from the age of 3 years, hypertension since the age of 16 years, multiple lipoma, repair of a complete atrioventricular canal defect at the age of 8 years, end-stage diabetic nephropathy presenting at the age of 30. An arteriovenous fistula was surgically created but she underwent renal transplantation at the age of 31 without prior dialysis. She had no exercise intolerance since her renal transplant, and had never experienced chest pain or discomfort.

On examination she had an arteriovenous fistula in her left upper arm, blood pressure of 140/90 mmHg, heart rate of 62 bpm, no edema or elevation of the jugular venous pressure, and equivalent diminution of peripheral pulses in the feet but no trophic skin changes. The apical impulse was left ventricular in type and the carotid pulses were unusually small and late peaking bilaterally. There was a loud harsh ejection systolic murmur radiating to the carotid arteries accompanied by a precordial systolic thrill, indicating the presence of left ventricular outflow tract obstruction. The electrocardiogram showed sinus rhythm, left axis deviation, QRS widening, and left ventricular hypertrophy with repolarization abnormalities consistent with severe aortic stenosis. A chest X-ray revealed moderate cardiomegaly and extensive intracardiac calcification, especially around the mitral valve annulus.

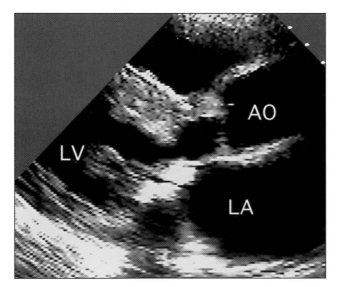

a

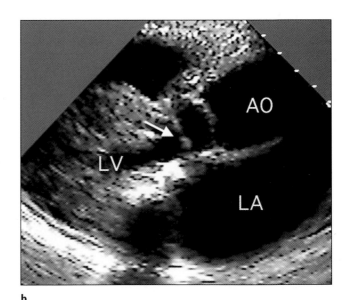

b

Figure 136.1
(a) Parasternal long-axis view in diastole. There is marked hypertrophy of the proximal interventricular septum and moderate hypertrophy of the other walls. An acoustic shadow is cast from the dense mitral annular calcification, present in both the anterior and the posterior annulus.
(b) Similar view in systole. The left ventricular cavity is obliterated. Sub-annular structures are again obscured by the annular calcium. A spicule of calcium (arrow) is seen in the left ventricular outflow tract.

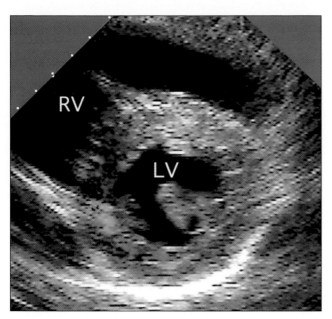

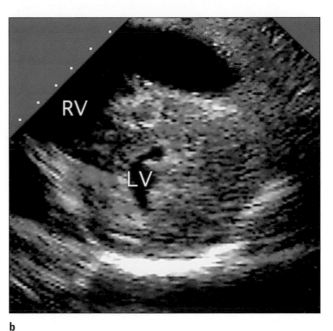

a   b

Figure 136.2
(a) Parasternal short-axis view in diastole. The marked left hypertrophy is demonstrated. The anterolateral papillary muscle is dominant. The cavity is small at end diastole.
(b) The cavity is nearly abolished at end systole.

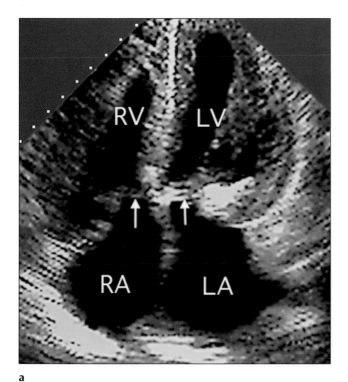

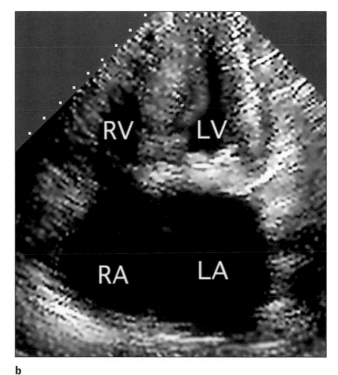

a   b

Figure 136.3
(a) Apical four-chamber view in diastole. A solid block of calcium obscures the anatomy of both mitral valve leaflets. There is biatrial enlargement and biventricular hypertrophy. Both atrioventricular valves arise from the interventricular septum at the same level (arrows). This is a clue that the patient has a surgically corrected endocardial cushion defect.
(b) In systole, the left ventricular cavity is a narrow slit. The apparent dropout of the interatrial septum is due to its parallel alignment with the ultrasound beam. The septum was intact.

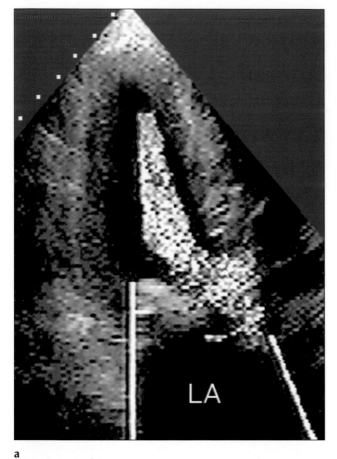

a

Figure 136.4

(a) Apical long-axis view of the left ventricle with color flow Doppler imaging in systole. Turbulent flow begins in the mid-cavity. The flow across the left ventricular outflow tract is narrowed and of high velocity, as well as being turbulent.
(b) Spectral display of continuous-wave Doppler across the left ventricular outflow tract. The peak velocity is over 5 m/s, indicating a peak greater than 100 mmHg (each calibration mark represents 1 m/s).
(c) Close-up image of the spectral pattern. There is a second late-peaking envelope with a peak velocity of approximately 3 m/s. This represents the intracavitary gradient that is caused by the near total cavity obliteration.

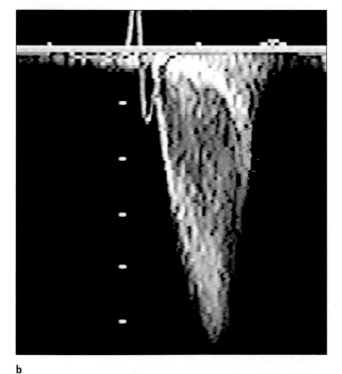

b

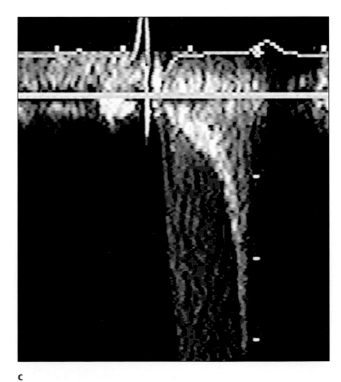

c

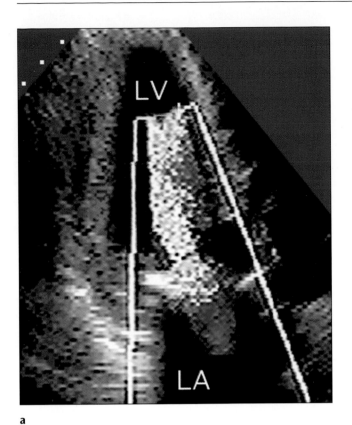

a

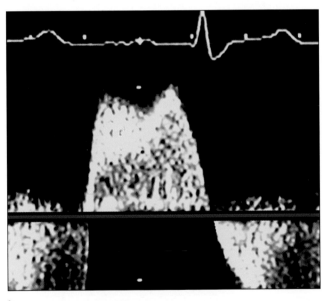

b

Figure 136.5

(a) Apical long-axis view in diastole with color flow Doppler imaging. The flow across the mitral valve is turbulent and of high velocity. Proximal flow convergence on the atrial side of the valve indicates significant mitral stenosis.

(b) Spectral display of continuous-wave Doppler across the mitral valve in diastole. The peak and mean gradient were obtained by digitizing the spectral envelope. The mitral valve area by the pressure half-time method was 1.2 cm^2 and the peak and mean gradients were 23 and 10 mmHg, respectively.

Discussion

A rare complication of surgical repair of complete atrioventricular canal defects is compromise of the left ventricular outflow tract. The 'goose neck deformity' of the left ventricular outflow tract may involve severe septal hypertrophy that causes dynamic outflow tract obstruction. The obstruction may become more severe over time as the left ventricle hypertrophies to normalize the increased load imposed by the obstruction. Abnormal mitral valve tissue may also obstruct left ventricular outflow.[1] Surgical procedures to correct the anomalies associated with complete canal defect may also inadvertently cause narrowing of the left ventricular outflow tract.[2] Echocardiography is essential in diagnosing this complication and following the progression.[3]

Residual mitral valve dysfunction after repair of a cleft leaflet has been well described. This patient had progressive mitral stenosis rather than recurrent regurgitation. Her single dominant papillary muscle indicates abnormal chordal attachments, and probably predisposed to development of obstruction after surgical closure of the cleft.

This patient had diabetic nephropathy, hypertension and secondary hyperparathyroidism so that she developed severe reactive hypertrophy, which further compromised an already narrowed outflow tract. The hyperparathyroidism resulted in the extensive organ calcification that involved the entire mitral annulus. It was hoped that restoration of her renal function, calcium and phosphate metabolism following renal transplantation might arrest the mitral annular calcification and alleviate the left ventricular outflow obstruction. In fact, the left ventricular hypertrophy continued to narrow the left ventricular outflow tract with progressive elevation of the left ventricular outflow tract peak systolic gradient. She was advised to undergo sub-aortic resection and probable mitral valve replacement, but declined because of potential compromise to her renal graft.

References

1. Ebels T, Meijboom EJ, Anderson RH, *et al.* Anatomic and functional 'obstruction' of the outflow tract in atrioventricular septal defects with separate valve orifices ('ostium primum atrial septal defect'): an echocardiographic study. Am J Cardiol 1984;54:843–7.

2. Van Arsdell G, Williams W, Boutin C, *et al.* Subaortic stenosis in the spectrum of atrioventricular septal defects. Solutions may be complex and palliative. J Thorac Cardiovasc Surg 1995;110:1534–41.

3. Reeder GS, Danielson GK, Seward JB, *et al.* Fixed subaortic stenosis in atrioventricular canal defect: a Doppler echocardiographic study. J Am Coll Cardiol 1992;20:386–94.

137

Aorto-pulmonary window

Martin St John Sutton MBBS
Susan E Wiegers MD

A 50-year-old woman was referred for an echocardiogram as part of an evaluation for lung transplantation for pulmonary hypertension that was believed to be primary. She had been short of breath for many years but had never sought medical attention until 2 years previously, when she had had a syncopal episode followed by a grand mal seizure. A workup for seizure activity included a chest X-ray, which demonstrated cardiomegaly and large proximal pulmonary arteries consistent with pulmonary hypertension. A two-dimensional echocardiogram showed enlarged right heart chambers, right ventricular hypertrophy, decreased right ventricular function and tricuspid regurgitation. The peak velocity of the tricuspid regurgitation indicated a pulmonary artery systolic pressure at systemic level. Her medical history was unremarkable except for a heart murmur that was detected at an elementary school medical examination, but was never followed up.

On examination there was mild central cyanosis with an oxygen saturation of 83% in room air at rest and minimal digital clubbing. Jugular venous pressure was elevated and she was in atrial fibrillation with a controlled ventricular rate of 78 bpm. There was a parasternal lift, indicating right ventricular hypertrophy, a holosystolic murmur, consistent with tricuspid regurgitation, and a loud pulmonary component to the second heart sound, indicating the presence of pulmonary hypertension. A chest X-ray showed an enlarged heart with dilated proximal pulmonary arteries. An electrocardiogram demonstrated sinus rhythm, right axis deviation, and right ventricular hypertrophy with strain.

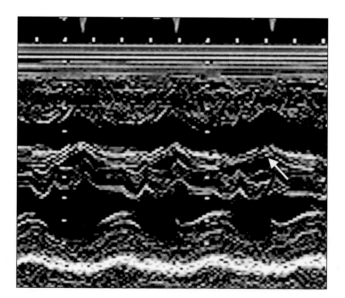

Figure 137.1
M-mode echocardiogram at the level of the mitral valve chords from the parasternal position. The right ventricle is hypertrophied and the cavity is enlarged. The echodensity within the right ventricle (arrow) is a hypertrophied septal band. Abnormal septal motion is present with a mid-diastolic posterior motion.

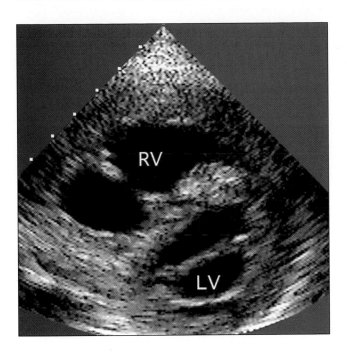

Figure 137.2
Parasternal short-axis view at the level of the mitral valve leaflets in diastole. The left ventricle is of normal size. Flattening of the interventricular septum is consistent with right ventricular volume overload. The right ventricular cavity is enlarged. Massive right ventricular hypertrophy is present. The free wall measures over 1.5 cm. The thickened septal band is also visible in this view.

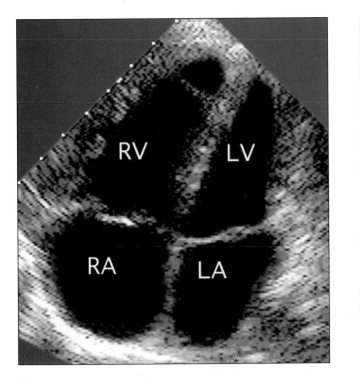

a

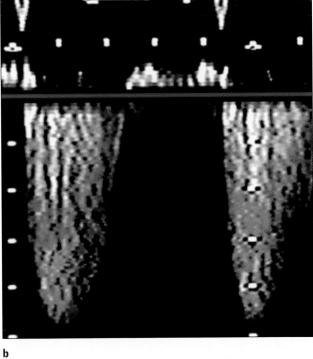

b

Figure 137.3
(a) The apical four-chamber view in systole demonstrates that the right ventricle is apex-forming. There is right ventricular hypertrophy and decreased right ventricular function. There was no evidence of an intracardiac shunt at atrial or ventricular level.
(b) Spectral display of continuous-wave Doppler across the tricuspid valve. The peak velocity is 4.8 m/s, which is diagnostic of systemic pulmonary pressures in the absence of pulmonary stenosis.

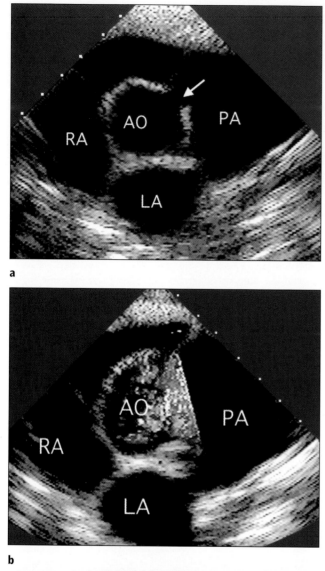

a

b

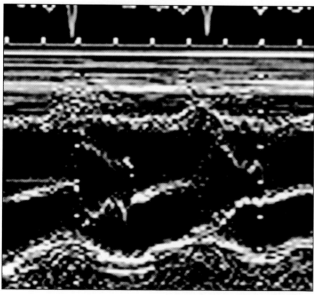

c

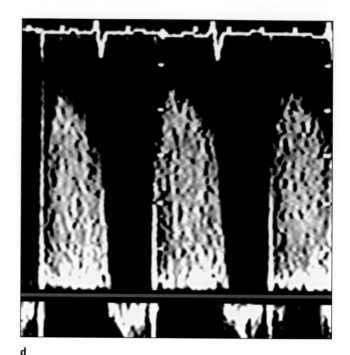

d

Figure 137.4

(a) The parasternal short-axis view at the level of the aorta showed normal aortic and pulmonary valves, excluding pulmonary stenosis as a cause of the right ventricular hypertrophy and dilatation. In addition, there was normal origin and anatomic relations between the great arteries. However, there is a defect in the wall between the aortic root and the pulmonary artery (arrow). This aortopulmonary window, which was completely unexpected and not previously diagnosed, is at least 8 mm in diameter. Considering that the aortic pressure is usually much greater than the pulmonary artery pressure, a very significant left to right shunt must have been present across this lesion. The pulmonary artery is severely dilated which is suggestive of severely elevated pulmonary artery pressures as well as adaptation to the shunt flow.

(b) Similar view with color flow Doppler imaging. There is low-velocity turbulent shunt flow between the aortic root and the pulmonary artery. The pulmonary artery and aortic pressures are nearly equal, which is why the flow has low velocity and is bidirectional.

(c) M-mode echocardiogram from the parasternal position. The dilatation of the pulmonary artery and right ventricular outflow tract has resulted in anterior displacement of the pulmonary valve which allows the two leaflets to be shown here. Although the motion is similar to that of the aortic valve, there is no right ventricular outflow tract anterior to this valve which rules it out as an aortic valve in a heart with normal great artery connections.

(d) Spectral display of continuous-wave Doppler across the pulmonary valve from the parasternal position. In diastole, pulmonary regurgitation reaches a peak velocity of 4.3 m/s which predicts a pulmonary diastolic pressure at systemic levels. In contrast, the systolic velocity is less than 1 m/s which again excludes pulmonary stenosis as a cause of the elevated right ventricular systolic pressures diagnosed from the velocity of the tricuspid regurgitation.

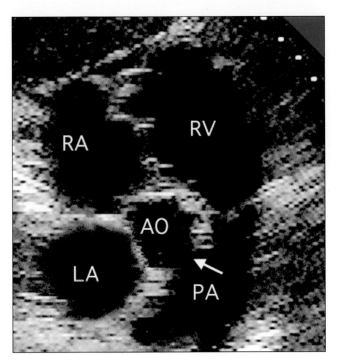

Figure 137.5
In the subcostal view of the short-axis of the aorta above the valve level there is a large defect (arrow) in the aorta. The interatrial septum is intact.

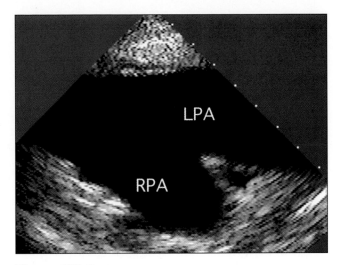

Figure 137.6
View of the pulmonary artery bifurcation from the parasternal short axis. This view is obtained by superior and medial angulation of the transducer from the parasternal short-axis view of the aortic root (similar to Figure 137.4a). Both the left (LPA) and right (RPA) branches of the pulmonary arteries are severely dilated.

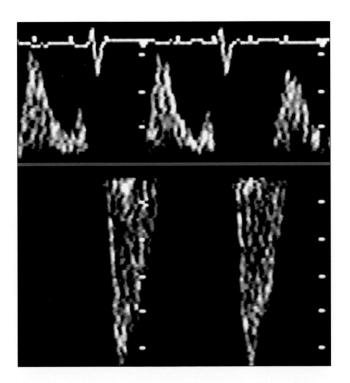

Figure 137.7
Spectral display of pulsed-wave Doppler in the descending thoracic aorta from the suprasternal notch. There is marked reversal of flow in diastole, although no aortic regurgitation was present. This is due to flow through the aorto-pulmonary window into the pulmonary artery in diastole.

Discussion

This patient was believed to have primary pulmonary hypertension and was being assessed for lung transplantation. In patients with clinical or echocardiographic evidence of pulmonary or right ventricular hypertension, a definitive etiology should be sought. Intracardiac shunting at atrial, ventricular, or great artery level must be excluded. In addition, subvalvular, valvular, and supravalvular pulmonary stenosis with an intact ventricular septum should also be excluded. Similarly, more complex structural anatomic anomalies should be looked for such as tetralogy of Fallot and pulmonary atresia. Echocardiography is of course key for the evaluation of the patient with pulmonary hypertension. Aorto-pulmonary windows are rare, but are usually easily diagnosed by echocardiography.[1]

A complete defect in the septation between the aorta and the pulmonary artery during embryogenesis results in truncus arteriosus. A partial defect leads to an aorto-pulmonary window.[2] Aorto-pulmonary windows are rarely encountered in adults. In this patient, the longstanding left to right shunt flow had resulted in the development of fixed pulmonary hypertension and right ventricular failure. This Eisenmenger's physiology was not recognized prior to the echocardiography. The patient underwent successful bilateral lung transplantation and patch closure of the defect between the great arteries with subsequent reverse remodelling of the right ventricle and restoration of nearly normal right ventricular contractile function.

References

1. Donaldson RM, Ballester M, Rickards AF. Diagnosis of aortico-pulmonary window by two-dimensional echocardiography. Cathet Cardiovasc Diagn 1982;8:185–9.

2. Steding G, Seidl W. Contribution to the development of the heart, Part II: morphogenesis of congenital heart diseases. Thorac Cardiovasc Surg 1981;29:1–16.

138

Tetralogy of Fallot

Martin St John Sutton MBBS
Susan E Wiegers MD

A 47-year-old woman was admitted as an emergency complaining of rigors and profuse sweating of one week's duration and transitory loss of speech. At the age of 6 years she had been noted to be centrally cyanosed and had squatting episodes. A clinical diagnosis of tetralogy of Fallot was made. She had a cardiac catheterization at 11 years which showed two ventricles at systemic pressure, a large muscular ventricular septal defect, severe pulmonary valvular stenosis with small central pulmonary arteries. She had a right Blalock–Taussig shunt placed, following which she was no longer cyanosed and improved symptomatically. Her parents did not consent to proceed to total correction on account of the mortality figure quoted. Over the past 5 years she had noted fatigue, increasing exercise intolerance due to dyspnea, and two near-syncopal episodes but no palpitations.

On examination she was febrile to 102°F, and centrally cyanosed with digital clubbing, splinter and conjunctival hemorrhages. Bilateral ankle edema and an elevated jugular venous pressure were also present. There was a palpable thrill over the upper left chest, a parasternal lift, a harsh systolic ejection murmur and a single second heart sound consistent with right ventricular outflow tract obstruction and an immediate diastolic murmur at the lower sternal border, indicative of pulmonary and/or aortic regurgitation. An electrocardiogram showed sinus rhythm and right bundle branch block. A chest X-ray demonstrated an enlarged heart with an upturned apex and pulmonary oligemia.

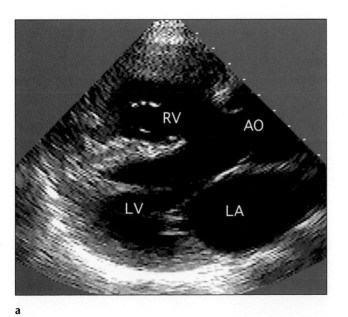

a

Figure 138.1
(a) Left parasternal long-axis view in systole demonstrates a normal-sized left ventricle with a large malalignment ventricular septal defect. The aorta over-rides the septum and the aortic root is enlarged. The right ventricle is hypertrophied. The mitral valve appears to be normal, the left atrium is mildly dilated, and the aortic leaflets are thickened.

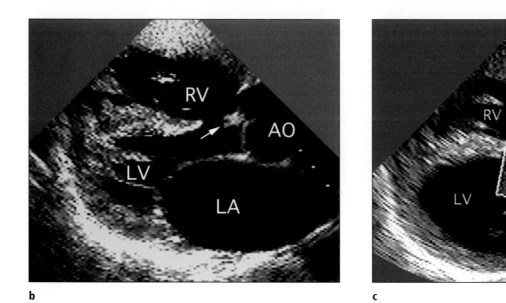

b   c

Figure 138.1
(b) A mass (arrow) is attached to the ventricular surface of the aortic valve. In diastole, it prolapses into the left ventricular outflow tract.
(c) Color Doppler imaging in systole. The left ventricular outflow (bottom arrow) is shown as red, moving towards the aortic valve in systole. In addition, low-velocity flow from the right ventricle (top arrow) crosses the ventricular septal defect and flows through the aortic valve and appears as blue flow as it moves away from the transducer towards the aortic valve.

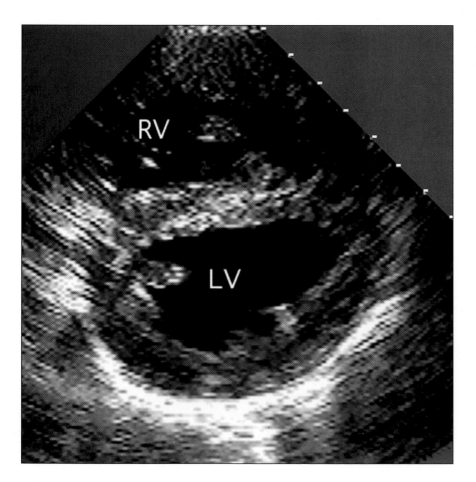

Figure 138.2
Parasternal short-axis view at the level of the papillary muscles in systole. The abnormal septal configuration indicates the presence of right ventricular pressure and/or volume overload. There is marked right ventricular free wall hypertrophy.

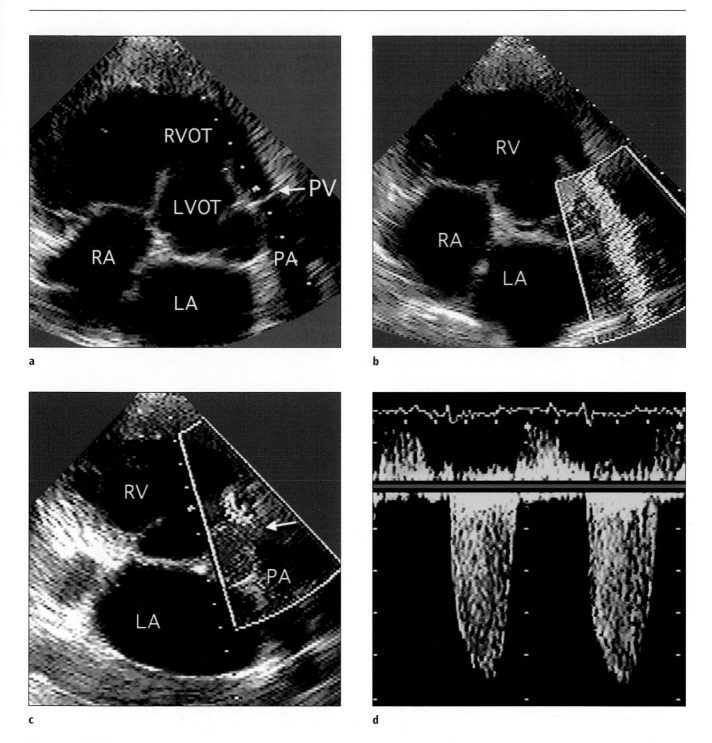

a

b

c

d

Figure 138.3

(a) Parasternal short-axis view at the base of the heart shows the large non-restrictive ventricular septal defect, which appears as an 'unroofed aorta'. The pulmonary valve (PV) leaflets are severely thickened, immobile, and stenotic. The right ventricular outflow tract and pulmonary artery are diminutive. Pulmonary valve motion was severely reduced in real time.

(b) Similar view with color flow Doppler in systole demonstrating the post-stenotic turbulence in the pulmonary artery.

(c) Diastolic image showing mild pulmonary insufficiency.

(d) Spectral display of continuous-wave Doppler across the right ventricular outflow tract and the pulmonary valve. The peak velocity is 4.4 m/s which corresponds to a peak gradient across the valve of 77 mmHg. It is not possible to define the separate contributions of the sub-valvular and valvular obstructions to this gradient.

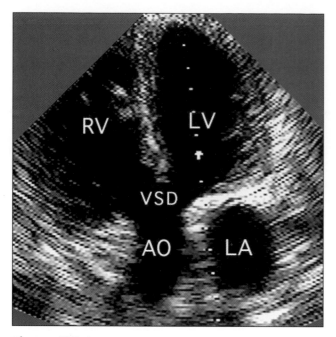

Figure 138.4
Apical four-chamber view with anterior angulation to reveal the large non-restrictive sub-aortic ventricular septal defect (VSD), the aorta over-riding the outlet septum and a dilated hypertrophied right ventricle that is larger than the left ventricle.

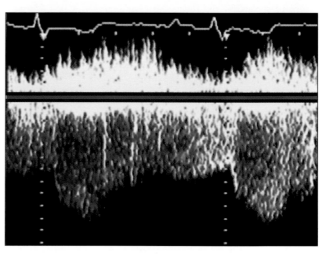

a

b

Figure 138.5
(a) Parasternal short-axis view at the base of the heart, with superior angulation to demonstrate the continuous color Doppler flow adjacent to the right pulmonary artery branch. This is flow through the Blalock–Taussig (BT) shunt.
(b) Continuous-wave Doppler tracing acquired from the suprasternal notch. There is continuous flow through the shunt into the pulmonary artery. The relationship of aortic to pulmonary artery pressure could not be determined, because the Doppler beam was not aligned with the direction of blood flow.

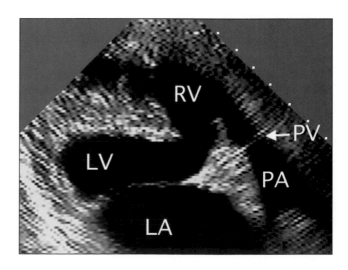

Figure 138.6
Off-axis view demonstrating that the malalignment of the aorta and the outlet septum accounts for both the ventricular septal defect and the right ventricular (RV) outflow obstruction.

Discussion

The diagnosis of tetralogy of Fallot is established unequivocally by a series of images that demonstrate a malalignment ventricular septal defect, pulmonary valvular stenosis, the aortic over-ride, and right ventricular hypertrophy. In this patient the finding of vegetations on the aortic valve leaflets and the presence of aortic regurgitation confirmed the clinical suspicion of endocarditis. The basic anatomic structural abnormality in tetralogy of Fallot is malalignment of the outlet septum which accounts for the infundibular and/or pulmonary stenosis and the sub-aortic ventricular septal defect[1] with secondary remodelling of both right and left ventricular chambers. This abnormality of the outflow septum allows tetralogy of Fallot to be distinguished from other non-restrictive ventricular septal defects with Eisenmenger physiology. Associated anomalies include right-sided aortic arch, anomalous coronary arteries, and absent left pulmonary branch artery. Coronary arteries should be carefully visualized on echocardiographic studies in patients with tetralogy of Fallot.[2] The right ventricular outflow tract may become so hypertrophied as to totally obstruct egress of blood from the right ventricle, constituting acquired pulmonary atresia.[3]

This patient was found to have *Streptococcus viridans* endocarditis. She responded to a 4-week course of intravenous antibiotics. She improved symptomatically on afterload reduction and plans to undergo total surgical correction. She will have intraoperative transesophageal echocardiography to assess the need for aortic valve replacement.

References

1. Gatzoulis M, Soukias N, Ho S, *et al.* Echocardiographic and morphological correlations in tetralogy of Fallot. Eur Heart J 1999;20:221–31.

2. Jureidini S, Appleton R, Nouri S. Detection of coronary artery abnormalities in tetralogy of Fallot by two-dimensional echocardiography. J Am Coll Cardiol 1989;14:960–7.

3. Geva T, Ayres N, Pac F, *et al.* Quantitative morphometric analysis of progressive infundibular obstruction in tetralogy of Fallot. A prospective longitudinal echocardiographic study. Circulation 1995;92:886–92.

139

Anomalous coronary artery from main pulmonary artery

Martin St John Sutton MBBS
Susan E Wiegers MD

A 31-year-old man was referred for investigation after a murmur was detected during a medical examination for life insurance. He had no symptoms of dyspnea, palpitations or syncope but had noticed intermittent aching in his chest unrelated to exertion or anxiety. There was no history of congenital or acquired heart disease in his immediate family and he had no risk factors for coronary artery disease. An electrocardiogram and chest X-ray were normal and he exercised for 14 min on a treadmill with a standard Bruce protocol without either symptoms or electrocardiographic abnormalities to suggest ischemia.

On examination he was normotensive and in regular rhythm with a resting heart rate of 62 bpm. There was no jugular venous distension or edema and peripheral pulses were equal bilaterally and normal. The apical impulse was normal and on auscultation there was a soft early diastolic murmur best heard in the pulmonary area. The electrocardiogram and chest X-ray were reviewed and were normal. A clinical diagnosis of mild pulmonary regurgitation was made.

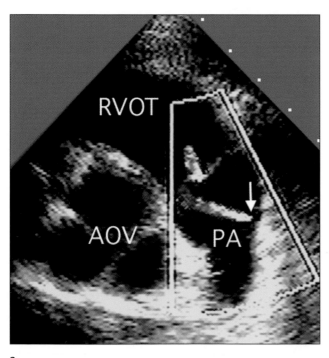

a

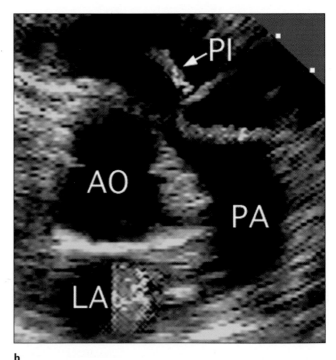

b

Figure 139.1
(a) Parasternal short-axis view of the aorta at the base of the heart in diastole with color flow Doppler imaging. There is a trivial jet of pulmonary insufficiency (PI). Just distal to the pulmonary valve, a low-velocity jet (arrow) enters the pulmonary artery (PA) from the right of the screen (patient's left). The origin of the left main coronary artery is seen in its usual anatomic location in the left sinus of Valsalva.
(b) Close-up of previous image. The aortic valve (AOV) is normal and closed in diastole. The abnormal jet is again visualized.

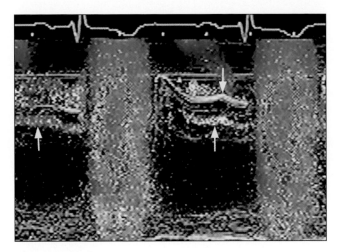

Figure 139.2
Color M-mode through the pulmonary valve (downward arrow) demonstrating the abnormal color jet (upward arrow). Color M-mode offers excellent temporal resolution. The color event is identified as holodiastolic.

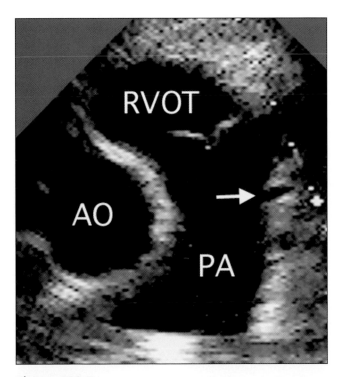

Figure 139.3
Close-up view of the proximal pulmonary artery (PA) from the parasternal position. The ostium of the aberrant coronary artery is visualized.

Discussion

The blood flow entering the main pulmonary artery in early diastole shown by color flow Doppler was from the anomalous origin of a small left circumflex coronary artery. Since the pressure in the pulmonary artery is lower than in the aorta, the anomalous coronary artery carries flow from left to left collaterals into the pulmonary artery. It is this reversed flow that is visualized emptying into the pulmonary artery in diastole. Coronary artery fistulous connections are usually to the ventricular chambers (coronary-cameral) or emanate from the left circumflex coronary artery to the bronchial circulation. If the entire left coronary artery originates from the pulmonary artery, there is reversed flow in the left coronary artery with evidence of left ventricular enlargement and severe contractile dysfunction with loss of R waves in the anterior precordial leads from extensive severe myocardial ischemia or infarction. Left ventricular contractile dysfunction is reversible if surgically corrected in the neonate. Echocardiography has been useful for establishing the diagnosis in asymptomatic patients and those with severe symptoms due to anomalous origin of the entire left coronary artery.[1,2]

In this patient, visualization of a normal left main ostium arising from the left sinus of Valsalva completely ruled out anomalous left coronary artery. Coronary arteriography subsequently confirmed the anomalous origin of a non-dominant left circumflex from the pulmonary trunk. Owing to the fact that this artery supplied an insignificant portion of the myocardium, the patient had no associated symptoms.[3] No therapy was undertaken and yearly treadmill stress tests for myocardial ischemia were advised.

References

1. Holley DG, Sell JE, Hougen TJ, *et al.* Pulsed Doppler echocardiographic and color flow imaging detection of retrograde filling of anomalous left coronary artery from the pulmonary artery. J Am Soc Echocardiogr 1992;5:85–8.

2. Jureidini SB, Nouri S, Crawford CJ, *et al.* Reliability of echocardiography in the diagnosis of anomalous origin of the left coronary artery from the pulmonary trunk. Am Heart J 1991;122:61–8.

3. Suzuki Y, Murakami T, Kawai C. Detection of anomalous origin of left coronary artery from pulmonary artery by real-time Doppler color flow mapping in a 53–year-old asymptomatic female. Int J Cardiol 1992;34:339–42.

140

Scimitar syndrome

Martin St John Sutton MBBS
Susan E Wiegers MD

A 26-year-old male heavy goods vehicle driver had two brief near-syncopal episodes, both of which occurred while driving. He sought medical advice in view of his occupation before applying for mandatory renewal of his special type of driving license. Neither episode was associated with any prodromal symptoms and on direct questioning he reported that he had never experienced chest pain or exercise intolerance but admitted to infrequent self-terminating palpitations, which he had had since early childhood. He had had no prior medical illness and no family history of congenital heart disease.

On physical examination he had dextrocardia, a normal apical impulse, normal heart sounds, without any additional sounds, and no cardiac murmurs. Electrocardiography showed a short PR interval and normal QRS duration and morphology. However, on a rhythm strip he sustained a short run of narrow complex tachycardia with ventricular rate of 280 bpm consistent with a bypass track. A chest X-ray showed dextrocardia with top normal cardiac size, a prominent right heart border, a small-volume right lung and a linear shadow close to the hilum of the right lung confined to the upper and middle zones.

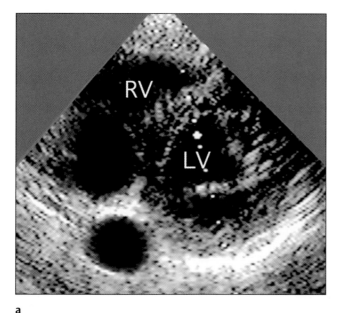

a

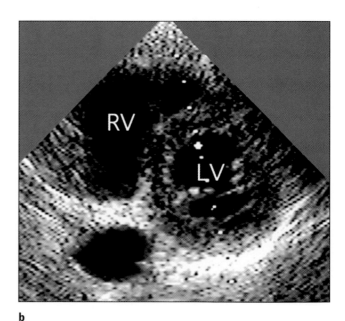

b

Figure 140.1
(a) Right parasternal short-axis view at the level of the mitral valve leaflets in diastole. The transducer has been placed at the fourth intercostal space in the right parasternal position. The left ventricle is of normal size. The right ventricle is dilated and mildly hypertrophied. The large vessel posterior to the right ventricle is the dilated inferior vena cava.
(b) Similar view in systole. The left ventricular function is normal, but the right ventricle remains enlarged in systole.

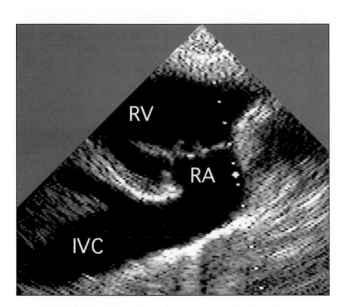

Figure 140.2
Off-axis right ventricular inflow view. The transducer is in a low right parasternal position and has been angulated medially and inferiorly. Only a portion of the right atrium is imaged in this view. It appears small, but this is due to foreshortening of the image. The inferior vena cava (IVC) is dilated at its attachment to the right atrium. The vessel that attaches to the inferior vena cava in this image could represent a hepatic vein, but was demonstrated on other images to be the anomalous pulmonary venous connection.

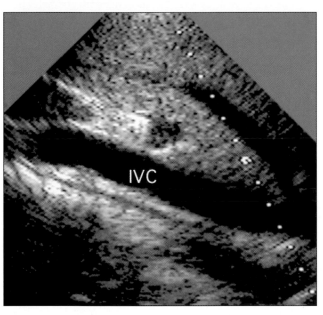

a

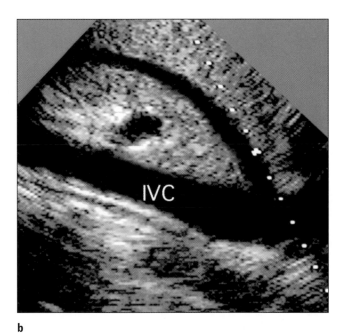

b

Figure 140.3
(a) Subcostal view of the inferior vena cava (IVC) as it transverses the liver. The distal inferior vena cava is of normal caliber, as opposed to the enlarged anastomosis to the right atrium that is demonstrated in Figure 140.2. There is an abnormal vessel imaged within the hepatic parenchyma.
(b) Lateral angulation from a similar subcostal view demonstrates an unusually large venous channel that is confluent with the inferior vena cava (IVC). This is the sub-diaphragmatic pulmonary venous drainage of part of the right lung and accounts for the enlarged right heart chambers.

Discussion

Anomalous pulmonary venous drainage is usually associated with sinus venosus atrial septal defects and less frequently with secundum atrial septal defects. Anomalous pulmonary venous drainage with either defect predominates in the right lung and also most commonly involves the right upper and/or right middle lobes. Drainage may be supracardiac, intracardiac, or infracardiac. In most patients the right heart chambers are enlarged from the increased pulmonary blood flow via the defect in the atrial septum and also from the anomalous pulmonary venous drainage. Dextrocardia or mesocardia is present in approximately 70% of patients. The result is hypoplasia of the right lung and abnormalities of the arterial supply to the right lung. In particular, the right main pulmonary artery may be smaller than the left main branch.[1] The anomalous veins are often visualized on transthoracic echocardiography.[2] Of patients with anomalous pulmonary venous drainage, 10–20% also have anomalies of systemic venous drainage. The most commonly associated systemic venous anomaly is a persistent left-sided superior vena cava that drains into the coronary sinus, which is obligatorily enlarged and can be recognized unequivocally by opacification with injection of contrast medium into the left cubital vein. In this patient, subsequent magnetic resonance angiography with gadolinium contrast enhancement demonstrated anomalous pulmonary venous drainage of the entire right lung to the inferior vena cava.

The scimitar syndrome is the name given to infracardiac drainage of pulmonary veins into the inferior vena cava. It may be more difficult to detect than other drainage because the site of attachment of the veins may be outside the echocardiographic window. Subcostal views are essential in the diagnosis. The anomalous vein is usually visualized as an abnormally large vessel that appears to run through the liver and attach to the inferior vena cava below the diaphragm. The vessel can be differentiated from a normal hepatic vein by its length and lack of branching. An abnormal flow pattern in the inferior vena cava, with monophasic flow and loss of reversal with atrial systole, can be a clue to the defect.[3] The partial anomalous drainage results in a left to right shunt. However, the shunt flow is rarely significant unless other defects, such as an atrial septal defect, are present.

The patient underwent successful electrophysiological radio-frequency catheter ablation of his bypass track, but did not pursue surgical correction of his anomalous pulmonary venous drainage.

References

1. Dupuis C, Charaf LA, Breviere GM, et al. The 'adult' form of the scimitar syndrome. Am J Cardiol 1992;70:502–7.

2. Shibuya K, Smallhorn JE, McCrindle BW. Echocardiographic clues and accuracy in the diagnosis of scimitar syndrome. J Am Soc Echocardiogr 1996;9:174–81.

3. Salazar J. Scimitar syndrome: five cases examined with two-dimensional and Doppler echocardiography. Pediatr Cardiol 1995;16:283–6.

141

Patent ductus arteriosus in a newborn

Martin St John Sutton MBBS
Susan E Wiegers MD

A 1-day-old full-term newborn male had a continuous murmur and was noted to have difficulty suckling on account of dyspnea believed to be due to development of congestive heart failure. He had episodes of arterial oxygen desaturation not fully responsive to inhibition of prostaglandin synthesis with indomethacin.

On examination there was mild hypoxemia, tachycardia, a wide pulse pressure, and a soft but continuous murmur audible best over the upper left chest consistent with a persistent patent ductus arteriosus.

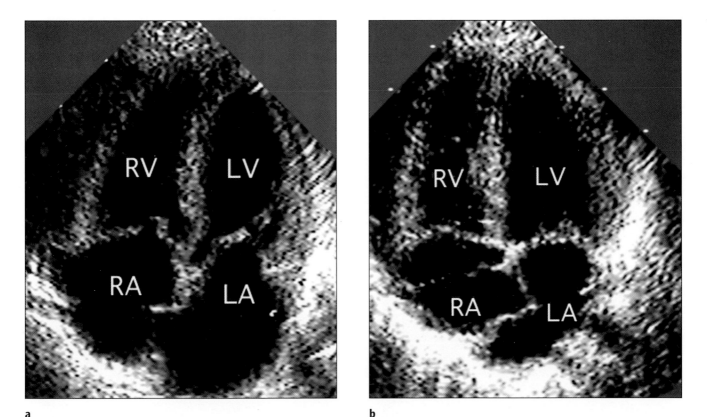

a

b

Figure 141.1
(a) Apical four-chamber view in early diastole. The left atrium is mildly dilated. The interatrial septum is highly mobile. The right ventricular wall thickness is nearly equal to that of the left ventricle, which is normal in a neonate.
(b) Similar view in late diastole. Note the Eustachian valve which runs across the floor of the right atrium to attach to the Thebesian vein of the interatrial septum at the level of the fossa ovalis. It is clear from this view that the interatrial septum is patent—also a normal finding in a 3-day-old baby.

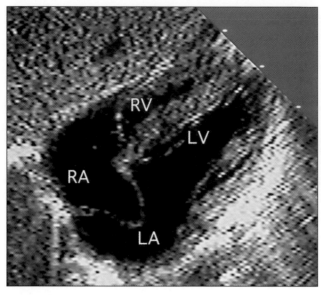
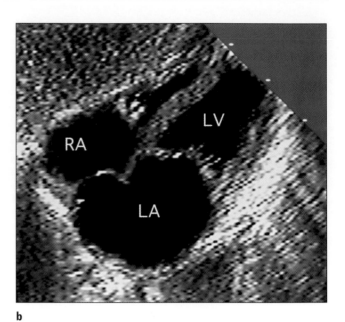

a

b

Figure 141.2

(a) Subcostal four-chamber view in diastole. The interatrial septum is almost aneurysmal. It is redundant and highly mobile throughout the cardiac cycle. Although this finding would be abnormal in a young child or adult, a percentage of neonates with this finding close the interatrial communication without residual abnormality in the septum.

(b) Similar view in systole. The left atrium is enlarged. The interatrial septum now bows into the right atrium.

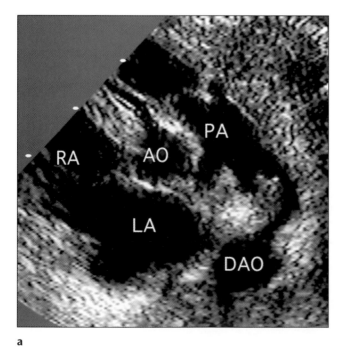

Figure 141.3

(a) Modified parasternal short-axis view at the base of the heart. The transducer has been angled superiorly and to the patient's left to image the pulmonary artery (PA). This image is easily obtained in the neonate, but is often difficult to achieve in the adult. The communication between the descending thoracic aorta (DAO) seen in short axis and the left pulmonary artery is clearly visualized. The diameter of the patent ductus arteriosus is on the order of the branch pulmonary arteries. The left pulmonary artery is the middle vessel, as the pulmonary artery appears to trifurcate at the site of the ductus. The proximal course of the right coronary artery is demonstrated from the origin in the right sinus of Valsalva as it runs anteriorly and rightwards.

a

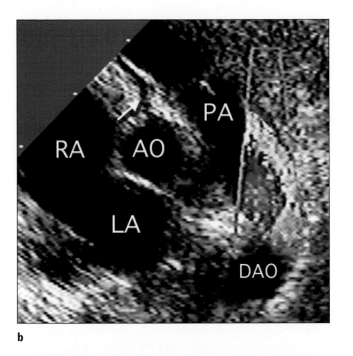

b

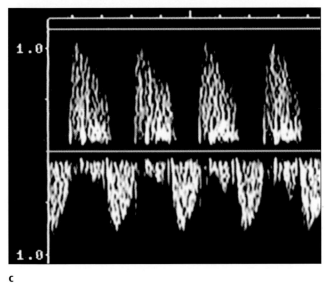

c

Figure 141.3

(b) Similar view with color Doppler flow imaging in diastole. The shunt flow between the descending thoracic aorta (DAO) and the left pulmonary artery (PA) runs along the lateral wall of the pulmonary artery. There is proximal flow convergence in the descending aorta as the jet enters the ductus. The right coronary artery (arrow) is again clearly visualized.
(c) Continuous-wave Doppler spectral display of flow through the patent duct. The pulmonary artery pressures in a neonate are nearly systemic. Thus the flow is bidirectional: antegrade blood flow during systole, and higher-velocity diastolic flow reversal into the pulmonary artery from the aorta. The low velocity of the flow reflects the low gradient between the two vessels.

Discussion

This infant had a large patent ductus arteriosus that was causing significant shunt flow. The ductus can usually be directly visualized in an infant. The reversed flow in the main pulmonary trunk can usually be detected by color flow and continuous-wave Doppler. These findings together with the dilated left atrium clinch the diagnosis. The ductus is always present immediately following birth, but shunting rapidly decreases and the duct normally closes within the first week of life. Echocardiography is far more reliable than clinical examination in detecting significant shunt flow.[1] Left atrial dilatation is a sign of significant shunt flow.[2] The modified parasternal short-axis view is easily achieved in neonates and is the best view for demonstrating the size and course of the ductus. Ductal size is an important predictor for the development of persistent patent ductus.[3] The parasternal short-axis is also usually the best view for Doppler assessment of ductal flow. However, the path of the ductus may be tortuous and the attachment can be variable, making the assessment of Doppler flow velocities less reliable. Diastolic reversal of flow in the abdominal aorta can be assessed by Doppler echocardiography and is also suggestive of patent ductus.

This infant was symptomatic and had a continuous murmur suggestive of patent ductus. The duct was relatively large and the left atrium dilated which was consistent with a hemodynamically significant shunt. Following additional indomethacin treatment the patent ductus arteriosus closed and color flow Doppler evidence of flow reversal was no longer demonstrable.

References

1. Davis P, Turner-Gomes S, Cunningham K, et al. Precision and accuracy of clinical and radiological signs in premature infants at risk of patent ductus arteriosus. Arch Pediatr Adolesc Med 1995;149:1136–41.

2. Phillipos EZ, Robertson MA, Byrne PJ. Serial assessment of ductus arteriosus hemodynamics in hyaline membrane disease. Pediatrics 1996;98:1149–53.

3. Kluckow M, Evans N. Early echocardiographic prediction of symptomatic patent ductus arteriosus in preterm infants undergoing mechanical ventilation. J Pediatr 1995;127:774–9.

142

Patent ductus arteriosus

Martin St John Sutton MBBS
Susan E Wiegers MD

A 41-year-old woman was referred for assessment of pulmonary hypertension and evaluation for lung transplantation. She had noticed slow but progressive reduction in exercise tolerance over approximately 10 years and had had two recent episodes of near-syncope, for which she had sought medical attention. She had had no seizure activity and could not identify any trigger for her near-syncope; in particular she had not experienced any palpitations, chest pain or diaphoresis. She had no family history of congenital or acquired heart disease and had no risk factors for heart disease. She had refused cardiac catheterization at the age of 17 years for investigation of a heart murmur, because she was asymptomatic and could exercise without difficulty. She had never used anorexigens and was believed to have primary pulmonary hypertension because she no longer had any murmur.

On examination there was no dependent edema, but there was an elevated jugular venous pressure with distinct 'a' and 'v' waves, mild central cyanosis and differential clubbing of the toes but not of the fingers. Her blood pressure and heart rate were within normal limits. There was a pectus carinatum and a left parasternal lift, indicating right ventricular hypertrophy. On auscultation there were no murmurs, but the pulmonary component of the second heart sound was loud, suggesting the presence of pulmonary hypertension. Respiratory excursion was symmetric and breath sounds were normal bilaterally. Electrocardiography demonstrated sinus rhythm, right axis deviation and right ventricular hypertrophy with repolarization abnormalities. A chest X-ray showed an enlarged heart and the pulmonary vascular markings suggested severe pulmonary hypertension with enlarged proximal pulmonary arteries.

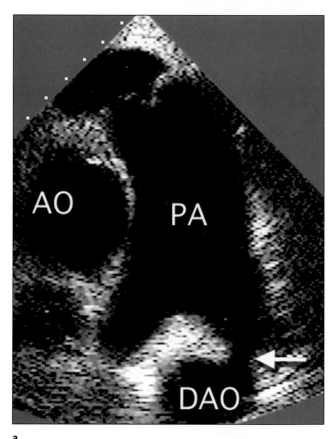

a

Figure 142.1

(a) In the left parasternal short-axis view of the aorta, the pulmonary artery (PA) is severely enlarged, as are the left and right branches. There is a normal-appearing pulmonary valve that closes early. A large connection (arrow) between the descending thoracic aorta (DAO) and the left pulmonary artery branch is visualized. This is a large patent ductus arteriosus. Originally, this must have allowed massive left to right shunt flow. With the development of Eisenmenger's physiology, the patient now has systolic pulmonary artery pressures that are higher than the systolic blood pressures.

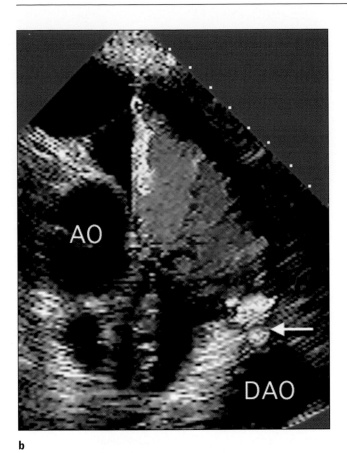

b

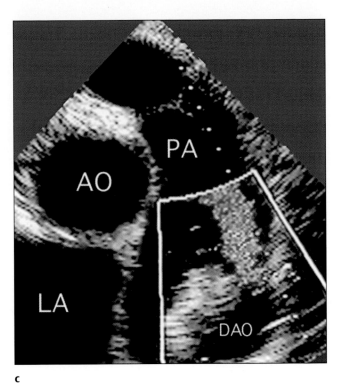

c

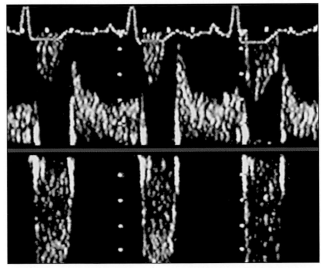

d

Figure 142.1

(b) Similar view in systole with color Doppler flow imaging. There is flow (arrow) from the pulmonary artery to the descending thoracic aorta (DAO) which is due to the suprasystemic pulmonary artery pressures. Proximal flow convergence is present on the pulmonary artery side of the defect.

(c) In diastole, a low-velocity color flow jet is visible as blood flows from the aorta into the left pulmonary artery.

(d) Spectral display of pulsed-wave Doppler in the patent ductus arteriosus. The sample volume has been placed in the mouth of the ductus on the pulmonary artery side. There is flow from the pulmonary artery into the aorta in systole. In diastole, the shunt reverses and the blood flows from the aorta into the pulmonary artery.

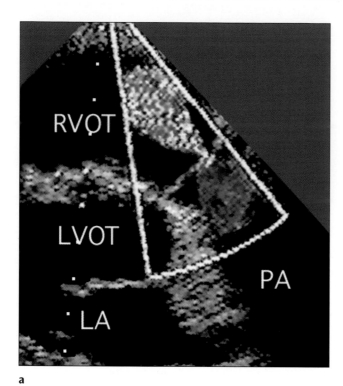

a

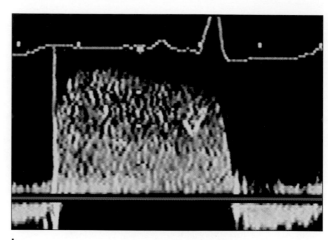

b

Figure 142.2
(a) Parasternal short-axis view of the pulmonary valve in diastole. The right ventricular outflow tract (RVOT) is dilated. There is a high-velocity turbulent jet of pulmonary insufficiency which arises from the pulmonary valve and extends into the right ventricular outflow tract.
(b) Spectral display of continuous-wave Doppler across the pulmonary artery in diastole. The pulmonary insufficiency jet has high velocity, reaching approximately 3.5 m/s in early diastole. Thus, the peak gradient between the pulmonary artery and right ventricle in diastole is 49 mmHg, which indicates a markedly elevated pulmonary artery diastolic pressure.

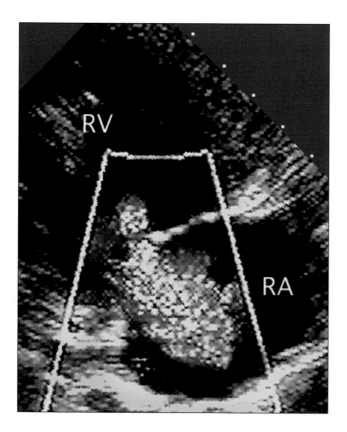

Figure 142.3
Right ventricular inflow view with color flow Doppler imaging from the parasternal position. There is a high-velocity turbulent jet in systole that extends into the right atrium. The jet of tricuspid regurgitation is broad at the level of the valve leaflets and its extent is consistent with moderately severe regurgitation.

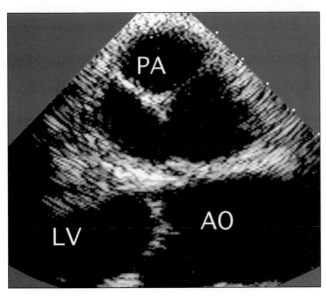
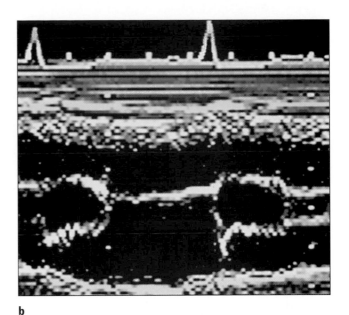

a   b

Figure 142.4

(a) Parasternal long-axis view, close-up of the pulmonary valve (PA) and the ascending aorta. The pulmonary valve has been anteriorly displaced by the dilatation of the pulmonary artery. It is unusual to visualize the pulmonary valve in short axis. However, the normal anatomic relationship is maintained with the pulmonary valve anterior to the aortic valve. The aorta and the pulmonary root are oblique to each other rather than parallel, as is seen in transposition of the great vessels.

(b) M-mode echocardiogram from the parasternal position. Premature systolic closure of the pulmonary valve is due to the severe pulmonary hypertension and right ventricular contractile failure.

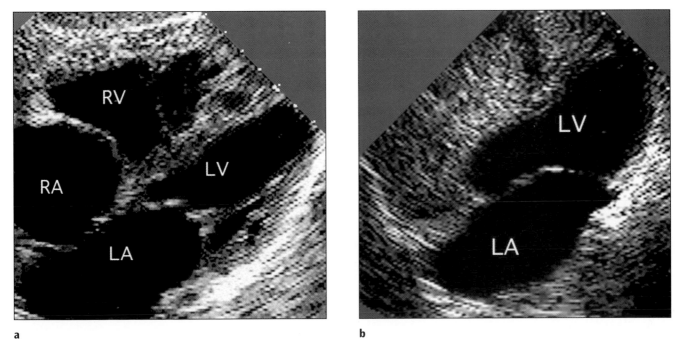

a   b

Figure 142.5

(a) Subcostal four-chamber view in late diastole. The right ventricle is apex forming and severely hypertrophied. The interatrial septum is intact.

(b) Similar view with injection of agitated saline into the right antecubital vein. The right atrium and ventricle are opacified by the microbubbles.

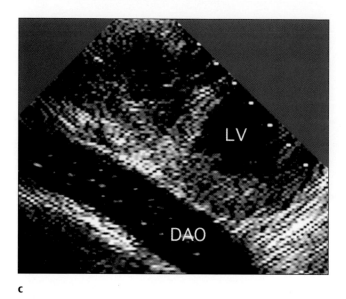

Figure 142.5

(c) Subcostal view of descending thoracic aorta (DAO) as it crosses the diaphragm. The pulmonary circulation normally filters out the microbubbles and no bubbles are visible in the left heart chambers. Microbubbles in the descending aorta confirm the diagnosis of patent ductus arteriosus with reversed shunting (Eisenmenger's syndrome).

c

Discussion

The diagnosis could have been made from the clinical history and examination of differential clubbing and the signs of pulmonary hypertension indicating the development of systemic pulmonary hypertension from an Eisenmenger reaction to a patent ductus arteriosus. There is echocardiographic evidence of systemic level pulmonary artery pressure from the reversed septal motion during systole, the severe right ventricular hypertrophy, and impaired contractile function with intact ventricular septum. It is imperative that patients with presumed primary pulmonary hypertension undergo echocardiography to rule out the presence of shunts that may lead to Eisenmenger's reaction and severe pulmonary hypertension.[1] The patent ductus is usually difficult to visualize, but was very large and easily seen in this patient. In addition, intravenous injection of agitated saline demonstrated a right to left shunt at duct level and retrograde passage of echo contrast into the descending thoracic aorta.[2]

Transesophageal echocardiography may be more sensitive for the diagnosis and can also be used to rule out a residual leak during closure.[3–5] This patient was listed for double lung transplant with surgical closure of the duct and awaits surgery.

References

1. Chen WJ, Chen JJ, Lin SC, et al. Detection of cardiovascular shunts by transesophageal echocardiography in patients with pulmonary hypertension of unexplained cause. Chest 1995;107:8–13.

2. Panetta C, Schiller N. Evidence of patent ductus arteriosus and right-to-left shunt by finger pulse oxymetry and Doppler signals of agitated saline in abdominal aorta. J Am Soc Echocardiogr 1999;12:763–5.

3. Shyu KG, Lai LP, Lin SC, et al. Diagnostic accuracy of transesophageal echocardiography for detecting patent ductus arteriosus in adolescents and adults. Chest 1995;108:1201–5.

4. Andrade A, Vargas-Barron J, Rijlaarsdam M, et al. Utility of transesophageal echocardiography in the examination of adult patients with patent ductus arteriosus. Am Heart J 1995;130:543–6.

5. Lavoie J, Javorski JJ, Donahue K, et al. Detection of residual flow by transesophageal echocardiography during video-assisted thoracoscopic patent ductus arteriosus interruption. Anesth Analg 1995;80:1071–5.

143

Corrected transposition of the great arteries

Martin St John Sutton MBBS
Susan E Wiegers MD

A 37-year-old woman developed palpitations for several minutes after a 10-km race and presented to the emergency room. She was normotensive and in sinus rhythm when examined, and the only abnormal finding was an apical pansystolic murmur. An outpatient two-dimensional echocardiogram was obtained which was reported to show mitral valve prolapse with mild mitral regurgitation. She was advised to take antibiotic prophylaxis against endocarditis before dental treatment. She remained asymptomatic for 10 years and then developed atypical chest pain during the latter part of a 6-km run.

She went directly to the emergency room, where an electrocardiogram showed no anterior forces; she was admitted to exclude acute myocardial infarction. Her medical history was unremarkable and she had participated in a vigorous exercise program without any dyspnea or chest pain.

Physical examination was noteworthy only for an apical pansystolic murmur radiating to the axilla with no apical displacement and no systolic click. The electrocardiogram showed sinus rhythm with first degree atrioventricular block and Q waves in precordial leads V1–V3.

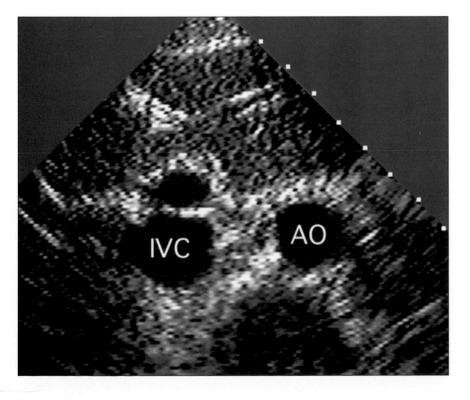

Figure 143.1
From the subcostal position, the transducer is angled directly to the spine to obtain this view. The inferior vena cava (IVC) and abdominal aorta (AO) are seen in short axis. The inferior vena cava and the liver are on the patient's right (on the left of the image) and the aorta and stomach are on the patient's left. This establishes normal abdominal visceral and atrial situs (situs solitus).

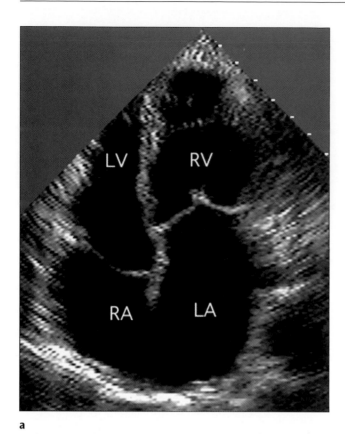

a

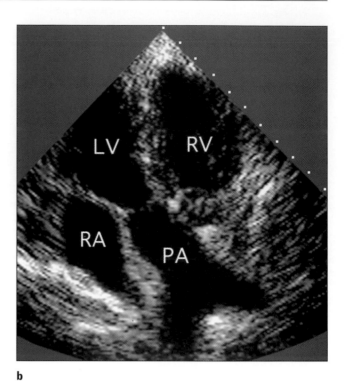

b

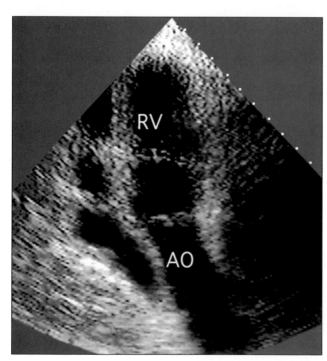

c

Figure 143.2

(a) Apical four-chamber view with the transducer in the standard position. The ventricle on the left of the screen contains the moderator band and its atrioventricular valve is apically positioned. These features identify it as a morphological right ventricle.

(b) Anterior angulation of the transducer demonstrates a great vessel with primary branching arising from the anatomic left ventricle which receives blood from the right atrium.

(c) Further anterior angulation from (b) demonstrates another great vessel, the aorta, which does not bifurcate. This vessel arises from the morphological right ventricle. The great arteries can be determined only by their pattern of primary branches, or by identification of the origin of the coronary arteries.

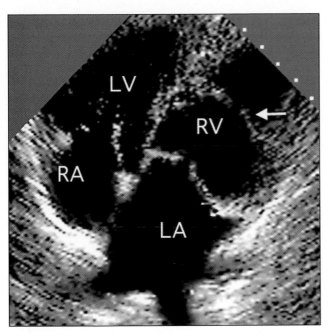
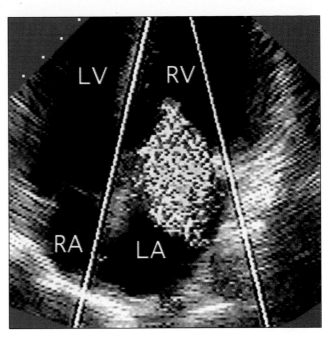

a   b

Figure 143.3

(a) The transducer has been moved to the right of the standard apical position. The moderator band in the morphological right ventricle is better seen. Again, apical displacement of the tricuspid valve plane confirms that the ventricle on the right of the screen is the right ventricle, in the usual location of the left ventricle. Three pulmonary veins can be seen entering the left atrium which flows into the right ventricle.

(b) Color Doppler imaging from the apical four-chamber view in systole. There is severe tricuspid regurgitation entering the left atrium. Since the right ventricle is the systemic ventricle (i.e. the aorta arises from it) the velocity of the tricuspid regurgitation was over 4 m/s.

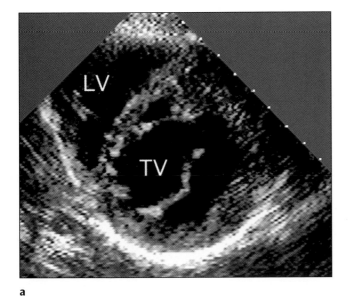
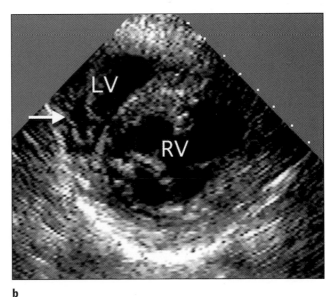

a   b

Figure 143.4

(a) Short-axis parasternal view at the level of the valve leaflets. As previously identified, the morphological right ventricle is the posterior ventricle. The three papillary muscles of the tricuspid valve are visible in this short-axis view. The posterior leaflet is small and not well imaged in this view. The anterior leaflet is seen on the anterior wall. The septal and posterior papillary muscles are adjacent to each other posteriorly.

(b) Similar short-axis view. The mitral valve (arrow) is visible in the left ventricle, which is compressed by the dilated right ventricle.

Discussion

Diagnosis of corrected transposition of the great arteries requires careful analysis of all of the anatomic connections of the heart. The apical four-chamber view demonstrates three key features, which become apparent when the two ventricles are examined individually and allow the diagnosis to be established. The apex of the normal heart is formed by the left ventricle, which has two papillary muscles, neither of which takes origin from the interventricular septum. The anterior mitral valve leaflet is continuous with the non-coronary sinus of the aortic valve and takes its origin from the interventricular septum 6–8 mm higher (closer to the base of the heart) than the septal leaflet of the tricuspid valve. The right ventricular septal and free wall surfaces are more coarsely trabeculated than the endocardial surface of the left ventricle. In addition, the moderator band, which conducts the terminal branches of the right bundle of Purkinje fibers to the free right ventricular wall, is easily visualized as a moderate-sized muscular tendon towards the apex of the right ventricle. The right ventricle contains the tricuspid valve and has its unique papillary muscular anatomy with insertion of chordae into the interventricular septum. Applying these criteria, it is clear in this patient's apical four-chamber view that the right ventricle is on the patient's left and the left ventricle is on the right, so that there is atrioventricular discordance. The right ventricle is the systemic ventricle and the tricuspid valve is moderately regurgitant with a decreased right ventricular contractile function. Ventricular–arterial discordance was demonstrated from the apical images.

The patient had been told in the past, at another institution, that she had mitral valve prolapse. This diagnosis was made erroneously on the original echocardiogram because the tricuspid valve in the systemic right ventricle was regurgitant and was misinterpreted as the mitral valve. The correct diagnosis is anatomically described as situs solitus with atrioventricular and ventriculoarterial discordance which is better known as congenitally corrected transposition of the great arteries. The course of blood is from the systemic veins to the right atrium to the left ventricle to the pulmonary artery and from the lungs to the left atrium to the right ventricle and to the aorta and systemic circulation. There is frequently systemic ventricular dysfunction and systemic atrioventricular valvular regurgitation which may progress with age, necessitating valve replacement. Intracardiac lesions that are associated with congenitally corrected transposition include ventricular septal defects and valvular and/or subvalvular pulmonary stenosis, neither of which were present in this patient.

In complex congenital heart disease it is important to determine atrial situs, atrioventricular and ventriculoarterial connections by identifying each chamber and artery by its internal anatomy.

The patient was reassured that her current condition did not necessarily preclude childbearing.[1] She was also advised that the tricuspid valvular regurgitation might eventually warrant valve replacement. Furthermore, cardiac transplantation could be considered if her ventricular function deteriorated severely.[2]

References

1. Connolly H, Grogan M, Warnes C. Pregnancy among women with congenitally corrected transposition of great arteries. J Am Coll Cardiol 1999;33:1692–5.

2. Carrel T, Neth J, Pasic M, et al. Should cardiac transplantation for congenital heart disease be delayed until adult age. Eur J Cardio-Thorac Surg 1994;8:462–8.

144

Transposition of the great vessels: Mustard intra-atrial repair

Martin St John Sutton MBBS

A 32-year-old woman was seen for routine yearly follow-up with no cardiac symptoms except for occasional short paroxysms of palpitations. Two days after birth she had been noted to be centrally cyanosed and underwent emergency cardiac catheterization, at which time the diagnosis was made of transposition of the great arteries with an intact ventricular septum and a patent ductus arteriosus that appeared to be closing. A balloon septostomy was performed after completion of the diagnostic catheterization which was associated with improvement in the arterial oxygen saturation to 71%. Five months later she underwent an intra-atrial Mustard procedure. Since that time she had developed normally

and had no cardiovascular symptoms except mild exercise intolerance and intermittent palpitations.

On examination she was not cyanosed or clubbed, and had an oxygen saturation of 96% in room air. She was in sinus rhythm with frequent ectopic activity and a normal blood pressure. There was a prominent 'v' wave in the jugular venous pulse, suggesting tricuspid regurgitation, and a marked parasternal lift and a holosystolic murmur at the lower left sternal border. She had mild hepatomegaly but no splenomegaly. Electrocardiography showed sinus rhythm, right axis deviation and right ventricular hypertrophy. A chest X-ray demonstrated cardiomegaly and a narrow supracardiac vascular pedicle.

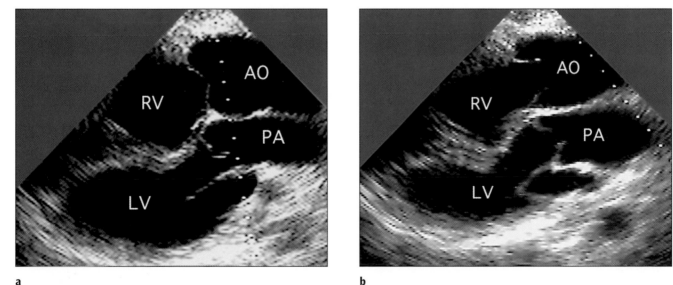

a   b

Figure 144.1
(a) Left parasternal long-axis view taken from a high second intercostal space. The anterior right ventricle is enlarged and hypertrophied with reversed septal motion. Two similar-sized great arteries are seen in their long axes, one anterior and the other posterior, travelling in parallel. It is not possible from this image alone to determine the identity of the great vessels. The left atrium is out of plane in this view.
(b) Similar view with the transducer angled posteriorly to image the left atrium. The bifurcation of the pulmonary artery is not seen in this view and cannot be identified with certainty. However, the parallel course of the great vessels is consistent with transposition.

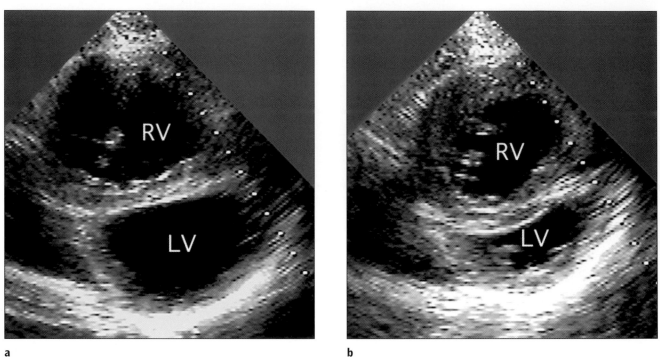

a

b

Figure 144.2
(a) Parasternal short-axis view at the level of the tips of the left ventricular papillary muscles. The right ventricle is circular in cross-section, larger than the left ventricle, and the septal configuration is reversed throughout the cardiac cycle. The three leaflets of the tricuspid valve are well seen in diastole.
(b) Similar systolic view. The right ventricular function is decreased and the septum moves paradoxically. The left ventricle is crescentic in both systole and diastole.

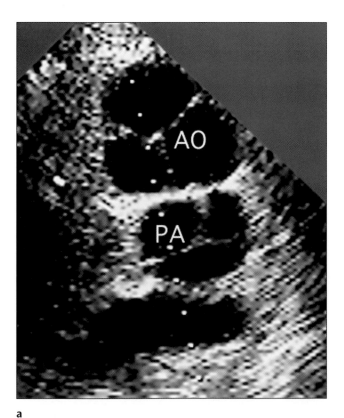
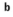

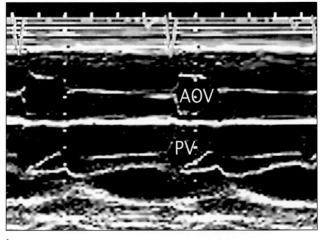

b

a

Figure 144.3
(a) Parasternal short-axis view at the base of the heart demonstrates two great vessels in short axis at valve level. The anterior great artery is the aorta, and posterior and leftwards (in reference to the patient) is the pulmonary artery, with the small left atrium behind it.
(b) M-mode echocardiogram from the parasternal position at the base, demonstrating the parallel position of the aortic and pulmonary valve roots.

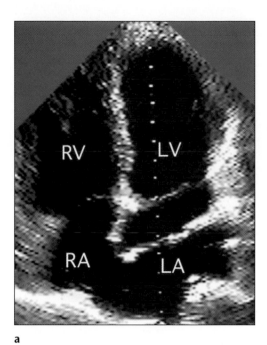
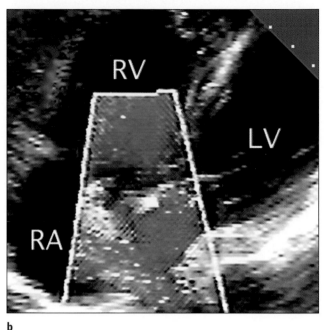

a   b

Figure 144.4
(a) In the apical four-chamber view the right ventricle is enlarged and apex-forming, but the feature of note is the intra-atrial baffle seen parallel to the mitral valve annulus. The surgically created baffle directs oxygenated blood from the pulmonary veins into the right atrium/right ventricle and to the aorta. The systemic venous blood is baffled into the left atrium/left ventricle and to the pulmonary artery without mixing with the pulmonary venous blood.
(b) Color flow Doppler demonstrates the inflow of blood from the pulmonary veins, across the baffle and into the right atrium and ventricle. The color jet has low velocity and is not turbulent, which is consistent with unobstructed baffle flow.

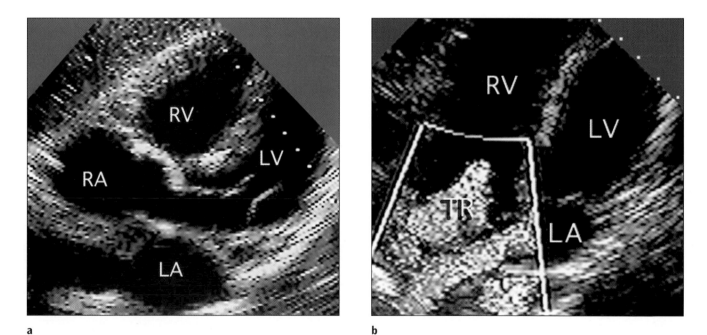

a   b

Figure 144.5
(a) Subcostal view of the systemic venous return from the inferior vena cava baffled to the left atrium without mixing with the oxygenated blood from the pulmonary veins.
(b) Color flow Doppler in systole demonstrates the systemic venous return from the superior vena cava entering the left atrium. Tricuspid regurgitation (TR) is present and appears to be moderate.

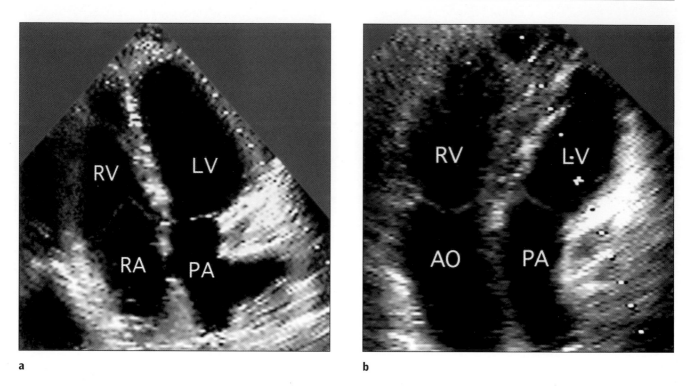

a   b

Figure 144.6

(a) Anterior angulation from the standard apical four-chamber view demonstrates the pulmonary artery, which is identified by its primary branching pattern, originating from the left ventricle. The bifurcation of the vessel eliminates the possibility that this is the aorta.

(b) Further anterior angulation and clockwise rotation shows the aorta arising from the right ventricle and the parallel course of the great vessels. The bifurcation of the pulmonary artery is not seen in this view.

Discussion

Transposition of the great arteries and associated anatomic defects are diagnosed by sequential chamber analysis, which includes identification of atrial situs, atrioventricular connections and ventricle–great artery connections. In this patient, there is normal situs and concordant atrioventricular connections but discordant ventricle–great artery connections. The great arteries cannot be identified by their position or their relation to each other. They can only be unequivocally identified by their pattern of branching.

This patient had previous corrective surgery. The Mustard procedure creates an intra-atrial baffle, which should be carefully examined by the use of color flow Doppler to demonstrate the pattern of systemic and pulmonary venous flow. Transesophageal echocardiography may be useful, even in the immediate postoperative period, to rule out pulmonary venous obstruction.[1] Patients who have undergone an atrial switch in the past have a good 15-year survival but face morbidity from the long-term complications of a systemic right ventricle and from arrhythmias and sudden death.[2] Abnormal function of the atrium after an atrial switch with loss of atrial contractility and contribution to cardiac output may decrease exercise tolerance in these patients.[3]

Survival in uncorrected transposition requires an obligatory shunt that is often at ventricular level. Coexistent outflow tract obstruction is also a frequently associated congenital lesion. Both of these well-known associated anomalies must be defined, and their importance assessed with echocardiographic imaging. An arterial switch at an early age is now the treatment of choice for this congenital abnormality. Nevertheless, patients who underwent an atrial baffle procedure in the 1960s through the 1980s are reaching adulthood in increasing numbers.

References

1. Kaulitz R, Stumper O, Fraser A, *et al*. The potential value of transesophageal evaluation of individual pulmonary venous flow after an atrial baffle procedure. Int J Cardiol 1990;28:299–307.

2. Birnie D, Tometzki A, Curzio J, *et al*. Outcomes of transposition of the great arteries in the era of atrial inflow correction. Heart 1998;80:170–3.

3. Reich O, Voriskova M, Ruth C, *et al*. Long-term ventricular performance after intra-atrial correction of transposition: left ventricular filling is the major limitation. Heart 1997;78:376–81.

145

Situs inversus, double-outlet right ventricle, atrial and ventricular septal defects

Martin St John Sutton MBBS
Susan E Wiegers MD

A 26-year-old man was referred for assessment and evaluation for heart and lung transplantation. He had been complaining of dyspnea, fatigue and recurrent episodes of near-syncope on mild to moderate exertion for several years. He had undergone repeated venesections for hyperviscosity syndrome consisting of leg cramps and extreme fatigue on only mild exertion and was currently requiring venesection every 3 weeks, with transitory symptomatic improvement. He had had a murmur detected at birth and was followed up until he was 2 years old, at which time he was noted to be slightly centrally cyanosed. A chest X-ray had revealed dextrocardia and a stomach on the right side. Cardiac catheterization soon afterwards demonstrated situs inversus and double-outlet right ventricle with a non-restricted ventricular septal defect.

On examination, he was centrally cyanosed with digital clubbing and an oxygen saturation of 81% in room air at rest. There was elevation of the jugular venous pressure and a prominent 'v' wave indicating the presence of tricuspid regurgitation. The apical impulse was unremarkable but there was a marked parasternal lift, suggesting right ventricular hypertrophy. On auscultation there was a soft holosystolic murmur heard optimally at the lower left sternal border which augmented with respiration and wide splitting of the second heart sound with a louder than normal pulmonary component to the second heart sound, suggesting pulmonary hypertension from a non-restrictive ventricular septal defect. Electrocardiography showed sinus rhythm, right axis deviation and right ventricular hypertrophy with repolarization abnormalities consistent with strain. A chest X-ray showed dextrocardia, situs inversus, cardiomegaly, and markedly enlarged proximal pulmonary arteries, suggesting pulmonary hypertension.

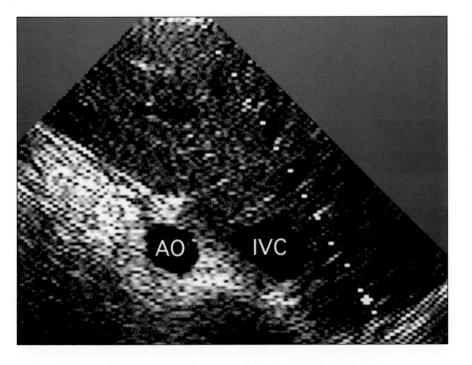

Figure 145.1
Transverse section through the abdomen, 2 or 3 cm below the xiphoid process. The transducer has been angled posteriorly to demonstrate the relationship between the inferior vena cava (IVC) and the abdominal aorta (AO). The inferior vena cava and the liver are on the patient's left (right of image). The abdominal aorta is on the right, indicating abdominal visceral inversion and atrial inversion.

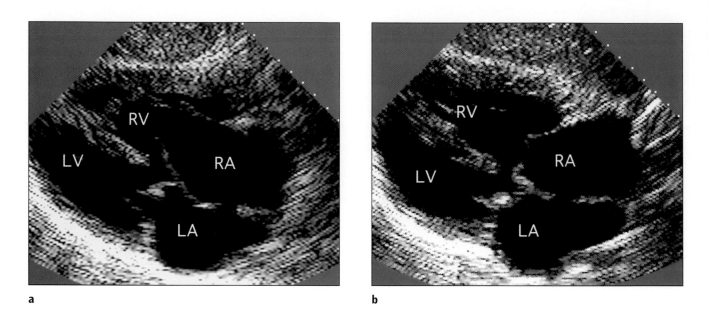

a b

Figure 145.2

(a) Subcostal four-chamber view in diastole. The apex points to the patient's right. The right ventricle (RV) is enlarged and hypertrophied. The moderator band is prominent. There are obvious defects in the upper interventricular and secundum atrial septa. There is biatrial enlargement with the right atrium being larger than the left. Both the mitral and the tricuspid valve medial leaflets are attached to the primum atrial septum. The mitral valve is thickened but is not stenotic.

(b) Biventricular systolic function is decreased.

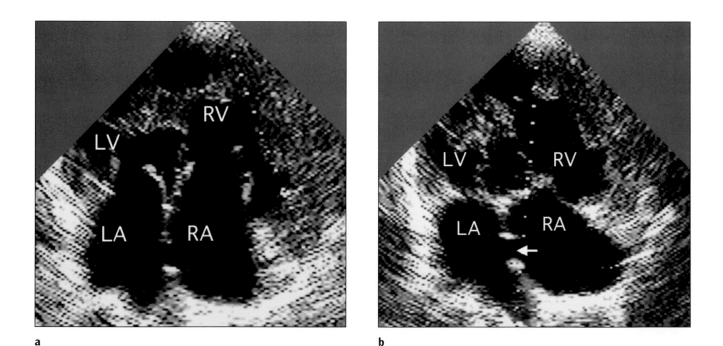

a b

Figure 145.3

(a) Right apical four-chamber view in diastole. The left ventricle is on the patient's right (on the left of the image). The right ventricle is heavily trabeculated and hypertrophied. The ventricular septal defect is partially masked in this view by the chordal insertions to the interventricular septum of the tricuspid valve.

(b) Similar view in diastole. The ventricular septal defect is again partially masked, this time by the chordal attachments of the thickened mitral valve to the crest of the interventricular septum. The secundum atrial septal defect (arrow) is clearly seen.

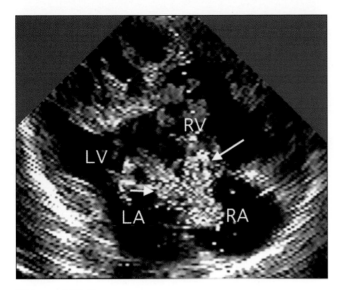

Figure 145.3
(c) Similar systolic view with color Doppler flow imaging. The mitral valve appears to be competent, as there is no significant jet of mitral regurgitation. However, there is moderate tricuspid regurgitation (longer arrow) and flow through the interatrial septal defect (shorter arrow).

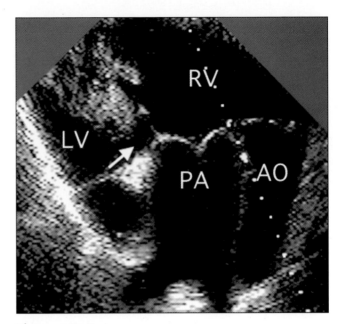

Figure 145.4
Anterior angulation of the transducer allows delineation of the ventricular septal defect (arrow) and the origin of the great vessels. Both arise from the morphological right ventricle. The aorta is more anterior and is of normal size. The pulmonary artery, identified by its primary branching pattern, is dilated. Its position is posterior and to the right of the aorta (left of screen).

Discussion

The complete diagnosis in this patient is situs inversus, double-outlet right ventricle, non-restrictive ventricular septal defect, secundum atrial septal defect and transposition of the great vessels. The systemic venous return reaches the right atrium and the right ventricle, wherein it mixes with pulmonary venous return to the left atrium which crosses the mitral valve and then the ventricular septal defect to reach the right ventricle. The aorta is not in close proximity to the ventricular septal defect (Taussig–Bing anomaly) and exits from the right ventricle. Careful delineation of situs and a segmental approach is strongly recommended when evaluating patients with complex abnormalities.[1,2] This patient's pulmonary circulation was unprotected and exposed to shunt flow and systemic pressures through the non-restrictive ventricular septal defect. He developed pulmonary hypertension at systemic level due to an Eisenmenger reaction to the intracardiac shunts. It is important in abdominal heterotaxy syndromes to undertake careful examination of the atrioventricular and ventriculoarterial connections to detect associated structural anomalies. The non-restrictive ventricular septal defect, which is easily visualized from every imaging plane, was the major cause of the irreversible pulmonary vascular disease, as there was no infundibular hypertrophy of sub-pulmonary outflow tract obstruction to protect the lungs. By the time the definitive diagnosis was made, pulmonary hypertension had developed so that surgical banding of the main pulmonary trunk and subsequent closure of the ventricular septal defect (in a two-stage procedure) was not possible. Early surgical correction of defects in patients with complex anatomy has been reported with acceptable mortality and good long-term survival.[3] Coronary artery anatomy should be delineated in patients for whom correction is planned, as the coronaries usually arise from the aortic sinuses.[4,5] This patient underwent successful heart and lung transplantation.

References

1. Huhta JC, Hagler DJ, Seward JB, *et al.* Two-dimensional echocardiographic assessment of dextrocardia: a segmental approach. Am J Cardiol 1982;50:1351–60.

2. Huhta JC, Smallhorn JF, Macartney FJ. Two dimensional echocardiographic diagnosis of situs. Br Heart J 1982;48:97–108.

3. Kleinert S, Sano T, Weintraub RG, *et al.* Anatomic features and surgical strategies in double-outlet right ventricle. Circulation 1997; 96:1233–9.

4. McKay R, Anderson RH, Smith A. The coronary arteries in hearts with discordant atrioventricular connections. J Thorac Cardiovasc Surg 1996;111:988–97.

5. Gordillo L, Faye-Petersen O, de la Cruz MV, *et al.* Coronary arterial patterns in double-outlet right ventricle. Am J Cardiol 1993;71:1108–10.

146

Repaired double-outlet right ventricle

Martin St John Sutton MBBS

A 24-year-old man was admitted complaining of fevers to 40°C, night sweats, nausea, profuse vomiting, palpitations, and orthostasis. His history was relevant in that a heart murmur had been detected at birth, and at 10 months he had had a cyanotic spell while feeding, and thereafter had had failure to thrive and shortness of breath. He had undergone cardiac catheterization which revealed a sub-aortic ventricular sepal defect, infundibular and pulmonary stenosis, and double-outlet right ventricle. The ventricular septal defect was closed, the infundibulum resected, and a pulmonary valvotomy performed, following which he had antibiotic prophylaxis for endocarditis prior to dental therapy. A year prior to this acute admission he had noticed progressive reduction in his exercise tolerance, shortness of breath, and sudden onset of self-terminating tachycardia associated with light-headedness, for which he could identify no trigger.

On examination, he was febrile, and hypotensive, with blood pressure of 85/60 mmHg and a heart rate of 116 bpm in regular rhythm. There was no elevation of the jugular venous pressure and no dependent edema. There were no cutaneous stigmata of endocarditis. Peripheral arterial pulses were present and equal bilaterally. There was a prominent right ventricular impulse and on auscultation a harsh ejection systolic murmur was audible maximally in the pulmonary area with a single second heart sound. Respiratory excursion was reduced over the right upper and midzone, over which there were coarse inspiratory and expiratory crackles. An electrocardiogram showed sinus tachycardia, first degree AV block right axis deviation, right bundle branch block and right ventricular hypertrophy. Telemetry demonstrated recurrent episodes of non-sustained ventricular tachycardia. A chest X-ray showed pneumonic consolidation of the right middle and upper lobes. Sputum and blood cultures both grew *Streptococcus pneumoniae*.

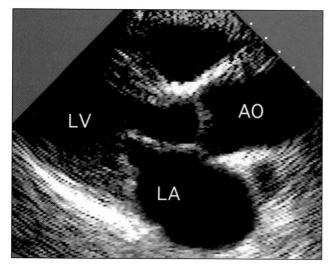
a

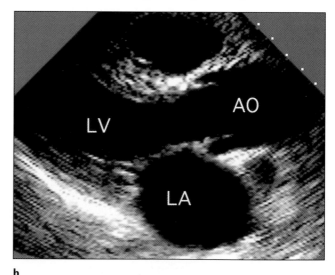
b

Figure 146.1
(a) Parasternal long-axis view in diastole. The maximum excursion of the mitral valve is severely curtailed and the leaflet is mildly thickened. The left atrium is mildly enlarged. The echo-bright portion of the proximal interventricular septum and anterior aortic wall is caused by the surgical patch used to close the ventricular septal defect in childhood.
(b) Similar systolic view. The aortic valve is normal. There is decreased left ventricular systolic function. Reversed septal motion consistent with elevated right ventricular pressure is also demonstrated.

512

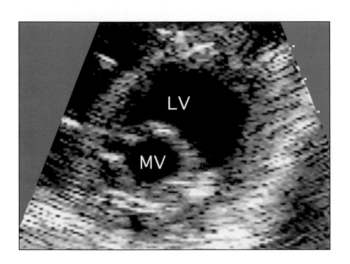

Figure 146.2
Parasternal short-axis view of the mitral valve orifice (MV). The view is off-axis in order to image the true orifice, which is not perpendicular to the left ventricular long axis. Planimetry in this view yielded a mitral valve area of approximately 1 cm^2. There is no commissural fusion. The stenosis is congenital rather than rheumatic in etiology.

Figure 146.3
(a) Parasternal short-axis view at the level of the aortic valve. The pulmonary artery (PA) is seen in long-axis. The bifurcation of the artery is seen and the great vessels have a normal anatomic relation to each other. The right ventricular outflow tract (RVOT) is hypertrophied. The pulmonary valve (PV) is thickened and there is a symmetric invagination of the pulmonary artery approximately 4 cm distal to the pulmonary valve. This is the site of greatest stenosis.
(b) Similar view with color flow Doppler imaging demonstrating turbulent flow in the pulmonary artery at the site of the supra-valvular obstruction.
(c) Similar color flow Doppler imaging in diastole. Significant pulmonary regurgitation was present. The retrograde flow causes a proximal flow convergence zone to be seen on the distal aspect of the supra-valvular stenosis.

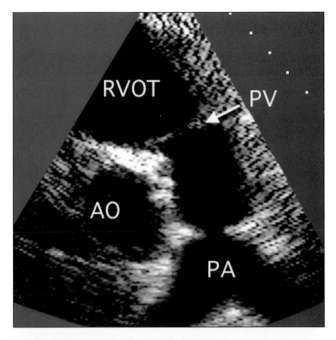

a

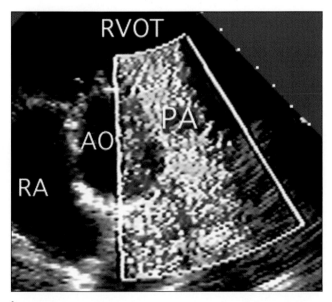

b

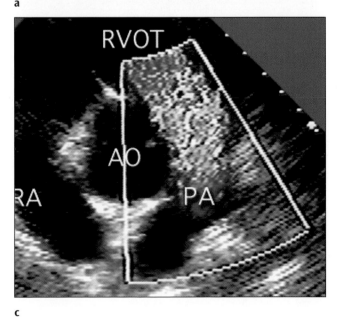

c

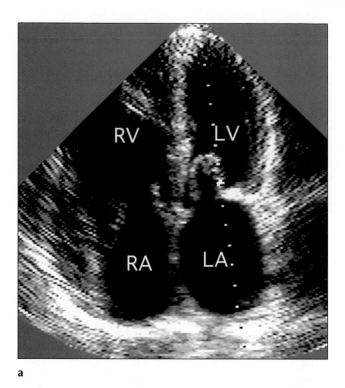

a

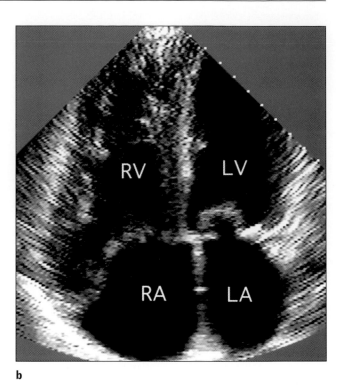

b

c

Figure 146.4
(a) Apical four-chamber view in diastole. The right ventricle is enlarged. The tricuspid and mitral annuli are co-planar. The congenitally abnormal mitral valve domes in diastole.
(b) Similar four-chamber view. The transducer has been moved medially to image the right ventricle more fully. The right ventricle is severely hypertrophied and is enlarged.
(c) Apical four-chamber view in diastole with color Doppler flow imaging. The turbulent transmitral flow suggests important mitral stenosis.

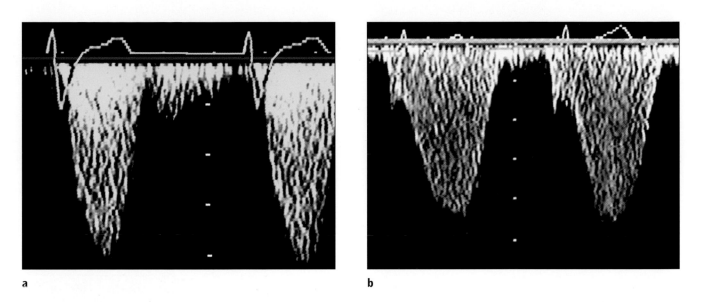

a   b

Figure 146.5

(a) Spectral display of continuous-wave Doppler across the pulmonary valve and supra-valvular obstruction. The peak velocity of 4.0 m/s predicts a peak gradient of 64 mmHg.

(b) Spectral display of continuous-wave Doppler across the tricuspid valve. The peak velocity is 4.3 m/s, which is equivalent to a gradient of 74 mmHg. Subtraction of the pulmonary gradient from the right ventricular systolic gradient gives an estimate of the pulmonary artery pressure distal to the stenosis of 10 mm Hg plus the right atrial pressure. Note the presystolic component of the tricuspid regurgitation which is due to first-degree atrioventricular block.

Discussion

Previous corrective surgery made full appreciation of the double-outlet right ventricle more difficult; however, the disposition of the great vessels was highly suggestive. The sub-aortic ventricular septal defect had been closed, but the aorta appeared to have been committed to the right ventricle originally. Echocardiography is essential in planning the repair in children to demonstrate the relationship of the ventricular septal defect to the great arteries and any intervening tissue such as straddling leaflets, which can cause obstruction after surgical repair.[1] In our patient, the echogenic pericardial patch was identified, but the residual problem was of right ventricular hypertension and consequent hypertrophy and dilatation due to main pulmonary artery stenosis. The unpredicted lesion in this patient was the dysmorphic mitral valve with important mitral stenosis.

The patient was treated with antibiotics and recovered with amelioration of his symptoms. The patient had an electrophysiological study that revealed an easily provoked monomorphic ventricular tachycardia with a rapid rate, indistinguishable from his clinical tachycardia. There is a high incidence of sudden death after repair of double-outlet right ventricle, presumably on the basis of susceptibility to malignant arrhythmias.[2] Therefore, the patient had an automatic implantable cardiac defibrillator (AICD) implanted and is currently waiting for reparative surgery to correct his right heart stenoses with planned replacement of the mitral valve.

References

1. Stellin G, Ho SY, Anderson RH, *et al.* The surgical anatomy of double-outlet right ventricle with concordant atrioventricular connection and noncommitted ventricular septal defect. J Thorac Cardiovasc Surg 1991;102:849–55.

2. Shen WK, Holmes DR Jr, Porter CJ, *et al.* Sudden death after repair of double-outlet right ventricle. Circulation 1990;81:128–36.

147

Tricuspid atresia

Martin St John Sutton MBBS
Susan E Wiegers MD

A 17-year-old woman was admitted via the emergency room with sudden onset of altered mental status, an expressive dysphasia and right faciobrachial weakness consistent with an acute dominant hemispherical stroke. In the emergency room she was deeply cyanosed with a hemoglobin level of 23.8 g/dl and an oxygen saturation of 73% on room air. She had a history of complex cyanotic congenital heart disease diagnosed at birth for which she had undergone cardiac catheterization at 3 months of age having failed to thrive. The diagnosis was tricuspid atresia, ventricular septal defect, rudimentary right ventricle, and an unobstructed right ventricular outflow tract with normally related great arteries. She had a pulmonary artery band performed to prevent development of pulmonary vascular disease soon after the cardiac catheterization. Her mother declined a Fontan procedure because of the high operative mortality quoted to her by the cardiac surgeon. From her early teens there was a progressive decline in her exercise capacity and deepening central cyanosis. During the 3 years prior to her stroke she had undergone intermittent venesections but had become hypotensive; she had a syncopal episode after venesection of one unit several months previously and the practice was discontinued.

On examination she was not able to communicate, because she was dysphasic and had an ipsilateral facial and right upper extremity weakness. She was centrally cyanosed with digital clubbing and an elevated jugular venous pressure with a normal blood pressure and in sinus rhythm. Peripheral arterial pulses were present and equal bilaterally. The apical impulse was hyperdynamic and there was a harsh ejection systolic murmur at the upper left sternal border. Her respiratory and alimentary systems were within normal limits. Electrocardiography showed sinus rhythm, left axis deviation and left ventricular hypertrophy. A chest X-ray showed mild cardiomegaly, right atrial enlargement, and a dilated proximal pulmonary artery with normal pulmonary vasculature.

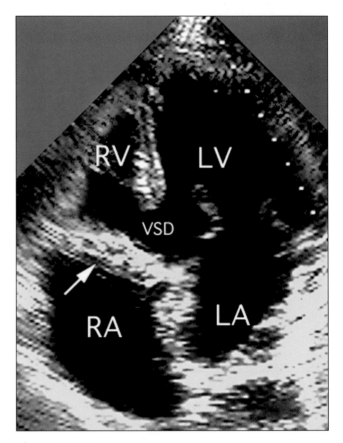

Figure 147.1

(a) Apical four-chamber view. The tricuspid valve (arrow) is atretic, being an imperforate band of fibrous tissue. The right atrium (RA) is enlarged, but the right ventricle (RV) is rudimentary. There is a non-restrictive ventricular septal defect (VSD) but the obligatory atrial septal defect is not visible in this frame. The size of the left ventricle is at the top limit of normal size. The mitral valve and left atrium are normal.

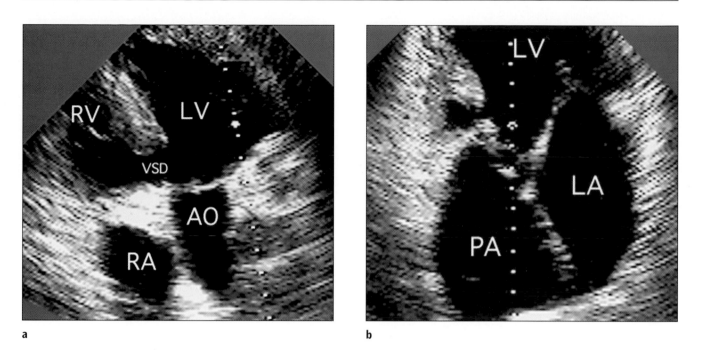

a   b

Figure 147.1
(b) Anterior angulation of the transducer permits visualization of the aorta arising from the left ventricle. The aortic valve was normal.
(c) Lesser anterior angulation shows the pulmonary artery taking origin from the left ventricle, as does the aorta. The ventricular septal defect and a small portion of the dysplastic right ventricle are visible on the left of the image (the patient's right). The surgically placed pulmonary artery band is immediately distal to the pulmonary valve. The main pulmonary artery distal to the band is severely dilated.

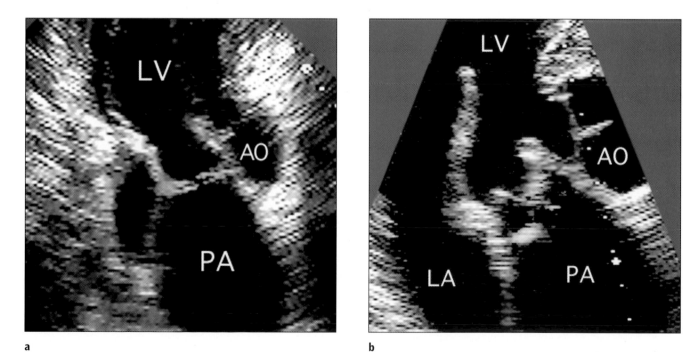

a   b

Figure 147.2
(a) Apical long-axis view of the left ventricle demonstrating double-outlet left ventricle. The aorta (AO) and the pulmonary artery (PA) arise in parallel from the left ventricle (LV). The pulmonary artery band is visible again in the proximal pulmonary artery.
(b) Close-up image of the pulmonary artery from the same view demonstrates both semilunar valves and the continuity between the anterior mitral valve leaflet and the pulmonary artery. The pulmonary artery band is not as clearly seen, but the post-stenotic dilatation is again appreciated.

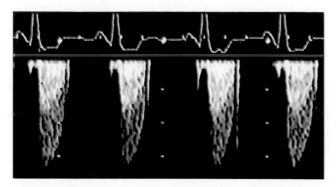

Figure 147.3
Spectral display of continuous-wave Doppler across the pulmonary valve and the pulmonary artery. The increased velocity is due to obstruction at the level of the band rather than the pulmonary valve. The peak velocity of 3 m/s (each calibration mark represents 1.0 m/s) indicates that the gradient between the left ventricular peak systolic pressure and the pulmonary artery pressure is only 36 mmHg. Therefore, the patient has significant pulmonary hypertension.

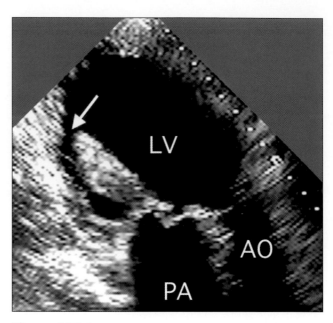

Figure 147.4
Apical four-chamber view with anterior angulation and slight clockwise angulation. A second muscular ventricular septal defect (arrow) is visible in the septum near the apex.

Discussion

This patient had tricuspid atresia presenting soon after birth with failure to thrive due to heart failure. The diagnosis of tricuspid atresia with ventricular septal defect and double-outlet left ventricle with an unprotected pulmonary circulation was made correctly at cardiac catheterization. Pulmonary artery banding was performed to protect against progressive pulmonary vascular disease. The apical two-dimensional echocardiographic images clearly show the anatomical defects in this patient. There is absence of the right atrioventricular connection as demonstrated by the echodense band in that region with no inflow from the right atrium to the right ventricle.[1] Systemic return reaches the only viable ventricle via a large secundum atrial septal defect that is not well seen in these images. The patient also has a rudimentary right ventricle, two ventricular septal defects, the residual stenotic pulmonary artery band, and the post-stenotic aneurysmal dilatation of the distal main pulmonary artery. The obligate shunting has resulted in cyanosis from birth.

Over the course of growing up, the pulmonary artery band had become insufficiently stenotic, so that her systolic pulmonary arterial pressure was only 36 mmHg less than left ventricular pressure (115 mmHg). Thus, the pulmonary artery pressure was 115 − 36 = 79 mmHg. The prolonged exposure to high flows at near systemic pressures had resulted in the development of fixed pulmonary hypertension. Two-dimensional and Doppler echocardiography can be used to assess the adequacy of banding as the patient ages.[2,3]

The patient's stroke syndrome was caused by interarterial thrombosis due to hyperviscosity syndrome and polycythemia. Endocarditis is also a consideration, based on her presentation, but there was no evidence of vegetations on echocardiography and blood cultures were negative. She made an almost complete recovery from her stroke with resolution of her dysphasia and only mild residual monoparesis of her right arm. She stabilized for a time, but died while listed for heart and lung transplantation.

References

1. Orie JD, Anderson C, Ettedgui JA, et al. Echocardiographic-morphologic correlations in tricuspid atresia. J Am Coll Cardiol 1995;26:750–8.

2. Jureidini SB, Alpert BS, Durant RH, et al. Two-dimensional echocardiographic assessment of adequacy of pulmonary artery banding. Pediatr Cardiol 1986;6:239–44.

3. Fyfe DA, Currie PJ, Seward JB, et al. Continuous-wave Doppler determination of the pressure gradient across pulmonary artery bands: hemodynamic correlation in 20 patients. Mayo Clin Proc 1984;59:744–50.

148

Complex cyanotic congenital heart disease

Susan E Wiegers MD

A 27-year-old English professor with complex cyanotic congenital heart disease presented to the emergency room with hypotension. She had been well until earlier in the day when she had noted mild shortness of breath and myalgias. She had become increasingly ill over the course of the afternoon and had several rigors prior to collapsing at home. She was brought to the emergency room where her blood pressure was 60 mmHg systolic, her pulse was 120 bpm and her room air oxygen saturation was 69%. She was awake but mildly confused and complaining of not being able to see. She was treated for presumed sepsis with broad-spectrum antibiotics and high-volume fluid resuscitation. She was treated briefly with pressor agents and her oxygen saturation increased to 75% on 100% inspired oxygen. She did not require intubation and recovered rapidly. Two of six sets of blood cultures grew *Streptococcus viridans*.

An echocardiogram was undertaken to attempt to detect the location of the endovascular infection. The patient was known to have dextrocardia with situs solitus. The heart was rotated to the right and the apex was in the right chest. The abdominal organs were in the usual anatomic arrangement with connection of the inferior and superior vena cava to the right atrium. The echocardiograms were obtained from the right parasternal and right apical locations.

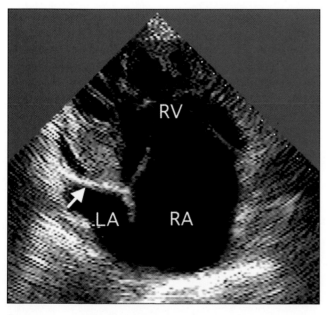

a

Figure 148.1

(a) Apical four-chamber view with the transducer oriented normally but positioned at the right apex. The atrioventricular valve, which is open in this diastolic frame, is the tricuspid valve. The right ventricle is severely enlarged and massively hypertrophied with dense trabeculations located within the cavity of the ventricle. The tricuspid valve leaflets themselves appear to be anatomically normal, but the annulus is severely dilated. The right atrium is enlarged. On the left of the screen, the left atrium communicates with the right atrium through a large atrial septal defect. The mitral annulus is co-planar with the tricuspid annulus but is imperforate (arrow). It is recognized as a dense line of tissue on the left of the screen adjacent to the tricuspid leaflets. The left ventricle is severely hypoplastic. The cavity of this small chamber is seen on the left of the screen, next to the right ventricle and apical from the mitral annulus. To summarize, it is clear from this image alone that the patient has mitral atresia, hypoplastic left ventricle and a large secundum atrial septal defect.

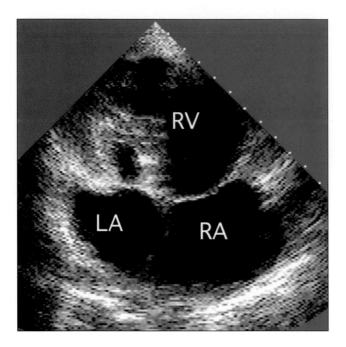

Figure 148.1

(b) Similar systolic view demonstrates that the right ventricular function is only mildly decreased, although it is difficult from a single view to estimate the function in this enlarged and asymmetric chamber. Despite the annular dilatation, the tricuspid valve does coapt. Only moderate regurgitation was present. The left ventricle is visible as a small circular chamber adjacent to the imperforate mitral annulus. The secundum atrial septal defect is visible between the left and right atria.

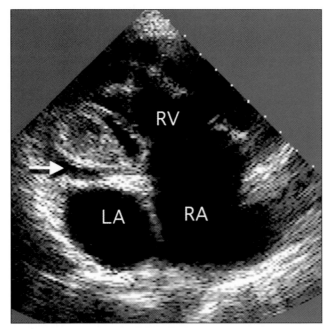

a

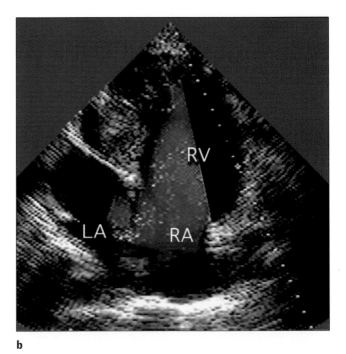

b

Figure 148.2

(a) Off-axis apical image of the hypoplastic left ventricle in short-axis (arrow). The left ventricle is a small circular chamber on the left of the image adjacent to the imperforate mitral annulus. The patient had a hypoplastic left ventricle as part of her congenital syndrome. Once again, in this diastolic frame the right ventricle is seen to be massively large and hypertrophied as it is the single functioning ventricle for this patient.

(b) A similar view with color flow Doppler imaging demonstrating flow from the left atrium across the interatrial septum into the right atrium and then into the right ventricular cavity.

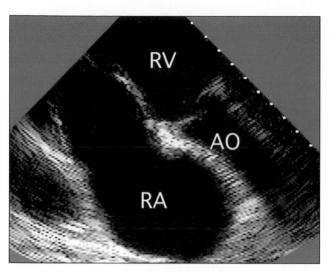

a

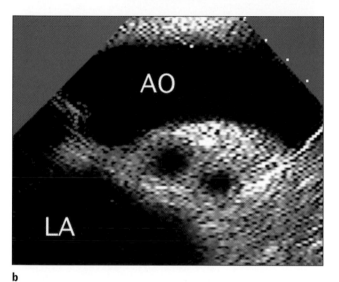

b

Figure 148.3

(a) Apical long-axis view of the right atrium and right ventricle. The tricuspid valve is open in diastole. A great artery arises from the right ventricle. Additional views confirm that this artery does not bifurcate and is the aorta rather than the pulmonary artery. The patient had transposition of the great arteries. This was necessary for survival after birth, owing to the hypoplastic left ventricle.

(b) High right parasternal view of the ascending aorta, which arises from the anatomic right ventricle. This view confirms that the vessel does not bifurcate and thus the patient has complete transposition of the great vessels. The aorta is the anterior structure but its connection to the right ventricle is poorly seen in this view. The aortic arch is left-sided in the normal anatomic position. Diminutive branch pulmonary arteries can be seen posterior to the aorta in this view. The patient had pulmonary atresia with hypoplastic right and left pulmonary arteries that were not confluent.

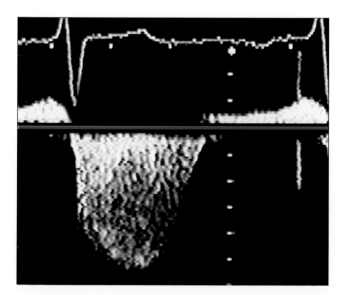

Figure 148.4

Spectral display of continuous-wave Doppler across the tricuspid valve regurgitation. Each calibration mark represents 1 m/s. The tricuspid valve is the systemic atrioventricular valve and the velocity of the regurgitation represented the patient's systolic blood pressure at the time of the study. The peak velocity of 5.2 m/s reflects a systolic gradient between the anatomic right ventricle and the anatomic right atrium of 110 mmHg.

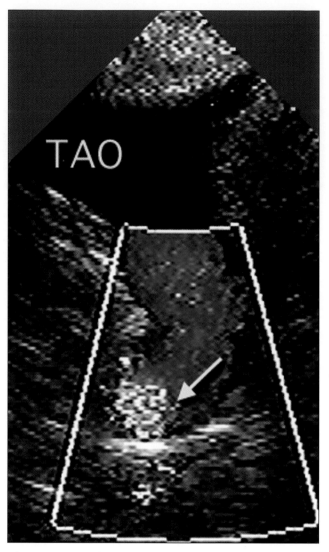

Figure 148.5
Suprasternal notch view with color flow Doppler imaging of the descending thoracic aorta, which was left-sided in this patient. The area of turbulent high-velocity flow in the descending thoracic aorta (arrow) represents the area of the Pott's anastomosis, which connected the descending thoracic aorta to the left pulmonary artery. The flow was continuous but the pressure gradient between the aorta and the pulmonary artery could not be assessed, because of the acute angle between the direction of flow and the ultrasound beam. The patient also has a Blalock–Taussig anastomosis between the right subclavian and the right pulmonary artery which could not be visualized. TAO, transverse aorta.

Discussion

This remarkable patient has survived to an unexpectedly advanced age with the following anatomy: situs solitus with dextrocardia; complete transposition of the great vessels with pulmonary atresia; mitral atresia; hypoplastic left ventricle and a large secundum atrial septal defect which is an obligate shunt for her. She has had two surgical procedures: a Blalock–Taussig anastomosis, which created a shunt between the right subclavian artery and the right pulmonary artery; and a Pott's anastomosis between the descending thoracic aortic and the left pulmonary artery. This confusing array of associated conditions has allowed her to survive. The circulation is as follows: the systemic venous return reaches the right atrium via a normally placed inferior and superior vena cava. The systemic return mixes with oxygenated blood from the pulmonary veins that empty into the left atrium and passes through the large secundum atrial septal defect into the right atrium. The mitral valve is imperforate, so that all of the blood that returns to the heart from the systemic venous circulation and from the pulmonary circulation crosses the tricuspid valve into the right ventricle. This is essentially a single ventricle, owing to the imperforate mitral valve and hypoplastic left ventricle. The blood is ejected from the right ventricle through the aortic valve into the aorta, which has a left-sided arch. Pulmonary circulation was present in infancy only through a patent ductus arteriosus. The two surgical shunts from the aorta to the pulmonary circulation now provide much of the patient's pulmonary artery flow. She also has large bronchial collateral vessels to the pulmonary circulation.

This patient has done exceptionally well, owing to a well-balanced pulmonary circulation that has prevented the development of severe pulmonary hypertension but has allowed enough pulmonary flow to enable the patient to be reasonably active. She participated in competitive sports as an adolescent.

The patient has an obligatory shunt of unoxygenated blood to the systemic arterial circulation and is cyanotic even at rest. She has, however, avoided many of the complications of cyanotic congenital heart disease. She has only mild scoliosis. She has been steadily employed since graduation from college. Several episodes of right ventricular failure have responded rapidly to diuresis and afterload reduction. This patient's episode of endocarditis could not be documented by echocardiography. There was no regurgitation across the aortic valve between the aorta and the right ventricle. The degree of tricuspid valvular regurgitation between the anatomic right ventricle and right atrium had not changed and the tricuspid valve did not appear different from previous studies. No definite vegetations were noted. It was therefore assumed that the endovascular infection was within one of her two surgically created shunts. Both shunts have high-velocity turbulent flow which predisposes to the development of endocarditis.[1,2] She was treated with 6 weeks of intravenous antibiotics with complete resolution of her symptoms and subsequently negative blood cultures. Four years later, she continues to be active and hemodynamically stable. Patients with congenital heart disease remain at high risk for endocarditis both before and after surgery. Dental care, antibiotic prophylaxis and a high index of suspicion for unusual sites of infection are important in the care of these patients.[3]

References

1. Morris C, Reller M, Menashe V. Thirty-year incidence of infective endocarditis after surgery for congenital heart defect. J Am Med Assoc 1998;279:599–603.

2. Turner S, Wyllie J, Hamilton J, *et al.* Diagnosis of infected modified Blalock–Taussig shunt by computed tomography. Ann Thorac Surg 1995;59:753–5.

3. Gersony W, Hayes C, Driscoll D, *et al.* Bacterial endocarditis in patients with aortic stenosis, pulmonary stenosis or ventricular septal defect. Circulation 1993;87(2 Suppl):I121–6.

149

Uniatrioventricular connection

Martin St John Sutton MBBS
Susan E Wiegers MD

A 29-year-old man had presented with central cyanosis and congestive heart failure soon after birth, and had undergone cardiac catheterization on day 2. He was diagnosed with situs solitus, univentricular connection to a morphological left ventricle, a rudimentary right ventricular chamber, non-restrictive ventricular septal defect and transposed great arteries. The pulmonary circulation was exposed to the systemic pressures and unprotected flows. Therefore, as soon as the diagnosis was made, the patient underwent banding of the main pulmonary artery approximately 1 cm above the pulmonary valve to reduce pulmonary blood flow and avoid pulmonary vascular disease. At 20 years of age, he had noticed diminished exercise tolerance and over the

next 3 years complained of progressive dyspnea, orthostasis and recurrent episodes of near syncope.

On examination he had digital clubbing, central cyanosis, and a heart rate of 46 bpm. His jugular venous pressure was elevated and he had mild bilateral ankle edema. There was a palpable precordial systolic thrill in the upper left parasternal region and a single second heart sound. A chest X-ray demonstrated marked cardiomegaly with pulmonary oligemia and the suggestion of a large systemic aorto-pulmonary collateral. Electrocardiography showed sinus bradycardia and left ventricular hypertrophy with repolarization abnormalities in the lateral leads.

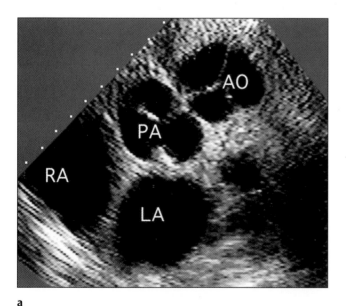

a

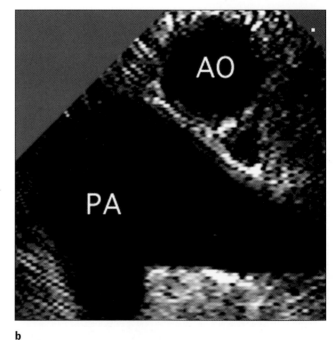

b

Figure 149.1

(a) Parasternal short-axis view at the base of the heart. The abnormal relationship of the great arteries is evident, since they are both seen in short axis. Both valves are trileaflet and appear anatomically normal. No coronary arteries are demonstrated in this view.
(b) The identification of the posterior great artery as the pulmonary artery is made by demonstration of its bifurcation. This view was obtained by superior angulation with slight clockwise rotation from the parasternal short axis. The pulmonary artery and its branches are severely dilated. This patient has levotransposition of the great arteries, since the aorta is anterior and to the left of the posteriorly positioned pulmonary artery (patient's left is to the right of the screen).

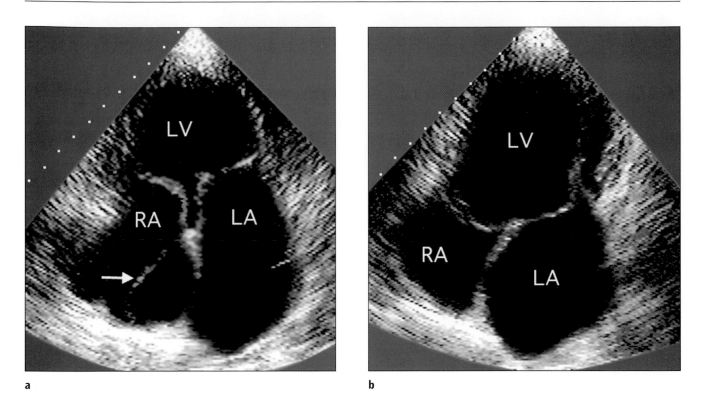

a   b

Figure 149.2
(a) Apical four-chamber view in diastole. The features to note are: there is biatrial enlargement, the septal leaflets of the right and left atrioventricular valves take origin from the interatrial septum primum at the same level, and both atria drain into a single ventricle. The single ventricle of left ventricular morphology is hypertrophied and has a globular shape. It lacks coarse trabeculations and a moderator band. The excursion of two atrioventricular valves is greatly exaggerated and, not surprisingly, they are both regurgitant. A Chiari network (arrow) is present in the right atrium
(b) Severely diminished systolic function is noted. The rudimentary right ventricle is not imaged in this view.

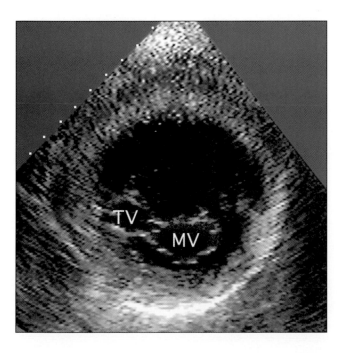

Figure 149.3
Parasternal short-axis view at the valve level. As was seen in the apical view, both atrioventricular valves enter the same enlarged, globular chamber. TV, tricuspid valve; MV, mitral valve.

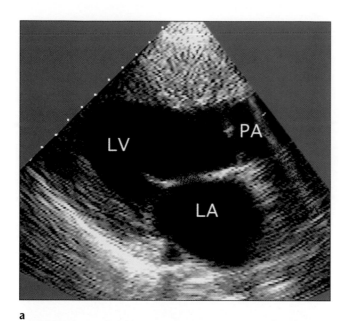

a

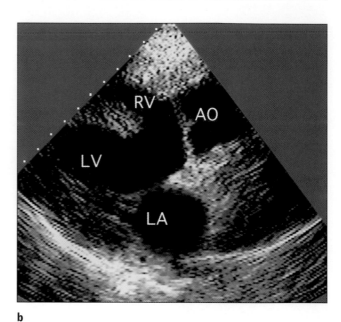

b

c

Figure 149.4

(a) Parasternal long-axis view showing the pulmonary artery (identified by its primary branching pattern in Figure 149.1) arising from the left ventricle. There is continuity of the mitral valve leaflet and the pulmonary artery. The pulmonary band is not well seen in this view.

(b) The transducer was moved up an intercostal space and to the patient's left to obtain an image of the anteriorly placed and left-sided aorta. The rudimentary right ventricle (RV) is also demonstrated in this view. The aorta over-rides the ventricular septum.

(c) The transducer was moved up another intercostal space and angled medially to obtain this view. The parallel course of the great vessels can be appreciated. The pulmonary artery band is now seen approximately 1 cm distal to the pulmonary valve.

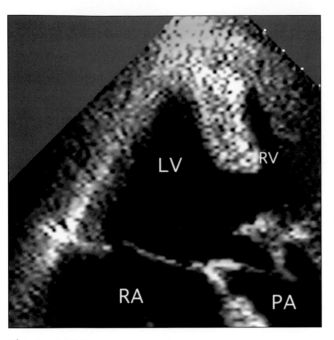

Figure 149.5
Off-axis apical image obtained by anterior angulation of the transducer from the standard apical image. The rudimentary right ventricle (RV) is more fully visualized. The pulmonary artery (PA) connection to the left ventricle is also clearly demonstrated. This great vessel was identified as the pulmonary artery from its primary branching pattern in previous views.

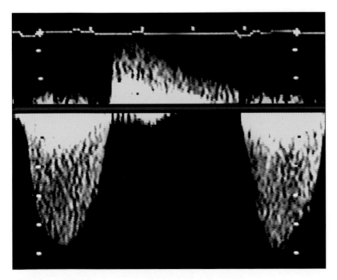

Figure 149.6
Continuous-wave Doppler velocity signal obtained across the pulmonary artery band, indicating a peak velocity of 5 m/s and thus a peak systolic gradient of 100 mmHg.

Discussion

Univentricular connection is readily demonstrable in the apical images and describes the intracardiac anatomy rather better than single ventricle because often the other ventricle, while rudimentary, can be identified. However, whether a rudimentary chamber constitutes a ventricle, or whether a ventricle should have an inlet and an outlet portion to be so designated, remains contentious. Two individual atrioventricular valves with similar origins are usually present. In general, those valves have greater than normal excursion and varying degrees of incompetence. The great arteries are most frequently transposed, as in this patient. Univentricular atrioventricular connections are four-fold more likely to be of the left ventricular type. Intracardiac shunts at atrial level, and pulmonary and infundibular stenosis are frequently associated with univentricular connection. Subaortic stenosis may also be present and further complicate attempts at surgical repair.[1] Symptoms are usually related in early life either to pulmonary oligemia or to excessive pulmonary blood flow; Doppler echocardiography can readily distinguish between the two, allowing specific interventional therapy to be determined.

This patient had a pulmonary artery band placed to protect the pulmonary circulation. This was successful, allowing him to survive to early adulthood without developing pulmonary hypertension. Definitive corrective surgery was not available at the time this patient was a child and even now has a high associated mortality.[2] Long-term ventricular failure due to the volume overload has been documented in patients with univentricular connections by stress echocardiogram.[3] Our patient refused consideration of heart transplantation and is maintained on medical therapy with continuous oxygen use.

References

1. O'Leary PW, Driscoll DJ, Connor AR, et al. Subaortic obstruction in hearts with a univentricular connection to a dominant left ventricle and an anterior subaortic outlet chamber. Results of a staged approach [see comments]. J Thorac Cardiovasc Surg 1992;104:1231–7.

2. Cochrane AD, Brizard CP, Penny DJ, et al. Management of the univentricular connection: are we improving? Eur J Cardio-Thorac Surg 1997;12:107–15.

3. Akagi T, Benson LN, Green M, et al. Ventricular function during supine bicycle exercise in univentricular connection with absent right atrioventricular connection. Am J Cardiol 1991;67:1273–8.

150

Truncus arteriosus

Martin St John Sutton MBBS
Susan E Wiegers MD

A 31-year-old man was admitted for heart and lung transplantation. He had been diagnosed as having tetralogy of Fallot as a school-aged child. He was deemed surgically uncorrectable at that time and was followed medically. He had been restricted symptomatically by shortness of breath during early childhood initially on moderate exertion, but in his late teens he was dyspneic even with mild exercise. He noticed progressive cyanosis, for which he was intermittently venesected from the age of 20 onwards, and this was accompanied by transitory symptomatic improvement.

On examination he was centrally cyanosed with marked digital clubbing and an oxygen saturation in room air of 78% at rest. There was elevation of the jugular venous pressure and marked dependent edema bilaterally. Peripheral pulses were bounding with a wide arterial pulse pressure. The apical impulse was forceful, suggesting left ventricular hypertrophy. On auscultation there was an ejection systolic murmur followed by an immediate holodiastolic murmur, both best heard at the upper left sternal border, and a single second heart sound. Electrocardiography showed sinus rhythm with biventricular hypertrophy. A chest X-ray revealed severe cardiomegaly, an absent pulmonary trunk and increased pulmonary vascularity consistent with an intracardiac shunt.

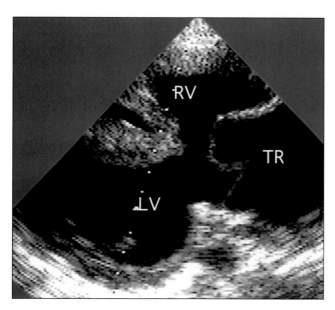 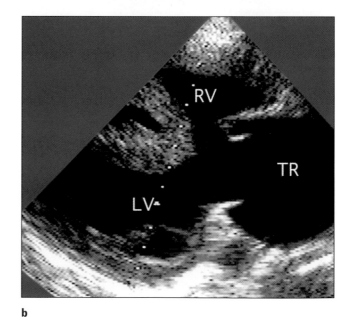

a   b

Figure 150.1
(a) Parasternal long-axis view in diastole. The very large truncus arteriosus (TR) and subtruncal ventricular septal defect are demonstrated. The severely dilated common arterial trunk measures over 7 cm in this view and over-rides the inlet portion of the interventricular septum. The mitral valve and left atrium are out of plane. There is severe right ventricular hypertrophy and the moderator band, which inserts onto the crest of the interventricular septum, is also hypertrophied. Left ventricular hypertrophy is also present.
(b) Similar view in systole. Left ventricular function is moderately decreased.

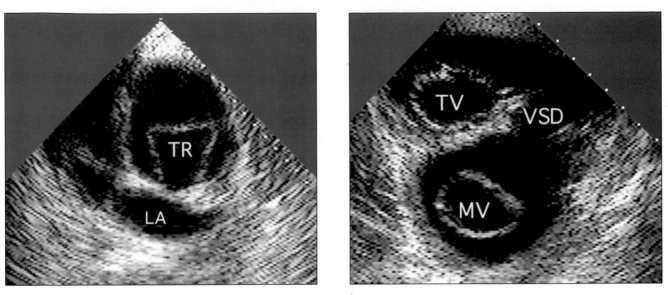

a   b

Figure 150.2
(a) Parasternal short-axis view of the truncus arteriosus (TR) with a trileaflet valve. The small left atrium (LA) is posterior to the truncal root. There is no evidence of a right ventricular outflow tract or pulmonary artery in their usual anatomic position.
(b) Parasternal short-axis view at the level of the mitral valve leaflets demonstrates enlarged chambers and the non-restrictive ventricular septal defect. Both the mitral valve (MV) and the tricuspid valve (TV) appear to be anatomically normal.

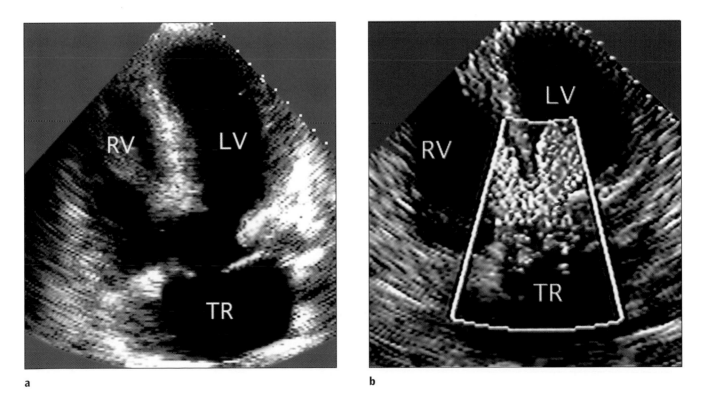

a   b

Figure 150.3
(a) Anterior angulation of the transducer from the four-chamber view demonstrates the very large truncus (TR) that arises from the ventricular mass and over-rides the interventricular septum. Both ventricles are hypertrophied and have diminished systolic function.
(b) Similar view in diastole with color flow Doppler imaging. The truncal valve is incompetent and the regurgitant jet passes equally into both ventricles. TR – truncus arteriosus.

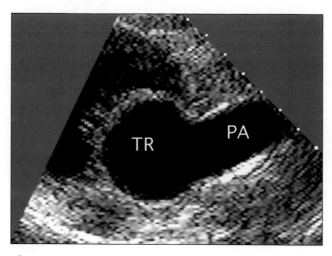

Figure 150.4
Short-axis image of the truncus arteriosus (TR) several centimeters above the truncal valve shows the common arterial trunk diameter to be much smaller. A single main pulmonary artery (PA) arises from it and passes to the patient's left. A bifurcation of this pulmonary artery could not be visualized.

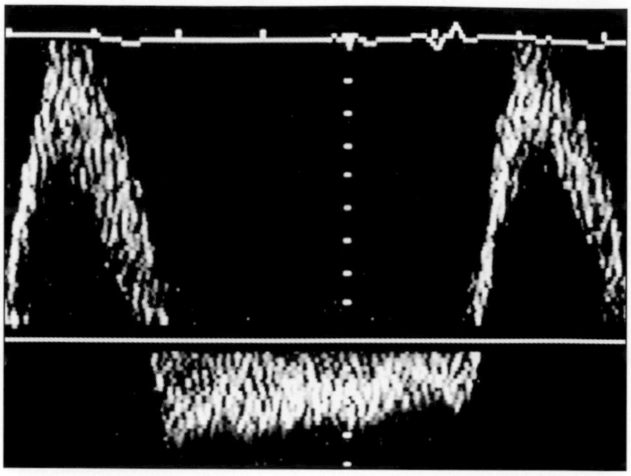

Figure 150.5
Spectral display of pulsed-wave Doppler with the sample volume in the ascending aorta distal to the origin of the pulmonary artery demonstrates diastolic flow reversal consistent with moderate truncal valve regurgitation. The transducer has been placed in the suprasternal notch to obtain this image. Diastolic flow below the baseline represents flow back towards the heart in diastole and may also represent diastolic run-off into the pulmonary artery.

Discussion

This patient exhibited all the clinical symptoms and signs of a truncus arteriosus with pulmonary vascular disease from unprotected increased pulmonary blood flow. The diagnosis can be made easily with two-dimensional echocardiography from a number of imaging planes. Diagnostically truncus arteriosus may be difficult to distinguish from tetralogy of Fallot. Both conditions have structural commonalities including a large great artery that over-rides the septum and a non-restrictive ventricular septal defect. If the origin of the pulmonary artery from the truncus is stenosed this can result in pulmonary oligemia, as occurs in tetralogy of Fallot. In a minority of patients with tetralogy or truncus arteriosus the aortic arch is right-sided. Furthermore, the main pulmonary artery in Fallot's tetralogy may be diminutive and the left pulmonary artery atretic which may make for diagnostic difficulties.

In this patient, the pulmonary artery was visualized arising from the truncus. The diagnosis of truncus arteriosus hinges upon demonstrating not only the absence of egress of blood from the right ventricle and the presence of an obligatory ventricular septal defect but also the origin of the pulmonary artery from the common arterial trunk. This is usually best visualized in short-axis imaging of the truncus above the truncal valve. The truncal valve is usually trileaflet as in this case but may be unicuspid, bicuspid or quadricuspid and is often regurgitant.[1] Significant truncal valve regurgitation impacts not only on survival but also on the likely success of surgical correction. Surgical correction of truncus arteriosus is currently being undertaken in neonates and infants with improved mortality rates.[2,3] Anomalous origin of the coronary arteries is a frequent association and must be diagnosed prior to surgery.[4] This patient had developed severe pulmonary hypertension from the unrestricted pulmonary flow. He underwent double lung and heart transplantation but died immediately postoperatively from multi-organ failure.

References

1. Fuglestad SJ, Puga FJ, Danielson GK, et al. Surgical pathology of the truncal valve: a study of 12 cases. Am J Cardiovasc Pathol 1988;2:39–47.

2. Pearl JM, Laks H, Drinkwater DC Jr, et al. Repair of conotruncal abnormalities with the use of the valved conduit: improved early and midterm results with the cryopreserved homograft. J Am Coll Cardiol 1992;20:191–6.

3. Barbero-Marcial M, Riso A, Atik E, et al. A technique for correction of truncus arteriosus types I and II without extracardiac conduits. J Thorac Cardiovasc Surg 1990;99:364–9.

4. Imamura M, Drummond-Webb JJ, Sarris GE, et al. Improving early and intermediate results of truncus arteriosus repair: a new technique of truncal valve repair. Ann Thorac Surg 1999;67:1142–6.

Index